Asbestos and Its Diseases

Asbestos and Its Diseases

Edited by

John E. Craighead, MD

Professor Emeritus and Former Chair
Department of Pathology
University of Vermont
Burlington, Vermont

Allen R. Gibbs, MB, ChB

Department of Histopathology
Llandough Hospital
Penarth, South Glamorgan
United Kingdom

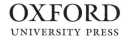

OXFORD
UNIVERSITY PRESS

2008

OXFORD
UNIVERSITY PRESS

Oxford University Press, Inc., publishes works that further
Oxford University's objective of excellence
in research, scholarship, and education.

Oxford New York
Auckland Cape Town Dar es Salaam Hong Kong Karachi
Kuala Lumpur Madrid Melbourne Mexico City Nairobi
New Delhi Shanghai Taipei Toronto

With offices in
Argentina Austria Brazil Chile Czech Republic France Greece
Guatemala Hungary Italy Japan Poland Portugal Singapore
South Korea Switzerland Thailand Turkey Ukraine Vietnam

Published by Oxford University Press, Inc.
198 Madison Avenue, New York, New York 10016

www.oup.com

Oxford is a registered trademark of Oxford University Press

Library of Congress Cataloging-in-Publication Data

Asbestos and its diseases / edited by John E. Craighead and Allen R. Gibbs.
p.; cm.
Includes bibliographical references.
ISBN 978-0-19-517869-2 (cloth: alk. paper)
1. Asbestosis.   2. Asbestos–Toxicology.   3. Asbestos–Health aspects.
4. Asbestos–Carcinogenicity. I. Craighead, John E. II. Gibbs, A. R.
[DNLM: 1. Asbestos–adverse effects. 2. Asbestosis–etiology.
3. Lung Neoplasms–etiology.   4. Occupational Exposure–adverse effects.
5. Pleural Neoplasms–etiology. WF 654 A7986 2008]
RC775.A8A75 2008
616.2'44–dc22   2007028381

9 8 7 6 5 4 3 2 1

Printed in the United States of America
on acid-free paper

In recognition of the late Irving J. Selikoff for his dedicated path-finding efforts to bring the health risks of asbestos exposure to the attention of labor, government, and the general public.

To the late Sir Richard S. Doll, whose painstaking rigorous analyses of disease and mortality rates transformed random clinical observations into concrete valid assessments of risk.

To the late Christopher Wagner, whose imaginative insightful observations in an obscure corner of sub-Saharan Africa resulted in the recognition of a subtle epidemic of an otherwise rare cancer attributable to amphibole asbestos exposure.

Preface

Friable crocidolite asbestos, in layers several feet thick, insulated the flight decks of aircraft carriers of the British Royal Navy during World War II. These vessels faired well, surviving relentless Kamikaze attacks in the Pacific. Alas, American vessels were not as well protected, although mountains of chrysotile and amosite asbestos were used in naval and merchant vessels during and after the war. The hulls and engine rooms, as well as miles upon miles of piping, and numerous mechanical components of these ships were lined by thick coats of heat and fire-resistant asbestos. We can only speculate as to what influence these precautions had on the survival of the Allies' war-time fleets and their crews.

During the construction of the New York's World Trade Center, spray-on asbestos was applied to the infrastructure of the lower 61 floors until public health dictates terminated insulation of the buildings with asbestos. Some architects predicted the dire effects of fire on the upper floors of the towers based on the relative capacities of substitutes to provide insulation. One can only wonder what effect, if any, asbestos insulation of the towers throughout might have had on the outcome of the tragedy of September 11, 2001.

Although once considered a miracle mineral, even the word—asbestos—now has ominous implications for all strata of our society. Incorporated in the past into over 3000 different industrial and consumer products, as well as in building materials and military equipment, opportunities for exposure continue to be ever present in our environment. Of all of us who are potentially exposed, blue collar workmen are at greatest risk.

Countless thousands of workers and servicemen in a wide variety of trades were disabled or have died consequent to the health effects of asbestos, and many more can be expected to be affected in years to come. Understandably, members of the general public still live in fear, and injured parties expect redress. As a consequence, litigation continues and financial awards in the billions have led to the bankruptcy of a number of Fortune 500 companies, and numerous smaller companies whose insurance was dissipated by court decisions and settlements.

The history of scientific inquiry into the causes of the diseases related to asbestos exposure can be traced to the early years of the 20th century when occupational health physicians first recognized the occurrence of asbestosis in textile workers. For the first three decades of the century, cases continued to appear as public health officials considered but failed to implement effective environmental control measures. World War II resulted in a dramatic increase in the use of asbestos in war ships and vehicles as well as in other instruments of war. Shortly after cessation of hostilities, the carcinogenic effects of asbestos were recognized, but another three decades passed before adequate controls were introduced by governmental dictates curbing the most egregious uses of asbestos in industrialized countries. By this time, the health impact of asbestos was manifest throughout the population in the form of asbestosis and lung cancer as well as the newly discovered and poorly understood cancer, malignant mesothelioma.

Although one might implicate our forefathers in this widespread, relentless medical catastrophe, it has been only in recent decades that science has appreciated the complexities of the problem and the long latencies before the asbestos-associated diseases appear clinically. After all these years, prevention remains the hallmark of disease control, inasmuch as modern treatments remain, to a large extent, futile.

Asbestos is not one but a family of naturally occurring fibrous silicates located in mineral deposits scattered worldwide. The physical and chemical properties of these various minerals not only influence their industrial uses but also dictate their pathogenicity. In this book, we first consider the characteristics of the unique fibrous minerals known as asbestos and their discovery. We then turn to a discussion of the major uses of these materials in the past. The epidemiology of the diseases asbestos causes and the risks associated with exposure are then discussed. Individual asbestos-associated diseases are considered in detail from the clinical, pathological, and pathogenic perspective in the context of approaches to diagnoses and treatment. Finally, we look at the history of regulatory efforts based on governmental actions, and the complex story of litigation related to the asbestos-associated diseases in the United States. Finally, projections for the future worldwide occurrence of the asbestos-related diseases are calculated in the context of the 21st century.

An outstanding team of internationally recognized experts have contributed to this comprehensive book. It would be remarkable if the various authors agreed on all of the issues considered herein, and for that reason, the editor has avoided arbitrating strongly held personal viewpoints, when and if scientific issues remain to be resolved. Similarly, We have avoided pruning the text to eliminate all redundancies, since the arguments of the contributors require the development of background information. Several popularized books and comprehensive articles have been written on the subject, particularly from the historical perspective. Thousands upon thousands of scientific papers and a few scientific texts also have addressed various facets of the story of asbestos-associated diseases. We have designed this tome to be comprehensive and a distillation of the enormous literature on the subject. This is not a text to be read cover to cover, and it is certainly not bedside reading at the end of a long day.

John E. Craighead, MD
Allen R. Gibbs, MB, ChB Coeditors

Contents

Contributors   xi

Chapter 1. From Cotton-Stone to the New York Conference:
            Asbestos-Related Diseases 1878–1965   3
            Bruce W. Case

Chapter 2. Mineralogy of Asbestos   23
            John E. Craighead, Allen Gibbs, and Fred Pooley

Chapter 3. Diseases Associated with Asbestos Industrial
            Products and Environmental Exposure   39
            John E. Craighead

Chapter 4. Epidemiology and Risk Assessment   94
            Graham W. Gibbs and Geoffrey Berry

Chapter 5. Molecular Responses to Asbestos: Induction of Cell
            Proliferation and Apoptosis Through Modulation of
            Redox-Dependent Cell Signaling Pathways   120
            Nicholas H. Heintz and Brooke T. Mossman

Chapter 6. Benign Pleural and Parenchymal Diseases Associated
            with Asbestos Exposure   139
            John E. Craighead

Chapter 7. Lung Cancer Associated with Asbestos Exposure   172
            Richard Attanoos

Chapter 8. Malignant Diseases of the Pleura, Peritoneum, and
            Other Serosal Surfaces   190
            Allen R. Gibbs and John E. Craighead

Chapter 9. Nonthoracic Cancers Possibly Resulting from Asbestos
            Exposure   230
            John E. Craighead

Chapter 10. Diagnostic Features and Clinical Evaluation of the
            Asbestos-Associated Diseases   253
            David Weill

Chapter 11. Radiological Features of the Asbestos-Associated
Diseases   269
Haydn Adams and Michael D. Crane

Chapter 12. Mineral Fiber Analysis and Asbestos-Related Diseases   299
Allen R. Gibbs and Fred Pooley

Chapter 13. US Governmental Regulatory Approaches and Actions   317
John E. Craighead

Chapter 14. Therapeutic Approaches to Malignant Mesothelioma   326
Harvey I. Pass, Stephen Hahn, and Nicholas Vogelzang

Chapter 15. Asbestos Exposure and the Law in the United States   346
Kevin Leahy

Chapter 16. Asbestos Exposure and Disease Trends in the 20th and
21st Centuries   375
Bertram Price and Adam Ware

Index   397

Contributors

HAYDN ADAMS, MB, BS, MRCP, FRCR   Consultant Radiologist, Department of Radiology, Llandough Hospital, Cardiff and Vale NHS Trust, Penarth, Glamorgan, United Kingdom

RICHARD ATTANOOS, BSc, MBBS, FRCPath   Consultant Pathologist, Department of Histopathology, Llandough Hospital, Cardiff and Vale NHS Trust, Penarth, Glamorgan, United Kingdom

GEOFFREY BERRY, MA, PhD   Emeritus Professor, School of Public Health, University of Sydney, New South Wales, Australia

BRUCE W. CASE, MD, MSc, D. Occup. Hygiene, FRCP(C)   Associate Professor of Pathology, McGill University, Westmount, Quebec, Canada

JOHN E. CRAIGHEAD, MD   Emeritus Professor, Department of Pathology, University of Vermont, Amelia Island, Florida

MICHAEL D. CRANE, MB BCh FRCP, FRCR   Consultant Radiologist, Department of Radiology, Llandough Hospital, Penarth, Glamorgan, United Kingdom

ALLEN R. GIBBS, MB, ChB, FRCPath   Consultant Histopathologist, Department of Histopathology, Llandough Hospital, Cardiff and Vale NHS Trust, Penarth, Glamorgan, United Kingdom

GRAHAM W. GIBBS, MSc, PhD, MRSC, ROH   Adjunct Professor, Department of Public Health Sciences, University of Alberta, Devon, Alberta, Canada

STEPHEN M. HAHN, MD   Professor and Chair, Department of Radiation Oncology, University of Pennsylvania, Philadelphia, Pennsylvania

NICHOLAS H. HEINTZ, PhD   Professor, Department of Pathology, University of Vermont, Burlington, Vermont

KEVIN L. LEAHY, Esq.   Partner, Brown McCarroll, LLP Austin, Texas

BROOKE T. MOSSMAN, PhD   Professor, Department of Pathology, University of Vermont, Burlington, Vermont

HARVEY I. PASS, MD, BA   Professor and Chief, Division of Thoracic Surgery, NYU Medical Center, New York

FREDERICK D. POOLEY, PhD   Research Professor, Division of Materials and Minerals, Cardiff School of Engineering, Cardiff University, Cardiff, United Kingdom

BERTRAM PRICE, PhD   President, Price Associates, Inc., White Plains, New York

NICHOLAS J. VOGELZANG, MD, FACP   Professor of Medicine and Director, Nevada Cancer Institute, Las Vegas, Nevada

ADAM WARE, PhD   Senior Researcher, Price Associates, Inc., White Plains, New York

DAVID WEILL, MD   Associate Professor, Division of Pulmonary and Critical Care Medicine, Stanford University, Stanford, California

Asbestos and Its Diseases

1

From Cotton-Stone to the New York Conference: Asbestos-Related Diseases 1878–1965

Bruce W. Case

No writer can divorce him or herself from his or her experience. My own began through the chance relocation of a classmate to a farm facing the tailings of the Jeffrey Mine outside the mining town of Asbestos, Province of Québec. I spent 6 months there with my friends and shared their concerns about possible health effects of the mine and its tailings. As a pathologist is not equipped by training to study such causal relationships, I undertook experimental work with asbestos at New York's Mount Sinai School of Medicine, where I met Drs Irving Selikoff and Arthur Langer. Langer, a mineralogist, first interested me in using lung fiber content as a means of assessing exposure, although it was in Montreal that I had the opportunity to put it into practice (Case and Sebastien, 1987). Returning to McGill, I studied epidemiology with Drs Corbett and Allison McDonald, Patrick Sebastien, Margo Becklake, and others who had done much of the most important research concerned with asbestos-related disease since the mid-1960s. One of our projects was conducted jointly with Dr Philip Enterline (McDonald, Case, Enterline et al., 1990) at the University of Pittsburgh, who was retiring as the director of the US EPA's Center for Environmental Epidemiology. I applied for his position and stayed in Pittsburgh for 3 years. While there, I met many of the other pioneers in the field, including the late Drs Thomas Mancuso and Christopher Wagner. We are all shaped by those with whom we either worked or interacted professionally. To the extent possible this chapter relates the historical facts as I have learned them through these associations.

Introduction

Commonly used minerals and industrial chemicals, like pharmaceutical agents, often evolve through a complex life-story. Initially, the "miracle" substance is believed to solve potentially any manner of problem. Second, the miraculous nature of the substance is found to have something in common with the "Emperor's new clothes" and the pendulum swings in the opposite direction. Finally, in most cases, the assets and liabilities are totaled up as a true understanding and, most importantly, a realistic expectation is reached after years of use and study.

This is surely the history of the minerals known as asbestos (Chapter 2). These fibrous minerals had undeniable usefulness, but some resulted in catastrophic and widespread human health effects. The minerals known as "asbestos" represent a group of naturally occurring fibrous silicates, defined commercially much more easily than as "minerals." There are only three asbestos types of major commercial importance—chrysotile, the most widely used, and only member of the magnesium-rich serpentine class, and the asbestos amphiboles "crocidolite" (fibrous riebeckite) and "amosite" (fibrous cumming-tonite-grunerite). The latter iron-rich fibrous silicates are just two of over 50 members of the amphibole group, most of which are obscure minerals of no economic importance.

Practically, exposure is often difficult to characterize (Chapters 3 and 4). First, asbestos mixtures are frequently used in industry—especially chrysotile with either amosite (eg, in thermal insulation) or crocidolite (eg, in asbestos cement pipe). Second, for miners and millers of chrysotile, talc, and vermiculite in some geographical locations, if not end-product users, exposures to "contaminant" noncommercial amphiboles are common.

An additional factor confounding a strict separation of minerals goes beyond "asbestos" but involves two separate classes of the amphiboles, which collectively make up a great percentage of the earth's crust. Amphiboles occur both in forms that are and are not fibrous. For those that are not fibrous (called "prismatic" or simply "nonasbestiform"), the United States Occupational Safety and Health Administration (OSHA) (1992) ruled that the "available evidence supports a conclusion that exposure to nonasbestiform cleavage fragments is not likely to produce a significant risk of developing asbestos-related disease." The distinction, however, is not a simple one; the problems were also noted by this author in the *British Journal of Industrial Medicine* (Case, 1991a). What is and what is not "asbestiform" tremolite would be less critical if those who advocate such a definition could show that there is a clear distinction between fiber and cleavage fragments from a disease-causing perspective. Unfortunately, this is not the case. The differences in structure between massive, acicular, and fibrous morphology are not "sharply defined but do represent points on a spectrum of structural forms." So-called cleavage fragments may, in a strict morphological sense, be fibrous in their microscopical appearance, and there is no convincing evidence that these 'fibers' are of no public health concern (Case, 1991a,b; American Thoracic Society, 1990).

Despite these difficulties, the best definition of "asbestos" is probably still the simplest: "A group of fibrous minerals that can be split longitudinally and have commercial uses" (Wagner, 1990). It originally was used for chrysotile, in the commercial sense, and "if this had been maintained and the other materials referred to as the amphibole fibres…confusion in assessing the risk hazard would not have occurred." According to the International Agency for Research on Cancer (IARC), "there remains taxonomic confusion and lack of a standard operating definition for fibers. 'Asbestos' is often inappropriately used as a generic, homogeneous rubric, and even when the asbestos fibre type is specified, its source is rarely stated" (Kane et al., 1996). Throughout the rest of this chapter and through this book, quotation marks around "asbestos" may not be used, but readers should keep these reservations in mind.

The grouping of the three commercial asbestos minerals is usually supplemented by the addition of the three "noncommercial" asbestiform amphiboles tremolite, actinolite, and anthophyllite, which are regulated in the United States. All, particularly the latter in Finland, have had some exploitation for commerce, although their principal health effects either have been recognized in environmental settings, or as occupational coexposures (sometimes variably referred to as "contaminants") with other minerals, including chrysotile, vermiculite, and talc.

The amphiboles extend far beyond the usual and regulated five, and their nonfibrous analogues are common. As noted, this has led to some difficulty in classification, but at least in theory all of the amphibole minerals do have a structural asbestos form. Some of these unregulated asbestiform amphiboles are occasionally present in situations of occupational or environmental exposure as health hazard. The classical examples are fibrous winchite and richterite that are components of the asbestos cocktail known as "Libby amphibole" from the infamous deposit at Zonolite Mountain in Libby, Montana (Bandli and Gunter, 2006; McDonald et al., 2004; Peipins et al., 2003; Sullivan, 2007). Recently, edenite was added to the list (Biggeri et al., 2004; Bruno et al., 2006; Travaglione et al., 2003).

This introductory chapter is meant to paint, with broad strokes, the first stages in the development of our knowledge of asbestos, especially our understanding of its human health effects. Experimental studies, both in vivo and in vitro, are referred to only incidentally. The latter may be of value in helping us understand mechanisms and possible treatment, but they are not helpful in quantitative risk assessment, despite the continued reliance of some national and international agencies on laboratory observations, at least for hazard evaluation (Chapter 5).

The asbestos story is a long one. If sheer numbers of scientific and nonscientific publications are a guide, we should know more about asbestos and its effects, and presumably have reached more consensus than we have for any other chemical or mineral. Yet, we clearly have not. While asbestos production and use have declined precipitously since the peak year of 1973 in the United States (Virta, 2003a) and 1977 (Abratt et al., 2004) in South Africa, it leveled out at about 2×10^6 tons per year in the 1990s and into the 21st century, a level just under 50% of the peak production in the mid decades of the last century. Western society has essentially stopped mining and using asbestos; commercial bans with some exceptions are in place or soon will be in all of the European Economic Community as well as in Australia, Argentina, and elsewhere; and mining has effectively ended in both the United States and Canada. The last American mine to close was in California in 2002 and the last Canadian mine is due to close permanently in Thetford Mines, Québec in 2008 (McDougall, 2007). Mining and product manufacture appear conversely to be increasing elsewhere, for example, in China, Kazakhstan, Russia, and Zimbabwe. As in other industries, cheap labor has made asbestos mining more viable in these economies.

Asbestos is commonly distributed in the earth's crust. According to the United States Geological Survey (USGS), asbestos (usually chrysotile but amphiboles as well, including crocidolite in Missouri among other places) has been found in 20 states and mined in 17 (Kisvarsanyi and Kisvarsanyi, 1989; USGS, 2001, 2006). In Canada, asbestos mining occurred in four of the ten provinces.

> There have been thousands of applications for asbestos. Most were viewed as practical solutions to difficult problems. For instance, asbestos helped make the braking systems in automobiles much more dependable, it enabled the production of inexpensive cement-based water-supply pipes, and despite the dire consequences to the installers, asbestos insulation made the warships of World War II much safer. (USGS, 2001)

The latter is often forgotten today, and what caused the asbestos group to be called "miracle minerals" was ironically the ability to protect and save lives. Similarly, in France, the first large Western country to "ban" asbestos—the Paris Metro Fire in 1903 took 84 lives and resulted in the use of the mineral in reconstruction. Asbestos in schools and other public buildings—in the recent past a source of great worry to parents and faculty alike (despite lingering questions about the degree and tremendous cost of remediation [Abelson, 1990; Berry, 1990])—was introduced to protect the occupants.

What, then, went wrong? It was a gradual realization of the diseases that resulted from exposure to these inherently toxic minerals (coupled with a reluctance of governments and industry to accept and act upon this knowledge). We see today a similar situation with the reluctance to accept the reality of global warming and its inevitable future consequences, compounded by the inaction of industry and government. Finally, and least inherently obvious, the sheer volume and complexity of knowledge about asbestos and its health effects, coupled with a failure to use the best available science in a timely and reasonable manner to protect health, has resulted in exposures of workers, which are unacceptable and yet avoidable. Unfortunately, as the so-called developed countries discontinue the mining and manufacturing of asbestos and asbestos products, they are replaced by developing countries, where labor is cheap and environmental standards are often poor. While much has been made of available substitutes for asbestos, in these countries one or more forms of asbestos itself is the substitute; only the sources have changed.

This introductory chapter is not meant to be comprehensive; the following chapters will outline individual diseases and their relation to exposures. My goal here is to set forth how we came to understand asbestos and its potential as a cause of disease. In this vein, it is important for the reader to understand that the initial observations may, in retrospect, receive more attention than they deserve; for example, the "first" observation that asbestos could cause lung cancer (LC), is far less important than the emergence of a general understanding of how, when, and under what circumstances LC could result from asbestos exposure—and, how both exposure and disease can be prevented in future. Date-by-date historical analysis is less important in this regard than the following two questions.

First, when did the first solid body of evidence (usually one or more epidemiological studies; or, occasionally a collection of cases in either a given geographical area or occupational group, so large that it effectively constituted what is known as either an ecological or prevalence study) emerge?

Second, and more difficult to determine, when did this evidence enter the known realm of "best available medical science"?

Even today consensus as to what questions have and have not been answered is difficult. It is important to understand that "consensus" is not "universal agreement," and is not quantifiable. One writer's consensus will be another's ongoing debate, although both should be informed by more than personal opinion. Evaluations of the most basic hazards do change over time, as can be seen by the recent reversal of the IARC's 1988 hazard evaluation for synthetic mineral fibers as "possibly carcinogenic to humans (Group 2B)" (for "glasswool," rockwool, and slagwool) (IARC, 1988). By 2002, however, epidemiological studies led the same body to conclude that "insulation glass wool, continuous glass filament, rock (stone) wool and slag wool are not classifiable as to their carcinogenicity to humans (Group 3)" due to the insufficiency of human evidence (IARC, 2002).

There is little we know now that we did not know 10, 20, or in many cases, 40 years ago, although there is much to be learned by the synthesis of past knowledge, and especially what we can do to prevent future disease. It is hoped that this chapter will inform on the evolution of knowledge about asbestos exposure and its hazards. In doing so, two points that were landmarks have been chosen as "beginning" and "end"—the beginning of chrysotile mining in the Province of Québec, Canada, and the New York Conference summarizing knowledge of asbestos health effects published in 1965 by the New York Academy of Sciences (Selikoff and Churg, 1965).

The Discovery and Beginnings of Asbestos

Although fibrous minerals resistant to heat have been known for centuries, and to a lesser degree for millennia, asbestos as a group of commercially useful fibrous minerals are a 20th-century phenomenon beginning principally in Canada, and to a lesser degree in South Africa and Italy, in the late 19th century. The history of earlier uses of asbestos is of academic interest and is well summarized by others (Browne, 1994; Virta, 2003a,b). A brief overview of the historical events in Québec, which are seldom described elsewhere, follows.

The discovery of asbestos in Québec was, without exception, of the mineral that we now know as chrysotile. The discovery of other fibrous minerals having some of the same commercial properties but different chemical and physical qualities came earlier in South Africa and later in Australia.

Two points are of note in the origins of the industry in Québec; first, the potential commercial value was quickly realized and second, arguments over money and "flips" in the ownership of mining land with rapidly accelerating prices quickly followed. Ironically, the first asbestos litigation, so much a concern today, actually took place shortly after the discovery.

Fortier (1983) reports that Logan, in his Canadian Geological Report of 1847, noted for the first time the presence of chrysotile in the Eastern Township region of Québec. This and previous observations in the Appalachian serpentine belt before the American Revolution were not accompanied by any realization of the commercial value of what was found. Mid-18th-century references were similarly ignored. A patent for a machine that could produce an asbestos lining for industrial machines was submitted in England in 1857. A London syndicate also became interested in extracting asbestos in the Italian Alps during the 1800s. The Patent Asbestos Manufacturing Company making asbestos-containing products was started there in 1871 (Fortier, 1983).

In 1860, the first asbestos specimens were extracted from a Québec riverbank. A specimen was shown in London at the International Exhibition of 1862. However, although a company for making asbestos-containing products was started in Québec in 1871, the find was not thought to be commercially worthwhile.

It is difficult to sort out the facts from the apocryphal as to the first meaningful discovery of commercial asbestos, but it is known that it was in the Thetford Mines area of Québec in the late 1870s, where "chrysotile was visible in some quantity in surface outcrops" (Smith, 1968). According to tradition, in 1876, a farmer named Joseph Fecteau stopped to rest for a few moments (Poulin, 1975) and discovered a rock having white filaments (pierre au cotton, literally cotton-stone). An eyewitness claimed that Fecteau was picking blueberries with friends, one of them named Onésime Gilbert walking ahead. According to this account, Gilbert saw a "vein which shone in the sun." "Come and see—I have found a gold mine," he related to the others, and soon all five were scraping pieces of chrysotile with their pocket knives to take home (Gilbert, 1955). And "white gold" was what he had indeed found: to this day the district encompassing the mining area is officially named Or Blanc (Fortier, 1983; Poulin, 1975; Smith, 1968).

Not long thereafter the find provided object lessons for the future. The local homesteader who owned the rights to the land, Robert Ward, was shown the material by Fecteau and excitedly took it to Québec City. University professors there told him it was worthless (the first, but not the last academic error about asbestos). Ward believed otherwise, and he sent samples to Boston where Brown relayed a more optimistic opinion. Ward bought the 218 acres he homesteaded from the Crown on May 13, 1878. Exactly 1 month later, he resold 100 acres to the Asbestos Packing Company of Boston for $4000—a windfall profit by 19th-century standards.

Then followed asbestos litigation! The Boston company sued Ward and won, claiming the original sale had mistaken one part of the lot for another. Eight years later, in 1888, the American company resold the land again to Bell Asbestos Company of London, England, for over £41,000; the next "flip" was to the Keasbey and Mattison Company— for $650,000, just 8 years later. Three trends were established: the British-American control of a Québec resource; the immense value of that resource; and the willingness to use the courts to get it. The latter two remain factors to the present day, although surely not in the way these 19th-century principals had anticipated.

The Period of Isolated Observations and the Emergence of Asbestosis as a Disease

As we shall see with the other asbestos-related diseases, asbestosis was first reflected in incremental accumulation of case reports and anecdotes. It is perhaps difficult in retrospect to understand why the definitive discovery of the disease took 40–50 years: after all, we now believe that 25 f/mL-years of exposure conveys, on average, a risk for causing disease in 1% of an exposed population (Dupre et al., 1984). While there is no way to know the exact exposures of the early miners, millers, and plant-workers in Canada, England, and the United States, it is reasonable to believe they must have been so high as to represent a multiple of this figure in a single year. Indeed, even as late as 1951, there were many reports on exposure in mines and factories that exceeded 30, 50, 75, or in one instance up to 2×10^8 particles per cubic foot—and while these figures are not directly translatable to f/mL, one would have to multiply by at least three, assuming all particles counted in a midget impinger were indeed "asbestos" (Liddell, 1991).

There is a latency period even for asbestosis, but few knowledgeable scientists would put it beyond 20 years at this level of exposure. So why were cases not seen by members of the medical profession—or at least, not reported until the 1920s and later? Some observers have tried to state otherwise but their analysis has been envisioned to be post hoc revisionism by those familiar with the times. The UK Inspectors of Factories and other regulators retained the confidence of labor unions, even receiving kind words from Karl Marx, who praised their work (Bartrip, 2001).

However, the immensely "dusty" environments were certainly known, and documented, and a "dusty" environment had long been known to be detrimental to health. There were certainly reports of pulmonary disease due to dust inhalation before the official recognition of asbestosis in 1930 (Merewether and Price, 1930), and probably before 1920. Silicosis was first officially compensated in Great Britain in 1925, but was recognized much earlier. Indeed, the importance of silicosis—and especially tuberculosis— may have confounded early knowledge of asbestosis just as tuberculosis later confused South African physicians when they encountered the first large geographical cluster of crocidolite-induced malignant mesothelioma (MM). In Québec, as elsewhere, there was confounding by tuberculosis and silicosis—in Thetford Mines the tuberculosis rate was almost twice that of the national rate, and the highest of any community in the Province (Cartier, 1949; Delisle and Malouf, 2004). Silicosis had earlier caused a "scandal" in a nearby community where many workers had died, and there was some overlap between those responsible for industrial hygiene in the two industries (as well as government policy). Nevertheless, by 1946, asbestosis was being compensated in Québec as well, although not in the absence of radiological evidence of the disease (Cartier, 1949).

Part of the problem may have been that asbestosis itself was a "new" disease. "At the beginning of the 20th century, the asbestos industry was so small that individual physicians never encountered a sufficient number of cases of asbestosis or LC to be alerted to the danger" (McCulloch, 2002). Even if they had, they lacked our current epidemiological tools to describe them in terms of risk; a concept that awaited the work of Sir Richard Doll in the 1950s.

The first recorded case reports of asbestosis and LC in Québec (Enterline, 1991; Enterline et al., 1978) are attributable to Desmeules and Sirois (1941). Of note, the authors "…considered it logical that, as has been assumed for silicosis, asbestosis represented a predisposing factor for pulmonary carcinoma." Given that the industry had started more than 50 years before, there were surely asbestosis cases much earlier.

The evolution of knowledge in the United Kingdom is emblematic. While it was generally established by 1930 (Merewether and Price, 1930) that asbestosis was known to be caused by exposure, the evidence had been accumulating for some time. Although some cite earlier reports, it is generally accepted that "the first medical paper on the subject appeared in 1924" (Bartrip, 2004). William Cooke, a pathologist, briefly described the case of a young woman who worked in the Rochdale textile plant in Lancashire, England, as a "rover." She had, in fact, been said to have suffered "asbestos poisoning" 2 years earlier, and there was an inquest when she died in 1924. Relying on archival material, Bartrip (2004) quotes Cooke as having testified that "mineral particles in the lungs originated from asbestos and were, beyond reasonable doubt, the primary cause of the fibrosis of the lungs and therefore of death." Cooke (1924) published his results the same year, but first used the term "asbestosis" in a 1927 report of the same case (Cooke, 1927). Between 1927 and 1930 a number of case reports appeared in the British and South African literature, and coincidentally it was in 1927 that a medical inspector was asked to ascertain "whether the occurrence of this disease in an asbestos worker was merely a coincidence, or evidence of a definite health risk in the industry." Merewether began immediately, and completed his investigation in October of 1929. He determined that a prolonged duration of exposure to "asbestos dust" at high concentration produced "definite occupational risk among asbestos workers as a class" (Merewether and Price, 1930).

The medical literature tended to differ from country to country (or language to language); first reports ranged from 1924 in the United Kingdom to 1941 in Québec to 1950 in Denmark (Frost, 1950).

It can be fairly said that by 1930, almost 50 years after the first Québec discovery, the "new" disease of pulmonary asbestosis was established, and the first of what were to be many decades of well-intentioned but ultimately unsuccessful approaches to dust control were put in place (Doll, 1955; Merewether and Price, 1930). As previously noted, we now know that as late as 1951, dust levels were so high that asbestosis was inevitable (Liddell, 1991). Even today, while mining and milling industries in most countries have controlled exposure to a point where asbestosis can be prevented, in some regions of the world such as in parts of China, conditions are believed to be sufficient to constitute an ongoing problem (Tossavainen et al., 2001).

The discovery of asbestos as causing asbestosis triggered increasing interest in the protection of those exposed. Progress was, however, incremental, with each generation lowering the limits on exposure promulgated by the one before and often declaring that the problem was thereby likely to be solved (Chapter 13).

Further complicating the asbestosis issue was its diagnosis—pathological, and especially clinical. The question of uniform pathological criteria for diagnosis was not addressed in early efforts. In 1982, a committee of the National Institute for Occupational Safety and Health (NIOSH) and the College of American Pathologists (Craighead et al., 1982) settled the issue. A scheme for both diagnosis and grading was offered, and although some (especially in the United Kingdom) have found it overly liberal in its lowest category it remains generally accepted.

Even so, clinical diagnosis was, and is, most important, as it would be contraindicated to biopsy lung simply to prove asbestosis unless another, treatable disease was seriously considered in the differential diagnosis. While criteria for the latter have changed over time, imaging techniques have always taken pride of place, with the International Union Against Cancer (UICC)/ILO B-reading schema being the "gold standard" until recently, despite possible inaccuracy and the potential for biased readings at the lower end (Gitlin et al., 2004; Chapter 11). Very recently, more advanced techniques (eg, high resolution CT scan) have been suggested as an improved diagnostic tool, but a uniform scheme analogous to the B-reader's chest x-ray has yet to be tested.

Regardless of the method used for diagnosis, most of those with asbestosis, both historically and today, neither had a tissue diagnosis of the disease nor any need of one. Even the crudest of x-rays would have been capable, coupled with clinical signs of unequivocal fibrosis in the lungs of many of the workers seen by Merewether or in later studies. These were patients with hundreds of f/mL-years of cumulative exposure who were likely to die of asbestosis or its complications. As the intensities of the exposures waned, the diagnosis increasingly became an issue. A related issue has been the ability to identify and quantify not only the presence and extent of asbestosis radiologically, but the degree of functional impairment implied by such a diagnosis coupled with measures of severity such as pathological grade and extent.

It was also discovered early on that asbestos could, indeed often did, cause pleural changes. Most often, these were relatively isolated, well-demarcated fibrotic lesions on the thoracic lining of the chest wall named "pleural plaques" (PP) (Chapters 6 and 11). They were recognized as markers of exposure and as such later became controversial as possible markers of asbestos-related disease risk probability, or harbingers of cancer. When calcified, PP were relatively easy to diagnose by chest x-ray, but if not they could be confused with unrelated tissue masses such as "fat pads." In addition, some observers referred to them as part of a spectrum of lesions called "pleural asbestosis." This is a term less confusing if confined to a much rarer true diffuse fibrosis of the pleura accompanying marked asbestos exposure and producing true restrictive lung disease (Chapters 6 and 10). It is better still avoided altogether; the use of the term, while acceptable if used carefully, always risks being confused with true pulmonary interstitial fibrosis caused by asbestos exposure. Other nonneoplastic but *clinically significant* pleural lesions have been described more recently (Constantopoulos et al., 1985, 1991; Peipins et al., 2003; Weis, 2001). Although there is still debate about the degree to which PP are "independent" markers of LC and MM risk in the populations in which they occur, there has never been any indication that any of the nonneoplastic pleural lesions can themselves transform into malignancies. Another error that is sometimes made by unwitting researchers is to assume that the recovery of fibers from such plaques, or even more egregiously from pleural tumor tissue, is a legitimate means of measuring asbestos "in the pleura"; by definition such new growths would not be the proper locations to look. Better means for evaluating the "actual" pleura should be relied upon (Boutin et al., 1996; Dumortier et al., 2002).

Asbestos and Malignancy: Early Observations (1930–1955)

During this period of time, a relationship between asbestos exposure and malignancy had not been established, but some astute observers raised the possibility. The initial basis for suspicion was LC reported in cases of asbestosis. As noted by Enterline (1991; Enterline et al., 1978), the first such published observation was by Wood and Gloyne (1934), who reported on two cases of LC (then a relatively rare malignancy) among 43 cases of asbestosis, but did not link either the latter disease or its cause with the malignancy. Gloyne (1935) indeed specifically rejected the hypothesis in a report of an additional two cases a year later; notably one case of presumptive "squamous carcinoma of the pleura" was also mentioned. The two cases were found incidentally at autopsy, in women workers at an asbestos plant. Because Wood and Gloyne rejected a causal relationship, the first statement in the literature reflecting causation is usually attributed to a single case report by Lynch and Smith (1935). They related the disease to "asbestosis" rather than asbestos exposure per se "by reason of chronic bronchial irritation...comparable with the current knowledge of the etiology of such tumors" (Enterline et al., 1978). In fact, the authors of both reports were nonetheless skeptical about such a relationship given the lack of what would today be called epidemiological and experimental animal evidence—the two modern cornerstones of hazard evaluation in risk assessment (Case and Mattison, 1991).

The self-published narrative literature review by Enterline et al. (1978) is extremely useful in assembling the isolated findings between 1934 and 1964 in context. It was initially designed to answer the question "does asbestosis predispose to lung cancer?" When the authors became convinced that the answer to that question had already been established in the affirmative (an answer that has subsequently been challenged) they turned their attention to a historical description of when and how this concept had developed, and included MM in their inquiries.

The first case reports of "pleural cancer" related to "asbestosis" seem clearly to have been from Germany (Wedler, 1943). Nazi Germany was, in fact, well ahead of the rest of the West in their assessment of dust-related diseases (and smoking), as well as in preventive measures and industrial hygiene (Proctor, 1999). Wedler noted three autopsy reports of asbestosis in asbestos plant-workers. Two of the three also had "pleural cancer." In addition, 14 cases of "lung or pleural cancer" were found in a review of 92 autopsies of patients with asbestosis.

In 1952, a short account by Cartier, a physician at the Industrial Clinic for the mines located in and around Thetford Mines, Québec, was appended to a long article published by Smith (Cartier 1952; Smith 1952). Cartier (1952) noted eight cases of LC among 4000 asbestos miners and millers over a 10-year period, two of which he called "pleural MM," the latter a term not yet in general use. Cartier was not impressed by the small number of LC, but the appearance of the rarer MM variant (thought at the time to be a form of LC) led him to speculate that these tumors might have an occupational origin. Other scientists attempted to persuade Cartier that the diagnosis was wrong and that the "mesotheliomas" were, in fact, bronchoalveolar carcinomas, perhaps denying Cartier an important place in history as the first outside wartime Germany to suspect that MM was a consequence of asbestos exposure. On the other hand, this author reviewed the original autopsy report of one of Cartier's two patients and interviewed the worker's then 80-year-old son, and indeed a differential diagnosis between "pleural MM" and "bronchoalveolar carcinoma" was considered by the reporting pathologist, since the tumor appeared to arise in a major bronchus. According to his son, the subject was an office worker who had been a very heavy smoker and whose office had been immediately adjacent to tremolite-rich chrysotile mines for almost 30 years. Cartier also later reported six LC cases found among 40 autopsy cases with asbestosis (Enterline et al., 1978; Cartier 1955), while seven cases were found among workers without asbestosis (denominator unknown). Although Cartier did not believe there was "...any statistical relationship of a cause (sic) relationship," his paper was soon overshadowed by the definitive epidemiological study of Doll (1955) that established asbestos once and for all as a cause of LC.

The Period of Discovery (1955–1965): Epidemiology in the Ascendancy

The period began with a publication by Doll (1955) representing the first true epidemiological study linking asbestos exposure to LC, and culminated with the publication of the Proceedings of the New York Conference in 1965 (Selikoff and Churg, 1965). What had been the subject of isolated case observations, editorial comments, and even some compensation law (as in Germany, the United Kingdom, and Canada) gave way to a methodical scientific approach that established once and for all that asbestos was a cause of LC and of MM. The details of how and when this did or did not occur remain controversial, but in retrospect it is clear that everything that followed built on the work of this time period. Hueper, who wrote about environmental lung cancer and air pollution and lung cancer from 1951 through three decades, summarized the case reports:

> Thus, there is at present a total of 80 cases of asbestosis cancer (sic) of the lung on record. (Hueper, 1956)

He further dismissed on epidemiological grounds Cartier's impression that eight lung cancers among a workforce of 4000 workers over 10 years would of necessity prove a lack of association, since the raw numbers failed to take into account what we would now call person-years of employment, dose-response relationships, any external comparison of population risk, or mortality (not to mention the fact that of 40 autopsied workers with asbestosis, six died with LC). Hueper was skeptical initially about the effects of smoking on LC. This was in fact not at all unusual; like Hueper even Doll had at first been predisposed to think of the rising tide of automobile exhaust-related exposures in the general population during the first half of the century as the most likely explanation (Doll, personal communication, 2004).

From this point on, it is no longer useful to speak of "case reports" and none will be mentioned further; case reports had been useful in asking questions, but they are rarely useful in answering them. As Enterline writes of Doll's 1955 landmark paper:

> The paper by Doll marked an end to widespread acceptance of purely clinical observations…and opened the way for contributions by epidemiologists and biostatisticians. (Enterline et al., 1978)

There was now a major scientific shift from case reports and speculation to a reliance on solid proof provided by modern analytical epidemiology. It was fitting that Doll, who essentially founded the science, was the first to apply it to asbestos (Doll, 1955). He had used epidemiological inquiry only a few years earlier to prove tobacco as the principal cause of LC. As Greenberg (1999) notes:

> This paper was based on the analyses of two sets of data. First, Doll reviewed the death registrations provided (from the Rochdale, England textile plant) files for 105 employees who had been subjected to Coroners autopsies from 1935 to 1952. He noted that of the 75 who had asbestosis, 15 also were affected with LC, and that of the 30 without asbestosis, only three had LC. Then he reviewed the mortality experience of 113 males who had been employed in the so-called "scheduled areas" 7 for 20 or more years.[1] Asbestos workers who were employed for 20 or more years in so-called "scheduled areas" suffered a risk of LC some 10 times higher than experienced by the age-matched members of the general population.

---

1 Scheduled as a hazardous area under the Asbestos Industry Regulations 1931 requiring dust control and medical supervision.

The concept of a population-based context was new to the study of occupational cancer in general, and its major contribution was to establish definitively the relationship between exposure and LC. While "asbestosis" was used as a marker of exposure, Doll never stated "asbestosis" per se to be the cause: it was work in exposed areas that Doll associated with lung cancer. Regrettably, although a landmark, Doll's study was not recognized by many at the time and had little immediate impact on contemporary thinking.

Doll's work was the first prospective epidemiological study concerned with asbestos; it was followed by a second in Canada (Braun and Truan, 1958) and a third in the United States (Mancuso and Coulter, 1963). The Braun and Truan (1958) study of asbestos miners was reported to be "negative," but this conclusion was questioned by Hueper at the time, and later by McDonald (1973). The 1963 study of Mancuso and Coulter "got it right." It showed that of almost 1.5×10^3 asbestos product manufacturing workers, 19 developed LC (vs five expected). They also found three "peritoneal cancers," two of which were proven to be MM. Again, the Mancuso and Coulter (1963) study went largely unrecognized by workers in the field.

By this time, however, the finding of MM in the asbestos-exposed was not something new. It had been established by the seminal report of the South African pathologist, Wagner, working closely with Sleggs, a physician who noted an unusual disease among patients in the Northern Cape Province crocidolite fields beginning in about 1956.

Asbestos, mainly crocidolite and amosite at first but later chrysotile as well, had been mined in South Africa commercially since the mid-1920s, and on a smaller scale intermittently for several decades before. The Cape Asbestos Corporation factory in London was constructed in 1916 (McCulloch, 2002). Production increased through 1950, although not to the same levels as with chrysotile in Québec. Understandably, early South African scientific study did not follow the rigorous epidemiological approach applied by McDonald and colleagues in Québec.

Wagner had firm roots in South Africa, where his father was a prominent geologist who had published a definitive text on the geology of South Africa in 1930. According to Wagner in 1950 "the South African Government Engineer realized that the mines were becoming much larger and producing more dust. He therefore persuaded the South African government to register all asbestos mines."[2]

Wagner noted that the government mining "Engineer" asked for "an investigation to be undertaken" to answer two questions: first, were the asbestos-related diseases being recorded in other countries also occurring in South Africa?; and second, if so, was there a difference between the fiber types in this regard? Wagner also noted that up to this time no environmental disease had been noted and the diagnosis of MM as a disease entity was "highly controversial," with many doubting its actual existence. Those who accepted it believed that the tumor was very rare and of unknown etiology. This was complicated again by the fact, as in Québec, that until the 1950s "cases of pleural effusion and pleural thickening would be diagnosed as being tubercular in origin." The latter condition was considered fatal, and in South Africa the "limited pathology services in the rural areas" ruled out most autopsies.[3]

Although South African medical scientists were studying pneumoconiosis, they had focused on silicosis in gold miners. Wagner joined the staff of the South African

2 The following background information is from the personal notes of the late J. Christopher Wagner as kindly furnished by Dr. Margaret Wagner in February of 2004.
3 The latter was not true in Québec where the autopsy rate in workers in studies after 1973 exceeded 50% and of MM cases 70%.

Pneumoconiosis Research Unit in 1952. Two years later, he was appointed "Asbestos Research Fellow," charged to answer the two questions posed by the government mining engineer. He obtained the lungs of every miner or miller who died and had been exposed to asbestos dust. "Dusting chambers" for animal experiments were also established.

In Kimberley, 200 miles distant, the physician, Sleggs, who was Superintendent of a tuberculosis hospital, had seen cases of "pleural tuberculosis" that did not respond to therapy. Puzzled, he turned for help to the surgeon Marchand and the young pathologist, Wagner, far away in Johannesburg. Wagner describes in his notes his first MM case:

> [O]n the 15th February, 1956, I examined the body of a black shower attendant, and diagnosed a MM, on the macroscopic appearance post-mortem. Because this was such a controversial diagnosis I called Professor Becker to come and see the post-mortem and he agreed that this might be a case of diffuse MM…appropriate histological stains, to confirm the diagnosis…were carried out.

At first, the link to crocidolite seemed tenuous; the first patients were "housewives, shepherds, farmers, lawyers, and insurance agents" (Wagner, 1965). A visiting American pathologist, Steiner, had seen such cases and not only agreed with the diagnosis but told Wagner that his team "had the largest collection of this vary rare tumour in the world." But as of 1957, they were unsure of the cause, positing theories of complications of tuberculosis, viral infection "on its own" (Epstein-Barr virus had been associated with Burkitt's lymphoma by this time), or radioactivity (thorium ore was present geologically in the same area). Wagner however clearly preferred as explanatory the "association with blue asbestos," mostly on geographical considerations. The first 16 cases all were from the same region and four worked in the asbestos industry. Some had Asbestos Bodies in the lungs. Wagner realized the importance of establishing the relationship:

> Two thoughts occurred in me: firstly that minor exposure to asbestos dust could lead to the development of a previously unrecognised but fatal tumour, and secondly that they might occur many years after the initial exposure.

He realized the implications, if he were correct, not only to industry workers but also for "risks to those living in the vicinity of the asbestos mines and mills." Industries importing asbestos would have to be warned, and "the whole industry put at risk," but at first (mid-1957) the official reaction of South African "authorities…was that there was not sufficient evidence to disturb the industry in South Africa and elsewhere."

Wagner was instructed that while on sabbatical leave from 1957, he should give a short paper on another subject at a Pneumoconiosis Conference in October of that year. "Discussion of MM was not to be included in talks on asbestos disease with the European authorities, unless there was a direct inquiry. They were not to be mentioned at open meetings."

On his sabbatical, Wagner had the opportunity to visit the Cape Asbestos factory in Barking (a factory and locale studied later by Newhouse and Thompson [1965]). He met the medical officer and the two managing directors, and they brought up the subject of MM. They were of the same mind as the South Africans,

> that the association between MM and asbestos dust was most unlikely…if I persisted I would be wasting my time and effort, and that the trail would come to a dead end. I stated that I thought the situation required further investigation. They agreed that…they would give me reasonable assistance, thus, allowing me to visit their mines and factories in South Africa.

Wagner next visited the plant physician in Rochdale, in early 1958, the site of the largest textile factory in the United Kingdom. He was interested but "another interest he had was in a series of carcinoma cases, that occurred in factory workers with long exposure to asbestos dust. The appearance of one case was suggestive of a MM and had actually been described as an endothelioma" (Bartrip, 2001). At Rochdale, Wagner repeated his findings and suspicions about the Cape MM and was met with the same response: "they did not accept that there was an association between MM and asbestos exposure. They thought it would be extremely foolhardy of me to continue...(but) they would not stand in my way, and would give me any reasonable assistance that I might request."

By the time he returned to South Africa in April of 1959, Wagner's colleagues had collected "a few more cases," and it was around this time that they had a breakthrough. Up until this time, many cases had not been asbestos-related, or so they had thought. In fact, *none* of the new cases since his departure "indicate(d) that there was any exposure to asbestos." Marchand now asked one new patient who was considered "suspicious of a MM" whether he had worked with or been exposed to asbestos dust. The reply was "No, but my father managed a small asbestos mine" (many of the early South African mines were quite small). As Wagner succinctly puts it, "We then realized that we had been asking the wrong questions. All the other cases were then reinterviewed."

The team then set out to reinterview all of their cases, or when they were deceased, their relatives:

The questions were more detailed, with full life histories. Emphasis was placed on:

(1) At any time had you lived in the vicinity of an asbestos mine or mill?
(2) Had your work brought you in contact with asbestos or the blue dust at any time?

With this new approach, a history of exposure to asbestos dust in every case was established. Some were women who had left the mining villages at a young age with tumor development as much as 50 years later; others had been at the school in the village of Kuruman, "which was opposite the asbestos mills and in the break-time they used to slide down the tailings dump."

Shortly thereafter, Wagner and colleagues were visited by Stewart, the head of cancer research at the National Institutes of Health in the United States and an international authority on the geographical distribution of cancer. Stewart convinced the director of the Pneumoconiosis Research Unit that Sleggs and Wagner should present a paper on their findings at an International Pneumoconiosis conference in Johannesburg in 1959.

As we tend to forget today, while industrial medicine was becoming well-established, asbestos as a problem was less a topic of discussion than many other hazards. At the conference, the main interests were silicosis and coal-workers' pneumoconiosis. One scientist, however, John Gilson, Director of the British Pneumoconiosis Research Unit, was curious. Wagner took Gilson to visit amosite and chrysotile mines (around neither of which the group had found any MM); Gilson suggested Wagner's team "must collect more cases and also monitor other asbestos fields." "It was most important to see if this was a disease localized to one mining area, or...a hazard localized to one wherever (sic) crocidolite had been processed." Gilson agreed to try to persuade the British Medical Research Council to "consider an investigation into the problem in that country...(and) agreed that we should submit a paper for publication...."

The now-famous paper (Wagner et al., 1960) was published that year. Nevertheless, Wagner believed that the "paper was first rejected because the leading British pathologist did not believe in the existence (sic) of MM." However, another pathologist, Gough, "was able to convince the editor that the paper should be published." As noted later by Wagner, by this time the authors had established an association with the Cape Asbestos fields in South Africa or the industrial use of asbestos in 32 of the original 33 patients with histologically proven pleural mesotheliomas (Wagner, 1965).

By the time of publication, 14 additional cases were added in a footnote and 1 year later, the number had risen to a total of 87, two of which were peritoneal MM. A potent carcinogen had been unmasked, and its handiwork was clearly not limited to those with occupational exposure but to those in their households and even in the general surrounding environment.

There are some today who minimize the work of Wagner et al. (1960) as "a series of case reports." While it was not a prospective cohort study of the nature of Doll's (1955) or Mancuso and Coulter's (1963), it was certainly epidemiological in nature:

> Thirty-three cases (22 males, 11 females, ages 31–68) of diffuse pleural MM are described; all but one have a probable exposure to crocidolite asbestos (Cape blue). In a majority this exposure was in the Asbestos Hills which lie to the west of Kimberley in Northwest Cape Province. The tumour is rarely seen elsewhere in South Africa.

This is a classical description of the ecological study design and a rare unequivocal result therefrom. From that time forth, it was impossible not to associate MM with crocidolite and its amphibole chemical brethren.[4]

The New York Conference of 1964: The Case Is Made, and the Tasks Ahead Made Clear

In 1964 physicians, scientists, industrial representatives, and public health officials worldwide gathered in New York City to consolidate the by then rapidly accumulating knowledge associating asbestos exposure with disease. It is impossible to overstate the importance of this conference (Selikoff and Churg, 1965). It was a rare meeting of the minds; a confluence of purpose which has not been equaled in the asbestos research field since. Greenberg describes it:

> Contributors to the (published) report, with its 705 pages of text, constituted a contemporary International Who's Who. Its contributions varied qualitatively and quantitatively, but overall it constituted an excellent compendium of the state of knowledge of the physical and health aspects of exposure to dusts containing asbestos. (Greenberg, 2003)

Among the experts participating were the two principal organizers, Selikoff and Gilson, as well as Timbrell who developed the UICC asbestos samples for animal experiments (Timbrell et al., 1968) and Berry (a coauthor of Chapter 4). Wagner's real interest was a program in experimental pathology, but Gilson asked him to serve as an emissary for the recruitment of asbestos researchers. He approached McDonald, new Chair of Epidemiology at McGill University. McDonald had other interests, but was persuaded to attend the 1964 New York meeting—his first experience with asbestos research, but not his last, for his later work set the standard for asbestos cohort studies.

It is perhaps unfair to single out three who contributed most to our knowledge of asbestos health effects—but if one did, the lot would include Selikoff in the United States, Wagner in the United Kingdom, and McDonald in Canada. They did so in

---

4 Wagner was awarded the Charles Mott price in 1985 for his pathfinding contribution to cancer research. Regrettably, the prize rekindled some animosity among the original investigators as to "who should have been credited with the original discovery": the obvious answer is that they all deserved credit; Sleggs for finding the cases, Marchand for sampling them, and Ian Webster for allowing Wagner to concentrate on his studies of asbestos as opposed to more "topical" matters such as silicosis. But Wagner was the pathologist who not only made the diagnoses of this very rare disease, but followed through with observations of geographic pathology which established—at the time—that crocidolite in the Northwest Cape (and in the original study *only* crocidolite in that area: not one case in other chrysotile, amosite, or even crocidolite areas) was related to MM.

different ways, in keeping with their individual characters. Looking back at the work, however, one sees a pattern well summarized by a chance remark to this author by Simonato of IARC—three scientific explorers among many whose work may have seemed to be "heading west and east, while unbeknownst to them they were all heading north." None was perfect, but Wagner's genius, McDonald's discipline, organizational skills, and energy, and Selikoff's gift for publicity made possible the progress of 40 years, as they and their colleagues sat down to discuss asbestos exposure and disease.

And what a discussion it was! Selikoff, simultaneously the diplomat and the publicist, is described by Greenberg as having "no compunction about using the media in an attempt to alert the public and legislators to the hazards of asbestos and the urgent need for its control. He was photogenic and looked the part of a solid conscientious scientist. Selikoff was good at exposition and a good source of 'sound bites' attractive to journalists." This did not endear him to his colleagues, including Doll, who described him in 2004 as "wicked" in the sense he would say one thing in a meeting and then walk out the door and say something completely different to the media. This was a calculated approach: Selikoff said to this writer on one occasion that he recognized the differences in the pathogenicity of fiber types, but "would never admit it publicly," as to do so in his mind would interfere with his ultimate goal, which he phrased 10 years later this way: "I'm only interested that human beings not be further exposed to asbestos" (Stone, 1991).

In 1964 Selikoff opened the conference presaging Simonato's later remark about confluent directions: "This journey...has branched into intertwining roads, including those of epidemiology, oncology, physical chemistry, physiology, experimental pathology, and many others. Those of us who have been exploring these roads, meet now at a common junction, to exchange experiences and perhaps ask helpful directions" (Selikoff, 1965). He went on to praise those that had come before like Merewether, Lynch, and Gloyne. He spoke of Cartier, Vigliani, and Vorwald (who were all present) as groundbreakers in the field, and had special words of thanks for the "resourcefulness and energy" of Gilson.

Gilson followed by giving a nuanced address comparing the ways in which asbestos had saved and continued to save lives through its fire-resistant and friction properties "set against the adverse effects of its use, with which this conference has been solely concerned.... We must all hope that this conference will lead to a much more systematic surveillance of all those exposed to asbestos...(but) Let us not delude ourselves that animal studies are an inadequate substitute for well-planned epidemiological investigations in man.... If we are right in concluding, on the evidence presented at this conference, that there are probably important differences in the biological effects of different fibers, we must exploit to the full any opportunities for the investigation of groups of individuals exposed to only one type of fiber" (Gilson, 1965).

The latter suggestion was, in fact, one of the major accomplishments of the conference, in setting out goals for such investigations. After the conference in October 1964, a working group was convened to "discuss evidence of an association between exposure to asbestos dust and cancer." Forty delegates from eight countries were involved, including Cartier and McDonald from Canada; Bohlig from East Germany; Elmes, Gilson, Harrington, Knox, McCaughey, and Wagner from the United Kingdom; Sluis-Cremer, Thompson, and Webster from South Africa; and Selikoff, Churg, Hammond, Enterline, Mancuso, and many others from the United States. Published simultaneously in the Proceedings of the New York Academy of Science (Selikoff and Churg, 1965) and in the British Journal of Industrial Medicine (UICC, 1965) as a "Report and Recommendations of the Working Group on Asbestos and Cancer" of the UICC's Geographical Pathology

Committee, the report proposed an agenda for research. Later in the document, the group got down to hard specifics; the Canadians, Russians, Italians, and Cypriots were to investigate chrysotile; the Finns, anthophyllite; the Americans, chrysotile and tremolite (which had been discovered at Zonolite Mountain, Montana in 1928, although we find no mention of this in the text); Australians, crocidolite (although no Australians were present at the meeting); and South Africans, crocidolite, amosite, and chrysotile.

It is of interest to note that the "Terms of Reference" list only MM for this task—perhaps it was thought that this was, as it indeed turned out to be, the clearest point of difference between fiber types in terms of disease etiology. The longer, detailed country-by-country recommendation also invokes "the importance of fibre type on the risk of developing asbestosis, LC, and MM and other tumors," but it is not clear why the task was expanded, especially since it is specifically noted that "Present evidence indicates that the associated LC is not limited to exposure to any one type of asbestos fibre.... In the case of MM, evidence from several countries suggests that exposure to crocidolite may be of particular importance, but it cannot be concluded that only this type of fiber is concerned with these tumours, and further investigation of this problem is needed."

It is difficult to describe either the scope or the importance of the 1964 meeting and its publication in 1965. Everything that had been known to that point was summarized and virtually everything that would later be investigated came up in the discussions. Only a small sampling is possible here, and the full volume is mandatory reading for any serious student of the subject.

The question of who should finance asbestos research was raised by Hueper, who complained as regards the study of Braun and Truan (1958) that it was "...regrettable that the original plan of having a recent epidemiological survey on...aspects of asbestos production in Canadian mines and mills to be undertaken under the aegis of the National Cancer Institute of Canada was not adhered to and this study was carried out as an industry-dominated venture which yielded highly controversial negative results" (Hueper, 1965). Hueper was especially concerned at the lack of publications from the "giant American asbestos industry" regarding "large-scale observations on the incidence, morbidity, and mortality rates of asbestosis and asbestos cancers" over the preceding decade, when reports from so many other countries had been forthcoming. He believed that the necessary raw data (number and variety of exposed workers; occurrence and incidence of the diseases) was "most fragmentary in all countries, (but) especially in the United States and Canada, one being the principal consumer of asbestos and the other the chief producer..." (Hueper, 1965).

As the conference showed, this was about to change; Selikoff, Churg, and Hammond, for example, reported on the insulators' experience in the United States (Selikoff et al., 1965), pointing out that asbestos insulation work had been largely ignored and the one previous American study in naval workers had been limited to "study of men with relatively short durations of exposure." The investigators pointed out the difficulties in studying such a group as opposed to miners or textile workers, multiple employers, repeated but "limited and intermittent" asbestos exposure, and the differing nature of insulation materials with respect to asbestos content.

At the end of the conference, there was genuine cause for enthusiasm. The problems of disease related to asbestos exposure would be fully investigated and the pathogenic mechanisms worked out. The means of exposure would be explored and tools for measurement and control developed. There would be worldwide cooperation in doing so. For a few years, this was indeed the case. The appearance on the scene of the MM made the problems both medically urgent and scientifically fascinating. Here was a disease that few had even seen until 10 years earlier, and in the preceding 5 years, an avalanche of knowledge had been forthcoming. The conference is notable not only for the work presented but for the frankness of the freewheeling discussions that provide us a window into the thought processes and professional relationships of the time.

Regrettably, a time like those few days in New York would never come again; egos, litigation, industrial concerns, and societal events would conspire to make this impossible. Indeed, a few years after the conference it becomes difficult to regard asbestos science as a unified and worldwide phenomenon, despite the best efforts of many.

The history of the discovery of asbestos-related diseases has been fraught with controversy brought about by conflicting ideologies and financial interests. Sometimes it is difficult to untangle the two; advocacy is and should be part of scientific inquiry, but it should never precede it. The very depth and extent of the literature on asbestos exposure and disease makes it possible for virtually any author or group of authors to "prove" almost any viewpoint, should that be their goal (rather than scientific inquiry aimed at testing a hypothesis). As we move into the 21st century, there are new challenges; these include the naturally occurring asbestos in our environment and its effects on resident populations, the toxic legacy of the past, and perhaps most importantly, the development of useful scientifically based means for surveillance, prevention, and treatment. It is to be hoped that the animosities of the past will be put aside in this effort, and that all involved in asbestos research will join in the "spirit of 1964."

References

Abelson PH. The asbestos removal fiasco. *Science.* 1990;247:1017.

Abratt RP, Vorobiof DA, White N. Asbestos and mesothelioma in South Africa. *Lung Cancer.* 2004;45(Suppl. 1):S3–S6.

American Thoracic Society. Health effects of tremolite. This official statement of the American Thoracic Society was adopted by the ATS Board of Directors, June 1990. *Am Rev Respir Dis.* 1990;142(6 Pt 1):1453–1458.

Bandli BR, Gunter ME. A review of scientific literature examining the mining history, geology, mineralogy, and amphibole asbestos health effects of the Rainy Creek igneous complex, Libby, Montana, USA. *Inhal Toxicol.* 2006;18:949–62.

Bartrip PW. *The way from dusty death: Turner and Newall and the regulation of occupational health in the British asbestos industry, 1890's–1970.* London: The Athlone Press; 2001.

Bartrip PW. History of asbestos related disease. *Postgrad Med J.* 2004;80:72–76.

Berry G. EPA and asbestos removal. *Science.* 1990;248:1595.

Biggeri A, Pasetto R, Belli S, et al. Mortality from chronic obstructive pulmonary disease and pleural mesothelioma in an area contaminated by natural fiber (fluoro-edenite). *Scand J Work Environ Health.* 2004;30:249–252.

Boutin C, Dumortier P, Rey F, Viallat JR, De Vuyst P. Black spots concentrate oncogenic asbestos fibers in the parietal pleura. Thoracoscopic and mineralogic study. *Am J Respir Crit Care Med.* 1996;153:444–449.

Braun D, Truan T. An epidemiological study of lung cancer in asbestos miners. *Arch Ind Health.* 1958;17:634.

Browne K. Asbestos in history. In: Parkes D. ed., *Occupational lung disorders.* Oxford: Butterworths-Heinemann; 1994:417–418.

Bruno C, Comba P, Zona A. Adverse health effects of fluoro-edenitic fibers: Epidemiological evidence and public health priorities. *Ann NY Acad Sci.* 2006;1076:778–83.

Cartier P. Contribution á l'étude de l'amiantose. *Arch Mal Prof.* 1949;10:589–595.

Cartier P. In discussion following paper by W. E. Smith entitled "Survey of some current British and European studies of occupational tumor problems". *Arch Ind Hyg Occup Med.* 1952;5:262–263.

Cartier P. Some clinical observations of asbestosis in mine and mill workers. *Arch Ind Health*. 1955;11:204.

Case BW, Sebastien P. Environmental and occupational exposures to chrysotile asbestos: A comparative microanalytic study. *Arch Environ Health*. 1987;42:185–191.

Case BW. On talc, tremolite, and tergiversation. Ter-gi-ver-sate: 2: To use subterfuges. *Br J Ind Med*. 1991a;48:357–359.

Case BW. Health effects of tremolite. Now and in the future. *Ann NY Acad Sci*. 1991b;643:491–504.

Case BW, Mattison DR. Risk assessment in pathology education. In: Craighead JE, ed., *Environmental and occupational disease: A state-of-the-art conference for pathology educators*. Bethesda, MD: Universities Associated for Research and Education in Pathology (UAREP); 1991:77–83.

Constantopoulos SH, Goudevenos JA, Saratzis N, Langer AM, Selikoff IJ, Moutsopoulos HM. Metsovo lung: Pleural calcification and restrictive lung function in northwestern Greece. Environmental exposure to mineral fiber as etiology. *Environ Res*. 1985;38:319–331.

Constantopoulos SH, Theodoracopoulos P, Dascalopoulos G, Saratzis N, Sideris K. Metsovo lung outside metsovo. Endemic pleural calcifications in the ophiolite belts of Greece. *Chest*. 1991;99:1158–1161.

Cooke WE. Fibrosis of the lungs due to the inhalation of asbestos dust. *Br Med J*. 1924;ii:147.

Cooke WE. Pulmonary asbestosis. *Br Med J*. 1927;ii:1024–1025.

Craighead JE, Abraham JL, Churg A, et al. The pathology of asbestos-associated diseases of the lungs and pleural cavities: Diagnostic criteria and proposed grading schema. Report of the Pneumoconiosis Committee of the College of American Pathologists and the National Institute for Occupational Safety and Health. *Arch Pathol Lab Med*. 1982;106:544–596.

Delisle E, Malouf P. *Le quatuor d'asbestos: Autour de la gréve de l'amiante*. Les Éditions Varia; 2004.

Desmeules R, Sirois A. Amiantose et cancers pulmonaires. *Laval Med*. 1941;6:7.

Doll R. Mortality from lung cancer in asbestos workers. *Br J Ind Med*. 1955;12:81–86.

Dumortier P, Rey F, Viallat JR, Broucke I, Boutin C, De Vuyst P. Chrysotile and tremolite asbestos fibres in the lungs and parietal pleura of corsican goats. *Occup Environ Med*. 2002;59:643–646.

Dupré JS, Mustard JF, Uffen RJ. *Report of the Royal Commission on matters of health and safety arising from the use of asbestos in Ontario*. Toronto: Ontario Ministry of the Attorney General; 1984.

Enterline PE. Changing attitudes and opinions regarding asbestos and cancer 1934–1965. *Am J Ind Med*. 1991;20:685–700.

Enterline, PE, Sussman N, Marsh GM. *Asbestos and cancer: The first thirty years*. Pittsburgh: Philip E. Enterline, 1978.

Fortier C. *Black Lake: Lac d'Amiante 1882–1992, tome 1—amiante et chrome des appalaches. Cent ans d'histoire*. Saint-Georges de Beauce (Québec), Ateliers Graphiti Barbeau. Tremblay Inc., 1983.

Frost J. Three cases of asbestosis. *Ugeskrift for Læger [Doctors' Weekly]* 1950;112:1284–1289.

Gilbert J. La version du seul témoin vivant des cinq découvreurs de l'amiante (translation: The version of the only living witness among the five discoverers of asbestos). L'Action Catholique. December 5:99–100 IN: Smith GW, 1968 (reproduction), 1955.

Gilson IJ. Man and asbestos. In: Selikoff IJ, Churg J, eds., *Biological effects of asbestos*. New York, NY: New York Academy of Sciences; 1965;132:9–11.

Gitlin JN, Cook LL, Linton OW, Garrett-Mayer E. Comparison of "b" readers' interpretations of chest radiographs for asbestos related changes. *Acad Radiol*. 2004;11:843–856.

Gloyne SR. Two cases of squamous carcinoma of the lung occurring in asbestosis. *Tubercle*. 1935;17:5.

Greenberg M. A study of lung cancer mortality in asbestos workers: Doll, 1955. *Am J Ind Med*. 1999;36:331–347.

Greenberg M. Biological effects of asbestos: New York Academy of Sciences, 1964. *Am J Ind Med.* 2003;43:543–552.

Hammond EC, Selikoff IJ. Discussion. *Ann NY Acad Sci.* 1965;132:600–601.

Hueper WC. A quest into the environmental causes of cancer of the lung. *Public Health Monogr.* 1956;36:1–54.

Hueper WC. Occupational and nonoccupational exposures to asbestos. *Ann NY Acad Sci.* 1965;132:184–195.

IARC. *IARC Monographs on the Evaluation of Carcinogenic Risks to Humans, Vol. 43, Man-Made Mineral Fibres and Radon.* Lyon, IARC; 1988.

IARC. *IARC Monographs on the Evaluation of Carcinogenic Risks to Humans, Vol. 81, Man-Made Mineral Vitreous Fibres.* Lyon, IARC; 2002.

Kane AB, Boffetta P, Saracci R, Wilbourn JD, Eds. *Mechanisms of fibre carcinogenesis.* IARC Sci Publ., Lyon, International Agency for Research on Cancer; WHO, 1996.

Kisvarsanyi G, Kisvarsanyi EB. Precambrian geology and ore deposits of the southeast Missouri iron metallogenic province. In: Brown VM, Kisvarsanyi EB, Hagni RD, eds., *"Olympic Dam-type" deposits and geology of Middle Proterozoic rocks in the St. Francois Mountains terrane, Missouri; Guidebook prepared for Society of Economic Geologists Field Conference,* Society of Economic Geologists Guidebook Series, 1989; 4:1–40.

Liddell F. Asbestos in the occupational environment. In: Liddell FK. ed., *Mineral fibres and health.* Boca Raton, Florida: CRC Press; 1991:79–88.

Lynch KM, Smith WA. Pulmonary asbestosis iii: Carcinoma of the lung in asbestos silicosis. *Am J Cancer.* 1935;24:56–61.

Mancuso TF, Coulter EJ. Methodology in industrial health studies: the cohort approach with special reference to an asbestos company. *Arch Environ Health.* 1963;6:210–220.

McCaughey WT. Asbestos and neoplasia: Diffuse mesothelial tumors. Criteria for diagnosis of diffuse mesothelial tumors. *Ann NY Acad Sci.* 1965;132:603–613.

McCulloch J. *Asbestos blues: labour, capital, physicians and the state in South Africa.* Bloomington, IN: Indiana University Press; 2002.

McDonald J. Cancer in chrysotile mines and mills. In: *Biological Effects of Asbestos. Proceedings of a Working Conference held at the International Agency for Research on Cancer.* Lyon, France: IARC/World Health Organization; 1973.

McDonald JC, Case BW, Enterline PE, et al. Lung dust analysis in the assessment of past exposure of man-made mineral fibre workers. *Ann Occup Hyg.* 1990;34:427–441.

McDonald JC, Harris J, Armstrong B. Mortality in a cohort of vermiculite miners exposed to fibrous amphibole in Libby, Montana. *Occup Environ Med.* 2004;61:363–366.

McDougall S. Deadline looms for smelter in Asbestos. *The Montreal Gazette 2007;* August 28:B1.

Merewether E, Price C. *Report on effects of asbestos dust on the lungs and dust suppression in the asbestos industry.* London: H.M.S.O.; 1930.

Newhouse ML, Thompson H. Mesothelioma of pleura and peritoneum following exposure to asbestos in the London area. *Br J Ind Med.* 1965;22:261–269.

OSHA. Occupational exposure to asbestos, tremolite, anthophyllite and actinolite. *Federal Register.* 1992;57:24310.

Peipins LA, Lewin M, Campolucci S, et al. Radiographic abnormalities and exposure to asbestos-contaminated vermiculite in the community of Libby, Montana, USA. *Environ Health Perspect.* 2003;111:1753–1759.

Poulin J-C. *La cité de l'or blanc: Thetford Mines 1876–1976.* Thetford Mines (Québec): Textes Nelson Fecteau; 1975.

Proctor R. *The nazi war on cancer.* Princeton, NJ: Princeton University Press; 1999.

Selikoff IJ, Churg J. Eds. *Biological Effects of Asbestos,* New York: Ann NY Acad Science; 1965;132. Selikoff IJ. Opening remarks. In: IJ Selikoff, J Churg, eds. *Biological Effects of Asbestos,* New York: New York Academy of Sciences; 1965:132:7–8.

Selikoff IJ, Churg J, Hammond EC. The occurrence of asbestosis among insulation workers in the United States. *Ann NY Acad Sci.* 1965;132:139–155.

Smith GW. *Bell asbestos mines Ltd. 1878–1967.* Thetford Mines (Québec): George Washington Smith; 1968.

Smith WE. Survey of some current British and European studies of occupational tumor problems. New York: A.M.A. *Arch Ind Hyg Occup Med.* 1952;5:242–263.

Sullivan PA. Vermiculite, respiratory disease, and asbestos exposure in Libby, Montana: Update of a cohort mortality study. *Environ Health Perspect.* 2007;115:579–85.

Stone R. No meeting of the minds on asbestos. *Science.* 1991;254:928–931.

Timbrell V, Gibson JC, Webster I. UICC standard reference samples of asbestos. *Int J Cancer.* 1968;3:406–408.

Tossavainen A, Kotilainen M, Takahashi K, Pan G, Vanhala E. Amphibole fibres in Chinese chrysotile asbestos. *Ann Occup Hyg.* 2001;45:145–152.

Travaglione S, Bruni B, Falzano L, Paoletti L, Fiorentini C. Effects of the new-identified amphibole fluoro-edenite in lung epithelial cells. *Toxicol In Vitro.* 2003;17:547–552.

UICC (International Union Against Cancer). Report and recommendations of the working group on asbestos and cancer. *Br J Ind Med.* 1965;22:165–171.

USGS (U. S. Geological Survey). Fact sheet: Some facts about asbestos, United States Department of the Interior. USGS Fact Sheet FS-012–01:1–4, 2001.

USGS (U. S. Geological Survey). Reported Natural Asbestos and Fibrous Amphibole(s) Occurrences in the Central United States. OPEN-FILE REPORT 2006–1211.

Virta RL. Worldwide asbestos supply and consumption trends from 1900 to 2000. U. S. Geological Survey, U.S. Department of the Interior. Open-File Report 03–83:1–59, 2003a.

Virta RL. Asbestos: Geology, mineralogy, mining, and uses. U. S. Geological Survey, US Department of the Interior, in cooperation with Kirk-Ohmer Encyclopedia of Chemical Technology, Wylie-Interscience. Open-File Report 02:1–28, 2003b.

Wagner JC, Sleggs CA, Marchand P. Diffuse pleural mesothelioma and asbestos exposure in the north western cape province. *Br J Ind Med.* 1960;17:260–271.

Wagner JC. Epidemiology of diffuse mesothelial tumors: Evidence of an association from studies in South Africa and the United Kingdom. *Ann NY Acad Sci.* 1965;132:575–578.

Wagner JC. Progress in etiopathogenesis of respiratory disorders due to occupational exposures to mineral and organic dusts. In: *VIIth International Pneumoconioses Conference*; Proceedings, 1990; PART I:22–24. Pittsburgh, Pennsylvania, DHHS (NIOSH) Publication No. 90–108.

Webster I. Mesotheliomatous tumors in South Africa: Pathology and experimental pathology. *Ann NY Acad Sci.* 1965;132:623–646.

Wedler HW. Lung cancer in asbestosis patients [uber den lungenkrebs bei asbestos.]. *Dtsch Arch Klin Med.* 1943;191:189–209.

Weis C. *Amphibole mineral fibers in source materials in residential and commercial areas of Libby pose an imminent and substantial endangerment to public health.* 2001. U.S. EPA. Denver, United States Environmental Protection Agency (Region VIII) 1–23.

Wood WB, Gloyne SR. Pulmonary asbestos: A review of one hundred cases. *Lancet.* 1934;2:1383.

2
Mineralogy of Asbestos

John E. Craighead, Allen Gibbs, and Fred Pooley

History

Naturally occurring fibrous minerals have been used by humans for more than 4500 years. Ancient writers referred to the incombustible properties of asbestos. Finnish archeological relics of pottery from 2500 BC contain anthophyllite, an amphibole also deposited sparely in accessible mineral seams in North America and elsewhere. The Romans quarried chrysotile and tremolite in the Alps. Marco Polo discovered asbestos mines in the Ural Mountains during his travels in the mid-13th century, and Peter the Great exploited these deposits commercially at the turn of the 18th century. Chrysotile was discovered in the Province of Quebec in the mid-1800s (Chapter 1) but the mineral had been recognized as a curiosity in the Appalachian Mountains of eastern North America before the American Revolution. The so-called blue asbestos, crocidolite, was discovered in naturally occurring outcrops in South Africa in 1815, but commercial exploitation awaited the end of the 19th century. "Brown" asbestos, discovered in the Transvaal Province in northeast South Africa in 1907, was mined commercially shortly thereafter. According to McCulloch (2002), medieval alchemists were said to believe asbestos grew on fire-resistant salamanders, the basis for the motif of the salamander surrounded by flames. The terms "incombustible linen," "rock floss," "mineral silk," "cotton stone," and "feathered alum" were variously used before this family of minerals was characterized scientifically. A number of additional general descriptors were applied to the mineral in the past, but the word asbestos derived from the Greek word "indestructible" is now the commercial, nonmineralogical term universally employed.

Mineralogical and Geological Features

Asbestos is a generic term for a family of fibrous silicate minerals with a crystalline structure. Although most mineralogists consider the approach to be too general and nonspecific, the United States Occupational and Health Administration (OSHA) published a definition of asbestos in the Federal Register (October 9, 1975) that serves as a pragmatic legal and regulatory description referring to the six quite uniquely different species of asbestiform minerals depicted in Figure 2.1. The asbestos crystal fragments evaluated by phase contrast microscopy (PCM) at a magnification of 450–500× were said to have the following dimensions: length >5 μm and a length to diameter ratio of 3 or greater, the ratio being known as the aspect ratio. Practical as it may be, the definition

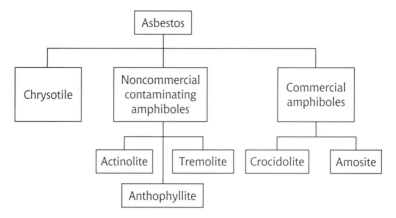

Figure 2.1 Mineralogical types of asbestos.

fails to emphasize the great diversity in lengths and breadths as well as the physical characteristics of the countless individual fibers that comprise these naturally occurring minerals and the commercial products derived from them. Another definition advanced by the American Society for Testing Materials is as follows: Asbestiform mineral fiber populations generally have the following characteristics when viewed by light microscopy:

1. Many particles with aspect ratios ranging from 20:1 to 100:1 or higher (>5 μm in length);
2. Very thin fibrils generally <0.5 μm in width; and
3. In addition to the mandatory fibrillar crystal growth, two or more of the following attributes:
   a. parallel fibers occurring in bundles;
   b. fibers displaying split ends;
   c. matted masses of individual fibers; and
   d. fibers showing curvature.

The minerals giving rise to asbestiform fibers have nonfibrous analogs that assume many crystalline configurations including shards (Figure 2.2).

The two major subfamilies of asbestos minerals are the serpentines and amphiboles, fibrous silicate minerals having distinctly unique physical characteristics and diverse geologic origins. It is unfortunate that modern society has chosen to use the all-inclusive term asbestos, for as discussed in detail elsewhere in this book, the various types differ dramatically in their biological characteristic and health importance. Only three of the asbestos types have been of commercial importance in most industrial countries—chrysotile, amosite, and crocidolite. Historically, over the period 1925–1975, between 90% and 95% of all asbestos used industrially was chrysotile; amosite comprised roughly 2%–3%, and crocidolite about 3% of the world's production. However, during the Second World War, large amounts of amosite were imported into the allied countries for the insulation of naval and merchant vessels as well as a diversity of war vehicles (Chapter 3).

Asbestos deposits occur in four types of rocks (Figure 2.3): Type 1—alpine type ultramafic rock, including ophalites and serpentinites containing chrysotile, and in some cases, minor amounts of tremolite, actinolite, and anthophyllite. Type 1 deposits are by far the most important and account for approximately 90% of the asbestos ever mined (Ross and Virta, 2001). Type 2—stratiform ultramafic intrusions containing chrysotile, and in some cases, minor amounts of tremolite, actinolite, and anthophyllite.

Asbestiform

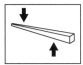 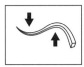 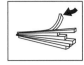

In the asbestiform habit, mineral crystals grow in a single dimension, in a straight line until they form long, thread-like fibers with aspect ratios of 20:1 to 1000:1 and higher, When pressure is applied, the fibers do not shatter but simply bend much like a wire, Fibrils of a smaller diameter are produced as bundles of fibers are pulled apart. This bundling effect is referred to as polyfilamentous.

Nonasbestiform

 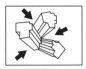 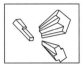

In the nonasbestiform variety, crystal growth is random, forming multidimensional prismatic patterns. When pressure is applied, the crystal fractures easily, fragmenting into prismatic particles. Some of the particles or cleavage fragments are acicular or needleshaped as a result of the tendency of amphibole minerals to cleave along two dimensions but not along the third. Stair-step cleavage along the edges of some particles is common, and oblique extinction is exhibited under the microscope. Cleavage fragments never show curvature.

Figure 2.2 Habits of asbestiform and nonasbestiform minerals. (Published with permission, Kelse and Thompson, 1989).

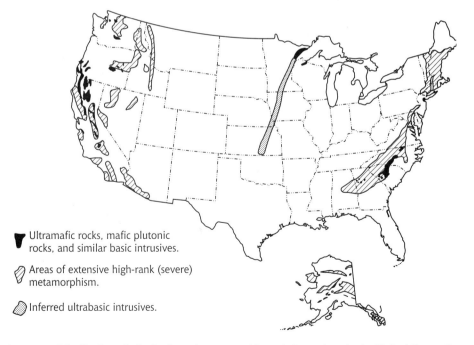

▼ Ultramafic rocks, mafic plutonic rocks, and similar basic intrusives.

▨ Areas of extensive high-rank (severe) metamorphism.

▨ Inferred ultrabasic intrusives.

Figure 2.3 Distribution of ultrabasic and metamorphic rock formations in the United States. In Hawaii, the types of mineral alteration that could lead to asbestos formation are restricted to the vicinity of volcanoes on the island of Oahu. (*Tectonic Map of North America*, US Geological Survey; Levine, 1978.)

Type 3—serpentized limestone containing chrysotile; Type 4—banded iron formations containing amosite and crocidolite.

While the amphiboles share certain crystal features, chrysotile is substantially different. For example, chrysotile tends to exist in the air as loosely adherent clumps or bundles of fibers, rather than as single fibers—this feature influences dramatically the aerodynamic properties of the material in the environment and its respirability. In contrast, amphibole fibers tend to occur singly, and thus, can be more readily transported deep into the lungs after inhalation. Each of the asbestos fiber types have different size ranges when airborne and in lung airways (Gibbs and Hwang, 1980; Pooley and Clark, 1980). The ability of inhaled asbestos fibers to produce a disease in both human and animals is well known. However, there remains some confusion as to which of the properties of these materials are primarily responsible for the initiation of the pathogenic response. Fine fibrous particle and some platy materials with a range of different chemical compositions can be carcinogenic, causing mesothelioma (MM), when instilled into the pleural or peritoneal cavities of animals, the degree of disease response being closely related to the length and diameter of the materials and, accordingly, the surface area (Stanton and Wrench, 1972). The carcinogenic potential of fibrous dust particles in animals increases with a decrease in fiber diameter, and it decreases with a reduction in length. The chemical nature of the mineral plays a lesser role in the malignant response in experimental animals (Davis, 1989; Timbrell, 1982). It is difficult to understand why the simple size parameter of asbestos fibers should be so strongly linked to the precipitation of disease. However, it is clear that it is necessary for fibers to be inhaled, deposited, and retained in the locations where subsequent disease occurs. The physical dimensions of the fibers dictate where they are most likely to deposit in the respiratory tract, whereas the durability of the particle determines retention (biopersistence) and the induction of malignant disease by fibers deposited near the serosal surfaces of the body.

The biopersistence of chrysotile and amphibole differ dramatically. Chrysotile is substantially less durable once inhaled into the respiratory tract, its half-life being measured in weeks and, at most, months. This feature relates to the susceptibility of the fiber to the acidic environmental condition of the lung. Mg^{2+} ions are leached from the chrysotile fiber, resulting in breakdown into constituent fibrils, with further degradation thereafter. The amphiboles exhibit this character to a much lesser degree. Although estimates differ, the half-life of amphiboles in the human lung is measurable in terms of decades, if not a lifetime.

Air Particulate Burdens and Respiratory Tract Response

Countless inorganic and organic particles are suspended in the air we breathe, even when measured distant from major sources of urban and industrial air pollution. There are estimated to be in one cubic meter of air, on the average, 1×10^5 particles in the 1–10 μm size range; 2×10^7 particles in the 0.1–1 μm range; and 3×10^8 particles in the 0.01–0.1 μm range (Cadle, 1966). A major proportion of these particles are generated from natural mineral deposits rather than from anthropogenic sources. Particles travel long distances in air. For example, dust generated in Sahara storms can be transported by prevailing winds to the Western Hemisphere and those originating in Asia regularly find their way across the Pacific to North America. Asbestos fibers have been found in Antarctic ice cores that originated more than 10 000 years ago, no doubt a reflection of the action of erosive forces on natural outcrops of the mineral over eons of time. Today, as in the distant past, asbestos particles in exceedingly low concentrations can be detected in the ambient atmosphere using ultrastructural approaches. Almost invariably, these fibers are relatively short, that is, <5 μm, and are not believed to be pathogenic. It is a credit to the efficiency of the defense mechanisms of our respiratory tract that these extraneous particles are eliminated continuously and do not accumulate in the lungs over a lifetime.

The depth of penetration of particles through the airways and their subsequent deposition in the lungs is dictated by the physical parameter referred to as aerodynamic diameter (Agency for Toxic Substances & Disease Registry, unpublished data, 2003). It is not their apparent size that solely determines deposition in the lungs, but their aerodynamic properties that incorporate both particle density and frictional drag. Aerodynamic diameter denotes the diameter of a sphere that has the same terminal velocity as the particle in question. This is a much studied property of dust particles used extensively to describe the capability of particles to penetrate and deposit in either the turbinates of the nasal cavities or the lung parenchyma (Lippman, 1990; Lippman et al., 1980).

Dust particles with aerodynamic properties allowing them to deposit in the lungs are referred to as respirable particles, although those that have properties that allow them to only deposit in the respiratory airways are referred to as "thoracic" in nature. As one might expect, the more respirable dust particles in air as measured by aerodynamic fractionation correlate closely with the occurrence of respiratory disease. The size ranges of airborne particles describe their behavior in the respiratory tract (Garrard et al., 1981; Gerrity et al., 1983). Movement of particles having an aerodynamic diameter greater than 1 μm is influenced mainly by inertial forces, whereas those less than 0.2 μm are transported by diffusion, and those between 0.2 and 1 μm are found to balance diffusional and gravitational forces. Sampling of particles in tissues is discussed in Chapter 12.

The aerodynamic properties of asbestos fibers closely depend upon the diameter of the fiber and only moderately on their length. The finer the fiber, the smaller the aerodynamic diameter, and its capacity to penetrate and deposit in the lung. Although, as noted above, the length of a fiber has only a minor influence upon its aerodynamic diameter, it does have a significant effect upon its ability to descend through the complex branching airways of the lung. In the major conducting airways, increases in fiber length will enhance the likely interception of particles as they travel deep into the lungs through the branching airways of decreasing size. This has the effect of limiting the size of asbestos fibers observed in human parenchymal tissue to approximately 30 μm in length. Where fiber length does have an important role to play in the pathogenesis of disease, it relates to the enhanced retention of particles at their site of deposition. The longer the fiber, the greater the probability that it will be retained at the site of deposition due largely to the inability of cellular defense mechanisms, for example, the alveolar macrophages, to eliminate particles that have extreme physical sizes. The retention of longer particles in lung tissue is elegantly demonstrated by the formation of ferruginous bodies (Chapter 6). Long particles are most probably an indication of a significant residence time of the fiber in the lung.

A comparison of how physical dimension influences respirability and deposition within the lung is pictured in Figure 2.4A and 2.4B. These illustrations represent the variation in the average dimension of amosite asbestos fibers observed in a sagittal section of lung. It can be seen in Figure 2.4A that the average diameter of fibers decreases from the center to the periphery, while Figure 2.4B illustrates the corresponding change in fiber length, which was found to increase from the center to the periphery. Retention near the periphery of the lung is therefore dictated by the ability of finer fibers to penetrate deeper and be retained on the basis of fiber length.

(A)

Amosite lung
Contours of average fiber diameter in microns

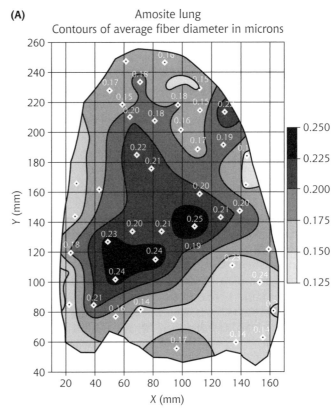

(B)

Contours of average fiber length in microns
(Particles >2 μm only)

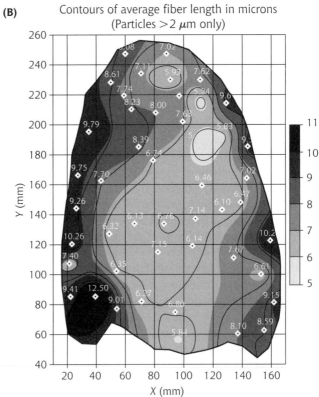

Figure 2.4 (A) Amosite lung contours of average fiber diameter in microns, (B) Contours of average fiber length in microns (Particles >2 μm only).

Occurrence and Physical-Chemical Properties of Chrysotile

Serpentine minerals are the source of commercial chrysotile and the noncommercial, nonasbestiform platy minerals, lizardite and antigorite. Seams of these minerals are insinuated in serpentine rock that is a metamorphic product of igneous origin. In localized deposits the serpentine has crystallized into fissures and cracks that developed during emplacement of the original magma. When sufficiently close to the surface in commercial amounts and quality, the minerals can be mined either by quarrying from vast open pits (Figure 2.5) or by deep mining where rich seams are followed in tunnels for relatively long distances underground. There are two distinct types of chrysotile deposits; one of the most common is the "cross" fiber deposit (Figure 2.6A), and the other is a "slip" fiber (Figure 2.6B). "Cross" fiber veins are formed in fractured serpentine with the fibers transversing a fissure at various angles to the wall rock, frequently perpendicular to it. In contrast, "slip" fiber veins are found in areas of intense sheering rather than

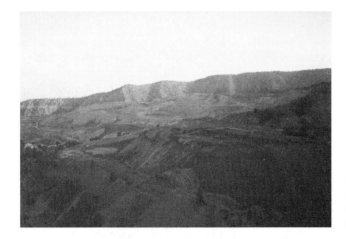

Figure 2.5 An open-pit chrysotile mine in the island of Cypress (courtesy of Benjamin E. Haglund, Esq.).

(A)   (B)

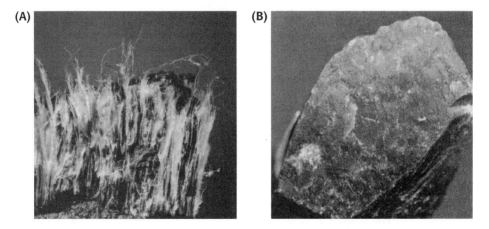

Figure 2.6 (A) "Cross" fiber and (B) "slip" fiber in serpentine rock. The layers of slip fibers are often thin and irregular in distribution along the cleavage plate. The cross seam ranges in highest from few millimeters to several centimeters. US Bureau of Mines Inf. Circular #8751, Department of Interior.

just fracturing, with the fibers occurring along the "slip" planes of the serpentine. As there are no physical constraints to the fiber length, "slip" fibers can be much longer than the "cross" fibers ($\geq$20 cm), but after processing the asbestos ore, extremely long fibers customarily break down to 1 cm or less. Another type of fiber is the "mass" fiber, which is probably related to the "cross" fiber and occurs as aggregates of disoriented bundles of chrysotile. A notable exception to the normal mode of occurrence of chrysotile is the fiber found in the New Idria serpentine located in central California, and at Stragan, Yugoslavia, generally referred to as Colinga fiber. These deposits consist of soft, powdery, pellet-like aggregates of chrysotile and are thought to be due to intensive crushing and pulverization during and after serpentization.

Deposits of chrysotile are found worldwide in geologic areas where serpentine has been formed. It is therefore a very common serpentine mineral. In certain environments it has a natural background induced by weathering and erosion of the serpentine rock. Commercially useful chrysotile asbestos has been mined in the past in North America (United States—Arizona, California, and Vermont), and Canada (Provinces of Quebec and British Columbia), in the Alps of Northern Italy, and the Island of Cypress. In Asia, chrysotile is mined commercially in the Urals of Russia, in Szechuan Province, and elsewhere in the People's Republic of China, Japan, and in central Kazakhstan. In Africa, it is located in Zimbabwe, Swaziland, and South Africa, whereas in Australia, chrysotile is found in the province of New South Wales. Chrysotile is also mined in central Brazil.

Typically, the ore contains substantially less than 10% chrysotile after removal from the mine site. The commercial product is semipurified by "cobbing," in which the rock is hand-picked from the mineral. It is then ball-milled to release the fibrous material. Subsequently, the mineral is separated from the accompanying rock debris by flotation and transit through a series of sluices. After oven drying, the end product is sieved into grades to separate fibers by length. In the past, the valuable long fibers were used in the manufacturing of textiles, whereas shorter particles, which are of less commercial value, were used, for example, in construction materials such as cement, joint compounds, and floor tile.

As might be expected, seams differ somewhat in the physical characteristics of the fiber. For example, the Colinga asbestos quarried in central California is composed of fibers that are almost exclusively less than 5 μm in length, although bundles of these relatively short fibers are commonly found in noncommercial amounts in nature. In contrast, the Cassiar mine in British Columbia produced in the past substantial quantities of high-quality "long" fibers measuring >5 μm in length. Elsewhere in North America and worldwide, commercial chrysotile deposits yield fibers of variable length, although in any one sample the majority of particles are less than 2 μm in length. Many, but certainly not all, commercial seams of chrysotile are located in proximity to noncommercial deposits of fibrous and nonfibrous amphiboles, tremolite, actinolite, and anthophyllite. Recently, still another asbestiform "contaminant" of chrysotile in the Western Alps was described (balangeroite [$(Mg, Fe^{2+}, Fe^{3+}, Mn^{2+})_{42}Si_{16}(OH)_{36}$]) (Groppo et al., 2005). Unfortunately, these amphiboles sometimes "contaminate" the chrysotile during mining and processing, as discussed elsewhere in this book. These so-called contaminates have the potential to produce MMs when introduced directly in large amounts into the body cavity or in rats experimentally, and some parties claim that they occasionally cause similar neoplasms in humans exposed to chrysotile in building materials and industrial products (Chapter 8). The subject of the purity of the finished product after milling and its carcinogenicity is a common topic of debate in the courtroom.

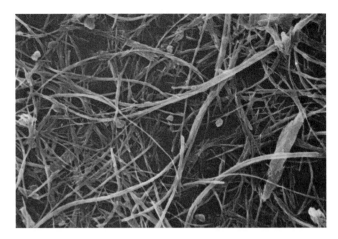

Figure 2.7 Scanning electron micrograph of chrysotile asbestos. Note the variation in length and breadth of individual one fiber. Characteristically, preparations are comprised of a heterogeneous accumulation of fibers, the majority of which are shorter than 5 μm. Industrial processing sieves chrysotile into 1 of 7 grades. The longest fibers are grade 1, and exceedingly short fibers are grade 7.

Chrysotile displays a characteristic physical structure, although as noted earlier, fibers differ substantially in length and width (Figure 2.7). Naturally occurring fibers are composed of uniform-sized subunit fibrils loosely bound together electrostatically by the ionic attraction of the Mg^{2+} (Figure 2.8). The fibrils that comprise the fiber tend to recombine to form aggregates. The size of the particles produced by crushing chrysotile are not uniform and the morphology varies with the intensity of manipulation of the sample and whether it takes place in a wet or dry state. It is rare to find reliable published data pertaining to the size of chrysotile particles. Published figures should be evaluated with skepticism inasmuch as dimensions are influenced by the techniques employed to prepare the particles for microscopical examination. Water and various chemicals, as well as body fluids, splay out the fibers and break them down into fibrils that average 0.1 μm or less in diameter. These "fragile" fibrils also tend to break down in the environment into shorter and shorter fibrils, until the residue is nondiscernable. Invariably, data on fiber dimension are subject to artifactual influences.

The chemistry of the serpentine group of minerals conform to the general formula $Mg_3Si_2O_5(OH)_4$. Major elemental substitutions of various cations (aluminum, calcium, chromium, copper, and platinum) are found in naturally occurring seams. The fibril of chrysotile is a network of alternating sheets of brucite and magnesium or $Mg(OH)_2$ forming parallel arrays (Figures 2.8 and 2.9). As a result of the imbalance in ionic composition of the sheets, they are rolled into a scroll configuration resembling the baker's jelly roll, thus exhibiting a tubular structure when examined by high resolution electron microscopy (Figure 2.10). In the lung, the fibers of chrysotile accumulate on the walls of airways and at bifurcations where they interact with the epithelial lining cells (Figures 2.11 and 2.12).

As a crystal, chrysotile contains about 13% water. While resistant to heat, the fibers are thermolabile at temperatures in the approximate range of 700–1000 °F, yielding a nonfibrous magnesium silicate known as forsterite. This product of pyrolysis is not pathogenic. Forsterite is found in the dust from used chrysotile containing brake shoes, and is formed as a result of the heat of friction (Chapter 3).

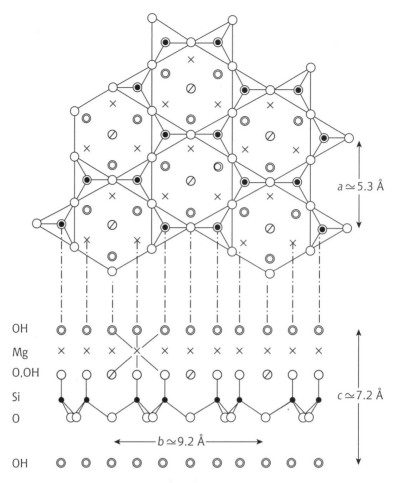

OH

Mg

O,OH

Si

O

$a \simeq 5.3$ Å

$c \simeq 7.2$ Å

$\longleftarrow b \simeq 9.2$ Å $\longrightarrow$

OH

Figure 2.8 Structural geometric chemical configuration of a chrysotile fiber and its constituent fibrils accounting for the crystalline nature of the particle and its relatively high water content.

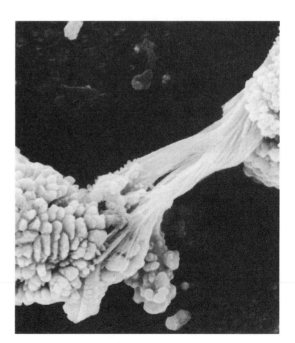

Figure 2.9 Scanning electron micrograph of chrysotile fiber with deposits of ferruginous materials. Note the twisted configuration of the fibrils comprising the fiber. It is rare for chrysotile to form asbestos bodies.

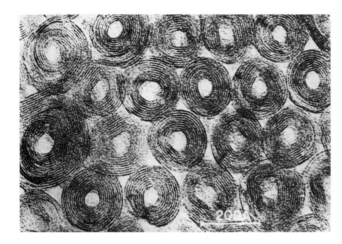

Figure 2.10 Fibers are annealed into subfibrils that do not readily break down because of the strong ionic attraction of the individual units.

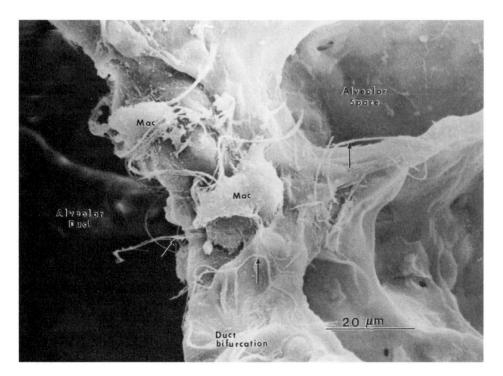

Figure 2.11 Scanning electron micrograph of the distal airway of the lung of a rat experimentally exposed by inhalation to chrysotile (arrow). Note the relative size of the fibrous particles and their interaction with the epithelium and macrophages (Mac) (courtesy of Arnold Brody, PhD).

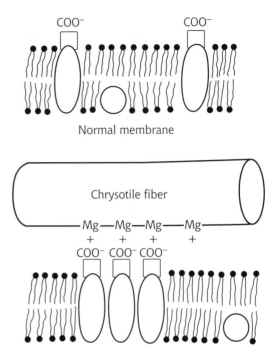

COO⁻   COO⁻

Normal membrane

Chrysotile fiber

Mg —Mg—Mg——Mg
 +   +   +   +
COO⁻ COO⁻ COO⁻

Figure 2.12 Diagrammatic depiction of the interaction of chrysotile (with its strong positive charge due to surface Mg^{2+}) and negative surface charge of cell membrane.

Occurrence and Physical-Chemical Properties of Amphiboles

Amphibole asbestos minerals have very similar crystalline structures and can only be distinguished readily on the basis of differences in their chemical composition—specifically, the cation constituents of the fiber. These minerals tend to form dust particles that are fibrous, straight, and rigid with parallel margins (Figure 2.13). Like chrysotile, the lengths and breadth of the fibers are quite variable, with the majority being short (<5 μm) (Figure 2.14). They show a tendency to be transported in the air singly rather than clumped together, as with chrysotile. Deposits of commercial amphiboles are found in three types of rocks: (1) unmetamorphized, the size sedimentary strata known as banded iron stone (amosite and crocidolite) such as those that occur in the Transvaal and Cape Provinces of South Africa, northwest Australia, and the highlands of the Bolivian Andes; (2) the so-called alpine-type ultramafic rock (anthophyllite), and tremolite; and (3) stratiform ultramafic intrusions (tremolite) that contaminate the surface soils with crocidolite and tremolite (Table 2.1). They are also located in such diverse areas of the world as eastern China, central Turkey, and Greece, where they have been associated with MM in the indigenous population, and central California in the United States, where their presence in outcrops and soils has been a topic of considerable public concern (but, as of yet, no demonstrable disease).

The amphiboles are important rock-forming minerals with perfect prismatic cleavage. They are a SiO_4 tetrahedra (sometimes with partial replacement of the silicon by aluminum). The chains are four tetrahedra wide, linked rigidly together at the base by cations in the form of octagons (Figure 2.15). These structures can be of great but variable length with the fibers running in parallel. This mineralogical characteristic is the basis for the extraordinary length of some fibers, accounting for their significant pathogenicity once

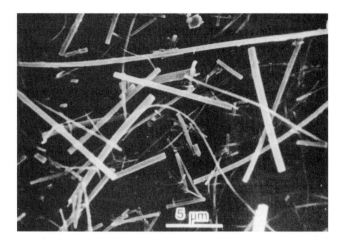

Figure 2.13 Scanning electron micrograph of amphibole asbestos. Note the variability in fiber length and breadth that is characteristic of these rod-like particles.

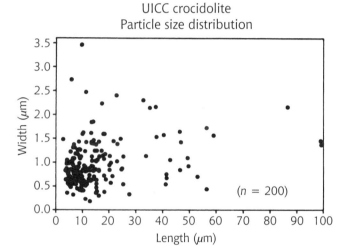

UICC crocidolite
Particle size distribution

($n = 200$)

Figure 2.14 Size distribution of the UICC crocidolite reference preparation. As noted, the majority of particles are less than 10 μm in length.

Table 2.1 Amphibole Asbestos Types and Nonasbestos Rock-Forming Counterparts

Asbestos	Nonasbestos Rock-Forming Counterpart	Chemistry
Crocidolite	Riebeckite	$Na_2Fe_3^{2+}Fe_2^{3+}Si_8O_{22}(OH)_2$
Amosite	Grunerite	$(Fe\text{-}Mg)_7Si_8O_{22}(OH)_2$
Tremolite	Tremolite	$Ca_2Mg_5Si_8O_{22}(OH)_2(\pm Fe)$
Anthophyllite	Antophyllite	$(Mg\text{-}Fe)_7Si_8O_{22}(OH)_{22}$
Actinolite	Actinolite	$Ca_2Fe_5Si_8O_{22}(\pm Mg)$

inhaled into the lung, and the formation of asbestos bodies (Figure 2.16). In contrast to chrysotile, the water content of the amphibole is relatively low and, compared to the particles of chrysotile, they are resistant to pyrolysis at temperatures less than 1000 °F.

Crocidolite, nominally referred to as "blue" asbestos because of the sea-blue naked eye appearance of the ore is the mineralogical term assigned to the fibrous habit of rie-beckite. Cummingtomite-grunerite is the technical term for the mineral that gives rise to the fibrous product known as amosite, nominally referred to as "brown" asbestos,

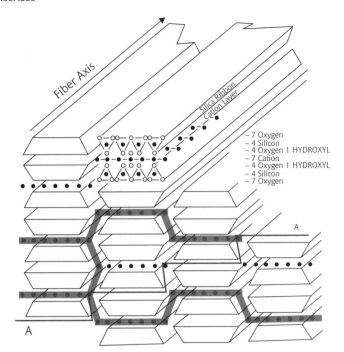

Fiber Axis

Silica Ribbon
Cation Layer

– 7 Oxygen
– 4 Silicon
– 4 Oxygen 1 HYDROXYL
– 7 Cation
– 4 Oxygen 1 HYDROXYL
– 4 Silicon
– 7 Oxygen

A

A

Figure 2.15 Ionic binding of amphibole fibrils with the solid line indicating potential fracture surfaces, thus forming thinner but long fibers.

an appearance attributed to the high iron content of the mineral. The name is derived from the acronym, AMSA (Asbestos Mines of South Africa). Thus, it is not a mineralogical term but one used in commerce. A major source of crocidolite commercially is the Cape Provinces of South Africa, particularly around Prieske on the Orange River, where underground mines account for most of the commercial product. However, outcrops of the mineral are distributed widely in the region of the mines, an area known as the blue hills because of the wide distribution of outcrops or crocidolite and its source mineral, riebeckite. Crocidolite from this area is known as "Cape blue" to distinguish it from the crocidolite found in the Transvaal fields in northeast South Africa. "Cape blue" asbestos differ from the Transvaal "blue" inasmuch as the latter contains varying quantities of amosite.

Similar iron stone formations are found in the crocidolite mining region of Western Australia near the community of Wittenoom in the Hammersley range of mountains. Of little commercial value are the crocidolite deposits located near Cochabanba in Bolivia and Lusaka, Zambia. These latter deposits are igneous in origin and mineralogically described as magnesio-riebeckite.

In the 1960s, fibrous cummingtonite grunerite was found in relatively high concentrations in the waters near the western terminus of Lake Superior in north central United States. The mineral was then discovered in tailings of taconite extracted from the nearby iron-ore-rich Mesabi range and discarded into the lake. A public outcry followed, and considerable research focused on the potential for this amphibole to cause disease in the regions' populus. Further study showed that the particles were relatively short ($<5\ \mu$m) and thus of no pathogenic significance. Epidemiological surveys in north central Minnesota have failed to demonstrate an increased prevalence of disease attributed to this minor amphibole component in taconite ores.

Commercial amosite is located only in the Transvaal where outcrops of mineralogical stratified rock consisting of ribboned reefs up to 10 feet in thickness course through the

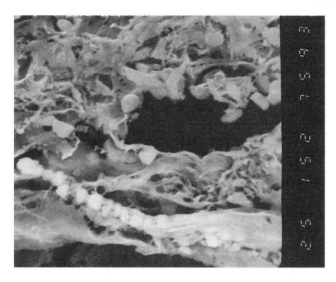

Figure 2.16 Scanning electron micrograph of lung revealing an asbestos body having an amphibole core. A small airway is surrounded by airspaces artifactually fragmented in preparation of specimen.

countryside vaguely giving the impression of the ribboned side of bacon. Geographically, the amosite deposits overlap those of crocidolite and, in some instances, both asbestos types are found together in the same mine. Amosite has also been found in Garhwal Himalaya and Chamoli, India, but these deposits are not commercially exploited to any great extent.

The underground mine deposits are extracted by cutting galleries at various subsurface levels along the reefs. Because asbestos is concentrated in the mine product, the arduous purification process required to extract chrysotile is not needed, although "hand cobbing" of crude ore continued to be done until the mines closed a few years ago. In the past, numerous small mines in surface outcrops were worked by entrepreneurial native residents.

Noncommercial deposits of asbestiform anthophyllite are found in many places in the world, particularly in precambrium rock. The name anthophyllite is derived from the Greek and means ambiguous. This, no doubt, refers to the range of common cations and trivalent metals found in the mineral. The only deposits of commercial significance are located in Finland, although outcrops have been found at scattered sites in the United States. Anthophyllite varies in configuration from asbestiform fibers to bladed and prismatic crystals. It commonly develops from regional metamorphism of ultrabasic rock and is frequently associated with talc and serpentine minerals. It does not occur in "cross" fiber seams but as fibrous masses with randomly oriented cubic blocks of fibers up to 3 cm in length, the fibers aligned parallel in each block. Overall, the anthophyllite fibers are relatively thick and crude, and as a result, rarely, if ever, cause MM.

Tremolite and actinolite asbestos are essentially products of metamorphic geologic activity. Mineralogically these two amphiboles are similar, but actinolite contains higher concentrations of iron. Tremolite is an early product of the thermal metamorphism of dolomites with silica impurities and is a contaminant of some industrial talc and vermiculite deposits. Of little industrial importance, fibrous tremolite is present in several countries in sufficient quantities for commercial exploitation, including Italy, Pakistan, Turkey, and South Korea. Tremolite, actinolite, and anthophyllite are not mined commercially in developed countries, although they are widely distributed in the earth's crust. These minerals are found in a wide range of geologic environments, and because of this diversity, tremolite and actinolite can occur in a variety of forms ranging from very fine, long fibers to shards or cleavage products with no apparent fibrous appearance.

Fluoroedenite is a mineral species detected near Biancavilla, a city in Sicily. It is locally linked with MM. It is a newly discovered member of the edenite-fluoroedenite series and similar in morphology and composition to minerals in the tremolite-actinolite series (Comba et al., 2003). The vermiculite ore in Libby, Montana contains approximately 4%–6% asbestiform amphibole (about 1/2 tremolite and 1/2 either winchite or richterite [or a mixture of both] in the tremolite series). Richerite is a sodic-calcific amphibole. Tremolite is a calcific amphibole as is edenite. The use of the term sodic or soda tremolite is to distinguish the fact that at least some of the mineral is sodium-rich. The pathogenic properties of these various mineral species is unknown. The amphibole asbestos constituents of the Libby, Montana vermiculite deposits are currently the subject of considerable investigation because of the relatively common occurrence of MM among miners.

References

Cadle RD. *Particles in the atmosphere and space.* New York: Reinbold; 1966.
Comba P, Gianfagna A, Paoletti L. Pleural mesothelioma cases in Biancavilla are related to a new fluoro-edenite fibrous amphibole. *Arch Environ Health.* 2003;58:229–232.
Davis JMG. Mineral fibre carcinogenesis: experimental data relating to the importance of fibre types, size, deposition, dissolution, and migration. In: Bignon J, Peto J, Saracci R, eds. *Non-occupational exposure to mineral fibres.* IARC Scientific Publication. 1989;90:33–45.
Garrard CS, Gerrity TR, Schreiner JF, Yeates DB. Analysis of aerosol deposition in the healthy human lung. *Arch Environ Med.* 1981;36:184–193.
Gerrity TR, Garrard CS, Yeates DB. A mathematical model of particle retention in the air spaces of human lungs. *Br J Ind Med* 1983;40:121–130.
Gibbs GW, Hwang CY. Dimensions of airborne asbestos fibres. In: Wagner JC, ed. *Biological effects on mineral fibres.* Vol. 1. IARC Scientific Publications. 1980;30:69–78.
Groppo C, Tomatis M, Turci F, et al. Potential toxicity of nonregulated asbestiform minerals: Balangeroite from the western Alps. Part I. Identification and characterization. *J Toxicol Environ Health.* Part A, 2005;68:1–19.
Kelse JW, Thompson CS. The regulatory and mineralogical definitions of asbestos and their impact on amphibole dust analysis. *Am Ind Hyg Assoc J.* 1989;50:613–622.
Lippman M, Yeates DB, Albert RE. Deposition, retention and clearance of inhaled particles. *Br J Ind Med.* 1980;37:337–362.
Lippman M. Effects of fibre characteristics on lung deposition, retention and disease. *Environ Health Perspect.* 1990;88:311–317.
McCulloch J. *Asbestos blues.* Bloomington, IN: Indiana University Press; 2002.
Pooley FD, Clark NJ. A comparison of fibre dimensions in chrysotile, crocidolite and amosite particles from samples of airborne dust and from postmortem lung tissue specimens. In: Wagner JC, ed. *Biological effects of mineral fibres,* Vol. 1. IARC Scientific Publications. 1980;30.
Ross M, Virta RL. Occurrence, production and uses of asbestos. In: Nolan RP, Langer AM, Ross M, Wicks FJ, Martin RF, eds. *The Health effects of chrysotile asbestos: Contribution of science to risk management decisions.* Can Mineral Spec Publ. 2001;5:79–88.
Stanton MF, Wrench C. Mechanisms of mesothelioma induction with asbestos and fibrous glass. *J Natl Cancer Inst.* 1972;48:797–821.
Stanton MF, Layard M, Tegeris A. Relation of particle dimension to carcinogenicity in amphibole asbestoses and other fibrous minerals. *J Natl Cancer Inst.* 1981;65:967–975.
Timbrell V. Deposition and retention of fibres in the human lung. *Ann Occup Hyg.* 1982;26:347–369.

3

Diseases Associated with Asbestos Industrial Products and Environmental Exposure

John E. Craighead

Introduction

Ramazzini fathered science's evolving understanding of the occupational diseases. In his 1713-pathfinding treatise, he stated

> Various and manifold is the harvest of diseases reaped by certain workers from crafts and trades that they pursue: all the profit that they get is fatal injury to their health. That crop generates mostly (from)...very fine particles inimical to human beings and induce particular diseases.

Almost 200 years later, Oliver (1902) noted when

> an individual is working in the dusty atmosphere of a factory for several hours a day, week...particles of dust immediately find their way into the finer bronchi, and subsequently into the pulmonary tissue itself. It is the repeated working in a dusty atmosphere that causes the trouble.

The history of asbestos-associated diseases recorded in the accompanying chapters of this book attest to the prophetic insights of these early seers. This chapter summarizes our current understanding of the health risks that are associated with employment in a diversity of industries where exposure is alleged to occur. More than 3000 different industrial products contain asbestos and it would be impossible to discuss many of the lesser uses. From the perspective of risk, all too often the physician and scientist are obliged to make assessments in the context of what has been learned from the study of more commonly used materials. Hence, the potential usefulness of these observations. Out of practical considerations, only selected published data is recorded here, but I have made every attempt to cite literature that meets a critical assessment of study design and analysis. The references provide a rich source of additional information. Countless unpublished laboratory analyses have been conducted in an attempt to quantify fiber release by industrial products under various work conditions. Much of this information has been developed for use in litigation and may be biased; accordingly, I have chosen not to include it in this chapter.

"Blue Collar" workers tend to move from shop to shop during the course of their careers. Union members often are assigned to different job locations on a daily basis.

Rarely is it possible for the investigator to envision exposures under these circumstances often based largely on recollections possibly tarnished by the passage of time and the prospect of successful litigation or compensation.

The mobility of workmen precludes critical epidemiological study and only on the rarest of occasions is reliable quantitative environmental exposure data available from the distant past. Job titles and descriptions are an unreliable basis for judging exposures and almost invariably workers move from task to task during the course of a work-day. A plumber is often a pipe fitter who also welds and strips gaskets. An automotive mechanic's chores are rarely limited to brake and clutch work. Bystander exposure is an ever present possibility.

Textile Mill Workers

The early history of asbestosis is largely a reflection of the use of asbestos in the manu-facturing of textiles immediately before and after the turn of the 20th century. The first recorded case in the medical literature was a 33-year-old man who had worked in the carding room of a London textile mill for 14 years. He died in 1900; a postmortem examination revealed extensive fibrosis of the lungs. Before his death, the patient volun-teered the insight that he was the only survivor among some ten men who had worked in the same shop. The implication was quite clear—his coworkers had suffered the same fate. The second medically recognized case associated with textile manufacturing was reported in the United Kingdom in 1924. Additional cases soon appeared and the epi-demic was documented retrospectively by Merewether (1930).

At the time, asbestos yarn was used to weave fire resistant fabric, or was braided together into rope for the packing used in plumber's valves and steam fittings. "Mattresses" stuffed with asbestos and felts were used to blanket steam engines and other heat-generating equipment. Apparently, a great many variations in manufactur-ing approaches developed and additives were introduced into fabrics that initially were predominantly cotton. As later studies showed, the manufacturing of asbestos textiles proved to be an exceedingly hazardous occupation whereas the users of the finished products were at considerably lesser risk. Initially, only a small proportion of the world's production proved suitable for spinning fibers since the long, flexible fibers of chrysotile were required. Short fibers comprise the bulk of the raw ore, but it is unsuitable for textile manufacturing. This form of chrysotile was used in millboard, sheeting, paper, and a plethora of other commercial items. In mills processing the crude ores, fibers are separated by sieving into various categories, on the basis of length. Since short fibers, $<5 \mu m$, comprise the majority of these particles in ore, they are relatively inexpensive in comparison to the more valuable long fiber products.

As South African amphiboles became commercially available during the early decades of the 20th century, crocidolite was incorporated into some textile products, largely as a minor constituent. The rigid, relatively inflexible fibers of amphibole were less useful than chrysotile. However, in the analysis of the public health epidemiological information, the confounding influence of amphiboles has proven to be an ever-present consideration. A report by Wagner et al. (1982) documents the results of fiber burden analyses on the lungs of workers in a textile factory that used small amounts of crocidol-ite and subsequently, greater amounts of chrysotile. Approximately 13% of deaths among the mill workers were due to malignant mesotheliomas (MM), presumably attributable to the crocidolite (Chapter 8). Analysis of lung tissue documented a heavy burden of crocidolite (Table 3.1).

Table 3.1 Lung Content of Chrysotile and Crocidolite Textile Workers in Comparison to Control Populations*

Study Group	No. in Study	Millions Fibers/g		% of Total Fibers	
		Chrysotile	Crocidolite	Chrysotile	Crocidolite
Subjects dying of MM	12	25	28	45	19
Exposed coworkers	12	55	24	57	26
United Kingdom 1976 (control series)	56	3	0.14	11	0.8
United Kingdom 1977 (consecutive postmortem examinations)	94	5	0.04	23	0.1

* Adapted from Wagner et al. (1982).

The details of textile manufacturing is beyond the scope of this review, but in the early years of the industry, it began with the crushing of crude, raw ore in the factory, followed by the "carding" of the asbestos and mixing it with cotton. The mix was spun, wound onto bobbins, twisted into yarn, and finally the end product was loomed. During each step, the worker was exposed. Dreessen et al. (1938) and Page (1937) published detailed descriptions of textile manufacturing in comprehensive reviews that consider the public health implications of the textile industry. On the basis of their comprehensive studies, Dreessen et al. (1938) developed the first recommendations for the control of workplace air concentrations of dust; they served as the official guideline in the United States for the subsequent 20-year period. It should be recalled that the association of lung cancers (LC) with asbestosis had only been reported in individual cases during the 1930s, and the role of asbestos in the genesis of MM was not a consideration at this time (Eglert and Geiger, 1936; Gloyne, 1935, 1936; Lynch and Smith, 1935).

Dust exposures in textile factories documented by Public Health Service surveys in the 1960s (Lynch and Ayer, 1966) yielded findings well within the threshold limit value established by Dreessen et al. (1938). Environmental sampling showed that the mean concentrations exceed the permissible amounts soon to be permitted by the Occupational Safety and Health Administration (OSHA) a decade later. In these studies, an estimate of the number of fibers ≥ 5 μm in length was attempted, but the conclusions are unconvincing. The ranges summarized in Table 3.2, to a large extent, represent values from factories where substantial differences in dust concentrations were found.

Several studies reported in the 1980s documented disease among textile workers whose employment began in the 1930s (Dement et al., 1983; McDonald et al., 1982, 1983; Peto et al., 1985). Comparison of observations is difficult because of differences in exposures and the approaches to analyzing results. However, several conclusions are warranted: (1) the overall mortality consequent to asbestosis was negligible, but the analysis did not address morbidity related to this disease; (2) the incidence of LC increased appreciably in exposed workers, largely in men and to a more limited extent, women, after 20 years of employment. Unfortunately, in these studies, smoking histories were not recorded; and (3) a low incidence of MM was documented, even after relatively short periods of employment, but to a large extent, these cases could be attributed to the use of small amounts of crocidolite in some factories. Of paramount importance, however, was the observation that the occurrence of LC in textile workers was

Table 3.2 Mean and Range of Asbestos Air Concentrations in Nine Textile Factories by Operation*

Work Activity	Mean[†]	Range[†]
Preparation	4.2	1.1–9.3
Carding	3.7	0.9–8.4
Spinning	3.6	1.1–10.3
Twisting	4.7	0.7–18.8
Winding	3.4	0.9–11.9
Weaving	2.5	0.7–9.8

* Adapted from Lynch and Ayer (1966).
[†] f/mL, phase contrast microscopy.

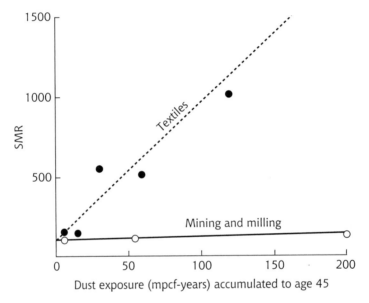

Figure 3.1 For unknown reasons, LC rates are substantially greater among textile workers than for chrysotile miners and millers (McDonald et al., 1983).

substantially greater than in chrysotile miners and millers with similar backgrounds of exposure. The formulae below illustrate the means for calculating relative risk (RR; McDonald, 1998).

Textile workers—So. Carolina	RR = 1 + 0.059 mpcf/yr.
Textile—Pennsylvania	RR = 1 + 0.051 mpcf/yr.
Miners & Millers—Québec	RR = 1 + 0.016 mpcf/yr.

mpcf = million particles per cubic foot.

It is clear from these analyses that the slope of the exposure-response line for LC in the textile industry is 50-fold steeper than the slope calculated for Québec miners and millers and friction product workers (Hughes, 1994; Figure 3.1). Despite considerable investigation, an explanation for these differences is wanting. It has been suggested that the mineral oils used to treat chrysotile in textile milling enhanced pathogenicity but experimental evidence to support this conjecture is lacking.

Until recent years garments made with asbestos fabric were widely used in industry and the military as well as by those responsible for fire control. Gibbs (1975) analyzed the airborne fibers 5 μm in length or greater in the breathing zone of workers wearing asbestos safety garments. At one factory where men wore asbestos-containing coats, hoods, and mittens, the concentrations of asbestos in the air ranged from 0.3 to 5.0 fibers/cm^3 (using phase contrast microscopy) and an 8-hour time-weighted concentration from 0.1 to 1.1 f/mL was calculated. At a second plant, the ambient air concentrations reached 9.9 to 26.2 f/mL and the 8-hour time-weighted average proved to be 4.7 f/mL. Variable numbers of these fibers were in the pathogenic range of $\geq$5 μm in length.

Shipbuilders and Navy/Merchant Marine Personnel

Naval architects began considering the use of asbestos for the insulation of oceangoing vessels early in the 1900s. Asbestos was utilized in increasing amounts in shipbuilding during World War I, but little documentation of its applications has been published. In 1934, a passenger vessel, the *SS Morro Castle*, burned at sea off New Jersey, resulting in a considerable loss of life. Inquires by the US Senate revealed the need for improved fire protection aboard ships and by 1938, the first US registered passenger vessel, the *SS Panama*, was commissioned with asbestos insulation aboard. At the time, naval vessels were launched with rigid weight limitations invoked by international treaties. It was soon discovered by naval architects that amosite asbestos pipe covering weighed 14 lbs per foot^3 with a temperature limit of 750 °F, whereas magnesia [$CaMg(CO_3)_2$] and magnesium oxide, the traditional insulations, weighed 16 lbs per foot^3 and had a temperature limit of 500 °F. Clearly, less weight for insulation translated into more armor, guns, and munitions as well as economies of fuel consumption. About ten different forms of insulation containing variable amounts of asbestos mixed with inorganic and organic binders were used aboard ships at the time. According to US Navy specifications in the 1940s, mixtures of chrysotile with amosite were customarily required, but a recent investigation of a mothballed World War II destroyer indicated that the amounts of amosite asbestos in boiler room insulation, in any one vessel, could range from 5% to 99%. Specifications differed elsewhere in the world and in the United Kingdom, crocidolite was incorporated into the mix, in part because of its availability but also because it was said to create less workplace dust. The extent to which crocidolite was used in shipyards in the United States during the war is unknown, but it was most probably a minimal proportion of the whole. Much more was used in shipyards in the British Isles. Since battle damaged allied vessels were often repaired and rehabilitated in eastern North American shipyards, we can assume that many workers were exposed to crocidolite as well as amosite and variable amounts of chrysotile (containing unknown amounts of tremolite contaminants; Marr, 1964).

In the United States, at the onset of the Lend Lease Program in the late 1930s, during the second term of F.D. Roosevelt, there were 8 naval and 24 private shipyards in the United States and in the territory of Hawaii with the capacity to build $\geq$2000 ton vessels. By the end of World War II, 99 additional yards and countless more contract shops contributed to the shipbuilding and repair effort! More than 5×10^3 merchant vessels and 1500 combat ships were launched during the 5 years of hostility (Fassett, 1948).

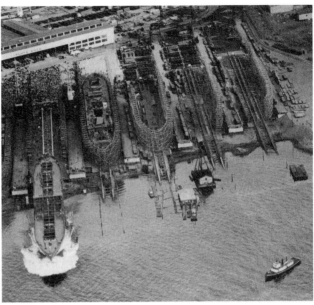

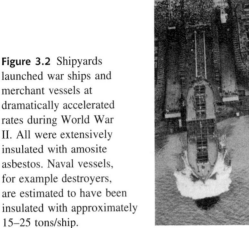

Figure 3.2 Shipyards launched war ships and merchant vessels at dramatically accelerated rates during World War II. All were extensively insulated with amosite asbestos. Naval vessels, for example destroyers, are estimated to have been insulated with approximately 15–25 tons/ship.

According to the analyses of Selikoff et al. (1979b), US shipyards employed about 7.5×10^4 men in the 1920s and 1930s. At the end of hostilities in 1945, 1.6×10^6 men and women were engaged in shipbuilding, an approximate 45-fold increase. Jobs were largely filled by unskilled workers with as many as 20% being women who left the household for wartime duty. Labor turnover was the norm, averaging 100% annually. Selikoff et al. (1979b) estimated that a total of 4.5×10^6 men and women were employed in shipyards during the World War II. These were the days when the national heroine was "Rosie the Riveter" who exemplified the war effort of the populus. It was the time when shipyards operated by the renowned automobile manufacture, H.J. Kaiser, on the west coast were launching a ship on a daily basis (Figure 3.2). One can only imagine the industrial anarchy that prevailed with inexperienced workers employed on an overtime basis, 50–60 hours per week. Since asbestos was accorded great value in the construction of seaworthy ships and because the health hazards associated with its use were thought by many to be negligible, extensive pollution of the workplace by asbestos was inevitable.

As noted above, the accepted permissible level of asbestos was based on the criterion established by Dreessen et al. (1938) from studies in textile mills (ie, 5 mpcf, million particles per cubic foot) equivalent to approximately 30 f/mL, an exceedingly high concentration considering today's OSHA standards (0.1 f/mL). Studies commissioned by the navy and conducted during the final years of the war by several of the country's most respected scientists (Fleischer et al., 1946) unfortunately contributed to the near universal apathy regarding the health effects of asbestos. These investigators reported a prevalence of asbestosis of only 0.29% among workers in four shipyards. Alas, the scientists were unaware of the protracted latency period required for the development of clinical asbestosis.

The use of asbestos felt for the insulation of turbines in naval vessels began in the mid 1930s. Pipe covering was a later development that soon found broad application in the engine rooms. Water repellant amosite felt, to prevent sweating by cold water pipes, was introduced in 1942. Pipe insulated with asbestos antiquated the use of wool and hair insulation that retained moisture and encouraged microbial growth and vermin. It was not long before block asbestos and pipe wraps with asbestos cloth attained universal usage. Often, pipes were covered by asbestos-containing cement, but friable asbestos often remained exposed on the surfaces of the boilers and piping. Nearly all the compartments of wartime ships were insulated with asbestos, although the concentrations in the boiler rooms and machine spaces were greatest. In the tight, poorly ventilated quarters of the smaller ships, such as destroyers and submarines, engine room attendants and sailors routinely came into physical contact with asbestos-containing materials. Repair work was particularly hazardous because large amounts of friable asbestos were released into the work environment when lagging was removed. In one study (Sheers and Coles, 1980), the mean value of 171 f/mL was found in a boiler room and 88 f/mL in an engine room during the removal of lagging. In the British Navy, crocidolite was sprayed on deckheads, bulkheads, and beneath the flight decks of aircraft carriers. Allegedly, some aircraft carriers were sufficiently top heavy that the risk of capsizing was a reality. In another reported study, removal of sprayed crocidolite was associated with a mean ambient air concentration of 345 f/mL (Sheers and Coles, 1980). A report by the US Maritime Commission noted "long after the vessel has been put to sea, flaking and cracking due to ships motions and vibrations are suspected of releasing asbestos into the surrounding space" (Nicholson et al., 1988).

Pleural and lung parenchymal disease associated with maritime shipyard employment was first recognized in the 1980s. As noted elsewhere (Chapter 6), pleural plaques (PP) and bilateral pleural thickening usually require a latency period of more than 10 years to become radiologically evident. Thus, the appearance of chest disease in the 1980s roughly corresponded to the time of maximal employment in wartime ship construction and repair (Selikoff et al., 1979a,b). Analyses by Sheers and Templeton (1968) correlate the presence of pleural disease with the severity of exposure. In continuously exposed shipyard workers, radiological studies demonstrated PP or pleural fibrosis (or both) in 28% of workers, whereas only 7% had evidence of asbestosis. The results of a radiological study of shipyard workers in the United States who were alive at least 20 years after first employment are summarized in Table 3.3. Smoking did not appear to influence the findings in this research (Ducatman et al., 1990; Selikoff et al., 1980), in contrast to observations in later studies (Chapter 6). A retrospective x-ray survey of more than 5000 men by Jones et al. (1984) revealed pleural abnormalities, primarily PP, in 26% of older merchant mariners with shipboard experience of >35 years. A similar survey by Selikoff et al. (1990) demonstrated parenchymal and pleural changes in 43% of long-term engine room staff with long histories at sea. Seamen with other duties aboard ship had a lower prevalence of asbestos markers.

On the basis of autopsy observations, Doll established in 1955 an association of LC with asbestos exposure. Epidemiological studies soon established a dosage relationship.

Within the period 1970 through 1978, four case-control studies were carried out in east coast communities that clearly established an association of employment in shipyards during World War II and the development of LC (Blot et al., 1978, 1980, 1981; Table 3.4). Similar observations on Pearl Harbor shipyard workers were reported by Kolonel et al. (1985; Table 3.5). In Bath, Maine, a geographically isolated shipbuilding community, 67% of the LC diagnosed during the 1970s occurred in current or former shipyard workers. As might be expected, the findings in these epidemiological studies are compromised since little information is available on job descriptions and thus the extent of asbestos exposure in members of the study groups.

Cases of MM were first reported among ship repairmen in Liverpool, England (Owen, 1964). Four years later, Harries (1968) discovered MM occurring in shipyard workers of

Table 3.3 Distribution of Small Opacities and Pleural Disease among Shipyard Workers*

ILO Classification Small Opacities[†] (Combined Perfusion)	Number Within Category					
	Active			Retired		
	Normal Pleura	Abnormal Pleura	Total	Normal Pleura	Abnormal Pleura	Total
0/-	0	0	0	0	0	0
0/0	9	2	11	3	3	6
0/1	12	10	22	15	6	21
1/0	10	13	23	11	12	23
1/1	33	31	64	16	34	50
1/2	5	3	8	2	6	8
2/1	3	1	4	3	10	13
2/2	2	3	5	4	16	20
2/3	0	0	0	0	1	1
3/2	0	0	0	2	0	2
3/3	1	1	2	1	0	1
3/4	0	0	0	0	0	0
Total	75	64	139	57	88	145

* Adapted from Selikoff et al. (1990).
[†] No large rounded opacities were observed.

Table 3.4 RR of LC Associated with Shipbuilding Employment*

Location in the United States	Years Cases Diagnosed	Total Sample	% of Male Population of Region Employed in Shipyards	Relative Risk[†]
Coastal Georgia	1970–1976	1057	21	1.6
Jacksonville, Florida	1976–1978	789	22	1.4
Tidewater, Virginia	1976	641	33	1.5
Bath, Maine	1974–1978	64	67	1.7

* Adapted from Blot (1978, 1980, 1981).
[†] Adjusted for cigarette smoking.

various trade categories. Small series of cases were soon reported from elsewhere in Great Britain (Edge, 1976; Fletcher, 1972; Sheers and Coles, 1980), the Netherlands (Stumphius, 1971), Italy (Puntoni et al., 1976), and Norfolk-Newport News (Tagnon et al., 1980). A dosage gradient was noted by Sheers and Coles (1980). Interestingly, the disease occurred predominantly in the pleural cavity, not in the peritoneum, suggesting exposure was less severe than in insulation factory workers (Chapter 8; Selikoff et al., 1965). Because shipyards were precipitously closed in 1945 after the cessation of hostilities, workers were usually lost to follow-up. Alas, no comprehensive epidemiological studies have been reported that address the incidence of disease arising from shipyard exposure. The difficulties inherent in such a study are magnified by the diversity of jobs held by shipyard workers and the high personnel turnover rates during the war. Nonetheless, limited information is available. For example, Tidewater, VA is a community where several large shipyards operated during

Table 3.5 Mortality from LC among Shipyard Workers Employed
15 Years or Longer by Latency Interval, Pearl Harbor, United States*

Latency Interval (yr)	Observed Deaths	Expected Deaths	SMR	95% CI
15–19	2	1.7	1.2	0.1–4.2
20–29	10	9.2	1.1	0.5–2.0
30+	22	13.2	1.7	1.0–2.5
Total	34	24.1	1.4	1.0–2.0

* Adapted from Kolonel et al. (1985).

Table 3.6 Incidence of MM, 1972–1978, among White
Male Residents of Tidewater, VA, According to Age*

Age (yr)	No. of Cases	No. of Cases Expected[†]	Incidence Rate (Cases/yr/10^3)
<40	0	1.3	0.0
40–49	5	2.3	1.5
50–59	18	3.6	6.2
60–69	25	5.3	14.1
70+	13	3.6	12.5
Total	61	16.1	2.7*

* Adapted from Tagnon et al. (1980).
† Age-adjusted rate using 1970 US populations based on estimated national incidence rates 1970–1976.

World War II. A MM incidence rate of 12.5 cases per year/10^5 members of the population was found in a survey conducted during the period 1972 through 1978 (Tagnon et al., 1980; Table 3.6). There has been no systematic effort by the US government to assess the incidence of asbestos disease, particularly MM, among navy personnel who devoted years of their life to service aboard ships during the war. In the view of the writer, this is an appalling social and scientific oversight! Those of us who read the depositions of former navy servicemen and shipyard workers who today suffer from MM repeatedly are reminded how often disease can be traced to a shipyard job or boiler room service aboard ships during the 1940s and 1950s. These cases continue to appear some 60 years after the war.

Insulators

In the early 20th century, shredded rope, wool felt, vegetable fibers and cork, as well as rock wool, diatomaceous earth, and cement were used in building insulation. Asbestos mixed with magnesia [$CaMg(CO_3)_2$] and/or magnesium oxide in a slurry of silicates was initially used as insulation material in the 1860s. Thereafter, various binders and substrates, including paper, were mixed with magnesia and either chrysotile or amosite, and to a much lesser extent, crocidolite. These products were introduced into commerce in the 1930s, but it was not until mobilization for war that amosite block and spray-on crocidolite became a significant component of building insulation. Fibrous glass was also used in commercial construction (Table 3.7; Balzer and Cooper, 1968).

Table 3.7 Approximate Composition of Insulation by Construction/Industry*

Type of Industry	Fibrous Glass (%)	Asbestos (%)
Commercial building	70	30
Heavy industrial building	30	70
Marine construction and repair	20	80

* Adapted from Balzer and Cooper (1968).

Table 3.8 Presumptive Asbestosis among Insulation Workers Based only on Chest X-Rays*

Latency (yr)	Abnormal X-Ray (%)	Asbestosis Grade (%)		
		1	2	3
0–9	10	10	0	0
10–19	44	42	2	0
20–29	72	45	22	5
30–39	87	53	25	9
40+	94	29	42	23

* Adapted from Selikoff et al. (1965).

Asbestosis in insulation workers was first reported by Merewether and his colleagues in the United Kingdom during 1934 and again somewhat later. A scant few additional cases were noted in the literature before the onset of World War II, but it was not until the cessation of hostilities that a flood of new cases were reported. During World War II, justifiable concern by naval officials served as the basis for the so-called Fleisher and Drinker study (Fleisher et al., 1946), the results of which lulled public health authorities to the conclusion that asbestosis was not an important risk for shipyard workers and naval personnel. It was recommended to continue the 500 mpcf regulatory criterion based on the Dreessen study of textile workers reported in 1938. Alas, the Fleisher study (1946) was flawed, largely because the extended clinical latency period for the disease asbestosis was not appreciated and LC and MM were not considerations at the time.

In 1965, Selikoff et al. reported the results of a chest x-ray survey of New York insulators. The strikingly high prevalence of radiological changes in the lung parenchyma of these workers correlated with the duration of employment (Table 3.8). Information on the presence of benign pleural disease in these workers was not reported. Although the duration of employment naturally paralleled advancing age, the authors chose to interpret their x-ray findings as an indication of asbestosis in the worker population. Subsequent observations in other cohorts of insulators have borne out the validity of their interpretation. The results of a morbidity study by Selikoff et al. (1979a) on a population of more than 1.7×10^4 union insulators from around the United States demonstrated a striking incidence of neoplastic disease in multiple organ systems. Alas, it is probable these data are not an accurate assessment of disease attributable to asbestos exposure. The diagnoses by the Selikoff group were on the basis of "Best Evidence" appraisals by the authors using mortality information such as death certificates from sources throughout the country. The US National Statistics were used as the basis for establishing the incidence of disease in a so-called "control" population. Possible risk factors such as diet, cigarette smoking, and alcoholic beverage use were not accorded consideration in the evaluation. The results of subsequent studies have not supported their conclusions regarding disease in organ systems, other than the lungs (Chapter 9).

Elmes and Simpson (1977) in Belfast, Jarvholm and Sanden (1998) in Sweden, and Balzer and Cooper (1968) in the United States San Francisco Bay area reported similar observations with respect to the occurrence of asbestosis. The latter authors (Balzer and Cooper, 1968) discovered asbestosis in 25% of the insulators they studied using chest x-rays, but the risk was doubtless higher, based on environmental sampling data.

The rampant flurry of new cases of asbestosis, LC, and MM that resulted from sustained exposures of building and shipyard insulators to asbestos in the 1940s has been followed by a smoldering epidemic of new cases resulting from exposure to in-place asbestos insulation in ships, commercial and public buildings, and even in the insulation heating systems of homes of unsuspecting average citizens. The impact of these sporadic and often unrecognized exposures defies calculation, but it is clearly evident in the case material evaluated by the writer. Data published by Roggli and Sanders (2000) provides some hint as to the magnitude of the problem.

Figure 3.3 illustrates an important point regarding the MM occurring in amphibole-exposed insulation workers. The data is consistent with observations published in 1964 by Selikoff that depicts the experience of insulation manufacturers in an amosite factory. Peritoneal MM were found to develop in workers with exceptionally high and prolonged exposures to amphibole asbestos, such as insulators (Chapter 8).

In the past, both crocidolite and chrysotile asbestos were widely used for spray-on applications in building construction.

In 1973, the US Environmental Protection Agency (EPA) banned the spraying of asbestos insulation within buildings (Figure 3.4). The US National Emission Standards for Hazardous Air Pollutants (NESHAP) regulations promulgated by the EPA now dictate asbestos removal before renovation of buildings is undertaken. Before that time, sheet metal installers and other workmen invariably were exposed to high concentrations of friable asbestos during building construction and renovation. For example, electricians and communication workers pulling wires through dead spaces in buildings and sheet metal workers installing heating and air-conditioning systems were at particular risk, since they often came into indirect contact with spray-on asbestos.

Vermiculite is a hydrated platy magnesium-aluminum-iron silicate that expands 8- to 12-fold into wormlike structures when heated (*Vermiculare* (L), to breed worms). It is mined from deposits scattered worldwide and has numerous applications in agriculture/ horticulture, construction, and in industry. In addition to its modest cost, vermiculite has insulating characteristics that make it exceptionally useful for home application. In its expanded form, the mineral is light and can be installed without difficulty into confining spaces such as residential attics.

The world's largest vermiculite quarries in northwest Montana have been mined for more than 50 years. Studies by the OSHA and independent investigators in the 1980s (McDonald et al., 2004) found asbestiform minerals in the ore bodies in concentrations ranging up to 6% (Chapter 2). The report describes MM occurring among 4.2% of workers allegedly attributable to exposure in the mines or mills of Libby, Montana. The Standard Mortality Rate (SMR) for LC was 2.4, not adjusted for smoking.

In recent unpublished studies by the EPA, bulk samples of commercial expanded vermiculite installed as insulation in residences were found to contain tremolite/actinolyte in concentrations as high as 2%. Disturbances to the "in-place" vermiculite created asbestos aerosols in which were found long fibers (>5 μm) in concentrations exceeding the contemporary OSHA limits.

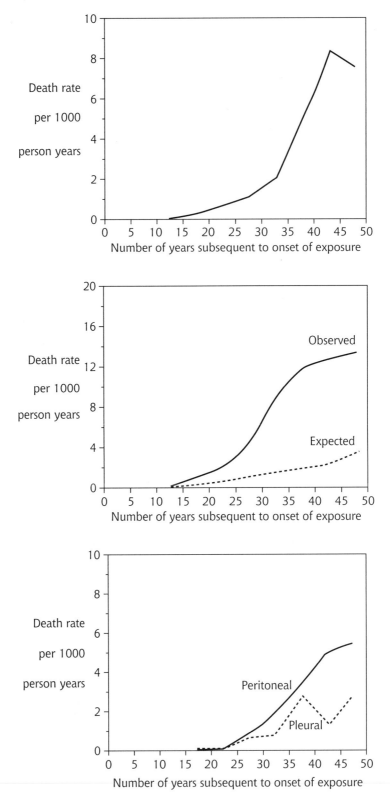

Figure 3.3 Comparative prevalence of pleural and peritoneal mesotheliomas among insulators can best be attributed to their heavy exposure to amphibole asbestos.

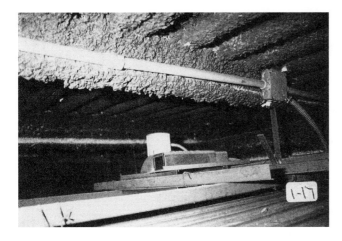

Figure 3.4 Spray-on asbestos was applied extensively in dead spaces of buildings; its use was banned in 1973 by the US Environmental Protection Agency.

Plumbers and Pipe Fitters

Plumbers and pipe fitters are responsible for the installation and maintenance of pipes and fixtures for water, gas, high-pressure steam and chemical transmission, as well as for drainage, sewage, heating, refrigeration, and air-conditioning systems. They may be at risk for exposure to a wide variety of potentially toxic and carcinogenic chemicals and gases, in addition to asbestos, in the diverse workplaces where they are employed. It is the rare plumber and pipe fitter who does not remove and replace insulation in the course of their daily activities.

Table 3.9 summarizes the results of two studies of plumbers that demonstrate a significant but modest increase in the occurrence of disease in various major organ systems. Although an increase in LC risk was found in this and other unpublished studies (Kaminski et al., 1980), the findings are inconclusive with regard to the possible role of asbestos in the pathogenesis of the neoplasm. The control populations were not comparable to the study group and smoking histories were not available. Moreover, plumbers and pipe fitters are said to smoke more than workers in other occupations (Levin et al., 1985; Walrath et al., 1985).

The data in Table 3.9 are limited to workers classified as plumbers, although job assignments are often flexible. When the occurrence of MM in a cohort of 7×10^3 plumbers was evaluated by Cantor et al. (1986), 16 cases were recorded in death certificates, whereas only two would have been expected. Thus, the RR was substantially elevated. A similar conclusion was reported by Teta et al. (1983) on the basis of a study of Connecticut insulators. These results must be qualified in view of the difficulties in establishing the diagnosis of MM definitively from death certificate data.

The apparent increase in the prevalence of lymphatic and hematopoietic is noteworthy (Table 3.9). If not an artifact, it may reflect exposure to chemicals in the workplace environment, although the possibility of an asbestos effect cannot be ruled out (Chapter 9).

Construction Workers

In the past, the construction industry accounted for more than 50% of the asbestos used in the developed countries of Europe and North America (Nicholson et al., 1982). Among the countless products manufactured and used by the industry were shingles and roofing felts,

Table 3.9 PMR for Plumbers in Two Death Certificate Studies

	*Kaminski et al. (1980)**	*Cantor et al. (1986)†*
All malignancy	1.27‡	1.27‡
Esophagus	2.75‡	—
Stomach	1.30	1.48‡
Large intestine	1.16	1.14
Lung, bronchus	1.29‡	1.38‡
Lymphatic and hematopoietic	1.46‡	1.80‡
Other lymphoid tissues	1.63‡	1.17
Nonmalignant respiratory disease	0.96	1.37

* Survey of 3369 white male deaths in 1971.
† Survey of 3491 male deaths, 1960–1979.
‡ Significant.

concrete pipe and sheet material, architectural panels and plenums, joint and taping compounds, heating system insulation, floor tile, electrical wire and cable, paints, and plumbing fixtures.Numerous opportunities for exposure to asbestos occur during the manufacturing of materials and equipment, transportation, and installation. In addition, workers are now involved in repair as well as in abatement (Lange et al., 1996) and demolition of existing structures, with the potential for "in-place" asbestos exposure continuing (Table 3.10).

Roughly, 7.8×10^6 workers are employed in various capacities in the construction industry. Using death certificate data, Robinson et al. (1995) recently reported the proportional mortality rate (PMR) among men employed 1984 through 1986 in 19 states. Mortality was significantly elevated for cancer of the esophagus, larynx, lung, and pleural cavity. Chronic pulmonary disease occurred commonly. Whether or not this was obstructive pulmonary disease or a restrictive condition attributable to dust exposures is not known, but it is highly likely that obstructive disease due to smoking was responsible for considerable disability. A survey of North Carolina construction workers who died between 1988 and 1994 (Wang et al., 1999) revealed a significantly increased mortality for cancer of the buccal cavities (PMR = 143), pharynx (PMR = 134), and lung (PMR = 113). Pneumoconiosis was also increased (PMR = 111). Unfortunately, the data in these two studies and an additional investigation by Stern et al. (2001) were not adjusted for smoking. It is difficult to assess what role, if any, asbestos might have played in the occurrence of disease in these populations, in part because information on exposure is lacking. Studies that provide insight into this question have been reported from Canada (McDonald and McDonald, 1980), Australia (Ferguson et al., 1987), and Sweden (Malker et al., 1985). In an Australian survey, 13% of the MM cases occurring during the study period 1980–1985 were among workers in the construction, maintenance, and demolition trades. An additional 2.6% of cases were categorized as plumbers. In a survey by McDonald and McDonald of MM occurring in North America, 13% were workers employed in the construction industry (excluding plumbers who accounted for an additional 6%). In the Swedish survey of Malker et al. (1985), 20% of the MM developed in workers nominally classified as construction tradesmen, including plumbers. The remarkable similarity in the outcomes of these three investigations emphasizes the consequential role asbestos played in the occurrence of MM among workers in the construction trades. Using referral material, largely from litigation, Roggli et al. (2002) diagnosed asbestosis in 17% of the construction workers he studied. In this investigation, histopathologic information was used; an approach that no doubt increased the sensitivity of the evaluation.

Table 3.10 Representative Exposure Levels, Absent Respiratory Protection, by Construction Activity*

Construction Activity	Representative Time-Weighted Average Exposure Levels (f/mL)
New construction	
A/C pipe installation	0.02 to 0.06
A/C sheet installation	≤0.15
Roofing felt installation	ND[†] to 0.6
Renovation/remodeling	
Drywall demolition	0.15 to 11
Remove built-up roofing	ND to 0.2
Remove flooring products	0.02 to 0.04
Routine maintenance: commercial/residential	
Remove/repair/replace ceiling tiles	0.02 to 1.4
Repair lighting	0.01 to 2.8
Other work above drop ceiling	0.01 to 2.8
Repair boilers	0.04 to 0.53
Repair plumbing	0.04 to <0.1
Repair roofing	ND to 0.3
Repair drywall	0.02 to 1.4
Repair flooring	0.02 to 0.04

* Adapted from HEI-AR (1991).
† ND: not detected.

Building Interior Workmen

In the past, an enormous variety of asbestos-containing materials were formally manufactured and distributed worldwide for applications to the floors, ceilings, and walls of commercial and public buildings and homes during construction and restoration. They include preformed floor tiling, molded wall, cement and Transite board products as well as compounds that are reconstituted for spray-on or hand application (such as drywall, joint and taping compounds, sealing material, plasters of various types, and textured paints). The products contained calcite (Ca carbonate), dolomite (Ca Mg carbonate), gypsum (plaster of Paris—$CaSO_4$), aluminum silicate clays, including kaolin and feldspar, and perlite (noncrystalline—SO_2), mica (a platy Al silicate), talc (a platy Mg silicate), and vermiculite (a platy biotite). To a substantial extent (up to 15% by weight), these commercial formulations contained short fibers (<5 μm) of chrysotile that served as a binder facilitating application. To the extent that traces of tremolite/actinolite were contaminants, it is believed that long fibers (>5 μm) would have been sieved out in the grading process. Some preparations of vermiculite and talc are known to contain contaminants of tremolite/actinolite and/or anthophyllite. And, some, but not all, Transite board, manufactured by Johns-Manville Corp., often but not invariably, contained crocidolite and/or amosite.

In recent years, concern has been raised regarding the health risks incurred by drywallers who, to a large extent, devote a substantial part of their workday to their trade. Before World War II, interior walls were usually covered by a lath mesh over which was applied a film of plaster, a time-consuming task requiring considerable manual skill.

The housing boom that followed the war prompted the development of new, less costly, manpower-efficient approaches. This was accomplished by the manufacturing of paneled wallboard installed by hanging the sheets over wall joists, and joining them by drywall compound and tape. After installation, drywall "finishers" prepared the surface for painting. The unions between the drywall sheets were pasted over with joint compound, commonly called "mud," to fill the joints and any defects in the drywall board. Drywall joint compound was applied as a wet paste, which was troweled into the drywall joints. Some commercial formulations were purchased as wet compounds, ready for installation, whereas others were dry and required mixing by the finisher. While the latter procedure required only minutes to accomplish, it was often a dusty activity. Once the drywall compound had dried and had become firm, it had the consistency and texture of chalk. The joint compound was then sanded or finished to create a smooth, uniform surface. This activity also generated a fine dust, although the evidence suggests that the particles of asbestos were, to a variable extent, encompassed by the drywall compound and not friable. Dry sanding was done using various mechanical approaches (Table 3.11). Wet wall sanding was an alternative to reduce the airborne dust concentrations, but was infrequently used by finishers. Plastering is now an occupation largely of historical importance since drywallers and tapers have done most of the interior building work since the late 1940s.

Epidemiological data addressing the health risks of drywalling and taping are lacking. Fischbein et al. (1979) conducted a preliminary radiological study of 110 drywallers, the majority of whom were smokers or ex-smokers. No information was available on their work history as a drywaller or in other trades. Fifty-one percent of the men studied after 20 years or more of employment were claimed by the investigators to have chest x-ray abnormalities which they chose to attribute to asbestos. One must question the validity of these quantitative conclusions, inasmuch as short particles of asbestos are not known to cause asbestosis, and the conclusion that asbestosis exists requires more definitive evidence than that utilized by the authors. To the extent that radiological changes were actually present, they could have reflected the effects of smoking and/or emphysema.

Systematic case-controlled cohort studies focused on drywallers have not been reported. Investigations of workers in related fields have demonstrated the anticipated increase in prevalence of LC and bladder cancer in populations of heavy smokers—painters (Steenland and Palu, 1999) plaster and cement masons (Stern et al., 2001).

Cases of MM presumably attributable to drywall and taping compound exposure have not been noted in surveys conducted in Australia (Ferguson, 1987), Sweden (Malker et al., 1985), and North America (McDonald and McDonald, 1980).

Table 3.11 Summary of Airborne Asbestos Fiber Concentrations (in Fibers >5 μm/mL) in the Drywall Taping Process Using Personal Air Sampling*

	Concentrations		
	Range	Mean	Median
Application	0.4–1.3	0.9	0.9
Mixing (dry powder)	9.0–12.4	11.2	12.2
Mixing (Premix)	1.2–3.2	2.4	2.3
Hand sanding	2.1–24.2	11.5	11.5
Pole sanding	1.2–10.1	4.3	4.0
Sweeping	4.0–26.5	12.1	7.7

* From Verma and Middleton (1980).

Floor Tile and Linoleum Installers and Removers

During the second half of the 20th century, asbestos-containing asphalt, vinyl, and mastic flooring manufactured by a number of suppliers were used extensively in developed countries of the western hemisphere and Europe. Consumption figures, however, are not available and little information exists on the number of workers involved full- or part-time in the installation and removal of these flooring materials. OSHA regulations dictated that all floor tile installed after 1980 be asbestos-free, although a final ruling for phaseout was invalidated by federal court action. Regardless, asbestos-containing floor tiling is no longer used in North America and Europe, but unknown amounts remain installed in buildings (in various stages of wear and disrepair) worldwide. In the past, composition flooring in sheets or tile squares contained up to 25% chrysotile asbestos encompassed by a binder. Thus, the asbestos was not friable, although polishing, sanding, and repetitious daily walking over the surface releases fibers in low concentrations (Murphy et al., 1971; Sebastian et al., 1982). Crossman et al. (1996) conducted a study of fiber release comparing ambient concentrations in room air in proximity to flooring using a variety of techniques commonly employed by workmen for removing tile in-place. The voluminous body of data provided in this report shows that small numbers of respirable fibers are released during removal. Using the EPA dictated AHERA (Chapter 13) procedures and analyzing fiber release by transmission electron microscopy, it was found that the ambient air concentration of fibers >5 μm at the work site was increased approximately twofold (avg $= <0.014$ f/mL) above background (avg $= <0.006$ f/mL). The number of asbestos "structures" <0.5 μm was roughly tenfold greater than those ≥ 5 μm or longer. Dry pneumatic removal of the tile yielded the highest airborne concentrations of the long fibers (mean $= 0.66$ f/mL). As might be expected, differences in values related to procedural approaches were substantial but did not alter consequentially the overall findings. One can conclude that the use of EPA recommended procedures substantially reduced the aerosols of long, presumably pathogenic fibers from the air at the work site. It would seem that well-intentioned prophylactic removal of asbestos flooring in homes and public buildings is an unnecessary precaution.

Asbestos-Cement Manufacturers and End-Product Users

In the past, asbestos was mixed with cement for use in the fabrication of pipe, sheet, and corrugated panels, as well as in construction products, such as roofing and shingles. Asbestos imparted tensile strength, durability and impact strength as well as heat and fire resistance. Roughly 10%–15% of the final mix contained asbestos, either chrysotile, crocidolite, amosite, or all three in various combinations, depending on the manufacturer and the intended application. In the mid-decades of the last century, the cement industry was the world's major consumer of asbestos, mainly chrysotile (Table 3.12). Untold numbers of workers were potentially exposed during the manufacturing and molding of the finished product, particularly in the cutting and drilling of asbestos-cement products. While asbestos-cement is no longer used in North America and Europe, it undoubtedly is still manufactured in some developing countries.

There are many different formulations of cement, but the most common is Portland in which limestone is a major constituent. Portland-Pozzolan cement also contains siliceous or aluminous materials and gypsum. Crystalline silica is a minor constituent of most cements, silicosis is not known to develop as a result of exposure to dust during the manufacturing or use of the finished product. Indeed, pneumoconiosis attributable to

Table 3.12 World Production of Cement, 1995 (Rounded Metric Tons $\times$ 10⁴)

China	41.0
Japan	9.2
United States	7.7
Russia	5.5
India	5.5
Others	52.2
World total (approximate)	119.6

nonasbestos-containing cement has not been reported. Weill et al. (1973) have provided us an overview of the manufacturing process:

> Bags of asbestos packed in a compressed form are delivered by boxcar and stored in the plant. Although improvements in packaging have been made, bags occasionally tear with subsequent dust emission. The bags of asbestos are opened, the block of fiber broken up and, finally, the conveyor is charged with the material. Asbestos fibers are "opened" by means of a blower and cyclone and, in the wet process, fibers are then discharged into a beater and mixed into the cement slurry. Silica enters a dry mix by way of a shaker.... After a series of transfers, a wet sheet is formed. Cutting of the wet sheet to an approximate size is not associated with significant dust production. The roughly sized sheets are then cured for a week and, after the sheet is considerably drier, it enters the punch press for more precise sizing and introduction of nail holes into the shingle.... Cutting of corrugated sheeting also results in the dust production. Final curing is performed in large autoclaves. Important dust exposures occur either early in the process where the fiber is unpacked, the conveyor loaded and fiber discharged into the beater, and later when the dry product is sawed or punched for sizing to commercial specifications.

In 1974, about 30% of the water distribution and sewer pipe sold in the United States contained asbestos (Meylan et al., 1978). In addition, it was used in chemical plants because of the cement pipe's resistance to acid and alkali, and other corrosives; it was also installed extensively as conduits for electrical and telephone wire and cable. Asbestos-cement sheet had a plethora of uses in building construction and manufacturing plants. Exposures to asbestos accrued during manufacturing and in the manipulation and cutting of the end product, particularly with power tools. According to an OSHA submission by the Asbestos Information Service, fiber concentrations assayed by PCM typically ranged from 1 to 2.5 f/mL (Daly et al., 1976) in the work place. Since manufacturing workers in the past were exposed for relatively prolonged periods of time, often in poorly ventilated and enclosed factories, the risk of developing an asbestos-associated disease would have been consequential. In contrast, the end-product users who would cut and drill pipes and sheet for relatively short periods of time during a workday were at a substantially lesser risk. It is difficult to assess the hazard associated with removal, but presumably, workmen carrying out demolition now use adequate respiratory protection equipment.

At times, concern has fomented regarding the possible risk for the development of digestive and urinary tract cancers in consumers of water distributed in municipal asbestos-cement pipe. In studies conducted in Connecticut, in the twin cities of Minnesota and in the Puget Sound region, no evidence of such an association was found (Cook et al., 1976; Mason et al., 1974; Meigs et al., 1980; Levy et al., 1976; Severson, 1979), although evidence suggesting a possible association accumulated in Canada (Cooper, 1979; Wigle, 1977).

Concern has also been voiced regarding the possible contribution of asbestos sheet, such as in roofing, to air pollution. Presumably, weathering of the sheet over an extended

Table 3.13 RR of LC in Cement Mill Workers*

	Chrysotile	Crocidolite	O/S	95% CI
Henderson and	+	?	2.31	1.29–3.81
Enterline (1979)	+	+	5.22	2.70–9.11
Lacquet et al. (1980)	+	+[†]	0.89	0.62–1.42
Clemmeen and	+	+[†]	1.72	1.26–2.29
Hjalgri-Jenson (1981)				
Albin et al. (1990)	+	+[†]	1.8	0.9–3.7
Finkelstein (1986)	+	+	3.87	2.61–5.53
Alies-Patin and	+	+	2.17	1.13–3.81
Valleron (1985)				
Hughes et al (1987)	+	+[†]	1.44	1.18–1.74
Thomas et al. (1982)	+	O	0.91	0.61–1.30
Ohlson and Hogstedt	+	O	1.23	0.61–2.19
(1985)				
Gardner et al. (1986)	+	O	0.92	0.64–1.27
Raffn et al. (1989)	+	+	1.8	1.54–2.1

* References provided in Gardner et al. (1986).
[†] Included amosite.
? Not Known.

period of time might be expected to release asbestos from its matrix into the environment. Helsen et al. (1989) studied chrysotile sheet that had been exposed to the elements for 51 years. They found the magnesium content of the asbestos fibers had been leached and replaced by calcium ions that theoretically were thought to line the surface of the fiber. Although the fibers resembled chrysotile ultrastructurally, they no longer had its elemental make-up.

As noted above, some asbestos-cement products contain chrysotile, and others crocidolite or amosite, whereas others contain more than one type. High concentrations of these fibers have been demonstrated in the lungs of deceased asbestos-cement workers (Albin et al., 1990). Gardner et al. (1986) summarized published data on the occurrence of LC among employees of factories manufacturing asbestos-cement. Updated information is summarized in Table 3.13. As one observes, considerable variability in the RR is found that no doubt can be attributed to the lack of adequate controls for smoking in many studies. Differences in the intensity of exposure, particularly to crocidolite and amosite, are other variables that require evaluation. No comparative information is available on the association of disease with dosage and the prevalence of asbestosis in the various study groups. However, in an autopsy study of cement workers who had been employed by the industry for an average of 15 years, 57 of 89 (64%) had ferruginous bodies, most probably asbestos bodies (AB), in the lung tissue and 16 (18%) had diffuse lung fibrosis histologically (Johansson et al., 1987; Magnani et al., 1998). Dust exposure in the factories studied by Weill et al. (1973) correlated with the presence of small irregular shadows in the lung fields by x-ray and respiratory symptomatology (Abrons et al., 1988; Finkelstein, 1986; Ohlson et al., 1985; Wollmer et al., 1987).

Asbestosis has not been reported among factory workers manufacturing cement containing chrysotile asbestos. In several recent investigations focused on cement mill workers, the occurrence of MM corresponded to the use of the commercial amphiboles alone or mixed with chrysotile (Albin et al., 1990—RR = 22.8; Giaroli et al., 1994—RR = 6.0; Neuberger and Kundi, 1990—RR ~ 5; Raffn et al., 1989—RR = 5.5). Finkelstein (1991) showed that the Doll and Peto formula known as "cubic residence-time" applies to cement factory workers. The formula proposes that "the MM incidence is increased (during) each period of exposure, by an amount proportional to the intensity and duration of that exposure, and to the cube of time (exposure) first occurred."

No increase in the prevalence of MM was noted in mills using chrysotile exclusively, but data allowing one to compare exposure dosages are not available for evaluation (Gardner et al., 1986; Hughes et al., 1987; Ohlson and Hogstedt, 1985).

Installers of asbestos-cement pipe are exposed to variable amounts of asbestos during the brief times they use mechanical saws and drills to custom cut the pipe. An industrial report in 1977 indicated 11–100 f/mL, with a geometric mean of 30 f/mL might be released during these times. Since the exposure durations are customarily short (ie, less than a few minutes) and generally occur out-of-door, the risk of developing disease as a consequence, specifically MM, would appear to be minimal.

Occupants of Public and Commercial Buildings

Concerns regarding asbestos contamination of the ambient air in public buildings, such as schools, municipal structures, and churches, erupted into a flurry of lawsuits in the United States during the 1980s. It is difficult to assess the basis for the tumult at the time, but it seemed to represent the consequence of an erupting nationwide concern regarding environmental pollution in general, but also the realization that spray-on asbestos in building insulation posed an unreasonable hazard (Sawyer and Spooner, 1977). In addition, it was also recognized that asbestos could be released from deteriorating heating systems and the insulation of poorly maintained buildings and ceilings, joint compounds, and asbestos flooring (Sebastien et al., 1982). In his 1977 report, Sawyer documented the presence of seemingly high concentrations of asbestos in sweepings from buildings (1.6 f/mL) and dry dust (4 f/mL) in a University library building.

Since the early 1980s, the assessment of the potential risk for occupants in public buildings has been the subject of considerable research (Burdett and Jaffrey, 1986; Byrom et al., 1969; Corn et al., 1991; Crump and Farrar, 1989; Lee et al., 1992; Price et al., 1992; Wilson et al., 1994). Table 3.14 documents the mineralogical types of asbestos-containing materials in more than 1200 buildings in New York City. While chrysotile was found exclusively in the majority of these structures, commercial amphiboles (amosite and crocidolite) were detected to a variable extent, roughly 10%. In this regard, it should be recalled that crocidolite was the major constituent of the product Limpit that was aggressively promoted and used in spray-on asbestos in building insulation as late as the 1960s.

Ambient air sampling of the public spaces, private homes, and public buildings has provided a sound basis for evaluating potential risks for occupants. These data show that the indoor and outdoor dust concentrations are roughly equivalent, leading to the conclusion that asbestos in buildings does not pose a hazard for occupants (Table 3.15).

Risks for custodial personnel, however, can prove to be consequential when and if asbestos-containing construction material is not encompassed by binders and/or is in a state of ill-repair. However, the risks for exposure are job-specific. Mlynarek et al. (1996) detected a mean 8-hour time-weighted average exposure of 0.03 f/mL > 5 μm during ceiling tile replacement with a maximum air concentration of 0 to 7 f/mL > 5 μm. In six public buildings studied by Wickman et al. (unpublished EPA project no. J1007468–2001), personal air sampling demonstrated an arithmetic mean

Table 3.14 Mineral Composition of Thermal Insulation Products Found in Some New York City-Owned Buildings and Structures*

	Nonasbestos Containing Thermal Products	Asbestos-Containing Thermal Products		
		Chrysotile Only	Mixed Asbestos Types	Amphibole Asbestos
N	466	470	276	52
Percent of all products	37	37	22	4

* Adapted from Table 4–5 from HEI-AR (1991).

Table 3.15 Average Building Airborne Asbestos Concentrations (Fiber > 5 μm/mL in the United States and the United Kingdom) Determined by Transmission Electron Microscopy Analysis*

	Indoor		Outdoor
	Asbestos Fibers >5 μm Long (f/mL)		Mean Concentration
Site	Range	Mean	Fibers >5 μm long (f/mL)
UK nonresidential buildings with ACM	ND to 0.0017	0.00032	0.00007
UK residences with ACM	ND to 0.0007	0.0004	0.0005
UK buildings without ACM	ND to 0.0007	0.00018	ND
US Residences with ACM	ND to 0.002	0.00023	ND
US Public buildings with damaged ACM	ND to 0.00056	0.00005	0.00010
US Public buildings with undamaged ACM	ND to 0.00028	0.00005	
US Schools with ACM	ND to 0.0016	0.0002	—

ACM = Asbestos-containing material; UK = United Kingdom; US = United States.
* Adapted from Table 4–10, from HEI-AR (1991).

concentration of asbestos structures (ie, free fibers, bundles, clusters, or matrices) of all sizes to be 9×10^{-4}/mL, with the highest amounts being 2.55×10^{-2} structures/mL. In an additional study recorded by Corn et al. (1994), personal exposure data during electrical/plumbing work ranged from 0 to 3.5×10^{-2} f/mL > 5 μm in length. Similar data on cable running proved to be 1×10^{-3} to 2.88×10^{-1} f/mL > 5 μm in length and 0.000 to 7.7×10^{-2} f/mL > 5 μm in workers engaged in heating, ventilation, and air-conditioning.

Papers presented at the Third Wave New York Academy of Sciences Conference in 1991 suggested that MM occurring in schoolteachers may have been consequent to classroom exposure (Anderson et al., 1991; Lilienfeld, 1991). The evidence supporting such a contention is weak and circumstantial at best. A case report from the United Kingdom is more compelling (Stein et al., 1989). These authors describe the case of an office worker who lacked a history of occupational or home exposure but died with a MM. Her lungs at autopsy contained amosite; the same mineral was found in the ceiling of the building in which she had worked for a substantial period of her adult life. Rosenman (1994) published the results of a mortality study of more than 800 New Jersey schoolteachers. A deficit for LC among white male teachers was found. None of the diseases customarily attributed to asbestos including MM were detected in this survey. It is noteworthy, however, that the number of participants in the study would have been insufficient to detect a low prevalence of MM in the population.

Workmen Using Gaskets and Packing

Space scientists continue to debate whether the elimination of asbestos from a rubber "O" ring on the Columbia Space Shuttle caused or contributed to its tragic destruction in 1986. We will never know! No asbestos-containing industrial product is more widely used than gaskets. The applications are countless. Although the EPA acted to prohibit the manufacture, importation, processing, and distribution of most asbestos-containing gaskets by 1994, the "phase-out" period for gaskets and packing "in-place" will no doubt extend for many years.

Numerous types and configurations of gaskets are installed in the plumbing of residential and commercial buildings, high-pressure steam lines, sewer systems, oil and chemical processing plants, pumps, automobiles, locomotives and railroad cars, and vessels of every size and configuration.

Although crocidolite was used experimentally to a limited extent in the past, as well as in a few commercial applications, in recent years chrysotile has been employed exclusively over a range of concentrations, but up to 70% in some gaskets. Asbestos provides tensile strength to binders of a great diversity of formulations, but it also adds heat resistance and protects against the corrosive effects of chemicals and solvents. Sheet gasket material is cut and molded for specific applications by workmen in the field. Precut gaskets are fabricated by manufacturers to address specific needs, either as a mixture of asbestos with a binder, or intermixed with spiral stainless steel mesh. Metal-jacketed gaskets consist of a mixture of compressed asbestos and filler covered with a thin, metal coat. Packing material, often in the form of woven rope, is used to fill spaces that do not conform to the laminated configuration of the gasket.

Table 3.16 documents asbestos release during the manipulating of sheet gaskets (Cheng and McDermott, 1991). One presumes that this study was done with dry materials, thus, potentially creating an opportunity for greater aerosolization of dust. Nonetheless, exceedingly low levels were found.

Conceptually, workmen might be expected to experience an exposure to asbestos in gaskets and packing during the cutting and installing of new gaskets and more importantly,

Table 3.16 Personal Air Sampling of Workers Exposed while Manipulating Sheet Gasket*

Procedure	Fibers/mL[†]
Cutting power shears/wheel cutter	0.017
Cutting with knife on lead surface	0.012
Cutting with saber saw	0.39
Cutting with power shears/wheel cutter	0.49

* Adapted from Cheng and McDermott (1991).
† Phase contrast microscopy.

the removal of defective gaskets, as well as during reconditioning and repair of pipes, valves, and equipment. Theoretically, there are countless opportunities for exposure to gasket and packing breakdown in the work place. However, from the perspective of exposures having health consequences, the asbestos is encompassed by the binding materials, and fiber release would be expected to *de minimis*. Moreover, the bulk of the released fibers would be expected to be relatively short (<5 μm) and thus, nonpathogenic.

These hypothetical considerations are borne out by the results of work site evaluations reported in the literature (Boelter, 2002; Cheng and McDermott, 1991; McKinnery and Moore, 1992; Peters and Peters, 1996; Spence and Rocchi, 1996) and numerous additional unpublished simulation studies (Environmental Profiles, 1998, 1999, 2004; Mangold, 1982 [personal communication]; Nolan and Langer, 1993 [privately published]).

In work by Spence and Rocchi (1996), both phase contrast microscopy (PCM) and transmission electron microscopy (TEM) were employed to document fiber release in relation to the difficulties encountered by the workmen in removing gaskets that had, or had not, adhered to the settings. While a range (0.04–0.24 f/mL) was detected by PCM after removal of a nonadherent gasket, in only 4 of 11 samples were asbestos fibers actually detected by TEM, and the highest concentration was 1.4×10^{-3} f/mL. As might be expected, these authors found numerous nonasbestiform dust fibers in the aerosols, raising an important question regarding the value of PCM analyses since this commonly employed monitoring procedure indiscriminately detects both nonasbestos and asbestos fibers (Chapter 12).

The EPA recommends creating "wet" conditions for work with gaskets to reduce aerosolization of fibers. Experiments vividly demonstrate the reduction in air concentrations of dust that results when water is applied to the worksite (Cheng and McDermott, 1991). An additional study compared fiber release during the installation and removal of gaskets and packing at an experimental simulated worksite under "dry" conditions. The results were comparable. A critical analysis of published data brings to light differences in analysis which would tend to inflate the values recorded in Table 3.17. Of greatest importance are the lack of data on fiber dimension and the frequent absence of information on the actual identity of the structures claimed to be asbestos. Until such data is available, the results of environmental sampling will be suspect. A reviewer of published and unpublished industrial hygiene studies should reasonably conclude that many of the fibers claimed to be asbestos in air samples are relatively short (<5 μm) and may, in fact, not be asbestos; thus, their health importance is doubtful.

The exposures documented by environmental sampling at various job sites no doubt do not represent the bulk of a workman's overall time on the job. Accordingly, exposure while manipulating gasket material must be averaged on a time-weighted basis with the time devoted to other activities elsewhere in the work setting. When this is done,

Table 3.17 Personal Air Sampling* of Workers Installing and Removing Gaskets and Packing[†]

	PCM	*TEM*[‡]
Gaskets	0.16–0.2	4.6/3.0
Packing	0.3/0.1	4.4/0.4

* Geometric mean of multiple determinations.
[†] Adapted from McKinnery and Moore (1992).
[‡] Fibers of all lengths.

I conclude that the overall exposures experienced by those who work with gaskets and packing are of no health consequence. However, no critical epidemiological studies have been reported that allow one to assess the health impact associated with the manipulation of gasket and packing materials.

Electricians

Countless different types of electrical wire and cable are supplied by manufacturers and distributors worldwide. Their fundamental structure is similar, there being a core of solid or woven metallic copper or aluminum wire as the electrical conductor insulated by a coat of Teflon, Neoprene, rubber, or plastic of variable thickness. Embedded in this matrix is a network of synthetic or vegetable fibers and variable amounts of chrysotile asbestos. Chrysotile provides tensile strength while allowing flexibility and provides resistance against heat and fire. Amphibole asbestos is not used, largely because the fibers contain iron (Chapter 2). Iron in the enveloping coat of an electrical wire would create magnetic fields, clearly an undesirable feature, resulting in loss of conductivity and the generation of heat.

Numerous experimental simulations of the workplace of an electrician, such as during the stripping, cutting, and abrading of the insulation material, have been carried out in various commercial test laboratories in an effort to document possible fiber release from damaged insulation material. As might be expected, these analyses have failed to demonstrate consequential increases in airborne concentrations of friable asbestos in the breathing zone of the electrician, no doubt in part because the fiber is encapsulated by the amorphous material that covers the conductor. Consistently, the values detected in various laboratories are substantially below the 1994 OSHA permissible exposure level (PEL) of 0.1 f/mL.

Electron microscopic studies of shredded wire insulation have shown chrysotile fibers to be encompassed by a coating of amorphous binder as seen in Figure 3.5 (Craighead, unpublished data). Clearly, the asbestos is not friable and thus, cannot be envisioned to be a hazard for the electrician.

Published health data on wire and cable manufacturing personnel are scant. Ward et al. (1994) conducted a mortality study of more than 9×10^3 men and women working at a World War II cable manufacturing company. This investigation of cancer mortality was compromised inasmuch as toxic concentrations of chlorinated naphthalene were present in the work environment (since the chemicals were used in the manufacturing of the cable insulation). Regardless, save for a modest increase in the standardized mortality rate (SMR) for LC, that is, in males, a SMR = 1.3 [95% CI = 115–147] and females, a SMR = 1.34 [95% CI = 0.93–166], no striking increase in cancer was found. Smoking information was not available for these workers, again negating the value of the study.

Electricians employed in shipbuilding and repair as well as in construction and building maintenance are at risk for asbestos-associated disease because their work often takes them into confined spaces in the bowels of ships and buildings where all too often, poorly maintained asbestos can be found. In addition, electricians work in proximity to insulators and in areas where sheet and spray-on asbestos were applied. In an uncontrolled, unregulated manner, they inadvertently come in contact with these materials behind plenums and enclosed spaces. In the course of their work, electricians pull wire through the infrastructure of a ship or building, a job that has been shown in some simulations to increase the airborne asbestos concentration some 500-fold above ambience. In the study of Keyes et al. (1991), several samples obtained during their investigation yielded 50/mL so-called "asbestos structures" as measured by transmission electron

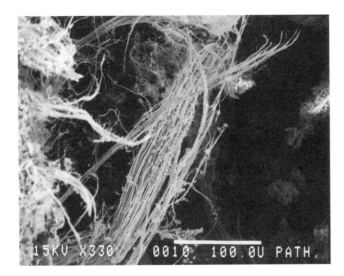

Figure 3.5 Scanning electron microscope illustration of the fibrous composition of the insulation of an electric wire exposed by abrasion, as when an electrician "strips" a wire. The chrysotile is embedded in amorphous polymers and resins of a variety of types and thus is not friable.

microscopy (although many of the "structures" probably were short and thus, particles of doubtful pathogenicity; Corn, 1992).

In the past, substantial exposure no doubt occurred during renovation when environmental controls were inadequate. In the study of Paik et al. (1983), air sampling suggested that roughly 60% of electricians received time-weighted average exposures exceeding 0.1 f/mL.

Selikoff et al. (1979b) claimed that 60% of the shipyard electricians they studied had radiological evidence of asbestosis. It is likely the liberal diagnostic criteria used by these investigators to establish the diagnosis of asbestosis, would not be accepted by all today. In a study by Hodgson et al. (1988), 25% of electricians who had worked as tradesmen for 20 years or longer had asbestosis diagnosed radiologically.

MM is known to occur with an increased frequency in electricians. Nine of some 211 (4%) deaths among a study group of more than 1.6×10^3 electricians who worked in English shipyards between 1940 and 1968, died with MM (Newhouse et al., 1985). In one study, a RR of 18 was found, whereas McDonald and McDonald (1980) calculated a RR of 2.8 for MM among North American shipyard electricians.

Studies of LC among electricians are difficult to evaluate because of the common use of tobacco products by these workers. A survey of more than 1800 electricians in Switzerland (Guberan et al., 1989) found a LC mortality risk of 0.95 for electricians, in comparison to the general Swiss population. In another study from New Zealand, electrical tradesmen were shown to have a RR of 0.88 (Pearce et al., 1989). In the United States, a study conducted by the National Cancer Institute demonstrated a RR of 1.1 for electricians (Zahm et al., 1989). It appears clear from these data that LC is not an asbestos-related problem among electricians. No doubt this reflects the limited and sporadic exposures these workers experience, wherein the amounts of asbestos in the work environment are insufficient to cause asbestosis.

Automotive Mechanics

Wood blocks were the brake shoe of choice on horse- and mule-drawn wagons of the 1800s. Later, leather nailed to wood was used as the abrasive surface. Iron brake shoes were developed for the railroads after Westinghouse air brakes were introduced in the late eighteen sixties. The first patent for the linings of railroad brakes was awarded in 1895—a composite of sawdust, iron, graphite, and linseed oil mixed with asbestos. At the turn of the century, some brakes were comprised of camel hair and cotton impregnated by various binding materials. Asbestos impregnated resins and asphalt brake shoes were perfected about this time, and molded asbestos brake linings were introduced in the 1920s. Crocidolite was evaluated to a limited extent experimentally, and on the brakes of railroad cars, but by 1910 chrysotile became the asbestos of choice for the manufacturing of molded brake linings (Table 3.18).

Now, brakes on automobiles, railroad locomotives, and cars use either shoes or discs, as stators and rotors (or both). They convert the kinetic energy of the moving vehicle to the heat of friction at the interface. The increase in temperature alters the microstructure of the molding as well as the physical and chemical properties of the chrysotile on the abrasive surface. At 250 °C (the approximate temperature reached during sporadic automotive braking), organic material begins to degrade and at 600 °C–780 °C, dramatic chemical and structural changes occur in the friction material. Dehydroxylation of chrysotile with the loss of the fiber's crystalline structure begins to take place at these temperatures.

At about 800° C–850° C, the residue is largely silica and a nonfibrous material known as forsterite ($2Mg^3[Si_2O_5](OH)_4 3Mg^2SiO_4 + SiO_2 + H_2O$) (Chapter 2). These temperatures are attained with heavy, high speed braking. Davis and Coniam (1973) and Weir and Meraz (2001) documented the physical changes in the dust released during braking. The heat-altered material contained fibrous particulates having a low aspect ratio, that is, length to breadth ratio, and the inorganic debris was encompassed, to a variable extent, by it (Jacko et al., 1973).

Tables 3.19 and 3.20 summarize information on chrysotile fiber release by disc and drum brakes at various vehicular velocities and deceleration rates and by the classification of the job in the workshop. While several considerations may dictate the absolute amounts, it is apparent that the concentrations are *de minimis* from the health perspective (Cha et al., 1983; Moore, 1988; Spencer et al., 1999; Williams and Muhlbaier, 1982). As illustrated in Figure 3.6, the fibers are relatively short (Yueng et al., 1999) and the majority of the chrysotile fibers are, in fact, loosely configured bundles of fibrils often encompassed, in part or in whole, by the incinerated binder materials of the brake shoe linings, or the pads of the disc brake (Weir et al., 2001). Table 3.21 shows the results of studies of the asbestos in the work environment of automotive maintenance personnel. Inconsequential amounts of asbestos are detected in the breathing zone of the workmen. Kauppinen and Korhonen (1987) estimated the 8-hour time weighted average (TWA)

Table 3.18 Brake Lining Composition*

Ingredient	Automobile	Truck
Asbestos (chrysotile)	55±	33±
Resins and polymers	28	48
Oxides and pigments	9	16
Metals	3	2
Carbon, graphite, etc.	5	1
Total	100%	100%

* Modified from Lynch (1968).

Table 3.19 Asbestos Emissions from Disc and Drum Brakes Monitored during Field Usage of Vehicle*

Velocity (km/hr)	Deceleration Rate (m/s)	% Asbestos[†] Mean
Disc brakes		
40	1.8	0.004
40	4.9	0.0087
64	1.2	0.016
64	1.8	0.049
64	2.5	0.038
64	4.9	0.027
65	0.3	0.025
88	1.8	0.051
Drum brakes		
40	1.8	0.015
40	2.5	0.0075
40	4.9	0.065
64	1.2	0.0068
64	1.8	0.013
64	2.5	0.0060
64	4.9	0.026
88	1.8	0.051

* Modified from Williams and Muhlbaier (1982).
[†] Presumptive, but unproven short particles of chrysotile.

Table 3.20 Asbestos Fiber Concentrations in the Work Place by Operation during Maintenance of Trucks and Buses*

	Asbestos Fiber Concentration f/mL[†]		
	Range	Median	Mean
Opening and brushing of brakes	<0.1–1.0	0.3	0.3
Cleaning of brakes by brushing	0.1–4.5	0.9	1.3
Cleaning of brakes with compressed air jet, enclosure and exhaust in use	0.2–3.0	0.7	1.2
Loosening rivets from brake linings	<0.1–1.6	0.2	0.3
Punching rivets into brake linings	0.1–3.5	0.4	0.7
Grinding of brake linings with machine, no exhaust	0.3–125	67	56
Grinding of brake linings with machine, exhaust in use	0.1–5.9	0.6	1.5
Bevelling edges of brake linings with file	0.1–0.9	0.3	0.4
Grinding of brake drums	0.1–0.3	0.2	0.2
Background to brake maintenance	<0.1–0.1	0.1	<0.1

* Modified from Kauppinen and Kerhonen (1987).
[†] Presumptive but unproven short particles of chrysotile.

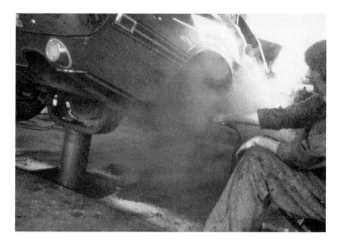

Figure 3.6 Dimensions of fibers of chrysotile in brake shoe dust (Yeung et al., 1999).

Table 3.21 Summary of Asbestos Exposure Monitoring Using Personal Air Samples*

Range for Duration of Sample Period (minutes)	Asbestos Concentration in Fiber/mL[†]		
	Median	Mean	Range
10–60	<0.02	<0.03	<0.01–0.15

* Adapted from Moore (1988).
† Exposure estimates reflect actual time-weighted averages for the sampling period during which brake service work was carried out, not the full 8-hour shift. Identity and length of particle not established.

exposure associated with various jobs. Their data and the findings of others (Cheng and O'Kelly, 1986; Hickish and Knight, 1970) show that the exposures sustained by brake shoe mechanics are inconsequential with regard to the amounts believed to be required to cause disease.

By evaluating the lungs for fibrous material, fiber burden analyses provide a semi-quantitative means for assessing exposures to asbestos. Butnor et al. (2003) examined the lung tissue of ten automotive mechanics with MM. In three cases, elevated concentrations of commercial amphibole asbestos were detected and in two of the three, there were increased numbers of AB. Chrysotile and the noncommercial amphiboles, tremolite, also were present in two of the cases that also exhibited elevated concentrations of commercial amphibole asbestos. It would appear that at least three of the ten cases had no evidence of industrial exposure other than garage work. The lack of chrysotile in the lungs does not exclude the possibility of exposure to elevated air concentrations of asbestos in the past because of the known relatively rapid clearance of chrysotile from the lungs.

In 1976, studies by Lorimer et al. and Rohl et al. indicated a risk to vehicular maintenance workers consequent to exposure to asbestos in brake shoe dust. These investigations provided background information not unlike the data summarized above, although overall the values they reported were somewhat higher than those noted by subsequent workers. The health data recorded suggested that pleural and parenchymal disease was occurring in mechanics, a conclusion not borne out by later observations of others. As an outgrowth of a presentation by Selikoff and his coworkers to federal officials, the then US Department of Health, Education and Welfare issued a widely circulated "Dear Colleague" letter calling to the attention of the medical community a "potential health hazard" along with

Table 3.22 SMR for Friction Product Workers ≥10 years of Employment

	McDonald et al. (1984)	Newhouse and Sullivan (1989)	Finkelstein (1989)
SMR	149*	107[†]	101[‡]
CV	(117–187)	(86–132)	ND[§]

CV = Coefficient of variation.
* Statistically significant increase.
[†] Males only.
[‡] Both sexes.
[§] Data not provided.

recommendations designed to protect workmen. This precipitous action by a governmental agency, in the absence of published, peer-reviewed data, created unrest in the public health community, and among the millions of men and women working in the automotive industry.

Meta-analyses (Goodman et al., 2004; Wong, 2001) have consistently failed to demonstrate a risk for the development of MM among garage mechanics. Cohort studies (Hansen, 1989; Jarvholm and Brisman, 1988; Nicholson et al., 1986; Rushton et al., 1983) and a case-control study of Hessel et al. (2004) have lead to similar conclusions. A report from Sweden (Jarvholm and Brisman, 1988) yielded an SMR of 127 for LC, suggesting a possible increased risk, but no compelling evidence of an increased incidence of MM was found. In a survey from Germany, Rödelsperger et al. (1986) found the RR for MM among mechanics was 0.87 (95% CI = 0.32–2.35). In a death certificate survey of 21 800 mechanics working in Denmark (Hansen, 1989), only one possible MM was found. A similar retrospective mortality study documented the possible occurrence of two MM cases among almost 2.2×10^4 mechanics. Analyses of garage workers by Rushton et al. (1983) failed to yield evidence to indicate an increased incidence of MM in these study populations.

LC in friction product workers has been evaluated in three critically conducted studies (Finkelstein, 1989; McDonald et al., 1984; Newhouse and Sullivan, 1989). Although the value of these studies is compromised by the lack of smoking histories and documentation of exposure, the results summarized in Table 3.22 shows that in only one of the three studies, excess mortality was noted. In a critical review of this report, Berry (1994) considered ancillary information that tends to negate the findings of McDonald et al. (1984). A few cases of MM were noted in these series, but it was concluded that no confirmed MM could be attributed to exposure to chrysotile in brake dust.

In a cohort study reported by Finkelstein (1989), laryngeal carcinoma was diagnosed in three men who had worked for longer than 20 years in the automotive industry. The resulting standardized mortality rate (SMR) was strikingly elevated, but in two other studies, no increase was noted. Again, the confounding effects of smoking may account for the discrepancies. Because of the rarity of this cancer, and the relatively small number of workers evaluated in the Finkelstein study, conclusions must be guarded.

In a recent literature review, it was concluded "the evidence did not support an increased risk of...lung cancer...." The meta-analysis by Goodman et al. (2004) calculated a RR of 1.07 (CI 95% = 0.88–131) for the studies he concluded were of the highest design quality in the meta-analysis and 1.17 (CI 95% = 1.01–1.36) for those considered to be of lesser quality.

Surveys evaluating the occupation of patients with LC have failed to demonstrate an increased risk for the development of LC and MM among automotive mechanics (Benhamou et al., 1988; Lerchen et al., 1987; Milne et al., 1983; Morabia et al., 1992).

Similar assessments have been undertaken to determine if an association was demonstrable between employment in the automotive trades and MM. None was found (Spirtas et al., 1994; Teta et al., 1983). In a study of disease occurring in New Hampshire gas station attendants and mechanics, the PMR for LC was 112 (CL = 82–153; Schwartz, 1987). Apparently no MM occurred in the study populations (Spirtas et al., 1994).

Individual case reports of MM occurring in automotive mechanics provide no compelling evidence of a causative association of exposure to brake shoe and clutch plate dust with disease (Huncharek et al., 1989a,b; Langer and McCaughey, 1982).

The issues considered here have recently been summarized in a comprehensive "state-of-the-art" review (Paustenbach et al., 2004).

A coarse kraft paper containing 10% crocidolite and 25% chrysotile asbestos was manufactured in the United States as an abrasive surface for at least some automobile automatic transmissions. The paper was bonded to the moving surfaces to provide friction. No published documentation is available on this subject. I am aware of a MM developing in a long-term transmission assembly worker whose job entailed the use of abrasives on component parts to remove excess paper residue before assembly of the finished product. No other exposures were known.

Railroad Workers

In the era of the steam locomotives, roughly a quarter of a million workmen were employed by railroads in the United States. Countless others worked on railroads worldwide.

> The railroad industry has long recognized its multitude of problems related to health. It is an integrated industry in the sense that it carries out all phases of the activities which go into transportation, which is its final product. It builds the roads, constructs the cars, paints the stations, even caters food for its passengers. Although engine building and car building of new equipment are (usually) done by independent companies and new road beds are (often) constructed by independent contractors, the maintenance of the railroad and its equipment involve the operating companies in nearly every task known to the basic manufacturer; thus, the railroad employee is exposed to nearly every kind of occupational hazard known to man. (Beard, 1965)

Exposure to asbestos was believed to occur in the manufacturing of locomotives and railcars and in the shops and round houses where repairs and reconditioning were carried out (Figure 3.7). Operating personnel aboard trains were considered by some to be at modest risk, and the track maintenance crews and yardmen were allegedly exposed to brake shoe dust and asbestos in tie shields. With the conversion of railroad locomotion to diesel in the early 1950s much of the concern regarding asbestos-related health risks abated, although litigation continues to focus today on the alleged risks associated with exposure to friction product breakdown in which the amounts of chrysotile are relatively low (<10%) in comparison to automotive brake shoes.

In the past, the boilers and piping of steam locomotives were extensively insulated with mixtures of amphibole and chrysotile, requiring locomotive and railcar manufacturers to apply block asbestos and magnesia "mud" containing either commercial amphiboles or chrysotile, or a mixture of both types, as was usual (ie, 15% asbestos + 85% carbonate of magnesia; Mancuso, 1983).

A few reports of MM occurring in railroad workers found their way into the literature before the 1980s (Cochran and Webster 1981; Greenberg and Davies, 1974; Huncharek, 1987; Lieben and Pistawka, 1967; Maltoni et al., 1991; McDonald and McDonald, 1980; Mostert, 1979; Nurmenen 1975; Ruttner, 1991; Webster et al., 1977). In 1983, Sepulveda and Merchant conducted a systematic radiological survey of a selected group of railroad

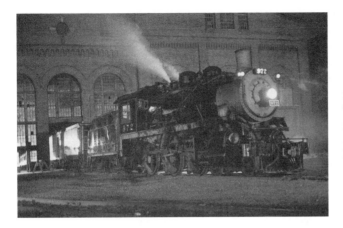

Figure 3.7 Steam locomotive underway. The boilers usually were insulated with mixtures of amosite and chrysotile. Periodic reconditioning of locomotives resulted in the contamination of the workplace with large amounts of friable asbestos.

Table 3.23 Radiological Abnormalities among Railroad Shop Workers by Job Category*

Job Description	Pleural Disease + Small Lung Opacities (%)
Boilermaker	33
Machinist	30
Car men	3
Sheet metal workers	2
Laborers	2
Electrician	13
Others	15

* From Sepulveda and Merchant (1983).

shop workers. Their findings, summarized in Table 3.23, demonstrate the strikingly high prevalence of pleural stigmata of asbestos exposure in railroad boilermakers and machinists. A similar high prevalence of PP associated with pulmonary functional abnormalities was reported by Hjortsberg et al. (1988a,b).

Asbestosis was rarely a clinical consideration in this study (2%) and functional lung changes were probably attributable to smoking. Using pulmonary function evaluations, Oliver et al. (1985) came to this conclusion, although 23% of the workers she studied had PP. Lundorf et al. (1987) found that 57% of maintenance and repair shop workers in Sweden had pleural or lung parenchymal changes attributable to asbestos.

Traditionally controlled epidemiological investigations of railroad workers have been difficult to conduct because of the diversity of their occupational activities and sites of employment, as well as poor documentation of possible exposures to asbestos. In 1983, Mancuso assembled a cohort of 197 machinists who were hired before 1935 and alive in 1956. It was possible to obtain death certificates on 132 of these workers. Of the 29 (22%) who had cancer, 10 were believed to have died of MM of the pleura with latency periods ranging from 33 to 55 years. There were no notations of asbestosis, and benign pleural disease; the high prevalence of LC was not remarkable for a population with a high proportion of smokers.

The following excerpts are from the statement of a machinist who worked in shops where railroad locomotives and cars were repaired (Mancuso, 1983):

First the boiler of the engine was stripped of the old asbestos lagging. In this procedure, the tinners took off the tin or jacket, exposing the boilers, and the tin off the fire boxes, exposing the old asbestos. Then the lagging men would come onto the engine to remove the asbestos. Big wooden wagons would be pulled up on each side of the boiler and the asbestos men would get on top of the boiler and on the running board and throw the asbestos into the wagons from a height of 10 to 25 feet. This created an enormous amount of dust.

Underneath the boiler, the men would just hand pass the asbestos to the wagon. The floor around the engine looked like a snow storm, it was completely white, there weren't any precautions to isolate this, (and) there were no precautions for ventilation.

The lagging men were usually snow white in color because their clothes were covered with asbestos. There were dozens of men of all crafts working under, and around the locomotives, that got asbestos on them.

The laggers would blow off the asbestos from the engine with an air hose to clean the boilers, to prepare for the work of the boilermakers and other crafts. The laggers would put on the new asbestos and the tinners would then climb on the engine and put tin over all the asbestos covering. The painters would come on and take the air hose and blow off all the pieces of asbestos lagging that the tinners had knocked off by applying the tin.

When the engine was moved out, the pit would be full of asbestos. The lagging men would get down in the pit and get out the big chunks of asbestos. Then the laborers would sweep it up and throw the little pieces in the scrap wagon. Every man in the shop, regardless of where he was, was exposed to it (asbestos) by the wind carrying it all over the shop—it settled on the lockers, on the men's tool boxes, it settled on the steel beams, it settled on everything.

The men putting on and taking off the asbestos were working on scaffolds that are placed around the engine. The machinist with the helpers would be working below underneath the scaffolding. They would strip the locomotives of the main rods attached to the wheels, drop the binders, take off the guides, crossheads and crankshaft, cylinder heads and valve heads, brake shoes, spring suspension.... This would happen on both sides of the engine for the same work is done on each side. When the men were working on the scaffold, it looked like after a snowfall. Some of the men would wear bandanas and pull them over their faces (like a bank robber) trying to keep them from inhaling the dust.

A case-controlled analysis using death certificates obtained on 87% of more than 1.5×10^4 railroad workers yielded a strong association of MM (OR 7:2) with the skilled trades and steam locomotive repair work. In contrast, engineers, firemen, and railcar workers who were deemed to have intermittent exposures had an OR for MM that was not significantly elevated (Schenker et al., 1986).

In the studies cited above, LC apparently was not a notable health problem. However, a detailed analysis of Swedish railroad shop workers exposed largely to chrysotile documented a LC SMR of 82 for workers employed for fewer than 30 years, but an SMR of 192 for those with employment records of 30 or more years. The confounding influence of smoking could not be assessed but was no doubt substantial (Ohlson et al., 1984).

Sheet Metal Workers

Sheet metal workers install ductwork for heating and air-conditioning systems in new and existing buildings. Often they work in "dead" spaces and behind plenums in the walls and above ceilings where spray-on asbestos had been applied, or where asbestos sheeting was installed in the past. It was estimated by Selikoff et al. (1965) that 50% of the high-rise buildings constructed before 1970 in the United States were insulated with asbestos. Much of the material would readily be disturbed by those working in closed spaces since the asbestos is not encased in a binder, and thus is friable. Asbestos dust concentrations of as high as 100 f/mL were found in the ambient air of work sites during spray-on installation operations by Drucker et al. (1987).

Table 3.24 Prevalence of Pleural and Lung Parenchymal Changes in New York Union Sheet Metal Workers in Relation to Duration of Employment*

Years of Union Membership	% Parenchymal Opacities[†]	% Pleural Fibrosis[‡]	Any X-Ray Abnormality in Thorax
≤10	2	1	3
11–20	7	4	10
>20	19	17	29

* Adapted from Michaels et al. (1987).
[†] Small irregular/rounded opacities.
[‡] 26% of total had PP.

About 40% of sheet metal workers are installers who risked exposure to asbestos in the various buildings where they work; fabricators, on the other hand, experience little or no exposure in the shops where they assemble ductwork. Although the opportunities for exposure to asbestos in recently constructed buildings now are few, many structures were built and insulated before 1970 and have yet to be renovated satisfactorily.

Michaels et al. (1987) conducted a comprehensive evaluation of sheet metal workers in New York. While less than a third of the eligible union members participated in the studies summarized in Table 3.24, the findings nonetheless provide some insight into the possible prevalence of asbestos disease in this worker population, particularly in relation to the duration of employment. Studies of this type have many intrinsic shortcomings that include (1) the incorporation of data on both fabricators and installers and thus, persons with markedly differing degrees of exposure; (2) the lack of lifetime employment information such as the subjects' prior jobs; (3) the lack of smoking data; (4) the inherent parallels of age and duration of employment; and (5) the uncritical interpretation of chest x-rays, which often lack objective evidence of an asbestos-associated disease such as PP. Regardless, 16% of a study population of more than 7×10^2 sheet metal workers were believed to have radiological changes characteristic of asbestosis.

Baker et al. (1985) carried out a similar study in Boston among union members. They found bilateral pleural disease in 51% of a study group population of almost 1.4×10^3 sheet metal workers. More than 70% had PP. A striking effect of smoking on the prevalence of plaques in the worker population was observed, a finding rarely discussed in the asbestos literature (Weiss et al., 1981; Chapter 6).

Chemical, Petrochemical, and Refinery Workers

Temperature control is the key to the efficient operation of chemical and petrochemical manufacturing plants and refineries. The typical facility has virtually miles of piping, usually insulated in the past with asbestos, often in a 15:85 percent ratio with a magnesia substrate. In addition, cracking coils, key to the function of a refinery, as well as the boilers and vats used in chemical plants, are extensively insulated. Countless valves and pumps with asbestos gaskets and packing are installed in these facilities. While construction of refineries and chemical plants requires teams of pipe fitters and plumbers (usually outside contractors) and dismantling is done by demolition specialists, the day-to-day maintenance of refineries and chemical plants is the responsibility of the factory's full-time staff.

In 1960, Eisenstadt and Wilson reported MM in two refinery foremen (57 and 58 years of age). The findings of AB in the lungs and PP in one of these workers at autopsy raised the concern of an asbestos etiology based on several sporadic case reports in the foreign literature at the time. This report predated the pathfinding publication of Wagner et al. (1960; Chapter 1).

Some 20 years later, a report by Lilis et al. (1980) suggested that workers in the oil refineries were developing an inordinate number of MM and LC. In conflict with this claim was the result of a meta-analysis of Wong (1986, 1989, 1995) that demonstrated an SMR of 77 (95% CI = 74–81) for LC in the operational and maintenance personnel of oil refineries. And, a retrospective cohort study of more than 2.1×10^4 refinery and chemical workers yielded an SMR of 91, although in this study, the potential latency period required for the development of disease was not carefully controlled and the population of workers was said to be "dynamic," that is, high turnover (Hanis et al., 1985). Thus, it is unlikely these latter data are reliable.

Gennaro et al. (1994) reported a MM SMR of 320 for workers with a median employment duration of 27.5 years at two Italian refineries. Their conclusions were challenged by Wong (1995) but supported by the work of Finkelstein (1996) who reported an OR of 24.5 (95% CI = 3.1–102) for MM, but an OR of only 0.88 for LC. Furthermore, they found an OR of 1.73 (95% CI = 0.83–3.6) for refinery workers, in comparison to other "blue collar" workers at the plant. These data suggested that the refinery workers, as a group, were at an increased risk for developing LC. An additional 5 year mortality study at a Texas refinery (Tsai et al., 1996) yielded a MM SMR of 469 (95% CI = 152–1093) and an SMR for LC of 178 (95% CI = 139–996). Statistically significant increases in the number of cases of MM were found in mortality studies of more than 1.9×10^4 refinery workers in several Gulf states (Lewis et al., 2000) and in a second study of more than 6×10^3 deceased long-term employees of refineries elsewhere in the United States (Gamble et al., 2000). This has not been a consistent finding in comprehensive investigations of refinery worker populations. No published information documenting benign pleural disease in these population groups exists.

Because workers in refineries and chemical plants are potentially exposed to a diversity of chemicals, possible unrecognized influences on the development of disease must be a consideration. For example, increases in the incidence of leukemia have found in some but not all studies of refinery workers (Dagg et al., 1992; Dement et al., 1998; Lewis et al., 2000; Marsh et al., 1991; Tsai et al., 1992). Nonetheless, the findings indicate that some workers experience sufficient exposure to amphibole asbestos to develop MM, but not necessarily LC.

Thermoelectric Power and Chemical Plant Workers

Studies focused on workers employed at thermoelectric power plants have, to a variable extent, consistently demonstrated increases in the incidence of MM (Boffetta et al., 1991; Bonnell et al., 1975; Crosignani et al., 1995; Forastiere et al., 1989; Hirsch et al., 1979; Imbernon et al., 1995; Lerman et al., 1990). The occurrence of LC is also reported to be increased but the smoking histories of the workmen were often not known. Thus, data on the incidence of LC possibly attributable to asbestos are open to skeptical interpretation. Useful quantitative information on the prevalence of pleural and parenchymal lung disease and malignancies attributable to power plant asbestos exposure are not reported.

A particularly illuminating 35-year experience at a Norwegian electrochemical plant that produced nitric acid was reported by Hilt and his colleagues (Hilt et al., 1985, 1987). These studies are particularly meaningful because exposure to crocidolite asbestos could be semiquantitated on the basis of the work assignments of the employees in a relatively

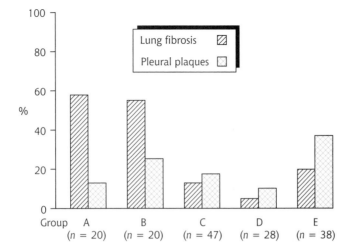

Figure 3.8 Thermoelectric power and chemical plant workers. (A) Twenty men who had mainly been employed in the fiber hut and who had experienced very heavy asbestos exposure; (B) Twenty men who had been heavily exposed when working regularly plugging the joints in the nitric acid towers, and who had also partly been in the fiber hut; (C) Forty-seven process operators from the nitric acid towers with mostly indirect exposure; (D) Twenty-eight process operators from the incinerator hall with mostly indirect exposure; and (E) Thirty-eight other maintenance workers from both the nitric acid towers and the incinerator hall with both moderate and indirect asbestos exposure.

stable work force. The details of the job assignments of the study group are worthy of careful consideration:

> Different types of asbestos were used for various purposes in the production of nitric acid. Large asbestos packings, mainly crocidolite, were used to pack the joints in the incinerators which combusted ammonia and nitrogen oxides. Maintenance work on the 79 incinerators was continuous. Considerable amounts of asbestos dust were generated in the warm dry atmosphere of the incinerator hall when old, dry packing material was renewed. Nitric acid was synthesized at the plant in…high outdoor granite towers which were plugged from top to bottom with a mixture of asbestos and waterglass.
>
> The workers who packed the joints and in particular, those who prepared the packing material in the so called 'fibre hut' were exposed to high concentrations of asbestos dust. Both serpentine and amphibole asbestos was used for this purpose. All other production and maintenance workers at the plant were indirectly exposed to asbestos. Reliable dust measurements at the plant were first carried out after 1970. According to the employees, working conditions had improved a great deal by that time. Consequently, these measurements cannot be considered representative of the working conditions in previous years.
>
> In addition to the exposure to asbestos dust the workers at the plant were also exposed to chemical agents such as nitrous gases, nitric acid vapours, and ammonia. (Hilt, 1987)

Nonmalignant chest disease among survivors after an approximate 56-year period of follow-up is summarized in relation to exposure history (Figure 3.8). Hilt (1987) compared his experience to the observations of Lilis et al., 1984 who documented clinical evidence of pulmonary fibrosis in 24% of the chemical workers they studied and PP in 14%. The type of asbestos evaluated in these studies is not known.

Table 3.25 shows the prevalence of selected cancers including MM in the Norwegian electrochemical plant workmen. The number of workers whose health experience could

Table 3.25 Standardized Incidence Ratio for Selected Cancer Forms during the Observation Period 1953–1988*†

Types of cancer	Lightly Exposed Group		Heavily Exposed Group	
	SIR	95% CI	SIR	95% CI
All cancers	91	60–131	186	121–272
Lung cancer‡	175	70–360	647	324–1.159
Pleural MM	4.065		8.621	
Stomach cancer	59	6–212	166	33–486
Colon cancer	85	8–305	285	57–836
Cancer of unknown origin	368	118–861	312	31–1.124
All other cancers	38	15–86	33	6–95

SIR = Standardized incidence rate.
* Comparative calculation, based on Norwegian national data.
† Adapted from Hilt et al. (1985).
‡ Smoking histories not known.

be incorporated into these calculations was rather small, thus, precluding an accurate assessment of risk. The "control" population was believed to be representative of the country as a whole, not a select subgroup comparable to the study group of workers.

Paper and Pulp Mill Workers

More than 1.3×10^7 tons of pulp paper, paper board and kraft paper are produced in the United States annually. Even greater amounts are manufactured in the northern tier, heavily forested regions of North America and Eurasia, as well as in selected sites in the southern hemisphere. In the United States, several hundred thousand workers are employed directly in paper manufacturing and countless others are involved in forestry and wood cutting.

Wood is converted to pulp after debarking and shipping by using either mechanical or chemical processes (or both), the latter being the most common. During processing, dioxins are released (recognized carcinogens in rodents). After removal of the lignin, the remaining cellulose pulp is bleached and a wide variety of additives (such as dyes, resins, starch, clays, talc, waxes, defoamers, bacteriostats, anticorrosives, and asbestos) are introduced according to specifications of the custom-made product. The concentration of the slurry is adjusted using steam-heated water and the residue extruded onto continuously moving, 10–20 foot wide, belts of felt. The process encourages rapid evaporation and drying resulting in the finished product. Papers are coated or further processed and then packaged on reels or spools for delivery to the customer.

Until the late 1970s, the paper industry was a major user of asbestos-containing felts employed in the rolling of paper pulp into the final product, that is, kraft cardboard, newsprint, or sheet paper. The felts were comprised of chrysotile asbestos woven into cotton belts more than 200 feet long and several feet wide. During the process, wet pulp is extruded onto the moving felt belts that were flushed with warm water. Concern has been voiced that workmen are exposed to friable asbestos when the belts break or tear during operation or when they are changed during routine maintenance. Presumably, chrysotile emanating from these felts might account for the MMs that have occasionally been observed in paper mill workers, but there is no epidemiological evidence to support such a thesis. An increase in the prevalence of PP or bilaterally symmetrical pleural thickening and/or asbestosis has not been demonstrated in paper mill workers.

Studies by Millette (1999) documented a substantial release of chrysotile fibers from swatches of asbestos-containing dryer felt that were handled or blown on by compressed air (60 psi) for 4–5 minutes. However, the manufacturing procedures do not require the blowing of compressed air on dryer felts. Thus, the study did not simulate work conditions in the mill. Subsequent testing of a number of samples of dryer felt from two different manufacturers by Lee (ca. 2000, personal communication) indicated that little or no asbestos was released during simulations carried out in a research paper mill facility at the Western Michigan University. Dryer felts in these studies contained 20%–50% water by weight. In these studies, the functional equivalent of background levels of asbestos was found in the ambient air surrounding paper mills. For example, the average yield of personal samplers indicated an exposure during the test of 3.2×10^{-3} f/mL, an inconsequential exposure.

Depending on their job, pulp and paper mill workers might come into contact with commercial amphibole asbestos in the insulation installed throughout paper mills. For example, some mill workers might experience an exposure equivalent to a plumber or pipe fitter. In some mills, Transite board panels were used on the walls of work areas. Preliminary epidemiologic investigations have associated several different malignancies with employment in pulp and paper mills, but a consistent pattern of disease has not become apparent. In an analysis of more than 1×10^3 paper mill employees in the state of New Hampshire, the number of cancers of the digestive tract and lymphopoietic system was increased in comparison to the overall incidence in the adult male population of the State (Schwartz, 1988). A similar increase was not found in woodcutters and loggers. An increase in the prevalence of a variety of common cancers among pulp and paper workers was found by Milham (1983) but the results lacked statistical significance. A study of 20 deceased pulp and paper workers showed a significant increase in the incidence of LC among long-term employees (Solet et al., 1989), but information on smoking was not always available. A more comprehensive investigation was reported by Jappinen et al. (1987) and Jappinen (1987) from Finland with similar findings. Mortality studies by Robinson et al. (1986) and Matanoski et al. (1998) show nonsignificant increases in the incidences of various cancers. No pattern or trend in the occurrence of any specific neoplasm was found.

Three studies have demonstrated an increased incidence of MM among pulp and paper workers, suggesting exposure to amphibole asbestos in the workplace (Band et al., 1997; Jarvholm et al., 1988a; Toren et al., 1996). The occupational histories and job descriptions of the affected workers were not published and the accuracy of the diagnosis was not established in most cases. As noted above, pulp and paper mill workers might be expected to experience exposure to commercial amphibole asbestos in the insulation installed throughout paper mills.

Several authors have noted the absence of any excess mortality from nonmalignant respiratory disease in paper mill workers (Coggon et al., 1997; Chan-Yeung et al., 1980; Ericsson et al., 1988; Ferris et al., 1967; Henneberger 1989; Jappinen, 1987; Jarvholm et al., 1988b; Matanoski et al., 1998; Thoren et al., 1989; Wong et al., 1996). In these studies, no evidence of asbestosis was noted.

Papers and cloth filters containing asbestos have been used in the beverage industry presumably to provide tensile strength to the filters. Attempts to associate the use of these products with disease have failed.

A unique paper product was manufactured in a factory in northeast United States during the 1950s for use in the preparation of the filters for cigarettes. In 1952, environmental monitoring in the factory documented air concentrations of 80 f/mL of crocidolite in the workplace air, a concentration substantially exceeding the permissible amounts at the time. Talcott et al. (1989) monitored the health outcomes of some 33 workers from 1953 until 1988. At that time, 28 (85%) of the men had died, a mortality rate exceeding the expected by 3- to 4-fold. Nineteen of the men died with cancer; 11 being LC and five MM. Five of these workers clinically were believed to have asbestosis but documentation was incomplete.

Cigarettes utilizing the asbestos-containing Micronite filters were widely advertised and distributed. In the early 1950s, it was estimated on the basis of sales figures that almost 1.2×10^9 cigarettes with filters were sold in the United States (Maxwell, 1989). No information exists on the health effects consequent to the presumptive inhalation of crocidolite asbestos by this means, although a few juries in the United States have seen fit to award damages to the smokers with MM. Alas, the scientific question remains unresolved.

In 1995, Longo et al. evaluated crocidolite fiber release by smoking machines from filtered cigarettes that had been stored for some 40 years. Analysis of the filters documented the presence of 10 mg of crocidolite per cigarette. On the basis of their experimental observations, the investigators calculate that a person smoking a pack a day would take into the respiratory tract more than 1.3×10^6 crocidolite fibers >5 μm during a single year. Analysis of lung tissue from several MM cases who alleged smoking cigarettes with Micronite filters failed to demonstrate increased lung burdens of crocidolite (Pooley F, ca. 1995, personal communication).

Iron, Steel, and Foundry Workers

Beginning in the second half of the 19th century, steel mills and foundries in industrialized countries employed hundreds of thousands of workers in a great diversity of occupations, often for relatively short periods of time.

Steel and iron manufacturing is a highly integrated industry. The process begins with the mining of coal and iron ore and ends with the fabrication of molded and rolled or cast products. Metallurgical coal is made by heating bituminous coal in ovens at temperatures exceeding 2000 °F, a process that drives off toxic gases (including carcinogenic polycyclic aromatic hydrocarbons and nitrosamines) yielding coke, a relatively pure form of carbon. The coke is then amalgamated at high temperatures with limestone and iron ore in a blast furnace where "pig" iron is made and formed into ingots (Figure 3.9). The waste by-product is slag that is dumped on "sterile" mountains near the mills. Ingots of "pig" iron are then transported to rolling and finishing mills where specialized products are formulated, often incorporating various metals and chemicals such as the addition of tin and zinc. From beginning to end, the mills operate at high temperatures and require the use of insulation for personnel protection and heat efficiency.

A comprehensive investigation of the mortality experienced of almost 6×10^4 mill workers in the greater Pittsburgh, Pennsylvania area was carried out for the period 1953 through 1963 by Redman et al. (1969), Mazumdar et al. (1975), and Rockette and Redmond (1976). Complex confounding influences affected the outcome of their analyses. These included (1) "the healthy worker effect" (that selects workers whose overall health status is sound and superior to members of the general population), (2) the influence of poorly characterized chemical exposures in the workplace environment, (3) the lack of information on the smoking habits of members of the study populations, and (4) the lack of documentation of asbestos exposure. Interestingly enough, no striking

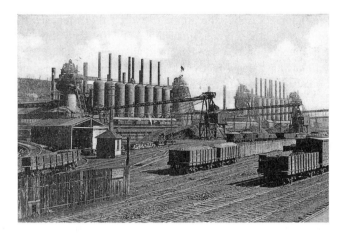

Figure 3.9 Bessemer converters extensively used in the steel manufacturing industry before and during World War II.

increase in disease attributable to asbestos was documented in these studies. Regardless, exposure to asbestos no doubt occurred among workers in some job categories in the steel mills. For example, the studies of Blot et al. (1983) revealed cases of asbestosis among pipe coverers working in steel mills. A significant increase in the incidence of lung and genitourinary cancer among coke oven workers was found. This association is well-documented and generally attributed to exposures to coal gases and tobacco smoke. In an overlapping study of steel workers in the Pittsburgh area, Radford (1976) noted an increased incidence of LC surprisingly in white, but not black workmen. He also documented increases in urinary bladder and renal cancer in the white workers. These effects can best be attributed to smoking possibly compounded by industrial exposures to polycyclic aromatic hydrocarbons and chromates. Among long-term steel workers, Blot et al. (1983) discovered an OR of 1.8 (95% CI = 1.2–2.8) for LC adjusting for smoking. These data support the conclusion that carcinogenic inhalants in the mill environment contributed to the development of LC.

In a survey of steel plant workers, Kronenberg et al. (1991) found evidence of pleural disease that they chose to attribute to asbestos exposure in 22% of a study group of almost 9×10^2 workers. A single MM was believed to have occurred in this population. Rocskay et al. (1996) noted pleural thickening by chest x-ray in 21% of ironworkers, and PP in 19% of steel mill workers. These reports provide only limited, sketchy information on the conduct of the investigations, including the results of critical analysis. The above data, although limited, suggest that asbestos exposure occurs among steel and ironworkers, but the findings do not attest to a high risk of either incapacitating or life-threatening disease.

Metal founding is an ancient craft in which ferrous and nonferrous metals are melted and molded. In the past, environmental controls in foundries were often limited to the tolerance of the worker and little dust control eventuated. According to Koskela et al. (1976), worker populations in the industry manifest high turnover rates (under the circumstances, not surprising). Dust in the foundries includes crude carbon particulates derived from coal, iron particulates, and to a variable extent, silica (used in the structuring of sand molds) and asbestos (used in the insulation of pipes and the lining of furnaces). Apparently talc is sometimes used in the molds as a "parting" agent, thus introducing the possibility of contamination with asbestiform minerals. Other silicates, alumina, mullite, sillimanite, magnesia, and spinel, on occasion, make up the particulate mix (Mattioli et al., 2002).

In foundries, airborne concentrations of polycyclic aromatic hydrocarbons repeatedly have been shown to be elevated (Gibson et al., 1983). Tossavainen (1990) lists additional constituents of the foundry environment considered to be carcinogenic.

Numerous epidemiological studies have consistently documented a high incidence of LC among foundry workers (Finkelstein and Wilk, 1990; Gibson et al., 1977; Tola et al., 1979; Palmer and Scott, 1981). Unfortunately, these retrospective surveys provide little or no information on the use of tobacco by the workers included in the study. In an investigation documenting the mortality experience of more than 8×10^3 foundry workers in the United States, Andjelkovich et al. (1992) found "no evidence…of a relationship between LC and foundry exposure." They attributed the LC in these workers to smoking. Decoufle and Wood (1979) failed to observe deaths due to pneumoconiosis in a mortality study of almost 3×10^3 foundry workers. One can conclude from these and numerous other epidemiological studies on steel and foundry workers that the high incidence of LC was caused by smoking, possibly confounded by exposure to polycyclic aromatic hydrocarbons of industrial origin. There is no concrete evidence to suggest that exposure to silica and asbestos lead to the development of LC in these settings. However, in the experience of the writer, MM certainly occurs among workers in some foundries. Although the incidence appears to be low, no systematic, epidemiological studies of this question have been reported.

Ferruginous bodies were demonstrated in the lungs of steel and foundry workers in pathological studies conducted by Churg and Warnock (1981) and Dodson et al. (1993). Earlier work has demonstrated a "benign" pneumoconiosis in foundry workers presumably consequent to exposure to iron oxides in the work environment (Hamlin and Weber, 1950). The writer has associated accumulations of iron particulates in the lungs of foundry workers with the formation of relatively spherical ferruginous bodies, crusted by spiculated surface deposit of biological iron. These structures are often termed siderotic bodies. A unique "mixed dust" pneumoconiosis was described by McLaughlin and Harding (1956) due to exposure in foundries to silica and mixtures of nonasbestos dusts, particularly hematite. Asbestos is not a component of the lesion.

In the analytical studies of Dodson et al. (1993), and Churg and Warnock (1981), ferruginous bodies having asbestos cores were found in the bronchoalveolar lavage and lung specimens of foundry workers, but a variety of additional nonasbestiform fibers and granules were discovered that formed the cores of ferruginous bodies. The composition of this core material is not clear. Fibers and shards of carbon, such as graphite, are often constituent. The diagnostic importance of differentiating these latter structures from AB is apparent, but as shown by these investigators, analytical TEM and x-ray spectrometry is required in order to obtain definitive evidence (Chapter 6).

Jewelry and Dental Laboratory Technicians

Anecdotal reports and a few incompletely documented cases in the literature identify jewelry manufacturers and dental laboratory technologists as candidates for asbestos-associated disease. Kern and Frumkin (1988) found PP in two long-term workers in a Rhode Island jewelry factory. The writer recently diagnosed a MM in a life-long Rhode Island jewelry technician whose husband, a coworker, had PP. No other source of exposure was identified. Asbestos-containing molds for molten metal were believed to be the source of exposure in all four cases. During a 15-year period, MM was documented in five New Mexico Native American silversmiths from an isolated pueblo of roughly 2×10^3 residents (Driscoll et al., 1988). Although amphibole asbestos insulated work tables were the presumptive source of exposure, the patients also participated in ceremonial dancing and allegedly whitened their leggings and moccasins with raw asbestos block. A calculated total of approximately 0.045 cases would have been expected in the tribal population during the elapsed 15-year period during which these cases occurred (Driscoll et al., 1988).

The writer has consulted on the two cases of dental laboratory technicians with MM, whose only presumed source of exposure was the molds used to prepare dental prostheses. A report documents two additional cases of MM—one in a dentist and the second in a technician (Reid et al., 1991). Apparently, chrysotile and crocidolite were used in periodontal dressings as well as in liners for casting rings and crucibles (Burnett, 1976; Brune and Beltesbrekke, 1980; Hazards of Asbestos in Dentistry, report by Council on Dental Therapeutics, 1996). Environmental studies are limited in detail and scope; they have failed to demonstrate increases in airborne friable asbestos in the laboratory during and after manipulation of asbestos linings for dental molds (Davis, 1995).

Abrasive Grinding Wheel Workers

Comprehensive and quantitative information is not available on the diverse uses of grinding wheels in industry and the number of manufacturers of abrasives worldwide. The wheels that contain asbestos customarily are comprised of two components: (1) an inner, nonabrasive support core usually containing chrysotile asbestos embedded in a resin binder; (2) the surface (annealed onto the support core) made up of a resin that is embedded with abrasives such as chipped industrial diamonds, carborundum, or cubic boron nitride. The selection of abrasive is based on the intended use of the wheel. During customary usage, the asbestos-containing support core is not abraded or damaged, and the operator sustains no exposure. Valid experimental information on asbestos fiber release by grinding wheels has not been published and epidemiological observations are not found in the literature.

Asbestos Exposures of Household and Community Residents

In a pathfinding study, Newhouse and Thompson (1965) claimed presumptive household exposure in 36 of 76 patients (47%) with MM in London, England. Their observation has been confirmed in numerous case series reported from North America and Europe (Anderson et al., 1976; Epler et al., 1980; Huncharek et al., 1989a; Li et al., 1978; Lilis et al., 1979; Joubert et al., 1991; Kilburn et al., 1985; Knishkowy and Baker, 1986; Schneider et al., 1996; Vianna and Polan, 1978). In a cohort study evaluating some 2×10^2 deaths among spouses of cement factory workers in Italy, Magnani et al. (1993) documented a SMR of 200 (95% CI = 96–369) for LC, and a SMR of 792 for pleural tumors, presumably MM. Detailed information on exposure and questions of diagnosis prevail. Accordingly, these cases invariably are subject to error, but there can be no doubt, domestic exposure occasionally results in MM among family members! The author had personal opportunities to consult on a number of such cases.

The typical story centers on either a husband or father who wore work clothes home on a regular basis, potentially contaminating his automobile and home environment. The patient was either a child who played with the father while he was still in his work clothes, or a spouse who shook out and laundered the work clothes, possibly assisted by a family member. In the cases reported by Newhouse and Thompson (1965), the mean age of first exposures was 18 years and on the average, the disease became symptomatic 38 years later. On occasion, two or rarely three members of the family of a shipyard worker, a pipe fitter or an insulator, or an asbestos factory worker developed MM. Lung fiber burden analyses have been reported in only a few cases. Although information on the duration and intensity of spousal exposures are lacking, it is clear they can accumulate substantial amounts of asbestos in their lungs (Table 3.26; Dodson et al., 2003). Household cases have not been reported to originate from workmen subject to modest occupational exposures, and to chrysotile asbestos.

Attempts to document disease among community members presumptively exposed to either asbestos in the environment or effluents from asbestos factories are fraught with methodological difficulties. The classical studies of Wagner and his associates in the Blue Hills region of South Africa (1991) document nonoccupational environmental exposure to crocidolite in 29 of 67 cases of MM known to have occurred from approximately 1956 to 1959. Residents of Wittenoom, Western Australia, a community where crocidolite was mined and milled for an approximate 23-year period, developed MM as a consequence of nonoccupational and nonspousal environment exposure (Hansen et al., 1998). A recent report (Luo et al., 2003) described the occurrence of PP in 20% of a population of rural residents residing in a remote region of the Province of Yunnan, China. MM occurred at the presumptive rate of 22 cases per year in a population estimated to be 6.8×10^4. Crocidolite asbestos was found in scattered patches of blue clay surface soil. Apparently, some of the residents of the region used the blue clay as building stucco. In addition, a "cottage" industry had developed in which crocidolite stoves were manufactured.

Figure 3.10 documents geographically the home residences of MM cases in New Orleans where for a period in the distant past, crocidolite tailings from a Johns-Manville Cement plant were used to surface driveways. The widespread occurrence of PP in Finland and regions of Eastern Europe are referred to in Chapter 6. While some of the Finnish cases resided in relative geographic proximity to an anthophyllite mine in central Finland, PP were also found among residents elsewhere in the country. MM has not been documented to develop in these nonoccupational residents of the country, a likely reflection of the limited capacity of anthophyllite to cause MM. Environmental tremolite exposures in Greece, New Caledonia, and Turkey have also been shown to result in MM (Goldberg et al., 1991; Langer et al., 1987).

Newhouse and Thompson (1965) found a striking cluster of cases of MM among those who resided within 0.5 miles of the London asbestos factory referred to above. These patients had not been exposed occupationally or in the home. The residents of communities surrounding Italy's largest cement factory have also experienced a significant

Table 3.26 Results of Fiber Burden Analysis ($\times 10^4$ Fibers) of Lung Tissue from Deceased Spouses with Mesothelioma and Presumptively Resulting from Household Exposure

	Amosite	Crocidolite	Chrysotile	Tremolite
Dodson et al. (2003)				
Patient a	2.6	—*	—	—
Patient b	—	52.2	—	—
Patient c	1.3	—	—	3.8
Huncharek et al. (1989b)	5.9		17.2	22
Craighead (unpublished)	0.1	—	—	—

* Less than detection level.

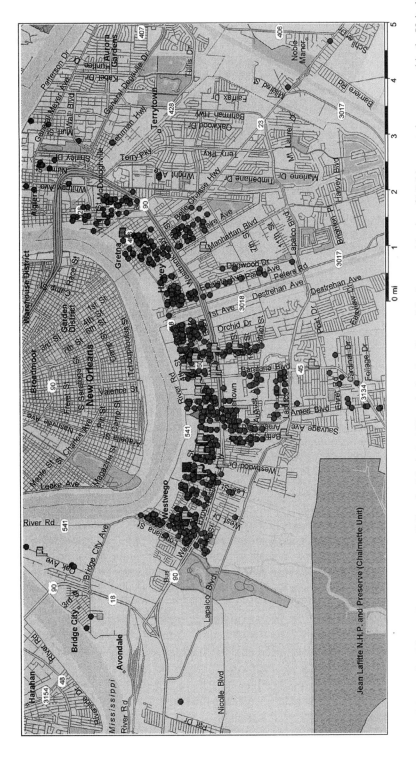

Figure 3.10 Marrero, Louisiana, a factory town paralleling the Mississippi River, is the site of one of the largest epidemics of MM known to have occurred in the United States as a result of environmental pollution, New Orleans is nestled in the river's loop. Marrero was the site of a long defunct Johns-Manville cement pipe factory that used crocidolite (triangle). Waste from the plant was distributed widely in the community to construct residential driveways, the location of which were plotted in a EPA survey (dots). During the 1990s MM developed in at least 19 community residents, and were brought to litigation. The patients had grown up in the neighborhood during the 1950s and 1960s and had no known occupational or domestic exposure to asbestos (flags). A Celotex factory using an unknown type of asbestos was located at the square. Its waste apparently was not used as fill in the community (illustration and background information graciously provided by Andre' Brossard, Jr Esq).

increase in the prevalence of MM (Magnani et al., 1991). A similar claim was made by Berry (1997) who studied communities surrounding the Johns-Manville factory in New Jersey that was said to have primarily used chrysotile for over 70 years of operation. However, it was not possible to exclude household exposure among family members with MM. Assuming the correctness of the author's observations, it is unlikely that chrysotile was the cause of the disease in these subjects.

References

Abrons HL, Petersen MR, Sanderson WT, Engelberg AL, Harber P. Symptoms, ventilatory function, and environmental exposures in Portland cement workers. *Br J Ind Med.* 1988;45:368–375.

Albin M, Jakobsson K, Attewell R, Johansson L, Welinder H. Mortality and cancer morbidity in cohorts of asbestos cement workers and referents. *Br J Ind Med.* 1990;47:602–610.

Alies-Patin AM, Valleron AJ. Mortality of workers in a French asbestos cement factory 1940–82. *Br J Ind Med.* 1985;42:219–225.

Anderson HA, Hanrahan LP, Schirmer J, Higgins D, Sarow P. Mesothelioma among employees with likely contact with in-place asbestos-containing building materials. *Ann NY Acad Sci.* 1991;643:550–572.

Anderson PH. GCA, Analysis of fiber release from certain asbestos products, Dec, 1982;132:75–80.

Anderson HA, Lilis R, Daum SM, Fischbein AS, Selikoff IJ. Household-contact asbestos neoplastic risk. *Ann NY Acad Sci.* 1976;271:311–323.

Andjelkovich DA, Mathew RM, Yu RC, Richardson RB, Levine RJ. Mortality of iron foundry workers. II. Analysis by work area. *J Occup Med.* 1992;34:391–401.

Baker EL, Dagg T, Greene RE. Respiratory illness in the construction trades. I. The significance of asbestos-associated pleural disease among sheet metal workers. *J Occup Med.* 1985;27:483–489.

Balzer JL, Cooper WC. The work environment of insulating workers. *Am Ind Hyg Assoc J.* 1968;29:222–227.

Band PR, Le ND, Fang R, et al. Cohort mortality study of pulp and paper mill workers in British Columbia, Canada. *Am J Epidemiol.* 1997;146:186–194.

Beard R. American Railroads Medical and Surgical Section Minutes (1965).

Benhamou S, Benhamou E, Flamant R. Occupational risk factors of lung cancer in a French case-control study. *Br J Ind Med.* 1988;45:231–233.

Berry G. Mortality and cancer incidence of workers exposed to chrysotile asbestos in the friction-products industry. *Ann Occup Hyg.* 1994;18:539–546.

Berry M. Mesothelioma incidence and community asbestos exposure. *Environ Res.* 1997;76:34–40.

Blot WJ, Morris LE, Stroube R, Tagnon I, Fraumeni JF Jr. Lung and laryngeal cancers in relation to shipyard employment in coastal Virginia. *J Natl Cancer Inst.* 1980;65:571.

Blot WJ, Harrington JM, Toledo A, Hoover R, Heath CW, Fraumeni JF Jr. Lung cancer after employment in shipyards during World War II. *N Engl J Med.* 1978;299:620–624.

Blot WJ, Brown LM, Pottern LM, Stone BJ, Fraumeni JF Jr. Lung cancer among long-term steel workers. *Am J Epidemiol.* 1983;117:706–716.

Blot WJ, Davies JE, Brown LM, et al. Occupation and the high risk of lung cancer in northeast Florida. *Cancer.* 1981;50:364–371.

Boelter FW. Airborne fiber assessment of dry asbestos-containing gaskets and packing found in intact industrial and maritime fittings. *AIHAJ.* 2002;63:732–740.

Boffetta P, Cardis E, Vainio H, et al. Cancer risks related to electricity production. *Eur J Cancer.* 1991;27:1504–1519.

Bonnell JA, Browker JR, Browne RC, Erskine JF, Fernandez RHP, Massey MO. A review of the control of asbestos processes in the Central Electricity Generating Board. Paper presented at: XVIII International Congress on Occupational Health; 1975; Brighton, England.

Brune D, Beltesbrekke H. Dust in dental laboratories. *J Prosth Dent.* 1980;44:211–215.

Burdett GJ, Jaffrey SA. Airborne asbestos concentrations in buildings. *Ann Occup Hyg.* 1986;30:185–199.

Burnett G. Substitute for asbestos in casting rings. *Brit Dent J.* 1976;141:171.

Butnor KJ, Sporn TA, Roggli VL. Exposure to brake dust and malignant mesothelioma: a study of 10 cases with mineral fiber analyses. *Ann Occup Hyg.* 2003;47:325–330.

Byrom JC, Hodgson AA, Holmes S. A dust survey carried out in buildings incorporating asbestos-based materials in their construction. *Ann Occup Hyg.* 1969;12:141–145.

Cantor KP, Sontag JM, Heid MF. Patterns of mortality among plumbers and pipefitters. *Am J Ind Med.* 1986;10:73–89.

Cha S, Carter P, Bradow RL. Simulation of automobile brake wear dynamics and estimation of emissions. SAE Technical Paper Series. Passenger Car Meeting, June 6–9, 1983; Dearborn, Michigan.

Chan-Yeung M, Wong R, MacLean L, et al. Respiratory survey of workers in a pulp and paper mill in Powell River, British Columbia. *Am Rev Respir Dis.* 1980;122:249–257.

Cheng VKI, O'Kelly FJ. Asbestos exposure in the motor vehicle repair and servicing industry in Hong Kong. *J Soc Occup Med.* 1986;36:104–106.

Cheng RT, McDermott HJ. Exposure to asbestos from asbestos gaskets. *Appl Occup Environ Hyg.* 1991;6:583–590.

Churg AM, Warnock ML. Asbestos and other ferruginous bodies. Their formation and clinical significance. *Am J Pathol.* 1981;102:447–456.

Cochran JC, Webster I. Mesothelioma in relation to asbestos fiber exposure. *S Afr Med J.* 1981;54:279–281.

Coggon D, Wield G, Pannett B, Campbell L, Boffetta P. Mortality in employees of a Scottish paper mill. *Am J Ind Med.* 1997;32:535–539.

Cook PM, Rubin IB, Maggiore CJ, Nicholson WJ. *X-ray diffraction and electron beam analysis of asbestiform minerals in Lake Superior waters.* International Conference on Environmental Sensing and Assessment 34(2):1–9, Las Vegas, NY; 1976.

Cooper RC, Tarter M, Kanarek M, et al. Asbestos in domestic water supplies in five California counties. Part II. Populations and tumor data base, EHS Publication #79–1, University of California, Berkeley; April, 1979.

Corn M, McArthur B, Dellarco M. Asbestos exposures of building maintenance personnel. *Appl Occup Environ Hyg.* 1994;9:845–852.

Corn M, Crump K, Farrar DB, Lee RJ, McFee DR. Airborne concentrations of asbestos in 71 school buildings. *Regul Toxicol Pharmacol.* 1991;13:99–114.

Corn M. Letter to the Editor re: article "Exposure to airborne asbestos associated with simulated cable installation above a suspended ceiling" by Keyes et al. 1991. *Am Ind Hyg Assoc J.* 1992;53:A232.

Council on Dental Therapeutics and Council on Dental Materials and Devices. Hazards of asbestos in dentistry. *JADA.* 1996;92:777.

Crosignani P, Forastiere F, Petrelli G, et al. Malignant mesothelioma in thermoelectric power plant workers in Italy. *Am J Ind Med.* 1995;27:573–576.

Crossman RN Jr, Williams MG Jr, Lauderdale J, Schosek K, Dodson RF. Quantification of fiber releases for various floor tile removal methods. *Appl Occup Environ Hyg.* 1996;11:1113–1124.

Crump KS, Farrar DB. Statistical analysis of data on airborne asbestos levels collected in an EPA survey of public buildings. *Regul Toxicol Pharmacol.* 1989;10:51–62.

Dagg TG, Satin KP, Bailey WJ, Wong O, Harmon LL, Swencicki RE. An updated cause specific mortality study of petroleum refinery workers. *Br J Ind Med.* 1992;49:203–212.

Daly AR, Zupko AJ, Hebb JL. Technological feasibility and economic impact of OSHA proposed revision to the asbestos standard, v. II. Roy F. Weston Environmental Consultants-Designers, prepared for Asbestos Information Association/North America, Washington, DC 1976.

Davis DR. Release of asbestos fibers during casting ring liner manipulation. *J Prosth Dent.* 1995;74:294–298.

Davis JMG, Coniam SW. Experimental studies on the effects of heated chrysotile asbestos and automobile brake lining dust injected into the body cavities of mice. *Exp Mol Pathol.* 1973;19:339–353.

Decoufle P, Wood DJ. Mortality patterns among workers in a gray iron foundry. *Am J Epidemiol.* 1979;109:667–675.

Dement JM, Hensley L, Kieding S, Lipscomb H. Proportionate mortality among union members employed at three Texas refineries. *Am J Ind Med.* 1998;33:327–340.

Dement JM, Harris RL Jr., Symons MJ, Shy CM. Exposures and mortality among chrysotile asbestos workers. Part II. Mortality. *Am J Ind Med.* 1983;4:421–433.

Dodson RF, O'Sullivan M, Corn CJ, Garcia JGN, Stocks JM, Griffith DE. Analysis of ferruginous bodies in bronchoalveolar lavage from foundry workers. *Br J Ind Med.* 1993;50:1032–1038.

Dodson RF, O'Sullivan M, Brooks DR, Hammar SP. Quantitative analysis of asbestos burden in women with mesothelioma. *Am J Ind Med.* 2003;43:188–195.

Doll R. Mortality from lung cancer in asbestos workers. *Br J Ind Med.* 1955;12:81.

Dreessen WC, Dallavalle JM, Edwards TI, Miller JW, Sayers RR. *A Study of Asbestosis in the Asbestos Textile Industry.* August 1938. Public Health Bulletin No. 241.

Driscoll RJ, Mulligan WJ, Shultz D, Candelaria A. Malignant mesothelioma: a cluster in a native American pueblo. *New Engl J Med.* 1988;318:1437–1438.

Drucker E, Nagin D, Michaels D, Lacher M, Zoloth S. Exposure of sheet metal workers to asbestos during the construction and renovation of commercial buildings in New York City. A case study in social medicine. *Ann NY Acad Sci.* 1987;505:230–244.

Ducatman AM, Withers BF, Yang WN. Smoking and roentgenographic opacities in U.S. Navy asbestos workers. *Chest.* 1990;97:810–813.

Edge JR. Asbestos-related disease in Barrow-in-Furness. *Environ Res.* 1976;11:244–247.

Eglert DS, Geiger AJ. Pulmonary asbestosis and carcinoma. *Am Rev Tuberc.* 1936;34:143–150.

Eisenstadt HB, Wilson FW. Primary malignant mesothelioma of the pleura. *J Lancet.* 1960; 80:511–514.

Elmes PC, Simpson MJC. Insulation workers in Belfast. A further study of mortality due to asbestos exposure (1940–75). *Br J Ind Med.* 1977;34:174–180.

Environmental Profiles, Inc. Report of Findings: exposure assessment: an evaluation of the contribution of airborne asbestos fibers from the replacement of gaskets and packing in Atwood & Morrill valves. EPI Project No. 23148, April 2004.

Environmental Profiles, Inc. Evaluation of asbestos exposures from asbestos containing gasket and packing materials. EPI Project No. 5195, January, 1999.

Environmental Profiles, Inc. Evaluation of the actual contribution of airborne asbestos fibers from the removal and installation of gaskets and packing material. EPI Project No. 8500, September, 1998.

Epler GR, FitzGerald MX, Gaensler EA, Carrington CB. Asbestos-related disease from household exposure. *Respiration.* 1980;39:229–240.

Ericsson J, Jarvholm B, Norin F. Respiratory symptoms and lung function following exposure in workers exposed to soft paper tissue dust. *Int Arch Occup Environ Health.* 1988;60:341–345.

Fasset FG Jr. *The Shipbuilding Business in the United States of America.* Vol 1. New York: Society of Naval Architects and Maine Engineers; 1948.

Ferguson DA, Berry G, Jelihovsky T, et al. The Australian mesothelioma surveillance program 1979–1985. *Med J Aust.* 1987;147:166–172.

Ferris BG, Burgess WA, Worcester J. Prevalence of chronic respiratory disease in a pulp mill and a paper mill in the United States. *Br J Ind Med.* 1967;24:26–37.

Finkelstein MM, Wilk N. Investigation of a lung cancer cluster in the melt shop of an Ontario steel producer. *Am J Ind Med.* 1990;17:483–491.

Finkelstein M. Pulmonary function in asbestos cement workers: a dose-response study. *Br J Ind Med.* 1986;43:406–413.

Finkelstein MM. Asbestos-associated cancers in the Ontario refinery and petrochemical sector. *Am J Ind Med.* 1996;30:610–615.

Finkelstein MM. Analysis of the exposure-response relationship for mesothelioma among asbestos-cement factory workers. *Ann NY Acad Sci.* 1991;643:85–89.

Finkelstein MM. Mortality rates among employees potentially exposed to chrysotile asbestos at two automotive parts factories. *Can Med Assoc J.* 1989;141:125–130.

Fischbein A, Rohl AN, Langer AM, Selikoff IJ. Drywall construction and asbestos exposure. *Am Ind Hyg Assoc J.* 1979;40:402–407.

Fleischer WE, Viles FJ Jr., Gade RL, Drinker P. A health survey of pipe covering operations in constructing naval vessels. *J Ind Hyg Toxicol.* 1946;28:9–16.

Fletcher D. A mortality study of shipyard workers with pleural plaques. *Br J Ind Med.* 1972;29:142–145.

Forastiere F, Pupp N, Magliola E, Valesini S, Tidei F, Perucci CA. Respiratory cancer mortality among workers employed in thermoelectric power plants. *Scand J Work Environ Health.* 1989;15:383–386.

Gamble JF, Lewis RJ, Jorgensen G. Mortality among three refinery/petrochemical plant cohorts. II. Retirees. *JOEM.* 2000;42:730–736.

Gardner MJ, Winter PD, Pannett B, Powell CA. Follow up study of workers manufacturing chrysotile asbestos cement products. *Br J Ind Med.* 1986;43:726–732.

Gardner MJ, Powell CA. Mortality of asbestos cement workers using almost exclusively chrysotile fibre. *J Soc Occup Med.* 1986;36:124–126.

Gennaro V, Ceppi M, Boffetta P, Fontana V, Perrotta A. Pleural mesothelioma and asbestos exposure among Italian oil refinery workers. *Scand J Work Environ Health.* 1994;20:213–215.

Giaroli C, Belli S, Bruno C, et al. Mortality study of asbestos cement workers. *Int Arch Occup Environ Health.* 1994;66:7–11.

Gibbs GW. Fibre release from asbestos garments. *Ann Occup Hyg.* 1975;18:143–149.

Gibson ES, Martin RH, Lockington JN. Lung cancer mortality in a steel foundry. *J Occup Med.* 1977;19:807–812.

Gibson ES, McCalla DR, Kaiser-Farrell C, et al. Lung cancer in a steel foundry: a search for causation. *J Occup Med.* 1983;25:573–578.

Gloyne SR. Squamous carcinoma of lung occurring in asbestosis: two cases. *Tubercle.* 1935;17:5–10.

Gloyne SR. Oat cell carcinoma of lung occurring in asbestosis. *Tubercle.* 1936;18:14–18.

Goldberg P, Goldberg M, Marne MJ. Incidence of pleural mesothelioma in New Caledonia: a 10-year survey (1978–1987). *Arch Environ Health.* 1991;46:306–309.

Goodman M, Teta MJ, Hessel PA, et al. Mesothelioma and lung cancer among motor vehicle mechanics: a meta-analysis. *Ann Occup Hyg.* 2004;48:309–326.

Greenberg M, Davies TA. Mesothelioma Register—1967–1968. *Br J Ind Med.* 1974;31:91–104.

Guberan E, Usel M, Raymond L, Tissot R, Sweetnam PM. Disability, mortality, and incidence of cancer among Geneva painters and electricians: a historical prospective study. *Br J Ind Med.* 1989;46:16–23.

Hamlin LE, Weber HJ. Siderosis: a benign pneumoconiosis due to the inhalation of iron dust. Part I: a clinical, roentgenological and industrial hygiene study of foundry cleaning room employees. *Ind Med Surg.* 1950;19:151–169.

Hanis NM, Shallenberger LG, Donaleski DL, Sales EA. A retrospective mortality study of workers in three major U.S. refineries and chemical plants. Part 1: comparisons with U.S. population. *J Occup Med.* 1985;27:283–292.

Hansen ES. Mortality of auto mechanics. A ten-year follow-up. *Scand J Work Environ Health.* 1989;15:43–46.

Hansen J, de Klerk NH, Musk AW, Hobbs MST. Environmental exposure to crocidolite and mesothelioma. *Am J Respir Crit Care Med.* 1998;157:69–75.

Harries PG. Asbestos hazards in naval dockyards. *Ann Occup Hyg.* 1968;11:135–145.

Health Effects Institute-Asbestos Research (HEI-AR). Asbestos in public and commercial buildings: a literature review and synthesis of current knowledge. Cambridge, MA, 1991.

Helsen JA, Van de Velde P, Kuczumow A, Deruyttere A. Surface characteristics of asbestos fibers released from asbestos-cement products. *Am Ind Hyg Assoc J.* 1989;50:655.

Henneberger PK, Eisen EA, Ferris BG Jr. Pulmonary function among pulp and paper workers in Berlin, New Hampshire. *Br J Ind Med.* 1989;46:765–772.

Hessel PA, Teta MJ, Goodman M, Lau E. Mesothelioma among brake mechanics: an expanded analysis of a case-control study. *Risk Anal.* 2004;24:547–552.

Hickish DE, Knight KL. Exposure to asbestos during brake maintenance. *Ann Occup Hyg.* 1970;13:17–21.

Hilt B, Langard, Andersen A, Rosenberg J. Asbestos exposure, smoking habits, and cancer incidence among production and maintenance workers in an electrochemical plant. *Am J Ind Med.* 1985;8:565–577.

Hilt B. Non-malignant asbestos diseases in workers in an electrochemical plant. *Br J Ind Med.* 1987;44:621–626.

Hirsch A, Di Menza L, Carre A, et al. Asbestos risk among full-time workers in an electricity generating power station. *Ann NY Acad Sci.* 1979;330:137–145.

Hjortsberg U, Orbaek P, Arborelius M Jr, Ranstam J, Welinder H. Railroad workers with pleural plaques: I. Spirometric and nitrogen washout investigation on smoking and nonsmoking asbestos-exposed workers. *Am J Ind Med.* 1988a;14:635–641.

Hjortsberg U, Orbaek P, Arborelius M Jr, Ranstam J, Welinder H. Railroad workers with pleural plaques: II. Small airway dysfunction among asbestos-exposed workers. *Am J Ind Med.* 1988b;14:643–647.

Hodgson MJ, Parkinson DK, Sabo S, Owens GR, Feist JH. Asbestosis among electricians. *J Occup Med.* 1988;30:638–640.

Hughes JM. Human evidence: lung cancer mortality risk from chrysotile exposure. *Ann Occup Hyg.* 1994;38:555–560.

Hughes JM, Weill H, Hammad YY. Mortality of workers employed in two asbestos cement manufacturing plants. *Br J Ind Med.* 1987;44:161–174.

Huncharek M, Muscat J, Capotorto JV. Pleural mesothelioma in a brake mechanic. *Br J Ind Med.* 1989a;46:69–71.

Huncharek M, Capotorto JV, Muscat J. Domestic asbestos exposure, lung fibre burden, and pleural mesothelioma in a housewife. *Br J Ind Med.* 1989b;46:354–355.

Huncharek P. Asbestos-related mesothelioma risk among railroad workers. *Am Rev Respir Dis.* 1987;135:983–984.

Imbernon E, Goldberg M, Bonenfant S, et al. Occupational respiratory cancer and exposure to asbestos: a case-control study in a cohort of workers in the electricity and gas industry. *Am J Ind Med.* 1995;28:339–352.

Jacko MG, DuCharme RT, Somers JH. Brake and clutch emissions generating during vehicle operation. Society of Automotive Engineers/Automobile Engineering Meeting; May 14–18, 1973; Detroit, MI.

Jappinen P, Hakulinen T, Pukkala E, Tola S, Kurppa K. Cancer incidence of workers in the Finnish pulp and paper industry. *Scand J Work Environ Health.* 1987;13:197–202.

Jappinen P. A mortality study of Finnish pulp and paper workers. *Br J Ind Med.* 1987;44:580–587.

Jarvholm B, Malker H, Malker B, Ericsson J, Sallsten G. Pleural mesothelioma and asbestos exposure in the pulp and paper industries: A new risk group identified by linkage of official registers. *Am J Ind Med.* 1988a;13:561–567.

Jarvholm B, Thoren K, Brolin I, et al. Lung function in workers exposed to soft paper dust. *Am J Ind Med.* 1988b;14:457–464.

Jarvholm B, Sanden A. Lung cancer and mesothelioma in the pleura and peritoneum among Swedish insulation workers. *Occup Environ Med.* 1998;55:766–770.

Järvholm B, Brisman J. Asbestos associated tumours in car mechanics. *Br J Ind Med.* 1988;45:645–646.

Johansson LG, Albin MP, Jakobsson KM, Welinder HE, Ranstam PJ, Attewell RG. Ferruginous bodies and pulmonary fibrosis in dead low to moderately exposed asbestos cement workers: histological examination. *Br J Ind Med.* 1987;44:550–558.

Jones RN, Diem JE, Ziskand MM, Rodriguez M, Weill H. Radiographic evidence of asbestos effects in American marine engineers. *J Occup Med.* 1984;26:281–284.

Joubert L, Seidman H, Selikoff IJ. Mortality experience of family contacts of asbestos factory workers. *Ann NY Acad Sci.* 1991;643:416–418.

Kaminski R, Stanislawczyk-Geissert K, Dacey E. Mortality analysis of plumbers and pipefitters. *J Occup Med.* 1980;22:183–189.

Kauppinen T, Korhonen K. Exposure to asbestos during brake maintenance of automotive vehicles by different methods. *Am Ind Hyg Assoc J.* 1987;48:499–504.

Kern DG, Frumkin H. Asbestos-related disease in the jewelry industry. Report of two cases. *Am J Ind Med.* 1988;13:407–410.

Keyes DL, Chesson J, Ewing WM, et al. Exposure to airborne asbestos associated with simulated cable installation above a suspended ceiling. *Am Ind Hyg Assoc J.* 1991;52:479–484.

Kilburn KH, Lilis R, Anderson HA et al. Asbestos disease in family contacts of shipyard workers. *Am J Pub Health.* 1985;75:615–617.

Knishkowy B, Baker EL. Transmission of occupational disease to family contacts. *Am J Ind Med.* 1986;9:543–550.

Kolonel LN, Yoshizawa CN, Hirohata T, Myers BC. Cancer occurrence in shipyard workers exposed to asbestos in Hawaii. *Cancer Res.* 1985;45:3924–3928.

Koskela R-S, Luoma K, Hernberg S. Turnover and health selection among foundry workers. *Scand J Work Environ Health.* 1976;2:90–105.

Kronenberg RS, Levin JL, Dodson RF, Garcia JGN, Griffith DE. Asbestos-related disease in employees of a steel mill and a glass bottle-manufacturing plant. *Ann NY Acad Sci.* 1991;643:397–403.

Lange JH, Lange PR, Reinhard TK, Thomulka KW. A study of personal and area airborne asbestos concentrations during asbestos abatement: a statistical evaluation of fibre concentration data. *Ann Occup Hyg.* 1996;40:449–466.

Langer AM, McCaughey WTE. Mesothelioma in a brake repair worker. *Lancet.* 1982;2:1101–1103.

Langer AM, Nolan RP, Constantopoulos SH, Moutsopoulos HM. Association of Metsovo lung and pleural mesothelioma with exposure to tremolite-containing whitewash. *Lancet.* 1987;i:965–967.

Lee RJ, Van Orden DR, Corn M, Crump KS. Exposure to airborne asbestos in buildings. *Regul Toxicol Pharmacol.* 1992;16:93–107.

Lerchen ML, Wiggins CL, Samet JM. Lung cancer and occupation in New Mexico. *JNCI.* 1987;79:639–645.

Lerman Y, Finkelstein A, Levo Y, et al. Asbestos related health hazards among power plant workers. *Br J Ind Med.* 1990;47:281–282.

Levin L, Silverman D, Hartge P, Hoover R. Smoking characteristics by occupational and industrial groups (abstract). *Am J Epidemiol.* 1985;122:537.

Levy BS, Sigurdson E, Mandel J, Laudon E, Pearson J. Investigating possible effects of asbestos in city water. *Am J Epidemiol.* 1976;103:362–368.

Lewis RJ, Gamble JF, Jorgensen G. Mortality among three refinery/petrochemical plant cohorts. I. 1970 to 1982 active/terminated workers. *JOEM.* 2000;42:721–729.

Li FP, Lokich J, Lapey J, Neptune WB, Wilkins EW Jr. Familial mesothelioma after intense asbestos exposure at home. *JAMA.* 1978;240:467–469.

Lieben J, Pistawka H. Mesothelioma and asbestos exposure. *Arch Environ Health.* 1967;14:559.

Lilienfeld DE. Asbestos-associated pleural mesothelioma in school teachers: a discussion of four cases. *Ann NY Acad Sci.* 1991;643:454–486.

Lilis R, Daum S, et al. Household exposure to asbestos and risk of subsequent disease. In: Lemen R, Dement J, eds. *Dusts and Disease,* Chicago: Pathotox Publishers, Inc.; 1979:145–156.

Lilis R, Lerman Y, Malkin J, Selikoff IJ. Interstitial pulmonary fibrosis: comparative prevalence and symptoms in insulation workers with over 30 years from onset of exposure.

In: VIth International Pneumoconiosis Conference Bochum, 1983, Vol. 2 Geneva: International Labour Organisation, 1984:697–715.

Lilis R, Daum S, Anderson H, Andrews G, Selikoff IJ. Asbestosis among maintenance workers. In: International Agency for Research on Cancer (IARC). Biological effects on mineral fibres. Lyon: IARC, 1980:795–810. IARC Scientific Publication; No. 30.

Longo WE, Rigler MW, Slade J. Crocidolite asbestos fibers in smoke from original Kent cigarettes. *Cancer Res.* 1995;55:2232–2235.

Lorimer WV, Rohl AN, Miller A, Nicholson WJ, Selikoff IJ. Asbestos exposure of brake repair workers in the United States. *The Mount Sinai J Med.* 1976;43:207–218.

Lundorf E, Aagaard MT, Andresen J, et al. Radiological evaluation of earlier pleural and pulmonary changes in light asbestos exposure. *Eur J Respir Dis.* 1987;70:145–149.

Luo S, Liu X, Mu S, Tsai SP, Wen CP. Asbestos related diseases from environmental exposure to crocidolite in Da-yao, China. I. Review of exposure and epidemiological data. *Occup Environ Med.* 2003;60:35–42.

Lynch JR, Ayer HE. Measurement of dust exposures in the asbestos textile industry. *Am Ind Health Assoc J.* 1966;27:431–437.

Lynch JR. Brake lining decomposition products. *J Air Pollut Control Assoc.* 1968;18: 824–826.

Lynch KM, Smith WA. Carcinoma of lung. *Am J Cancer.* 1935;21:56–61.

Magnani C, Terracini B, Ivaldi C, et al. A cohort study on mortality among wives of workers in the asbestos cement industry in Casale Monferrato, Italy. *Br J Ind Med.* 1993;50:779–784.

Magnani C, Borgo G, Betta GP, et al. Mesothelioma and non-occupational environmental exposure to asbestos. *Lancet.* 338:1991.

Magnani C, Mollo F, Paoletti L, et al. Asbestos lung burden and asbestosis after occupational and environmental exposure in an asbestos cement manufacturing area: a necropsy study. *Occup Environ Med.* 1998;55:840–846.

Malker HSR, McLaughlin JK, Malker BK, et al. Occupational risks for pleural mesothelioma in Sweden, 1961–1979. *JNCI.* 1985;74:61–66.

Maltoni ET. Mesotheliomas due to asbestos used in railroads in Italy. *Ann NY Acad Sci.* 1991;643:347–367.

Mancuso TF. Mesothelioma among machinists in railroad and other industries. *Am J Ind Med.* 1983;4:501–513.

Mangold CA. The actual contribution of Garlock asbestos gasket materials to the occupational exposure of asbestos workers, October, 1982.

Marr WT. Asbestos exposure during naval vessel overhaul. *Am Ind Hyg Assoc J.* 1964;25:264–268.

Marsh GM, Enterline PE, McCraw D. Mortality patterns among petroleum refinery and chemical plant workers. *Am J Ind Med.* 1991;19:29–42.

Mason TJ, McKay FW, Miller RW. Asbestos-like fibers in Duluth water supply. Relationship to cancer mortality. *JAMA.* 1974;228:1019–1020.

Matanoski GM, Kanchanaraksa S, Lees PS, et al. Industry-wide study of mortality of pulp and paper mill workers. *Am J Ind Med.* 1998;33:354–365.

Mattioli S, Nini D, Mancini G, Violante FS. Past asbestos exposure levels in foundries and cement-asbestos factories. *Am J Ind Med.* 2002;42:363.

Maxwell JC. *Historical sales trends in the cigarette industry.* Richmond, VA: Wheat, First Securities, Inc.; 1989.

Mazumdar S, Lerer T, Redmond CK. Long-term mortality study of steelworkers. *J Occup Med.* 1975;17:751–755.

McDonald AD, Fry JS, Woolley AJ, McDonald JC. Dust exposure and mortality in an American chrysotile asbestos friction products plant. *Br J Ind Med.* 1984;41:151–157.

McDonald AD, McDonald JC. Malignant mesothelioma in North America. *Cancer.* 1980;46:1650–1656.

McDonald AD, Fry JS, Woolley AJ, McDonald JC. Dust exposure and mortality in an American factory using chrysotile, amosite, and crocidolite in mainly textile manufacture. *Br J Ind Med*. 1982;39:368–374.

McDonald AD, Fry JS, Woolley AJ, McDonald J. Dust exposure and mortality in an American textile plant. *Br J Ind Med*. 1983;40:361–367.

McDonald JC, Harris J, Armstrong B. Mortality in a cohort of vermiculite miners exposed to fibrous amphibole in Libby, Montana. *Occup Environ Med*. 2004;61:363–366.

McDonald JC. Unfinished business: the asbestos textiles mystery. *Ann Occup Hyg*. 1998;42:3–5.

McKinnery WN, Moore RW. Evaluation of airborne asbestos fiber levels during removal and installation of valve gaskets and packing. *Am Ind Hyg Assoc J*. 1992;53:531–532.

McLaughlin AIG, Harding HE. Pneumoconiosis and other causes of death in iron and steel foundry workers. *AMA Arch Ind Health*. 1956;14:350–378.

Meigs JW, Walter SD, Heston JF, et al. Asbestos cement pipe and cancer in Connecticut 1955–1974. *J Environ Health*. 1980;42:187–191.

Merewether ER. The occurrence of pulmonary fibrosis and other pulmonary affections in asbestos workers. *J Ind Hyg*. 1930;12:198–222.

Meylan WM, Howard PH, Lande SS, Hantchett A. Chemical market input/output, analysis of selected chemical substances to assess sources of environmental contamination. Task III. Asbestos. Syracuse Resource Corporation, U.S. EPA, Washington, DC, August 1978.

Michaels D, Zoloth S, Lacher M, Holstein E, Lilis R, Drucker E. Asbestos disease in sheet metal workers: II. Radiological signs of asbestosis among active workers. *Am J Ind Med*. 1987;12:595–603.

Milham S. Occupational mortality in Washington State 1950–1979. Cincinnati: US Department of Health and Human Services, 1983. NIOSH No. 83–116.

Millette JR. Microscopical studies of the asbestos fiber releasability of dryer felt textile. *Microscope*. 1999;47:93–100.

Milne KL, Sandler DP, Everson RB, Brown SM. Lung cancer and occupation in Alameda County: a death certificate case-control study. *Am J Ind Med*. 1983;4:565–575.

Mlynarek S, Corn M, Blake C. Asbestos exposure of building maintenance personnel. *Regulatory Toxicol Pharmacol*. 1996;23:213–224.

Moore LL. Asbestos exposure associated with automotive brake repair in Pennsylvania. *Am Ind Hyg Assoc J*. 1988;49:A12–A13.

Morabia A, Markowitz S, Garibaldi K, Wynder EL. Lung cancer and occupation: results of a multicentre case-control study. *Br J Ind Med*. 1992;49:721–727.

Mostert C. Asbestosis and mesothelioma on the Rhodesia Railway. *Cent Afr J Med*. 1979;25:72–74.

Murphy RL, Levine BW, Al Bazzaz FJ, Lynch JJ, Burgess WA. Floor tile installation as a source of asbestos exposure. *Am Rev Respir Dis*. 1971;104:576–580.

Neuberger M, Kundi M. Individual asbestos exposure: smoking and mortality—a cohort study in the asbestos cement industry. *Br J Ind Med*. 1990;47:615–620.

Newhouse ML, Oakes D, Woolley AJ. Mortality of welders and other craftsmen at a shipyard in NE England. *Br J Ind Med*. 1985;42:406–410.

Newhouse ML, Thompson H. Mesothelioma of pleura and peritoneum following exposure to asbestos in the London area. *Br J Ind Med*. 1965;22:261–269.

Newhouse ML, Sullivan KR. A mortality study of workers manufacturing friction materials: 1941–86. *Br J Ind Med*. 1989;46:176–179.

Nicholson WJ, Holaday DA, Heimann H. Direct and indirect occupational exposure to insulation dusts in United States shipyards. *Occup Med*. 1988;74:37–47.

Nicholson WJ, Perkel G, Selikoff IJ. Occupational exposure to asbestos: population at risk and projected mortality—1980–2030. *Am J Ind Med*. 1982;3:259–311.

Nicholson WJ, Daum SM, Lorimer WV, et al. Investigation of health hazards in brake lining repair and maintenance workers occupationally exposed to asbestos. [NIOSH Contract

210–77-0119]. Environmental Sciences Laboratory, Mt. Sinai School of Medicine of the City University of New York, 1986.

Noble BS. Asbestos exposures during the cutting and machining of asbestos cement pipe. Report prepared by Equitable Environmental Health, Inc., March 16, 1977.

Nolan RP, Langer AM. Report on the chrysotile fibers released from the manipulation of asbestos packings. November 30, 1993.

Nurmenen M. The epidemiological relationship between pleural mesothelioma and asbestos exposure. *Scand J Work Environ.* 1975;1:128–137.

Ohlson C-G, Bodin L, Trydman T, Hogstedt C. Ventilatory decrements in former asbestos cement workers: a four year follow up. *Br J Ind Med.* 1985;42:612–616.

Ohlson C-G, Hogstedt C. Lung cancer among asbestos cement workers: a Swedish cohort study and a review. *Br J Ind Med.* 1985;42:397–402.

Ohlson CG, Klaesson B, Hogstedt C. Mortality among asbestos-exposed workers in a railroad workshop. *Scand J Work Environ Health.* 1984;10:283–291.

Oliver T. Dangerous Trades, E.P. Dutch & Co., New York, 1902; 271.

Oliver LC, Eisen EA, Green RE, Sprince NL. Asbestos-related disease in railroad workers: a cross-sectional study. *Am Rev Respir Dis.* 1985;131:499.

Owen WG. Diffuse mesothelioma and exposure to asbestos dust in the Merseyside area. *Br Med J.* 1964;2:214.

Page RT. A study of dust control methods in an asbestos fabricating plant. *Public Health Reports.* 1937;52:1713–1727.

Paik NW, Walcott RJ, Brogan PA. Worker exposure to asbestos during removal of sprayed material and renovation activity in buildings containing sprayed material. *Am Ind Hyg Assoc J.* 1983;44:428–432.

Palmer WG, Scott WD. Lung cancer in ferrous foundry workers: a review. *Am Ind Hyg Assoc J.* 1981;42:329–340.

Paustenbach DJ, Finley BL, Lu ET, Brorby GP, Sheehan PJ. Environmental and occupational health hazards associated with the presence of asbestos in brake linings and pads (1900 to present): a "state-of-the-art" review. *J Toxicol Environ Health Part B.* 2004;7:33–110.

Pearce N. Analytical implications of epidemiological concepts of interaction. *Int J Epidemiol.* 1989;18:976–980.

Peters GA, Peters BJ, eds. *Asbestos health risks*, Vol. 12, *Sourcebook on Asbestos Diseases.* 1996 (Michie).

Peto J, Doll R, Hermon C, Binns W, Clayton R, Goffe T. Relationship of mortality to measures of environmental asbestos pollution in an asbestos textile factory. *Ann Occup Hyg.* 1985;29:305–355.

Price B, Crump KS, Baird EC III. Airborne asbestos levels in buildings: maintenance worker and occupant exposures. *J Exposure Analysis Environ Epidemiol.* 1992;2:357–374.

Puntoni R, Valerio F, Santi L. Il mesotelioma pleurico fra i lavoratori del porto di Genova. *Tumori.* 1976;62:205.

Radford EP. Cancer mortality in the steel industry. *Ann NY Acad Sci.* 1976;271:228–238.

Raffn E, Lynge E, Juel K, Korsgaard B. Incidence of cancer and mortality among employees in the asbestos cement industry in Denmark. *Br J Ind Med.* 1989;46:90–96.

Ramazzini B. *Diseases of Workers*, 1713, Republished 1964 by Hafner Publishing Company, New York and London, p. 15.

Redmond CK, Smith EM, Lloyd JW, Rush HW. Long-term mortality study of steelworkers. III. Follow-Up. *J Occup Med.* 1969;11:513–521.

Reid AS, Causton BE, Jones JSP, Ellis IO. Malignant mesothelioma after exposure to asbestos in dental practice. *Lancet.* 1991;338:696.

Robinson C, Stern F, Halperin W, et al. Assessment of mortality in the construction industry in the United States, 1984–1986. *Am J Ind Med.* 1995;28:49–70.

Robinson CF, Waxweiler RJ, Fowler DP. Mortality among production workers in pulp and paper mills. *Scand J Work Environ Health.* 1986;12:552–560.

Rockette HE, Redmond CK. Long-term mortality study of steelworkers. X. Mortality patterns among masons. *J Occup Med.* 1976;18:541–545.

Rocskay AZ, Harbut MR, Green MA, Osher DL, Zellers ET. Respiratory health in asbestos-exposed ironworkers. *Am J Ind Med.* 1996;29:459–466.

Rödelsperger K, Jahn H, Brückel B, Manke J, Paur R, Woitowitz HJ. Asbestos dust exposure during brake repair. *Am J Ind Med.* 1986;10:63–72.

Roggli VL, Sanders LL. Asbestos content of lung tissue and carcinoma of the lung: a clinicopathologic correlation and mineral fiber analysis of 234 cases. *Ann Occup Hyg.* 2000;44:109–117.

Roggli VL, Sharma A, Butnor KJ, Sporn T, Vollmer RT. Malignant mesothelioma and occupational exposure to asbestos: a clinicopathological correlation of 1445 cases. *Ultrastruct Pathol.* 2002;36:55–65.

Rohl AN, Langer AM, Wolff MS, Weisman I. Asbestos exposure during brake lining maintenance and repair. *Environ Res.* 1976;12:110–128.

Rosenman KD. Causes of mortality in primary and secondary school teachers. *Am J Ind Med.* 1994;25:749–758.

Rushton L, Alderson MR, Nagarajah CR. Epidemiological survey of maintenance workers in London Transport Executive bus garages and Chiswick Works. *Br J Ind Med.* 1983;40:340–345.

Ruttner JR. Mesothelioma in Swiss railroad workers. *Ann NY Acad Sci.* 1991;643–646.

Sawyer RN, Spooner CM. Sprayed asbestos-containing materials in buildings: a guidance document. EPA-450/2–78-014 (OAQPS No. 1.2–094), 1977.

Schenker MB, Garshick E, Munoz, Woskie SR, Speizer FE. A population-based case-control study of mesothelioma deaths among US railroad workers. *Am Rev Respir Dis.* 1986;134:461–465.

Schneider J, Straif K, Woitowitz HJ. Pleural mesothelioma and household asbestos exposure. *Rev Environ Health.* 1996;11:65–70.

Schwartz E. A proportionate mortality ratio analysis of pulp and paper mill workers in New Hampshire. *Br J Ind Med.* 1988;45:234–238.

Schwartz E. Proportionate mortality ratio analysis of automobile mechanics and gasoline service station workers in New Hampshire. *Am J Ind Med.* 1987;12:91–99.

Sebastien P, Bignon J, Martin M. Indoor airborne asbestos pollution: from the ceiling and floor. *Science.* 1982;216:1410–1412.

Selikoff IH, Churg J, Hammond EC. The occurrence of asbestosis among insulation workers in the United States. *Ann NY Acad Sci.* 1965;132:139–155.

Selikoff IJ, Hammond EC, Seidman H. Latency of asbestos disease among insulation workers in the United States and Canada. *Cancer.* 1980;46:2736–2740.

Selikoff IJ, Hammond EC, Seidman H. Mortality experience of insulation workers in the United States and Canada, 1943–1976. *Ann NY Acad Sci.* 1979a;330:91–116.

Selikoff IJ, Lilis R, Levin G. Asbestotic radiological abnormalities among United States merchant marine seamen. *Br J Ind Med.* 1990;47:292–297.

Selikoff IJ, Lilis R, Nicholson WJ. Asbestos disease in United States shipyards. *Ann NY Acad Sci.* 1979b;330:295–311.

Selikoff IJ, Nicholson WJ, Lilis R. Radiologic evidence of asbestos disease among ship repair workers. *Am J Ind Med.* 1980;1:9–22.

Sepulveda MJ, Merchant JA. Roentgenographic evidence of asbestos exposure in a select population of railroad workers. *Am J Ind Med.* 1983;4:631.

Severson RK. *A Study of the Effects of Asbestos in Drinking Water on Cancer Incidence in the Puget Sound Region* [master's thesis]. Seattle, WA: Biomathematics Group, University of Washington, 1979.

Sheers G, Coles RM. Mesothelioma risks in a naval dockyard. *Arch Environ Health.* 1980;35:276.

Sheers G, Templeton AR. Effects of asbestos in dockyard workers. *Brit Med J.* 1968;3:574–579.

Solet D, Zoloth SR, Sullivan C, Jewett J, Michaels DM. Patterns of mortality in pulp and paper workers. *J Occup Med.* 1989;31:627–630.

Spence SK, Rocchi PSJ. Exposure to asbestos fibres during gasket removal. *Ann Occup Hyg.* 1996;40:583–588.

Spencer JW, Plisko MJ, Balzer JL. Asbestos fiber release from the brake pads of overhead industrial cranes. *Appl Occup Environ Hyg.* 1999;14:397–402.

Spirtas R, Heineman EF, Berstein L, et al. Malignant mesothelioma: attributable risk of asbestos exposure. *Occup Environ Med.* 1994;51:804–811.

Steenland K, Palu S. Cohort mortality study of 57,000 painters and other union members: a 15-year update. *Occup Environ Med.* 1999;56:315–321.

Stein RC, Kitajewska JY, Kirkham JB, Tait N, Sinha G, Rudd RM. Pleural mesothelioma resulting from exposure to amosite asbestos in a building. *Respir Med.* 1989;83:237–239.

Stern F, Lehman E, Ruder A. Mortality among unionized construction plasterers and cement masons. *Am J Ind Med.* 2001;39:373–388.

Stumphius J. Epidemiology of mesothelioma on Watcheren Island. *Br J Ind Med.* 1971;28:59.

Tagnon I, Blot WJ, Stroube RB, et al. Mesothelioma associated with the shipbuilding industry in coastal Virginia. *Cancer Res.* 1980;40:3875–3879.

Talcott JA, Thurbert WA, Kantor AF, et al. Asbestos-associated diseases in a cohort of cigarette-filter workers. *N Engl J Med.* 1989;321:1220–1223.

Teta MJ, Lewinsohn HC, Meigs JW, Vidone RH, Mowad LZ, Flannery JT. Mesothelioma in Connecticut, 1955–1977: occupational and geographic associations. *J Occup Med.* 1983;25:749–756.

Thoren K, Jarvholm B, Morgan U. Mortality from asthma and chronic obstructive pulmonary disease among workers in a soft paper mill: a case referent study. *Br J Ind Med.* 1989;46:192–195.

Tola S, Koskela R-S, Hernberg S, Jarvinen E. Lung cancer mortality among iron foundry workers. *J Occup Med.* 1979;21:753–760.

Toren K, Persson B, Wingren G. Health effects of working in pulp and paper mills: malignant diseases. *Am J Ind Med.* 1996;29:123–130.

Tossavainen A. Estimated risk of lung cancer attributable to occupational exposures in iron and steel foundries. In: Vainio H, Sorsa M, McMichael AJ, eds. *Complex Mixtures and Cancer Risk.* Lyon: International Agency for Research on Cancer (WHO), IARC; 1990:363–367.

Tsai SP, Dowd CM, Cowles SR, Ross CE. A prospective study of morbidity patterns in a petroleum refinery and chemical plant. *Br J Ind Med.* 1992;49:516–522.

Tsai SP, Waddell LC Jr, Gilstrap EL, Ransdell JD, Ross CE. Mortality among maintenance employees potentially exposed to asbestos in a refinery and petrochemical plant. *Am J Ind Med.* 1996;29:89–98.

Verma DK, Middleton CG. Occupational exposure to asbestos in the drywall taping process. *Am Ind Hyg Assoc J.* 1980;41:264–269.

Vianna NJ, Polan AK. Non-occupational exposure to asbestos and malignant mesothelioma in females. *Lancet.* 1978;1:1061–1063.

Wagner JC. The discovery of the association between blue asbestos and mesothelioma and the aftermath. *Br J Ind Med.* 1991;48:399–403.

Wagner JC, Berry G, Pooley FD. Mesotheliomas and asbestos type in asbestos textile workers: a study of lung contents. *Br Med J.* 1982;285:603–606.

Wagner JC, Sleggs CA, Marchand P. Diffuse pleural mesothelioma and asbestos exposure in the North West Cape Province. *Br J Ind Med.* 1960;17:260–271.

Walrath J, Rogot E, Murray J, Blair A. *Mortality patterns among U.S. veterans by occupation and smoking status.* Bethesda, MD: DHHS (PHS); 1985. NIH Publication No. 85-2756.

Wang E, Dement JM, Lipscomb H. Mortality among North Carolina construction workers, 1988–1994. *Appl Occup Environ Hyg.* 1999;14:45–58.

Ward EM, Ruder AM, Suruda A, et al. Cancer mortality patterns among female and male workers employed in a cable manufacturing plant during World War II. *JOM.* 1994;36:860–866.

Webster I, Cochrane JWC, Solomon A. Pneumoconiosis in non-mining industries on the Witwaterand. *S Afr Med J.* 1977;51:261.

Weill H, Waggenspack C, Bailey W, Ziskind M, Rossiter C. Radiographic and physiologic patterns among workers engaged in manufacture of asbestos cement products. A preliminary report. *J Occup Med.* 1973;15:248–252.

Weir FW, Meraz LB. Morphological characteristics of asbestos fibers released during grinding and drilling of friction products. *Appl Occup Environ Hyg.* 2001;16:1147–1149.

Weir FW, Tolar G, Meraz LB. Characterization of vehicular brake service personnel exposure to airborne asbestos and particulate. *Appl Occup Environ Hyg.* 2001;16:1–8.

Weiss W, Levin R, Goodman L. Pleural plaques and cigarette smoking in asbestos workers. *J Occup Med.* 1981;23:427–430.

Wickman AR, Roberts DW, Hopper TL. Exposure of custodial employees to airborne asbestos. Technical report for U.S. EPA under EPA project No. J1007468–01-0.

Wigle D. Cancer mortality in relation to asbestos in municipal water supplies. *Arch Environ Health.* 1977;32:185–190.

Williams RL, Muhlbaier JL. Asbestos brake emissions. *Environ Res.* 1982;29:70–82.

Wilson R, Langer AM, Nolan RP, Gee JBL, Ross M. Asbestos in New York City public school buildings—public policy: is there a scientific basis? *Regul Toxicol Pharmacol.* 1994;20:161–169.

Wollmer P, Eriksson L, Jonson B, et al. Relation between lung function, exercise capacity, and exposure to asbestos cement. *Br J Ind Med.* 1987;44:542–549.

Wong O, Ragland DR, Marcero DH. An epidemiologic study of employees at seven pulp and paper mills. *Int Arch Occup Environ Health.* 1996;68:498–507.

Wong O. Malignant mesothelioma and asbestos exposure among auto mechanics: appraisal of scientific evidence. *Regul Toxicol Pharmacol.* 2001;34:170–177.

Wong O, Raabe GK. Critical review of cancer epidemiology in petroleum industry employees, with a quantitative meta-analysis by cancer site. *Am J Ind Med.* 1989;15:283–315.

Wong O, Morgan RW, Bailey WJ, Swencicki RE, Claxton K, Kheifets L. An epidemiological study of petroleum refinery workers. *Br J Ind Med.* 1986;43:6–17.

Wong O. Pleural mesothelioma in oil refinery workers. *Scand J Work Environ Health.* 1995;21:301–309.

Yeung P, Patience K, Apthorpe L, Willcocks D. An Australian study to evaluate worker exposure to chrysotile in the automotive service industry. *Appl Occup Environ Hyg.* 1999;14:448–457.

Zahm SH, Brownson RC, Chang JC, Davis JR. Study of lung cancer histologic types, occupation, and smoking in Missouri. *Am J Ind Med.* 1989;15:565–578.

4

Epidemiology and Risk Assessment

Graham W. Gibbs and Geoffrey Berry

Introduction

In this chapter we consider the magnitudes of risk for the development of asbestosis, malignant mesothelioma (MM), and lung cancer (LC) resulting from exposure to different airborne concentrations of asbestos. Information on risk is obtained from epidemiological studies. The risk analysis requires three components; first, the level of exposure, second, cases that have occurred, and third, factors that might confound or modify the exposure-response relationship. Information concerning LC is generally good as it is usually possible to establish cause of death even in retrospective studies initiated several decades ago. Although cases of MM may have been overlooked by pathologists in the past (30 or more years ago), ascertainment of new cases has greatly improved. In contrast, exposure assessments are invariably difficult; estimates, of necessity, often depend on extrapolation into the past and there are uncertainties in measurements. These arise from changes in instrumentation and sampling strategies. For example, in North America, it has been necessary to convert measurements made with instruments such as the Midget Impinger (Ayer et al., 1965; Gibbs and LaChance, 1974) and in the United Kingdom, Thermal Precipitator (HEI-AR, 1991) and in South Africa, Konimeters and Thermal Precipitators (Gibbs and DuToit, 1979) to "Membrane Filter Phase Contrast Microscopy equivalents" with the associated limitations of such conversions. In the past, there was often a lack of systematic sampling, and vague "guestimates" of early exposure were made (Rogers, 2001). Consequently, exposure-response relationships (that may be qualitatively valid within a study because relative exposure levels are reasonable) can be invalid for comparisons between studies because absolute exposure levels are incorrect.

Risk estimates are needed to establish criteria for the protection of workers. They are also required to estimate the number of cases likely to occur in future years (Chapter 16). This involves extrapolating exposure-response relationships forward in time. It involves uncertainties about the relationship between disease incidence and time since exposure, particularly for lengths of follow-up beyond the range of epidemiological data. Risk estimates are also required when exposures are low to assess the possible impact of environmental exposure. This involves extrapolation of exposure-response relationships in situations where exposure was heavy to much lower levels of exposure. This is critical when addressing the question—is there a threshold below which the risk is zero?

Asbestosis results from exposure to high concentrations of friable asbestos, generally over long durations (Merewether and Price, 1930). Therefore, it is not likely to be found in members of the general population. For example, among New Orleans cement workers, the risk of asbestosis related to cumulative exposure. However, there was little evidence for a risk of asbestosis below 30 f/mL-yrs (Weill, 1994), that is, 30 years of exposure at 1 f/mL, or 1 year of exposure at 30 f/mL. The concentrations of fibers in the ambient air of public buildings and homes containing asbestos are many orders of magnitude less (HEI-AR, 1991) (Chapter 3).

In risk assessments, estimates based on data from animal models are sometimes used. In such instances, human risks are inferred, occasionally unjustifiably. However, animal and cell systems have been valuable in providing insight into potential disease mechanisms, as well as the importance of biopersistence and fiber dimension in carcinogenicity and fibrogenicity. They have also resulted in models to screen for fibrogenicity and carcinogenicity. The usefulness of animal studies for determining risk is limited because of (1) poor characterization of the test material (ie, composition and dimensions), (2) methods of administration, (3) large differences in the solubility and biopersistence of the minerals (Bernstein et al., 1999, 2003; Oberdoerster, 1994), (4) enormous differences in dosage quantitated by fiber number when equal masses of the various fiber type are administered (Dunnigan and Muhle, 1994), (5) large differences in life expectancy between humans and animals (important when investigating long latency diseases) (Davis, 1994), and (6) results from animal systems have, in some cases, contradicted observations in humans. Many of these factors were evaluated in relation to carcinogenicity by a working group of the World Health Organization (WHO, 1992). Accordingly, possibly with rare exceptions, animal studies do not provide a reliable basis for estimating human health risks resulting from asbestos exposure and will not be considered further here.

Risk of Asbestosis

Evaluation of the risk for the occurrence of asbestosis is of interest from two standpoints: (1) initial attempts by the US Public Health Services (USPHS) to derive risk estimates for standard setting used an Impinger method to relate dust exposure to asbestosis (Dreesen et al., 1938); (2) the standard for asbestosis in the United Kingdom in the 1960s was the first attempt to set a standard based on a fiber count using a Phase Contrast Membrane Filter method.

In the United Kingdom, the hygiene standard for chrysotile was based on radiological and clinical changes in textile workers. In that case, basal rales and radiological changes were related to the duration of employment and to the number of years a worker was exposed to an estimated amount of dust. Rales, in the basal and lower areas of the lung, were an indication of a response to exposure. The radiological changes considered as possibly related to asbestosis were increased "general opacity in the lower lobes, blurring of the cardiac outline, pleural thickening, and adhesions." Measurements of dust in the textile industry between 1952 and 1966 were made using the Thermal Precipitator.[1] Between 1961 and 1966, the so-called Long Running Thermal Precipitator was used

---

1 The Thermal Precipitator is an instrument that draws fibers at a rate of 5–7 mL per minute between two cover slips. The particles are deposited on the slides as a result of being repelled by a hot wire and those particles with a length:diameter ratio between about 5 and 100 μm are counted on the light optical microscope.

which gave fiber counts similar to those obtained using the Membrane Filter method. The relationship between average Long Running Thermal Precipitator counts in 1961, and counts obtained by the Thermal Precipitator in 1960, were used to derive Membrane Filter Fiber Equivalent concentrations in f/mL. A review committee expressed the standard as follows:

> [A] proper and reasonable objective would be to reduce the risk of contracting asbestosis to 1% of those who have a lifetime's exposure to the dust. …asbestosis…means the earliest demonstrable effects on the lung…It is probable that the risk of being affected to the extent of having such early clinical signs will be less than 1% for an accumulated exposure of 100 f/cc for 25 years or 10 f/cc for 10 years. (*Br Occup Hyg Soc.*, 1968)

The levels were expressed as the number of f/mL greater than 5 μm in length as determined by the "Standard Membrane Filter Method."

Although exposure estimates and the standard were subsequently modified, the approach clearly laid out the fact that there was a finite risk and defined the estimate of that risk. This contrasted with the approach used by the American Conference of Governmental and Industrial Hygienists (ACGIH, 1992–1993) in the United States, which was far less quantitative, indicating that

> Threshold limit values (TLV) refer to airborne concentrations of substances and represent conditions under which it is believed that nearly all workers may be repeatedly exposed day after day without adverse health effects. Because of wide variation in individual susceptibility, however, a small percentage of workers may experience discomfort from some substances at concentrations below the threshold limit; a smaller percentage may be affected more seriously by aggravation of pre-existing condition or by development of an occupational illness.

Interestingly enough, the Committee on Hygiene Standards in the United Kingdom also examined the 1938 data of the USPHS. They showed that a satisfactory fit of the data was obtained that gave a risk of 1% for an exposure of 50 years estimated at 25 particles/mL as measured using the Midget Impinger. A risk of 1% was thought to involve a reduction of the count to 6 particles/mL.[2]

Since the 1960s, there have been several other studies that have examined the relationship between exposure and the occurrence of clinical and radiological *asbestosis*. In the Province of Quebec, radiological changes were examined for some 1.5×10^4 chrysotile miners and millers. The x-rays were read by a panel of six who independently used a then newly devised UICC/ILO classification. Exposure was estimated using Midget Impinger counts (Rossiter et al., 1972). In a later study, the exposure of each individual was converted to f/mL (ie, Membrane Filter equivalent concentration) and the best available information used to assess exposures. This was important because side-by-side samples taken with Midget Impingers and Membrane Filters showed poor correlation (Gibbs and LaChance, 1974). However, within a particular mine or part of a mine or mill, there was a much better relationship. Therefore, by a detailed evaluation of each job location, the most reliable estimates of exposure were made. The relationship between exposure estimates and radiological changes for workers ranging in age from 60 to 69 were estimated by Liddell et al. (1982).

---

2 In the Midget Impinger method, air is drawn through a liquid (in this case ethyl alcohol). The dust collected is allowed to settle in a cell (eg, haemocytometer cell) for a known time before the particles are counted. At the magnification at which particles are counted, only particles with diameters greater than about 1 μm are recorded.

The prevalence was not higher in smokers compared to nonsmokers as noted

Prevalence (%) 1/0 or more (UICC/ILO criteria) = 21.0 + 0.00210 (f/mL-yrs).

Prevalence (%) 2/1 or more (UICC/ILO criteria) = 5.1 + 0.00086 (f/mL-yrs).

This means that for radiological changes of 1/0 or more, there was a 0.2% increase in prevalence of asbestosis per 100 f/mL-yrs increase in exposure.

The reason for the high intercepts (age or the low specificity of minor degrees of paren-chymal change) is not fully explained. In another study comparing the risks from exposure to chrysotile derived from so-called "cross" and "slip" seams (Chapter 2), the limitation of being cross-sectional was avoided. The intercept for small opacities 1/0 or greater was about 20% but the slope was 4% per 100 f/mL-yrs. There was no difference between men exposed to "slip" and "cross" fibers (McDonald et al., 1984). The prevalence of 1/0 radiological changes, or more, in asbestiform tremolite exposed workers was 5%–10% per 100 f/mL-yrs. That study also found high intercepts unaffected by age and smoking (McDonald et al., 1986).

The original 1968 British Occupational Hygiene Society standard provided a 1% risk of radiological changes related to asbestosis for an exposure of 130 f/mL-yrs based on data from the textile industry. In a later and more complete study of the relationship between exposure and *asbestosis* at the same textile factory, Berry et al. (1979) reported a prevalence of 1% "possible asbestosis" at a cumulative exposure of 55 f/mL-yrs. They noted that cumulative exposure may not be the most appropriate measure, and that the prevalence may be greater when the same cumulative exposure is accumulated over more years. The prevalence of radiological or other evidence of asbestosis in Quebec miners and millers (Rossiter et al., 1972), the US (Dreessen et al., 1938) and the UK textile industry workers (Acheson and Gardner, 1979) were compared by McDonald (1984). Although such comparisons were difficult as prevalence studies likely underestimate risk, he concluded that after an exposure of 2 f/mL for 40 years asbestosis might be evident in about 5% of textile workers and 0.5% of production workers. Thus, textile workers were at higher risk. In this comparison, the Canadian and the US exposure data were converted from Midget Impinger to Membrane Filter fiber counts.

As far as mortality from pneumoconiosis is concerned, Liddell et al. (1984) reported the Relative Risk (RR) increased in parallel with the index of exposure expressed in f/mL-yrs, indicating that the fiber-equivalent estimate (ie, converted from particle counts) related to rates of death from asbestosis. The line fitted to the data was:

$$RR = 1 + 0.00647 \text{ f/mL-yrs.}$$

Risk of Malignant Mesothelioma

Amosite and crocidolite exposure are now well established as being associated with increased risks of MM (Table 4.1).

Wagner et al. (1960) first reported an increased risk of MM in persons working and living in the vicinity of crocidolite mines in Northern Cape Provinces, South Africa (Chapter 1). This finding established MM as a definite disease and crocidolite as the cause. It also showed that domestic and general environmental exposure to crocidolite could increase the risk of mesothelioma. Since then, MM has been reported in Australian crocidolite miners and millers (Armstrong et al., 1988), in manufacturers of crocidolite filter paper (Talcott et al., 1989), in gas mask workers (Acheson et al., 1982; McDonald and McDonald, 1978; McDonald et al., 2006), and in railroad brake manufacturers (Berry and Newhouse, 1983) among others (Chapter 8). The risks of MM in these crocidolite-exposed workers are reflective of the pathogenic potency of the mineral, even in workers where it has been claimed that the crocidolite exposure was minimal or rare. For example, a study of lung tissue burdens in insulation workers in the United States revealed that all had amosite in them but four of seven patients with MM had only crocidolite in their lungs (Kohyama and Suzuki, 1991). A recent study has shown that the concentrations of crocidolite in lung tissues of mesothelioma from Cape Province were relatively low (Nolan et al., 2006).

Amosite has been linked to an increased risk of MM in mining (Sluis-Cremer et al., 1992) and manufacturing (Levin et al., 1998; Seidman et al., 1986), shipyard employment, and naval/merchant marine service (Chapter 8).

Anthophyllite is believed to increase MM risk, but the risk is much lower than with the other amphiboles.

Table 4.1 MM Occurrence in Selected Study Populations Worldwide by Fiber Type

Study Cohort	Total # at Risk	Dead #	Dead %	Proportion of Mortality (%)
Crocidolite				
Gas mask manufacture—Canada (McDonald and McDonald, 1978)	199	56	28	16.1
Gas mask manufacture—United Kingdom (Acheson et al., 1982)	757	219	29	2.3
Gas mask manufacture—United Kingdom (McDonald et al., 2006)	772	632	82	10.3
Mining—Australia (Berry et al., 2004)	6908	2549	37	9.1
Mining—South Africa (Sluis-Cremer et al., 1992)	3430	423	12	4.7
Paper manufacturing (Talcott et al., 1989)	35	28	80	17.8
Amosite				
Factory—United States (Seidman et al., 1986)	820	528	64	2.7
Factory—United Kingdom (Acheson et al., 1984)	5969	422	7	1.2
Mining—South Africa (Sluis-Cremer et al., 1992)	3212	648	20	0.6
Factory—United States (Levin et al., 1998)	1130	315	28	1.9
Mixed fiber types				
Insulation workers—United States (Selikoff et al., 1979a)	632	478	6	7.9
Insulators—Sweden (Jarvholm and Sanden, 1998)	248	86	35	8.1
Insulators—North America (Selikoff and Seidman, 1991)	17,800	4951	28	9.2
Dockyard workers—United Kingdom	6292	1043	7	3.0
Shipyards and insulators—United States (Selikoff et al., 1979b)	440	79	18	10.1
Male factory workers—United Kingdom (Newhouse and Berry, 1979)	4600	775	17	5.9
Female factory workers—United Kingdom (Acheson et al., 1982)	992	225	23	9.3

(Continued)

Table 4.1 (Continued)

Study Cohort	Total # at Risk	Dead #	Dead %	Proportion of Mortality (%)
Tremolite				
Vermiculite mining—United States (McDonald and McDonald, 2002, 2004)	406	285	70	4.2
Anthophyllite				
Miners—Finland (Karjalainen et al., 1994)	999	503	50	0.8
Miners—Finland (Meurman et al., 1994)	735	137	19	2.9
Chrysotile				
Miners and millers—Canada (McDonald et al., 1997)	9780	8009	82	0.47
Thetford	5041	4125	82	0.61
Asbestos	4031	3331	85	0.2
Factory	708	553	78	0.9
Mining—Italy (Piolatto, 1990)*	1058	427	40	0.46
Textile plant (Hein et al., 2007)[†]	3072	1961	64	0.15
Factory (Weiss, 1977)	264	66	25	0
Cement plant (Thomas et al., 1982)	1970	351	18	0
Gas mask filter—United Kingdom (Acheson et al., 1982)	570	177	31	1[‡]
Friction materials—United States (McDonald et al., 1984)	3641	1267	35	0
Friction materials—United Kingdom (New house and Sullivan, 1989)	13,450	2577	19	0[§]

* Amphibole fibers have been milled at this mine.
[†] Some amphibole fibers have been found in the lungs of workers from this plant.
[‡] This case was also considered to have been exposed to crocidolite at another factory. There was also an excess number of persons with cancer of the ovary at the plant. These were considered by the authors to be possible additional cases of MM.
[§] There were 13 MM in total; 11 had contact with crocidolite; of the two working with chrysotile, 1 diagnosis uncertain, 1 work history was not well established.

While there are deposits of asbestiform tremolite and asbestiform actinolite that have been exploited on a limited scale in various parts of the world (Chapter 2), there have been no systematic long-term studies of these workers. However, increased rates of MM are reported in countries where persons have been exposed environmentally and domestically (Case, 1991; Luce et al., 2000). McDonald and colleagues (2002, 2004) studied workers in a Montana mine where asbestiform *tremolite* (sodic tremolite) was associated with vermiculite ore. As noted earlier, they found a high risk of MM and concluded that the carcinogenic potency of this asbestiform mineral was similar to crocidolite.

In the province of Quebec, chrysotile has been produced from mines located in and around the towns of Thetford Mines, Asbestos, Black Lake, and East Broughton (Chapter 2). Studies of Quebec chrysotile miners and millers reported since the early 1970s have consistently shown an increased risk of MM (McDonald et al., 1997). However, since some workers had high concentrations of asbestiform tremolite in their lungs (Rowlands et al., 1982) the question arose as to whether the MM were caused by chrysotile or by the *congruent*, tremolite. It has now been shown that the increase in MM risk is manifest only in chrysotile mines, where workers are also exposed to fibrous tremolite (Gibbs, 2001;

McDonald and McDonald, 1995; Rowlands et al., 1982). The risk of MM is higher among the miners and millers in the chrysotile mines at Thetford, compared with those working in the mines at Asbestos. The contamination by fibrous tremolite was higher in the mines at Thetford than at Asbestos as reflected in the lung tissue burdens of men working in these mines (McDonald and McDonald, 1995). Further, in the mines at Thetford, there was a higher risk of MM for the miners and millers in a localized area of five mines, compared with the ten other mines in the region (McDonald and McDonald, 1995, 1997). This corresponds to a fourfold difference in the concentration of tremolite in the lungs of miners in the two areas who died of causes other than MM. Thus, the relatively rare cases of MM are mainly (or perhaps wholly) a result of amphibole contamination. A conclusion that the MM is related to tremolite exposure is consistent with the finding of extremely low rates of the tumor in so-called downstream, that is, secondary industries in which only processed chrysotile is used. The levels of exposure to fibrous tremolite in these industries would be expected to be much lower than encountered by miners and millers. It is even possible that the exposures to tremolite were not the result of low concentration to contaminants of the ore, but resulted from exposure of miners working through rock strata containing tremolite (Gibbs, 2001). Though this remains speculative, it is supported by the high proportion of the MM at Thetford who were miners as opposed to millers.

Since fibrous tremolite can cause MM and is more durable than chrysotile, it is not surprising that there is a risk of MM when miners and millers are exposed to chrysotile ore contaminated with fibrous tremolite from congruent seams or dykes. Nonetheless, the risk associated with pure chrysotile exposure is still a matter of debate in some quarters.

MM has been shown to be associated with exposure to erionite, a fibrous zeolite (Baris et al., 1987; Wagner et al., 1985) and there is limited evidence that the tumor occurs among those exposed to fibrous fluoredenite amphibole (Comba et al., 2003).

Proportional Mortality Ratio (PMR) provides a useful way of comparing the risks for a relatively rare tumor (Table 4.1). However, a justifiable criticism of PMR is that the values increase steeply with the length of follow-up. Hence, comparisons between studies must be made at similar time intervals after first exposure. As would be expected, the severity of exposure influences risk and thus, the PMR. One way to overcome this criticism is to relate risk to level of estimated exposure as done by Hodgson and Darnton (2000) (Table 4.2). They produced models to estimate risks that were nonlinear. The experience of workers in the various industrial sectors listed in Table 4.1 is consistent with the differences in risk depicted in Table 4.2. The study cited in Table 4.2 includes workers with known exposure to chrysotile only, except that the table includes workers at a South Carolina textile plant where crocidolite yarn was used for some years and also includes workers at the Italian Balengero mine where some crocidolite was milled. The risks of MM from exposure to asbestiform tremolite were not determined by Hodgson and Darnton. However, as mentioned earlier, McDonald et al. (2002) reported 285 deaths in a cohort of 406 vermiculite miners exposed to an average concentration of 18 f/mL and 12 MM for a PMR of 4.2%.

Based on their analyses Hodgson and Darnton (2000) reported that the relative MM causing potencies of the commercial asbestos types, crocidolite, amosite, and chrysotile, were in the ratio of 500:100:1, respectively. This estimate assumed that the commercial chrysotile may be *contaminated* by tremolite. More recently, in a draft report prepared for the Environmental Protection Agency, Berman and Crump (2004) concluded that the best estimate of the potency coefficient for chrysotile may be less than 1/750th of that of the amphiboles and "the possibility that pure chrysotile is non-potent for causing mesothelioma cannot be ruled out by the epidemiology data." Yarborough (2006) in a detailed review concluded that, "the review of 71 asbestos cohorts exposed to free asbestos does not support the hypothesis that chrysotile, uncontaminated by amphibolic substances, causes mesothelioma."

Table 4.2 Risk of MM per f/mL-yrs (Adjusted for Age at First Exposure)*

	Expected Mortality per f/mL-yrs (%)
Crocidolite	
United States	0.68
Australia	0.48
South Africa	0.59
Total crocidolite	0.51
Amosite	
United States	0.12
South Africa	0.06
Total amosite	0.10
Chrysotile	
Men—United States[†]	0.0130
Women—United States	0
Italy[†]	0.0025
Canada	0.0009
United States	0
Total chrysotile	0.0010
Total mixed (amphibole and chrysotile)	0.021

* Reported by Hodgson and Darnton (2000)—Occupational Cohorts.
[†] Some crocidolite used.

Hodgson and Darnton (2000) considered only cohort studies. A hospital-based case-control study of MM was reported by Iwatsubo et al. (1998). The RRs were 1.2 (95% CI = 0.8–1.8) for cumulative exposure of 0.001–0.49 f/mL-yrs, 4.2 (95% CI = 2.0–8.8) for 0.5–0.99 f/mL-yrs, 5.2 (95% CI = 3.1–8.8) for 1–9.9 f/mL-yrs, and 8.7 (95% CI = 4.1–18.5) for 10 or more f/mL-yrs. These authors were careful to point out that estimates of cumulative exposure were based on the *subjectivity* of five occupational hygienists who classified jobs in terms of probability, frequency, and intensity of exposure, in the absence of measurements; they expressed the measure inside quotation marks ("f/mL-years"). They did not identify fiber types. They also noted, "The pattern of a dose-response relation is more doubtful at low doses because the uncertainties of exposure evaluations are highest for low doses."

In the general population, not all cases of MM can be attributed to established asbestos exposure. The annual risk of such background of MM cases has been estimated 1–2 per million population (McDonald and McDonald, 1994) and the lifetime risk as about 140–200 per million (HEI-AR, 1991; Hughes and Weill, 1986) or 360 per million based on 1980–2000 US women (Price and Ware, 2004).

Risk of Lung Cancer

Exposure to the commercial amphiboles, amosite, crocidolite, anthophyllite, and chrysotile as well as asbestiform tremolite (soda tremolite) increase LC mortality. For the purposes of risk assessment, it is necessary to relate the observed increase in risk to quantitative measures of exposure. This has been done by many investigators. However, two systematic examinations of large numbers of studies have been carried out in recent years by Lash et al. (1997) and Hodgson and Darnton (2000). Both performed meta-analyses of exposure-response relationships between the RR of LC and cumulative exposure to asbestos. The general differences in approach were as follows:

Lash et al. included 15 cohorts, and fitted the linear dose-response model within each cohort:

$$RR = A(1 + kd)$$

where A is an intercept term, that is the RR for zero exposure, k is the slope, or increase in RR per unit of exposure, and d is the cumulative exposure (f/mL-yrs).

On the other hand, Hodgson and Darnton included 17 cohort studies and fitted the average dose-response effect estimated for each cohort that they defined as

$$R_L = \frac{100 \times (\text{SMR} - 1)}{X}$$

where SMR is the ratio of observed (O) to expected (E) LC deaths for the whole cohort, and X is the mean exposure (f/mL-yrs) of the cohort. R_L is the slope of the relationship and is the percentage excess risk per unit of exposure. That is

$$RR = 1 + \frac{R_L d}{100}$$

The intercept, RR for zero exposure, was taken as 1.

Because Lash et al. (1997) fitted exposure-response relationships within each study, they were able to estimate the intercept, as well as the slope, of the relationship. Hodgson and Darnton (2000) included studies in which only the average exposure was available and assumed that the intercept was unity in order to estimate the slope. On the surface, this might appear to be a reasonable choice because zero exposure would not give rise to an increase in risk. In actual fact, the intercept is quite often not equal to unity because the LC death rates of the reference population may not correspond to the LC death rates of the workers (in the absence of exposure owing to local factors or differences in risk factors such as smoking levels between the workforce and the reference population) (Liddell and Hanley, 1985). The relationship between the slopes in the two formulations is

$$R_L = 100k$$

The cumulative exposure (d) at which the RR (RR = 2) is doubled

$$d(RR = 2) = \frac{100}{R_L} = \frac{1}{k}$$

Lash et al. (1997) concentrated on process (Table 4.3). On the basis of this analysis, they concluded that the risk of LC increases with the degree of processing of the asbestos (ie, as the asbestos moves from mining/milling environment to be incorporated into cement products and textiles, or other manufactured products).

In contrast, Hodgson and Darnton (2000) concentrated on fiber type (Table 4.4) and they found the highest risk was for the amphiboles, crocidolite, and amosite, with a much lower risk for chrysotile, and an intermediate risk for persons exposed to mixed amphibole and chrysotile dusts.

Table 4.3 Estimates of *k* for LC (Increase in RR of LC per f/mL-yrs of Exposure) by Industry from the Meta-Analysis*

	k	*d*(RR = 2)
All studies	0.0026	385
Mining and milling	0.00025	4000
Cement products	0.0034	294
Textile manufacturing	0.0077	130

* From Lash et al. (1997).

Table 4.4 Values of R_L for LC (the Percentage Excess Risk of LC per f/mL-yrs of Exposure) by Fiber Type from the Meta-Analysis*

	R_L	*d*(RR = 2)
Crocidolite	4.2	24
Amosite	5.2	19
Chrysotile	0.062	1613
Mixed	0.47	213

* From Hodgson and Darnton (2000).

The results obtained by these researchers may be compared for the 11 studies common to the two meta-analyses (Table 4.5). When the studies with a R_L of zero are excluded, the range of values is over two orders of magnitude. For six of the studies (nos. 5, 6, 7, 8, 10, and 11) the two meta-analyses gave similar values, and for all the intercepts in the analysis of Lash et al. (1997) were close to unity. However, for some of the other studies, there were large differences. For four of these (1, 2, 4, and 9) the intercepts were greater than 1.5 and correspondingly the slopes defined by Lash et al. (1997) were much less than those found by Hodgson and Darnton (2000). The opposite occurred for study no. 3 where the intercept was only 0.5. In addition, there were only 21 LC deaths in study no. 2 and no reliable exposure-response relationship fits (the 95% confidence interval given by Lash et al. (1997) for 100*k* is from 0 to 25). It is not surprising that the results from the two approaches differ.

The overall conclusions of the analyses also differ in part because of the studies cited in the analyses. Lash et al. (1997) included two chrysotile-mining populations, which meant that once this industry was taken into account, there was no possibility of finding an effect in mining because of fiber type. Hodgson and Darnton included two chrysotile mines, two crocidolite mines (Australia and South Africa), and an amosite mine (South Africa). Of the 19 subgroups analyzed by Hodgson and Darnton (2000), there were three with exposure to crocidolite, two to amosite, five to chrysotile, and nine with mixed exposure to chrysotile and amphibole. For two of the 15 cohorts included by Lash et al. (1997), an exposure-response relationship could not be fitted. One was the Montana vermiculite mine with *contaminating* tremolite. Of the other 12, one involved exposure to amosite, four to chrysotile, and seven mixed exposures to both chrysotile and amphibole, of which five were exposures predominantly to chrysotile. There was less variation in fiber type between the studies included by Lash et al. (1997), compared with those used by Hodgson and Darnton (2000), and consequentially, there was less opportunity to explore differences in effect between fiber types.

Table 4.5 Values of R_L (the Percentage Excess Risk per f/mL-yrs of Exposure) from the Meta-Analyses for the 11 Cohort Studies in Common to the Two Analyses*

			Lash et al.	
		Hodgson and		
Study No	*Reference*	*Darnton R_L*	*100k*	*Intercept*
1	US insulation factory (Seidman et al., 1986)	5.8	0.88	3.3
2	Canada asbestos cement plant (Finkelstein, 1984)	5.2	0.69	3.5
3	US textile factory (McDonald et al., 1983b)	0.8	3.6	0.5
4	German asbestos cement factory (Neuberger and Kundi, 1990)	0.45	0	2.1
5	UK textile factory (men; Peto et al., 1985)	0.37	0.41	1.1
6	US retirees (to 1980 Enterline et al., 1987; to 1973 Henderson and Enterline 1979)	0.21	0.25	1.5
7	US asbestos cement (plant 1; Hughes et al., 1987)	0	0.066	0.9
8	US textile factory (men; Dement et al., 1994)	4.6	2.4	1.3
9	US friction products plant (McDonald et al., 1984)	0.8	0	1.6
10	Canada chrysotile miners and millers (to 1992, Liddell et al., 1997; to 1989, McDonald et al., 1993)	0.06	0.02	1.2
11	Italy chrysotile miners (Piolatto et al., 1990)	0.03	0.02	1.0

* Hodgson and Darnton (2000) and Lash et al. (1997).

As far as chrysotile is concerned, it has been shown that chrysotile can be processed with no detectable increase in LC. This was demonstrated by the study of 1.35×10^4 workers manufacturing friction products at a factory in the north of England (Newhouse and Sullivan, 1989). More important, this population was studied during two time periods; there was no increase in risk of LC during the follow-up periods and when the response to exposure was examined, there was no statistically significant trend. Moreover, at no point on the exposure-response curve was the risk statistically different from zero (Berry and Newhouse, unpublished data). There were 229 LC deaths among men in the follow-up group with an SMR of 103 (95% CI = 90–118) including 143 deaths in the follow-up to 1979 with an SMR of 103 (95% CI = 86–121). Among women, there were 12 LC deaths in the follow-up to 1986 with an SMR of 57 (95% CI = 29–99) including six deaths in the follow-up to 1979 with an SMR of 53 (95% CI 19–116).

Both meta-analyses discussed above included only cohort studies. There have been three case-control studies reported that investigate the relationship between LC and occupational or environmental exposure. Jöckel et al. (1998) included over 1×10^3 LC cases in a study from Germany. For men exposed to asbestos for more than 940 hours the RR of LC was 1.45 after allowing for smoking. The data for the men were analyzed in more detail with respect to exposure by Pohlabeln et al. (2002). Cumulative exposures were estimated from job histories and exposure levels estimated by a panel of industrial hygienists based on their own experience and rules used for compensation in Germany. They found a RR of 1.94 (95% CI = 1.1–3.4) for those with exposure exceeding 10 f/mL-yrs adjusting for smoking. The results "cannot…be interpreted as the effect of the actual cumulative asbestos dose inhaled, as the expert assessment is necessarily imprecise in the absence of any measurement."

A second case-control study (Gustavsson et al., 2000) included all cases of LC in men aged between 40 and 75 years occurring over the period 1985 and 1990 in Stockholm. Of the LC cases, 93% had died at the time of data collection; as a result, information on occupational exposure and smoking was provided by next-of-kin. Two groups of controls were used; a population control and a group matched by mortality. The latter group was included to check for possible bias due to the high proportion of cases for whom information was only available from next-of-kin. Since risk estimates were similar, the two groups of controls were combined. For those with the highest quartile of cumulative exposure (>1.5 f/mL-yrs) the RR of LC was estimated as 1.68 (95% CI = 1.15–2.46), adjusting for smoking and other occupational exposures. A dose-response analysis gave an estimated increase in LC risk of 14% per f/mL-yrs. In a second paper (Gustavsson et al., 2002), the RR at a cumulative dose of 4 f/mL-yrs was estimated to be 1.9 (95% CI = 1.3–2.7) and the estimated cumulative exposure with a RR of 2 was 5 f/mL-yrs (95% CI = 2–50).

A third case-control study was published by Kreienbrock et al. (2001). The main aim of this study was to investigate the association between residential radon exposure and LC, but asbestos exposure was also recorded as a potential confounder. The RR for asbestos exposure was estimated as 1.7 (95% CI = 1.4–2.0) adjusting for smoking. Data from this study was analyzed further by Hauptmann et al. (2002) combining data from the studies of Jöckel et al. (1998) and Kreienbrock et al. (2001). The RR for asbestos exposure was 1.8 (95% CI = 1.2–2.6) for a group with cumulative exposure between 18 and 49 f/mL-yrs, and 2.6 (95% CI = 1.8–3.7) for exposure of 50 or more f/mL-yrs.

These three case-control studies failed to distinguish between amphibole and chrysotile asbestos exposures, and exposure estimates were based on expert opinions (in the absence of measurement data). The two studies conducted in Germany indicate a RR of 2 at between about 10 and 100 f/mL-yrs. For the Swedish study (Gustavsson et al., 2002), the cumulative exposure RR of 2 was estimated to be only 5 f/mL-yrs (although the upper limit of the CI was 50 f/mL-yrs). For whatever reasons, the estimates of risk at low exposure levels from this study are inconsistent with those from a wide range of other studies.

As more evidence accumulates, it is appropriate to review again the exposure-response relationships by combining the new evidence, including information from case-control studies. The findings of these three case-control studies do not alter the earlier conclusions. However, it is important to remember that the studies incorporated in the analyses by Hodgson and Darnton (2000) and by Lash (1997), were based on work histories obtained from records and exposures. Thus, extrapolations into the past were, in large parts, based on measurements of varying degrees of completeness. These three recent studies were not. While the more recent work provides additional evidence, they do not replace the earlier evidence. There is clearly a need for investigations of workers or others from occupations or situations in which documented exposures were lower than in many of the historical cohorts. As in the past, defining study populations and ascertaining cases is relatively easy, but assessing their exposures remains enigmatic.

In studies of occupationally exposed cohorts, confounding will occur when and if there is an association between the severity of exposure to asbestos and the amount of smoking. While this can be dismissed in some cases, by estimating the impact smoking could have on LC risk (Axelson, 1978), lack of smoking information may be a limiting factor in the estimation of LC risk for those exposed to asbestos.

Uncertainties in Risk Estimates

As with all studies involving humans, there are uncertainties. These mainly relate to three key variables: (1) disease outcome, that is, health or biological effect (or a surrogate for that effect), (2) exposure or dose (or a surrogate for the dose or exposure), and (3) confounding factors that otherwise influence the exposure-response relationship.

Disease Outcomes

As noted earlier the usual measure of LC is a death certification. Data for LC have gener- ally been found to be reasonably reliable. However, there are potential biases since workers may have a greater chance of being autopsied. In some studies, *best evidence* appraisals of the cause of death are used. Hodgson and Darnton (2000) chose to use death certificate evidence for their LC analyses to correspond to the reference population rates based on death certificates. Studies using *best evidence* LC data are likely to overestimate risk. In the case of MM, Hodgson and Darnton (2000) used *best evidence* as in the past, the diagnosis of MM was not coded on death certificates. This is acceptable when a reference population is not being used to estimate an expected number of cases. In fact, errors may occur when reference rates for rare diseases are used, especially if the reference popula- tion is not large. When MM was first recognized as a unique tumor, diagnosis presented a major problem. Diagnosis greatly improved when panels of expert pathologists and newer diagnostic techniques were introduced (Consensus Report, 1997; McDonald et al., 1973). Asbestosis is a pathological diagnosis. To carry out studies in life, it is necessary to have clinical criteria, but these have differed in various studies. Pulmonary function studies require standardization and data from appropriately selected reference populations also must be used. Even chest auscultation (a highly subjective clinical observation) can be standardized (Murphy and Sorensen et al., 1973). There is a well-known relatively high degree of variability in the evaluation of chest x-rays. Thus, studies should not be based on single reader's findings. If pathological specimens are used for diagnosis, criteria for diagnosis should be standardized and the pathologist kept *blind* as far as possible. For epidemiological purposes, radiological readings should be done *blind* and an appropriate number of positive and negative films included for evaluation.

Exposure Assessment

The evaluation of exposure is complex but a key consideration in risk assessment. Unfortu- nately, all too often, it is the *weak link* inasmuch as reliable quantitative information is often not available. A variety of technical approaches have been used in various studies to assess airborne dust concentrations (AIA, 1982, 1987; Cralley et al., 1972; Gibbs and LaChance, 1974; HEI-AR, 1991; Richards, 1994; Skidmore and Dufficy, 1983; WHO, 1997).

Since the introduction of the Membrane Filter method in the late 1960s, there have been several changes in the methodology. These changes introduced significant differ- ences in fiber counts. Rickards (1994) reported a concentration of 100 f/mL using the Thermal Precipitator that was converted to 400 f/mL using the Early Membrane Filter method. This figure became 800 f/mL when eyepiece graticule counting was established and changed to 1.6×10^3 f/mL when triacetin clearing of the membrane filter was replaced by acetone clearing. When modern quality control methods and sample density rules were introduced, the fiber concentration became 3200 f/mL.

Host and Environmental Considerations

The third category of parameter influencing risk estimates includes smoking, as well as other host and environmental variables. Selikoff et al. (1968) first reported a synergistic effect between asbestos and smoking in the causation of LC, and this observation was confirmed by Berry et al. (1972). In a later follow-up Berry et al. (1985) found that "overall nonsmokers have a RR of LC due to asbestos exposure 1.8 times that of smokers." More recently, Liddell (2001a) concluded, "the RR of LC from asbestos exposure is about twice as high in nonsmokers as in smokers." His conclusion was not without controversy since in another review, Lee (2001) stated, "asbestos exposure multiplies risk of LC by a similar factor in nonsmokers and smokers." The work of Liddell (2001a) was extended by Berry and Liddell (2004) who concluded, "The excess RR for LC from asbestos exposure is about three times higher in nonsmokers than in smokers," and "If interactions are present the RR from exposure changes only slightly between light and heavy smokers, but is higher (in the former than the latter). The RR estimated from epidemiological studies of a mixed population of nonsmokers and smokers applies to smokers."

In some areas, radon in homes is elevated. While debated, radon and radon daughters are now established carcinogens (Darby et al., 1998). This factor has not been generally taken into account in asbestos risk estimations.

The effect of not taking confounding, or modifying factors into account could lead to either an underestimation or an overestimation of the risk ascribed to asbestos, but an overestimation of risk is more likely, since in practice coexposures tend to correlate positively.

Thresholds of Risk

There are levels of exposure below which asbestosis resulting from exposure does not occur, but estimates of thresholds differ. It is debated whether there is a threshold below which there is no increase in risk of LC and MM (Browne and Gibbs, 1998). A linear dose-response relationship between RR and exposure is often used as "a widely accepted and scientifically reasonable compromise rather than an established scientific principle" (HEI-AR, 1991). Hodgson and Darnton (2000) noted that "direct statistical confirmation of a threshold from human data is virtually impossible," and used a non-threshold model. Browne (2001) criticized these authors, while Liddell (2001b), noted, "nonlinearity is extremely difficult to detect epidemiologically, especially at low levels of exposure."

While it might seem prudent for regulators to assume a linear risk through zero in the absence of proven evidence, it is argued that such an assumption is contrary to what is known about the interaction of asbestos with the respiratory tract. For example, not all fibers in the air are inhaled or penetrate into the lung. It is necessary for fibers to get to the pleura to cause disease, some fibers dissolve and are eliminated and the majority deposit proximally in the respiratory tract. Fibers are coated by biological fluids that may serve to protect the lung. There are DNA repair mechanisms that provide protection in the event genetic damage occurs. Taken together, it is highly improbable that there is a finite risk at close to zero exposure and it seems reasonable to conclude that thresholds exist.

Table 4.6 Epidemiological Studies of MM in Friction Product Workers

	Relative Risk (95% CI)	
Study Reference Source	*Wong, 2001*	*Goodman et al., 2004*
United States (McDonald and McDonald, 1980)	0.91 (0.39–2.13)	0.91 (0.35–2.34)
Canada (Teschke et al., 1997)	0.8 (0.20–2.30)	0.8 (0.20–2.30)
United States (Teta et al., 1983)	0.65 (0.08–5.53)	0.65 (0.08–5.53)
Germany (Woitowitz and Rodelsperger, 1994)	0.87 (0.46–1.64)	0.87 (0.43–1.70)
Spain (Agudo et al., 2000)	0.62 (0.17–2.25)	0.62 (0.11–2.36)
United States (Spirtas et al., 1994)	1.00 (0.60–1.60)	0.82 (0.36–1.80)*
Denmark (Hansen, 1989)[†]	—	0.8 (0.4–1.5)

* Updated in Hessel et al., (2004).
[†] Personal communication to Goodman et al.
From Wong (2001) and Goodman et al., (2004).

There is evidence to support the existence of at least a practical threshold for chrysotile that is a level at which risk is undetected (Browne and Gibbs, 1998). In addition to the studies in which the risks were zero in Table 4.2, there are other studies in which there is no evidence of chrysotile-related MM (Tables 4.1 and 4.6). Berry and Newhouse (1983) and Newhouse and Sullivan (1989) found no chrysotile-related MM in a study involving friction product manufacturing workers followed from 1946 to 1986. They did find crocidolite-related MM. Similar arguments could be made concerning chrysotile and LC. In a study of friction product manufacturers by Berry and Newhouse (1983), there was, as noted earlier, no significant increased in risk of LC with increasing exposure. There is no evidence that automobile brake mechanics (Table 4.6) are at an increased risk of MM due to their work with brake materials manufactured with chrysotile. A proportional mortality study by Hodgson et al. (1997) showed no increase in RR of MM in garage mechanics (PMR approximately 0.33) and Registry studies (Malker et al., 1985; Jarvholm and Brisman, 1988) also failed to show any increased risk. Leigh and Driscoll (2003) claimed increased risk based on a series of cases recorded in the Australian MM Register, but a systematic controlled study has not been carried out. The Registry contains extensive details on cases over about a 20-year period, but does not record details on a comparison population. Misclassification of exposures has also been reported (Kelsh et al., 2007). These factors severely limits conclusions.

There have been two meta-analyses of brake maintenance studies. Wong (2001) carried out such an analysis (Table 4.6) and found an overall RR of 0.90 (CI = 0.66–1.23). Goodman et al. (2004) also carried out a meta-analysis in which studies were classified into two tiers based on quality. The six studies conducted by Wong (2001) were in their top two tiers as well as studies by Hansen (1989) and Hessel et al. (2004). No evidence of an increased risk of MM was found. Wong (2006) reported further on the issues to consider in interpreting the automotive mechanic study result and concluded that automechanics do not have an increased risk of mesothelioma as a result of their brake and clutch work.

Lung cancer risk was evaluated by Goodman and his associates. For tier I and tier II studies the RR were 1.07 (95% CI = 0.88–1.31) and 1.17 (95% CI = 1.01–1.36), and for those studies controlled for smoking, the RR = 1.09 (95% CI = 0.92–1.28). Although some studies showed a small increase in risk of LC among motor vehicle mechanics, the data on balance do not support a conclusion that LC is related to asbestos exposure. Motor vehicle mechanics are exposed to potential lung carcinogens other than asbestos. Laden et al. (2004) concluded, "When examined in aggregate, the evidence did not support an increase in risk of either LC or MM among male automobile mechanics occupationally exposed to asbestos from brake repair."

Among 1.1×10^4 Quebec chrysotile miners and millers born 1891–1920, there was not a single MM case among workers employed for less than 2 years. This is also indicative of a threshold. Exposure levels were extremely high (reaching and exceeding 100 f/mL). In addition, there was no increase in the risk of LC below about 300 mppcf-years of exposure (McDonald et al., 1993). Above that level of exposure, the risk increased in parallel with exposure.

In a recent paper, Price and Ware (2004) argued that the time pattern of cases of MM in women "supports the existence of a threshold exposure and a quantifiable background rate." This argument was based on the observation that the age adjusted MM incidence rate for women had remained fairly constant between 1980 and 2000 at about 4 cases per million per year, corresponding to a lifetime risk of 360 per million.

Peritoneal MM and Chrysotile

Chrysotile asbestos does not increase the risk of peritoneal MM. In studies of Quebec chrysotile miners and millers, MM originating in the peritoneal cavity are not known to have occurred. In other industries where chrysotile was used exclusively, peritoneal MM rarely, if ever, has been diagnosed (Table 4.7). In the analyses by Hodgson and Darnton (2000), the ratio of the slopes for peritoneal and pleural MM were between 2.4 and 3.2, with the risks of peritoneal MM and pleural MM being identical at about 90 f/mL-yrs for crocidolite and 55 f/mL-yrs for amosite. Thus, peritoneal MM appears to develop only when exposure to amphiboles is high (Table 4.1). It seems reasonable to conclude that fibrous tremolite as a "contaminant" is rarely, if ever, found in chrysotile ore in concentrations adequate for exposures to cause primary peritoneal MM.

Predicting Incidence

As shown earlier, the risk of MM depends on (1) the fiber type and its dimensions, (2) duration of exposure, (3) interval of time since first exposure, (4) age at exposure, and (5) rate of elimination of fibers from the lungs. On the basis of estimates made over the past two decades, it is now established that the risk of MM increases with time since first exposure by the power of 3–4.

Equations expressing the relationship between MM incidence I and exposure level C, exposure duration d and time since first exposure t have been derived. The simple model is $I(t) = kC(t^{3.2} - (t - d)^{3.2})$ where $t > d$, k = constant, C = fiber concentration; t = time since start of exposure; d = duration of exposure (Hughes, 1989). The predicted incidence rate depends on the constants k, which have been developed by various authors.

An extension to this model that takes the rate of elimination of fibers from the body into account was suggested by Berry (1991, 1995, 1999). He found that crocidolite is slowly eliminated from the lung at a rate of 10%–15% a year (Berry, 1999).

In this model $I(t) = ce^{-\lambda(t-w)}(t - w)^3$ for $t > w$, where $I(t)$ = incidence at time t since the start of exposure, $c = afd$, where a is a constant; f is the fiber concentration, d = duration of exposure, and λ = elimination rate. Ignoring the lag period, this simplifies to

$$I(t) = ce^{-\lambda t} t^3$$

Table 4.7 Pleural and Peritoneal MM in Chrysotile-Exposed Populations

Study Population	Fiber Type(s)	# Exposed	# Dead	# Pleural	# Peritoneal	% Peritoneal
Mining (McDonald et al., 1997)	Chrysotile (tremolite contamination)	9780	8009	38	0	0
Mining (Piolatto et al., 1990)	Chrysotile but some amphibole milled at mine.	1058	427	2 (Pleural "cancer")	0	0
Textile plant (Hein et al., 2007)	Chrysotile, but also some amphiboles used at various times	3072	1961	3 (But site not specified)		
Textile plant (McDonald et al., 1983a,b)	Chrysotile, but also some amphiboles used at various times	2543	863	0	1 (Not confirmed by autopsy)	
Products factory (Weiss, 1977)	Chrysotile	264	66	0	0	0
Cement plant (Thomas et al., 1982)	Chrysotile and crocidolite before 1935	2970	351	2 (But exposed in period when crocidolite used)	0	0
Friction products (McDonald et al., 1984)	Chrysotile	3641	1267	0	0	0
Friction products (Newhouse and Sullivan, 1989)	Chrysotile, but crocidolite used in two specific time periods	13,450	2577	13 (None related to chrysotile exposure)	0	0
Gas mask workers (Acheson et al., 1982)	Chrysotile	570	177	(Reportedly also exposed to crocidolite)*	0	0
Cement manufacturing workers (Hughes et al., 1987)	Chrysotile and crocidolite	6931	2143	10	0	0
Cement products plant (Gardner et al., 1986)	Chrysotile	2167	486	(Not considered to be linked to exposure at the plant)*	0	0
Cement products plant (Ohlson and Hogstedt, 1985	Predominantly chrysotile	1176	220	0	0	0
Textile plant (Peto et al., 1985)	Chrysotile and crocidolite	3211	1113	11	0	0
Asbestos cement plant (Raffn et al., 1989)	Chrysotile only until 1946 then amphiboles introduced	8580	1346	12	1	0.07

* Peritoneal mesothelioma occurred in a man who was also exposed to asbestos at another factory.

Applying both the simple model and the elimination model, Berry (1991) used the observed number of MM to 1986 to predict the numbers of MM expected to occur at the Australian Wittenoom crocidolite mine and mill during the period 1987–2000. There was a good agreement with the observed number of cases when the prediction was based on the elimination model (Berry et al., 2004). However, the predictions based on the simple model were over estimates, thus indicating it is important to take the elimination of asbestos from the lungs into account when predicting MM risks.

Risk after Environmental Exposure

While most of the adverse health effects following exposure to asbestos are suffered by those exposed occupationally, there is no doubt that MM occurs after nonoccupational amphibole asbestos exposure (Wagner et al., 1960; Nolan et al., 2006; Newhouse and Thompson, 1965).

Reid et al. (2007) reported 67 MM cases in a cohort of over 4.8×10^3 residents of Wittenoon, Western Australia who had never worked for a mining company.

There have been several efforts to estimate risks due to the various asbestos types. Nicholson (1986), whose work was used by the USEPA, developed values of K_L, the fractional increase in LC risk per f/mL-yrs for 14 cohorts. These data were examined in the HEI-AR (1999) report. It was concluded that the analysis was subject to substantial errors. The estimates based on the various studies by Nicholson are shown in Table 4.8. When examined in relation to industry, it is immediately obvious that the values for the textile sector are different from the others. It is also evident that sectors of industry using large quantities of amphibole are different from nontextile sectors not using amphibole. Thus, risk estimates for LC are likely to be unreliable if fiber types are not taken into account.

The extent to which the US Environment Protection Agency (EPA) 1986 model (Nicholson, 1986) predicted MM (Camus et al., 2002) and LC risk was examined by in a study of women living in two Quebec chrysotile asbestos mining communities over the period 1970–1989. The average cumulative exposure after conversion to an occupational equivalent exposure of 40 hours per week was estimated to be 105 f/mL-yrs. The EPA model for MM, based on risk parameters derived from mixed fiber exposures, predicted that there should be 150 cases (range 30–750) of MM in the Quebec town of Asbestos. In fact, there was one peritoneal MM observed. On the basis of the same model, it was predicted that 500 (range 500–2500) MM would occur in the town of Thetford. In fact, 10 pleural MM were found. The Environmental Protection Agency models were clearly inappropriate for this situation because of the difference in MM risk between chrysotile and amphibole. Hodgson and Darnton (2000) estimated that the risk of MM would be 9×10^{-4} per f/mL-yrs for Quebec chrysotile miners and millers. Using this model and assuming linearity, the risk of MM would have been 0.0009 cum exp = 0.09%, which means that less than one death from MM would be predicted to occur at Thetford and at Asbestos, respectively. Hence, the Hodgson and Darton (2000) estimates appear to be close to reality in this situation.

As far as LC was concerned, there were 71 observed deaths due to LC, compared with 71.4 expected (Camus et al., 1998). Predictions based on an Environmental Protection Agency model (RR = 1 + 0.01 cum exp) gave a RR of 2 and 146 LC deaths (an excess of 75). Again, it is evident that the model was inappropriate. When the risk estimate for the Quebec mining and milling industry reported by Hodgson and Darnton was applied using their model (RR = 1 + 0.0006 cum exp), the predicted RR was 1.06, an indication

Table 4.8 K_L Factor Estimated by Various Organizations and Including the Values Proposed by Nicholson for EPA

Study	Percent Increase in Lung Cancer per f/mL-yr					Fibre Types/Sector
	EPA	CPSC	NRC	ORC	HSC	
Dement et al. (1983b)*	2.8	2.3	5.3	4.2		Chrysotile (some amphibole)/textile
McDonald et al. (1983a)	2.5				1.25	Chrysotile (some amphibole)/textile
Peto et al. (1985)	1.1	1.0	0.8	1.0	0.54	Chrysotile (also amphibole)/textile
McDonald et al. (1983b)	1.4					Mixed/textile
Berry and Newhouse (1983)	0.058	0.06		0.058		Chrysotile (some amphibole) friction
McDonald et al. (1984)	0.010					Chrysotile/friction
McDonald et al. (1980)	0.06	0.06	0.06	0.02–0.046		Chrysotile/mining
Nicholson et al. (1979)	0.17	0.12	0.15			Chrysotile/mining
Seidman et al. (1986)	4.3	6.8	9.1			Amosite/insulation
Amphibole	0.75	1.0	1.7	1.0		Mixed/insulation
Henderson and Enterline (1979)	0.49	0.50	0.3	0.069		Mixed fiber/products
Weill et al. (1979)	0.53	0.31				Chrysotile (some amphibole)/ asbestos cement
Finkelstein (1983)	6.7	4.8		4.2		Mixed/asbestos products
Newhouse and Berry (1979)						
Males			1.3			Mixed/asbestos products
Females			8.4			Mixed/asbestos products

* Estimate for textiles from Hein et al., 2007 = 1.98% per f/mL-yr.
Modified from HEI-AR (1991).

that 76 workers would die of LC (ie, an excess of 5 LC deaths). The risk estimate based on the work of Lash et al. (RR = 1 + 0.00025 cum exp) gave a RR of 1.025 predicting 73 LC deaths (ie, an excess of 2 LC deaths). Both these estimates are in agreement with the observations of Camus et al. (1998). Whether or not there is an actual excess risk of LC deaths at such low levels of RR is unknown, but highly doubtful.

Risk at Low Exposure

The environmental exposure situations considered in the previous section were not of a low order of magnitude. They demonstrate that exposure to crocidolite asbestos in a non-occupational setting can result in MM. They also show that in the case of chrysotile, the MM risk for the general population even in a community where even today persons are nonoccupationally exposed to chrysotile (Marier et al., 2007) is absent or nondetectable.

This conclusion is supported by a review of 123 MM cases in South Africa where it turned out that 23 had worked in a Cape crocidolite mine, 3 at the Penge amosite mine, 3 on mines producing Transvaal amosite and crocidolite, and 1 on a Transvaal crodicolite mine and 22 that resulted exclusively from environmental exposure of which 20 had environmental exposure to Cape crocidolite. The authors noted that there was a paucity of cases linked to amosite and no convincing case to chrysotile (Rees et al., 1999). There are situations in which appreciable proportions of the population may be exposed to low levels through the widespread use of asbestos. One such example arises when asbestos cement products are used in building construction. Since asbestos cement often incorporates some amphibole, one must ask what the consequent risk is to those who occupy office buildings and schools. Exposure levels are typically low. HEI-AR (1991) calculated an average value of 5×10^{-4} f/mL for schools containing asbestos cementitious materials, and 2×10^{-4} f/mL for exposure in public buildings. In both cases higher values (of 10 times these levels) occurred in 5% of schools or buildings studied by the Environmental Protection Agency. These data contrast with the current permissible occupational exposure for all fiber types in the United States of 0.1 f/mL.

There have been several attempts to estimate the risk at such low levels (ie, Doll and Peto, 1985; HEI, 1991; Hodgson and Darnton, 2000; Hughes and Weill, 1986; Nicholson, 1986) and all depend on extrapolation of exposure-response relationships derived from occupational settings to much lower levels. Hughes and Weill estimated that there would be five extra deaths per million among school children (0.6 LC, 4.4 MM) owing to 6 years' exposure to mixed fibers at a concentration of 1×10^{-3} f/mL. HEI-AR (1991) predicted between 6 and 60 lifetime premature cancer deaths per million school children exposed from age 5 to 18 years to levels of 5×10^{-4} to 5×10^{-3} f/mL, and 4 to 40 premature cancer deaths after exposure in a public building from age 25 to 45 years to levels of 2×10^{-4} to 2×10^{-3} f/mL. Hodgson and Darnton (2000) considered lifetime risks (to age 80 years) short-term exposure (up to 5 years) from age 30 for different levels of exposure to the different fiber types. For a cumulative exposure of 1.0×10^{-2} f/mL-yrs to crocidolite, the best estimates were 20 deaths due to MM per 1×10^5 workers exposed (range from 2 to 100 for the lowest to the highest estimates), and for amosite the corresponding estimates were 3 (range <1–20). For LC attributable to amphibole exposure, the lifetime risk was estimated to be in the range of <1–3 excess LC deaths per 1×10^5. The estimated risks for chrysotile were much lower and probably insignificant with the highest arguable estimate being one case of MM per 1×10^5 persons exposed, and a lower risk for bronchogenic carcinoma. These calculations yield theoretical numerical data, based on extrapolations and do not address biological considerations of disease mechanisms.

Future Risk of MM

The long lag time (so-called latency period; Chapter 8) between exposure and the occurrence of MM dictates that there are occupational groups in which deaths due to MM are still occurring today. Clinicians and pathologists in practice now are reminded of this fact all too often. Several investigators have attempted to predict the number of MM likely to occur in the future either for a specific occupational group such as the miners and millers at Wittenoom (Berry, 1991; de Klerk et al., 1989), or in national populations (ie, Leigh and Driscoll, 2003 for Australia; Peto et al., 1999 for Europe; Price and Ware, 2004 for the United States; Segura et al., 2003 for the Netherlands). Several problems influence the calculation of estimates of the number of MM that will occur in the future worldwide, as discussed in detail in Chapter 16.

References

ACGIH (1992–1993). *Threshold Limit Values for Chemical Substances and Physical Agents and Biological Exposure Indices.* Cincinnati OH.

Acheson ED, Gardner MJ. The ill effects of asbestos on health. In: *Asbestos: Final Report of the Advisory Committee Vol. 2.* London: HMSO; 1979:7–83.

Acheson ED, Gardner MJ, Pippard EC, Grime LP. Mortality of two groups of women who manufactured gas masks from chrysotile and crocidolite asbestos: a 40 year follow-up. *Br J Ind Med.* 1982;39:344–348.

Acheson ED, Gardner MJ, Winter PD, Bennett C. Cancer in a factory using amosite asbestos. *Int J Epidemiol.* 1984:13:3–10.

Agudo A, Gonzalez CA, Bleda MJ, et al. Occupation and risk of malignant pleural mesothelioma: A Case-Control study in Spain. *Am J Ind Med.* 2000;37:159–168.

AIA (Asbestos International Association) (1979: Amended 1 January 1982). AIA Health and Safety Publication Recommended Technical Method No 1 (RTM1).

AIA: AIA Health and Safety Publication Recom mended Technical Method No 1A (RTM1A). Dust monitoring strategy for individual exposure assessment, 1987.

Armstrong BK, de Klerk NH, Musk AW, Hobbs MST. Mortality in miners and millers of crocidolite in Western Australia. *Br J Ind Med.* 1988;45:5–13.

Axelson O. Aspects on confounding in occupational health epidemiology. *Scand J Work Environ Health.* 1978;4:98–102.

Ayer HE, Lynch JR, Fanney JH. A Comparison of Impinger and Membrane filter techniques for evaluating air samples in asbestos plants. *NY Acad of Sci.* 1965;132:274–287.

Baris I, Simonato L, Artvinli M, et al. Epidemiological and Environmental Evidence of the Health effects of exposure to erionite fibers: A four year study in the Cappadocian Region of Turkey. *Int J Cancer.* 1987;39:10–17.

Berman DW, Crump KS. *Final Draft: Technical Support Document for a protocol to assess asbestos related risk. Prepared for the Office of Solid Waste and Emergency Response.* Washington: US Environmental Protection Agency; 2004.

Bernstein DM, Rogers R, Smith P. The biopersistence of Canadian chrysotile asbestos following inhalation. *Inhal Toxicol.* 2003;15:1387–1419.

Bernstein DM, Rogers RA, Thevenaz P. The inhalation biopersistence and morphologic lung disposition of pure chrysotile asbestos in rats. Presented at: 7th International Symposium on Particle toxicology; October 13–15, 1999; Maastricht, Netherlands.

Berry G, Liddell FD. The interaction of asbestos and smoking in lung cancer—a modified measure of effect. *Ann Occup Hyg.* 2004;48:459–462.

Berry G, Newhouse ML. Mortality of workers manufacturing friction materials using asbestos. *Br J Ind Med.* 1983;40:1–7.

Berry G, de Klerk NH, Reid A, et al. Malignant pleural and peritoneal mesotheliomas in former miners and millers of crocidolite at Wittenoom, Western Australia. *Occup Environ Med.* 2004;61:1–3.

Berry G, Gilson JC, Holmes S, Lewinsohn HC, Roach SA. Asbestosis: a study of dose-response relationships in an asbestos textile factory. *Br J Ind Med.* 1979;36:98–112.

Berry G, Newhouse ML, Antonis P. Combined effect of asbestos and smoking on mortality from lung cancer and mesothelioma in factory workers. *Br J Ind Med* 1985;42:12–18.

Berry G, Newhouse ML, Turok M. Combined effect of asbestos exposure and smoking on mortality from lung cancer in factory workers. *Lancet.* 1972;2:476–479.

Berry G. Environmental mesothelioma incidence, time since exposure to asbestos and level of exposure. *Environmetrics.* 1995;6:221–228.

Berry G. Models for mesothelioma incidence following exposure to fibers in terms of timing and duration of exposure and the biopersistence of the fibers. *Inhal Toxicol.* 1999;11:111–130.

Berry G. Prediction of mesothelioma, lung cancer and asbestosis in former Wittenoom asbestos workers. *Br J Ind Med.* 1991;48:793–802.

British Occupational Hygiene Society. Hygiene standards for chrysotile asbestos dust. *Ann Occup Hyg.* 1968;11:47–69.

Browne K, Gibbs GW. Chrysotile asbestos-thresholds of risk. In: Chiyotani K, Hosoda Y, Aizawa Y, eds. *Advances in the Prevention of Occupational Respiratory Diseases.* Elsevier Science BV, 1998:304–309.

Browne K. The quantitative risks of mesothelioma and lung cancer in relation to asbestos exposure (letter to editor). *Ann Occup Hyg.* 2001;45:327–329.

Camus M, Siemiatycki J, Meek B. Non-occupational exposure to chrysotile asbestos and the risk of lung cancer. *NEJM.* 1998;338:1565–1571.

Camus M, Siemiatycki J, Case BW, Desy M, Richardson L, Campbell S. Risk of mesothelioma among women living near chrysotile mines vs US EPA asbestos risk model: preliminary findings. *Ann Occup Hyg.* 2002;46(Suppl. 1):95–98.

Case BW. Health effects of tremolite. *Ann NY Acad Sci.* 1991;643:491–504.

Comba P, Gianfagno A, Paoletti L. Pleural mesothelioma cases in Biancavilla are related to a new fluoroedenite fibrous amphibole. *Arch Environ Health.* 2003;58:229–232.

Consensus report. Asbestos, asbestosis, and cancer: the Helsinki criteria for diagnosis and attribution. *Scand J Work Environ Health.* 1997;23:311–316.

Cralley LJ, Ayer HE, Amoudru C, et al. Evaluation of asbestos exposures in the working environment. *Ind Med.* 1972;41:28–30.

Darby A, Whitley E, Silcocks P, et al. Risk of lung cancer associated with residential radon exposure in south-west England: as case-control study. *Br J Cancer.* 1998;78:394–400.

Davis JM. Other diseases in animals. In: Gibbs GW, Valic F, Browne K, eds. *Health Risks Associated with Chrysotile Asbestos. Ann Occup Hyg.* 1994;38:399–426.

de Klerk NH, Armstrong BK, Musk AW, Hobbs MS. Predictions of future cases of asbestos-related disease among former miners and millers of crocidolite in Western Australia. *Med J Aust.* 1989;151:616–620.

Doll R, Peto J. *Asbestos: Effects on Health of Exposure to Asbestos.* London: Health and Safety Commission, HMSO; 1985.

Dreessen WC, Dalla Valle JM, Edwards TI, et al. A study of asbestosis in the asbestos textile industry. *Publ Hlth Bul, Washington,* No 241, 1938.

Dunnigan J, Muhle H. Discussion. In: Gibbs GW, Valic F, Browne K, eds. *Health Risks Associated with Chrysotile Asbestos. Ann Occup Hyg.* 1994;38:399–426.

Enterline PE, Hartley J, Henderson V. Asbestos and cancer: a cohort followed up to death. *Br J Ind Med.* 1987;44: 396–401.

Finkelstein MM. Mortality among employees of an Ontario asbestos-cement factory. *Am Rev Respir Dis.* 1984;129:754–761.

Gardner MJ, Winter PD, Pannett B, Powell CA. Follow-up study of workers manufacturing chrysotile asbestos cement products. *Br J Ind Med.* 1986;43:726–732.

Gibbs GW, DuToit RSJ. Environmental considerations in surveillance of asbestos miners and millers. In: Selikoff IJ, Hammond EC, eds. *Health Hazards of Asbestos Exposure. Ann NY Acad Sci.* 1979;330:163–178.

Gibbs GW, LaChance M. Dust-fibre relationships in Quebec Chrysotile Industry. *Arch Environ Health.* 1974;28:69–71.

Gibbs GW. Health effects associated with mining and milling chrysotile asbestos in Quebec and the role of tremolite. In: *The health effects of chrysotile asbestos: Contribution of Science to Risk-Management Decisions.* The Canadian Mineralogist Special publication 5; 2001:165–175.

Goodman M, Teta MJ, Hessel PA, et al. Mesothelioma and lung cancer among motor vehicle mechanics: a meta-analysis. *Ann Occup Hyg.* 2004;48:309–326.

Gustavsson P, Jakobsson R, Nyberg F, Pershagen G, Järup L, Schéele P. Occupational exposure and lung cancer risk: a population-based case-referent study in Sweden. *Am J Epidemiol.* 2000;152:32–40.

Gustavsson P, Nyberg F, Pershagen G, Schéele P, Jakobsson R, Plato N. Low-dose exposure to asbestos and lung cancer: dose-response relations and interaction with smoking in a population-based case-referent study in Stockholm, Sweden. *Am J Epidemiol.* 2002;155:1016–1022.

Hansen ES. Mortality of Auto Mechanics. A ten year follow-up. *Scand J Work Environ Health.* 1989;15:43–46.

Hauptmann M, Pohlabeln H, Lubin JH, et al. The exposure-time-response relationship between occupational asbestos exposure and lung cancer in two German case-control studies. *Am J Ind Med.* 2002;41:89–97.

HEI-AR (Health Effects Institute-Asbestos Research). *Asbestos in public and Commercial Buildings.* Cambridge MA: Health Effects Institute; 1991.

Hein MJ, Stayner LT, Lehman E, Dement JM. Follow-up study of chrysotile textile workers: cohort mortality and exposure-response. *Occ Environ Med.* 2007;64:616–625.

Henderson VL, Enterline PE. Asbestos exposure: factors associated with excess cancer and respiratory disease mortality. *Ann NY Acad Sci.* 1979;330:117–126.

Hessel PA, Teta MJ, Goodman M, Lau E. Mesothelioma among brake mechanics: an expanded analysis of a case-control study. *Risk Analysis.* 2004;24:547–552.

Hodgson JT, Darnton A. The quantitative risks of mesothelioma and lung cancer in relation to asbestos exposure. *Ann Occup Hyg.* 2000;44:565–601.

Hodgson JT, Peto J, Jones JR, Matthews FE. Mesothelioma mortality in Britain: Patterns by Birth Cohort and Occupation. *Ann Occup Hyg.* 1997;41: 129–133.

Hughes JM, Weill H, Hammad YY. Mortality of workers employed in two asbestos cement manufacturing plants. *Br J Ind Med.* 1987;44:161–174.

Hughes JM, Weill H. Asbestos exposure—quantitative assessment of risk. *Am Rev Respir Dis.* 1986;133:5–13.

Hughes JM. *The Derivation and use of Asbestos Risk estimates.* In: *Proceedings—Symposium on Health Aspects of Exposure to Asbestos in Buildings 14–16 December 1988.* Cambridge: Harvard University; 1989:267–277.

Iwatsubo Y, Pairon JC, Boutin C, et al. Pleural mesothelioma: dose-response relation at low levels of asbestos exposure in a French population-based case-control study. *Am J Epidemiol.* 1998;148:133–142.

Jarvholm B, Brisman J. Asbestos associated tumours in car mechanics. *Br J Ind Med.* 1988;45:645–646.

Jarvholm B, Sanden A. Lung cancer and mesothelioma in the pleura and peritoneum among Swedish insulation workers. *Occup Environ Med.* 1998;55:766–770.

Jöckel K-H, Ahrens W, Jahn I, Pohlabeln H, Bolm-Audorff U. Occupational risk factors for lung cancer: a case-control study in West Germany. *Int J Epidemiol.* 1998;27:549–560.

Karjalainen A, Meurman LO, Pukkala E. Four cases of mesothelioma among Finnish anthophyllite miners. *Occup Environ Med.* 1994;51:212–215.

Kelsh MA, Craven VA, Teta MJ, Mowat FS, Goodman M. Mesothelioma in vehicle mechanics: is the risk different for Australians? *Occup Med.* 2007;57(8):581–589.

Kohyama N, Suzuki Y. Analysis of asbestos fibers in lung parenchyma, pleural plaques and mesothelioma tissues of North American Insulation workers. *Ann NY Acad Sci.* 1991;643:27–52.

Kreienbrock L, Kreuzer M, Gerken M, et al. Case-control study on lung cancer and residential radon in Western Germany. *Am J Epidemiol.* 2001;153:42–52.

Laden F, Stampfer MJ, Walker AM. Lung cancer and mesothelioma among male automobile mechanics: a review. *Rev Environ Health* 2004;19:39–61.

Lash TL, Crouch EA, Green LC. A meta-analysis of the relation between cumulative exposure to asbestos and relative risk of lung cancer. *Occup Environ Med* 1997;54:254–263.

Lee PN. Relation between exposure to asbestos and smoking jointly and the risk of lung cancer. *Occup Environ Med* 2001;58:145–153.

Leigh J, Driscoll T. Malignant mesothelioma in Australia, 1945–2002. *Int J Occup Environ Hlth.* 2003;9:206–217.

Levin JL, McLarty JW, Hurst GA, et al. Tyler asbestos workers: mortality experience in a cohort exposed to amosite. *Occup Environ Med.* 1998;55:155–160.

Liddell D. The quantitative risks of mesothelioma and lung cancer in relation to asbestos exposure (letter to editor). *Ann Occup Hyg.* 2001b;45:329–335.

Liddell FD, Hanley JA. Relations between asbestos exposure and lung cancer SMRs in occupational cohort studies. *Br J Ind Med* 1985;42:389–396.

Liddell FD, Gibbs GW, McDonald JC. Radiological changes and fiber exposure in chrysotile workers aged 60–69 years at Thetford Mines. *Ann Occup Hyg.* 1982;26:889–898.

Liddell FD, McDonald AD, McDonald JC. The 1891–1920 cohort of Quebec chrysotile miners and millers: development form 1904 and mortality to 1992. *Ann Occup Hyg.* 1997;41:13–36.

Liddell FD. The interaction of asbestos and smoking in lung cancer. *Ann Occup Hyg.* 2001a; 45:341–356.

Liddell FDK, Thomas DC, Gibbs GW, McDonald JC. Fiber exposure and mortality from pneumoconiosis, respiratory and abdominal malignances in chrysotile production in Quebec 1926–1975. *Ann Acad Med.* 1984;13(Suppl.): 340–344.

Luce D, Bugel I, Goldberg P, et al. Environmental exposure to tremolite and respiratory cancer in Caledonia. A case-control study. *Am J Epidemiol.* 2000;151:259–265.

Malker HS, McLaughlin JK, Malker BK, et al. Occupational risks for pleural mesothelioma in Sweden. *J Natl Cancer Inst.* 1985;74:561–566.

Marier M, Charney W, Rousseau R, Lanthier R, Raalte JV. Exploratory sampling of asbestos in residences near thetford mines: the public health threat in Quebec. *Int J Occup Environ Health.* 2007;13:386–397.

McDonald AD, McDonald JC. Malignant mesothelioma in North America. *Cancer.* 1980;46:1650–1656.

McDonald AD, McDonald JC. Mesothelioma after crocidolite exposure during gas mask manufacture. *Environ Research.* 1978;17:340–346.

McDonald AD, Case BW, Churg A, et al. Mesothelioma in Quebec chrysotile miners and millers: Epidemiology and Aetiology. *Ann Occup Hyg.* 1997;41:707–709.

McDonald AD, Fry JS, Woolley AJ, McDonald JC. Dust exposure and mortality in an American chrysotile textile plant. *Br J Ind Med.* 1983a;40:361–367.

McDonald AD, Fry JS, Woolley AJ, McDonald JC. Dust exposure and mortality in an American factory using chrysotile, amosite, and crocidolite in mainly textile manufacture. *Br J Ind Med.* 1983b;40:368–374.

McDonald AD, Magner D, Eyssen G. Primary Malignant Mesothelial Tumors in Canada. A pathologic review by the mesothelioma panel of the Canadian Tumor Reference Centre. Asbestos-Related Health Research Publications 1965–1984, Vol. 1, pp. 869–876, 1973.

McDonald J, McDonald A. Mesothelioma: is there a background? In: Bignon J, Jaurand M-C, eds. *The Mesothelial Cell and Mesothelioma.* New York, Basel, Hong Kong: Marcel Dekker; 1994:37–45.

McDonald JC, McDonald AD. Chrysotile, tremolite and carcinogenicity. *Ann Occup Hyg.* 1997;41:699–705.

McDonald JC, McDonald AD. Chrysotile, tremolite and mesothelioma. *Science.* 1995;267:775–776.

McDonald JC, Gibbs GW, Oakes D. Radiographic response to cumulative chrysotile fiber exposure in production workers 8–29 years after first employment. School of Occup Hlth, McGill University, Montreal, Canada, Abstract 26.2, 1984; 219.

McDonald JC, Harris J, Armstrong B. Cohort mortality study of Vermiculite miners exposed to fibrous talc: an update. *Ann Occup Hyg.* 2002;46(Suppl. 1):93–94.

McDonald JC, Harris J, Armstrong B. Mortality in a cohort of vermiculite miners exposed to fibrous amphibole in Libby, Montana. *Occup Environ Med.* 2004;61:363–366.

McDonald JC, Harris JM, Berry G. Sixty years on: the price of assembling military gas masks in 1940. *Occup Environ Med.* 2006;63:852–855.

McDonald JC, Liddell FD, Dufresne A, McDonald AD. The 1891–1920 birth cohort of Quebec chrysotile miners and millers: Mortality 1976–88. *Br J Ind Med.* 1993;50:1073–1081.

McDonald JC, Sebastien P, Armstrong B. Radiological survey of past and present vermiculite miners exposed to tremolite. *Brit J Ind Med.* 1986;43:445–449.

McDonald JC. Aspects of the Asbestos Standard. School of Occup Hlth, McGill University, Montreal, Quebec Canada. *Occup Lung Disease*, J. Ber, L. Gee, W. Keith, C. Morgan and

Stuart M. Brooks (eds.). Raven Press, New York. Asbestos-Related Health Research Publications 1965–1984, Vol. 2, 1984; 139–149.

Merewether ERA, Price CW. *Report on Effects of Asbestos Dust on the Lungs and Dust Suppression in the Asbestos Industry.* London, HMSO, 1930.

Meurman LO, Pukkala E, Hakama M. Incidence of cancer among anthophyllite asbestos miners in Finland. *Occup Environ Med.* 1994;51:421–425.

Murphy RLH, Sorensen K. Chest auscultation in the diagnosis of pulmonary asbestosis. *J Occup Med.* 1973;15:272–276.

Neuberger M, Kundi M. Individual asbestos exposure: smoking and mortality—a cohort study in the asbestos cement industry. *Br J Ind Med.* 1990;47:615–620.

Newhouse ML, Berry G. Patterns of mortality in asbestos factory workers in London. *Ann NY Acad Sci.* 1979;330:53–60.

Newhouse ML, Sullivan KR. A mortality study of workers manufacturing friction materials: 1941–1986. *Br J Ind Med.* 1989;46:176–179.

Newhouse ML, Thompson H. Mesothelioma of pleura and peritoneum following exposure to asbestos in the London area. *Br J Ind Med.* 1965;22:261–269.

Nicholson WJ, Selikoff IJ, Seidan H. Long-term mortality experience of chrysotile miners and millers in Thetford mines, Quebec. *Ann NY Acad Sci.* 1979;330:11–21.

Nicholson WJ. Airborne Asbestos Health Assessment Update. US Environmental Protection Agency, EPA-600/8–84/003F. Office of Health and Environmental Assessment, US Environmental Protection Agency, Washington DC, 1986.

Nolan RP, Ross M, Nord GL, et al. Asbestos fiber type and mesothelioma risk in the Republic of South Africa. *Clay Science.* 2006;12 Supplement 2:223–227.

Oberdoerster G. Macrophage-associated responses to chrysotile. In: Gibbs GW, Valic F, Browne K, eds. *Health Risks Associated with Chrysotile Asbestos. Ann Occup Hyg* 1994;38:399–426.

Ohlson CG, Hogstedt C. Lung cancer among asbestos cement workers. A Swedish cohort study and a review. 1985; 42:397–402.

Peto J, Decarli A, La Vecchia C, Levi F, Negri E. The European mesothelioma epidemic. *Br J Cancer.* 1999;79:666–672.

Peto J, Doll R, Hermon C, Binns W, Clayton R, Goffe T. Relationship of mortality to measures of environmental asbestos pollution in an asbestos textile factory. *Ann Occup Hyg.* 1985;29:305–355.

Piolatto G, Negri E, La Vecchia C, Pira E, Decarli A, Peto J. An update of cancer mortality among chrysotile asbestos miners in Balangero, Northern Italy. *Br J Ind Med.* 1990;47:810–814.

Pohlabeln H, Wild P, Schill W, et al. Asbestos fiber years and lung cancer: a two phase case-control study with expert exposure assessment. *Occup Environ Med.* 2002;59:410–414.

Price B, Ware A. Mesothelioma trends in the United States: an update based on surveillance, epidemiology, and end results program data from 1973 through 2003. *Am J Epidemiol.* 2004;159:107–112.

Raffn E, Lynge E, Juel K, Korsgaard B. Incidence of cancer and mortality among employees in the asbestos cement industry in Denmark. *Br J Ind Med.* 1989;46:90–96.

Reid A, Berry G, De Klerk N, Hansen J, Heyworth J, Ambrosini G, Fritschi L, Olsen N, Merler E, Musk AW. Age and sex differences in malignant mesothelioma after residential exposure to blue asbestos (crocidolite). *Chest.* 2007;131:376–382.

Rees D, Goodman K, Fourie E, Chapman R, Blignaut C, Bachhmann MO, Myers J. Asbestos exposure and mesothelioma in South Africa. *S Afr Med J.* 1999;89:627–634.

Rickards AL. Levels of workplace exposure. *Ann Occup Hyg.* 1994;38:469–475.

Rogers A. An evaluation of the exposure criteria and lung fiber burden associated with the Helsinki Criteria and its applicability to Australia. Dust Diseases Board of New South Wales Research Report, November, 2001.

Rossiter CE, Bristol LJ, Cartier PH, et al. Radiographic changes in chrysotile asbestos mine and mill workers of Quebec. *Arch Environ Health.* 1972;24:388–400.

Rowlands N, Gibbs GW, McDonald AD. Asbestos fibres in the lungs of chrysotile miners and millers-a preliminary report. *Ann Occup Hyg.* 1982;26:411–415.

Segura O, Burdorf A, Looman C. Update of predictions of mortality from pleural mesothelioma in the Netherlands. *Occup Environ Med.* 2003;60:50–55.

Seidman H, Selikoff IJ, Gelb SK. Mortality experience of amosite asbestos factory workers: dose-response relationships 5 to 40 years after onset of short-term work exposure. *Am J Ind Med.* 1986;10:479–514.

Selikoff IJ, Seidman H. Asbestos-associated deaths among insulation workers in the United States and Canada, 1967–1987. *Ann NY Acad Sci.* 1991;643:1–14.

Selikoff IJ, Hammond CE, Seidman H. Mortality experience of insulation workers in the United States and Canada, 1943–1976. *Ann NY Acad Sci.* 1979a;330:91–116.

Selikoff IJ, Hammond EC, Churg J. Asbestos exposure, smoking, and neoplasia. *JAMA.* 1968; 204:106–112.

Selikoff IJ, Lilis R, Nicholson WJ. Asbestos disease in United States shipyards. *Ann NY Acad Sci.* 1979b;330:295–311.

Skidmore JE, Dufficy CL. Environmental history of a factory producing friction material. *Bt J Ind Med.* 1983;40:8–12.

Sluis-Cremer GK, Liddell FDK, Logan WPD, Bezuidenhout BN. The mortality of amphibole miners in South Africa 1946–1980. *Br J Ind Med.* 1992;49:566–575.

Spirtas R, Heineman EF, Bernstein L, et al. Malignant mesothelioma: attributable risk of asbestos exposure. *OEM.* 1994;51:804–811.

Talcott J, Thurber W, Kantor A, et al. Excess lung cancers and mesotheliomas in a cohort of manufacturers of asbestos-containing cigarette filters. *N Engl J Med.* 1989;321:1220–1223.

Teschke K, Morgan MS, Checkoway H, et al. Mesothelioma surveillance to locate sources of exposure to asbestos. *Can J Publ Health.* 1997;88:163–168.

Teta MJ, Lewinsohn HC, Meigs JW, Vidone A, Mowad LZ, Flannery JT. Mesothelioma in Connecticut. *JOM.* 1983;15:749–756.

Thomas HF, Benjamin IT, Elwood PC, Sweetnam PM. Further follow up study of workers from an asbestos cement factory. *Br J Ind Med.* 1982;39:273–276.

Wagner JC, Skidmore JW, Hill RJ, Griffiths DM. Erionite exposure and mesothelioma in rats. *Br J Cancer.* 1985;51:727–730.

Wagner JC, Sleggs CA, Marchand P. Diffuse pleural mesothelioma and asbestos exposure in the Northwestern Cape Province. *Br J Ind Med.* 1960;17:260–271.

Weill H. Asbestos-Cement. In: Gibbs GW, Valic F, Browne K, eds. *Health Risks Associated with Chrysotile Asbestos. Ann Occup Hyg.* 1994;38,399–426.

Weill H, Hughes J, Waggenspack C. Influence of dose and fiber type on respiratory malignancy risk in asbestos cement manufacturing. *Am Rev Resp Dis.* 1979;120:345–354.

Weiss W. Mortality of a cohort exposed to chrysotile asbestos. *JOM.* 1977;19:737–740.

WHO. *Validity of Methods for Assessment of Carcinogenicity of Fibres.* Copenhagen, Denmark: WHO Regional Office; 1992.

WHO. *Determination of Airborne Fibre Number Concentrations. A Recommended Method, by Phase Contrast Optical Microscopy (Membrane Filter Method).* Switzerland, Geneva: WHO Publications; 1997.

Woitowitz H-J, Rodelsperger K. Mesothelioma among car mechanics. *Ann Occup Hyg.* 1994;38:635–638.

Wong O. Malignant mesothelioma and asbestos exposure among auto mechanics: appraisal of scientific evidence. *Reg Toxicol Pharmacol.* 2001;34:170–177.

Wong O. The interpretation of occupational epidemiologic data in regulation and litigation: studies of auto mechanics and petroleum workers. *Reg Toxicol Pharmacol.* 2006;44:191–197.

Yarborough CM. Chrysotile as a cause of mesothelioma: an assessment based on epidemiology. *Critical Rev Toxicol.* 2006;36:165–187.

5

Molecular Responses to Asbestos: Induction of Cell Proliferation and Apoptosis Through Modulation of Redox-Dependent Cell Signaling Pathways

Nicholas H. Heintz and Brooke T. Mossman

Introduction

For many years reactive oxygen species (ROS) and reactive nitrogen species (RNS) were viewed primarily as toxic byproducts of cellular metabolism or environmental insults. It is now widely recognized that ROS and RNS act as dose-dependent second messengers in cell-signaling pathways that control cellular processes as diverse as proliferation, migration, and programmed cell death (apoptosis). As *asbestos* is a commercial designation for a number of mineral fibers with distinct morphological, physical, and chemical properties, there is considerable impetus to dissect the effects of individual fiber types on cell-signaling pathways in the target cell populations that contribute to the pathogenesis of respiratory and pleural diseases.

Through surface chemistry or physical interactions with cells, asbestos fibers perturb the metabolism of ROS and RNS, and thereby influence redox-dependent signaling pathways. Recently, the patterns of activation, subcellular location, and duration of cellular signals have been shown to have profound effects on posttranslational protein modifications and gene expression that control cell function. Hence, the extent and duration of activation of signaling pathways elicited by specific fiber types likely represent critical determinants in cell responses such as acute injury, induction of proliferation, and apoptosis. With advanced imaging techniques that provide an avenue for studying responses at the single cell level, and gene expression profiling that provides access to complex patterns of responses in cells and tissues, a more complete understanding of the molecular responses to distinct types of asbestos is emerging. A detailed understanding of cell signaling responses to asbestos cells may provide a rationale for prevention and therapeutic intervention in asbestosis and asbestos-induced cancers.

Cell-Signaling Pathways

Mammalian cells depend upon the extracellular environment, and a wide variety of conditions, including temperature, nutrients, growth factors, hormones, and cell-to-cell contact, are important in maintaining homeostasis. The status of intracellular processes, such as energy utilization, rates of protein and RNA synthesis, protein folding, nucleotide pools, mitochondrial function, and organization of the cytoskeleton are also critical in maintaining normal cell function. Signals emanating from extracellular cues or intracellular processes impinge on targets that act as receivers, which then transduce information to effector molecules that govern cellular responses (Figure 5.1). In general, the specificity of a signal is dictated by the selectivity of the receiver. Most often signals are amplified as they course through a pathway, providing for increased sensitivity. Integration between pathways is accomplished by signaling proteins or diffusible factors that occupy regulatory nodes in multiple pathways, a process termed *crosstalk*. Positive and negative feedback loops modulate the intensity and duration of responses, and for every activation mechanism (eg, phosphorylation by a protein kinase) there is a corresponding

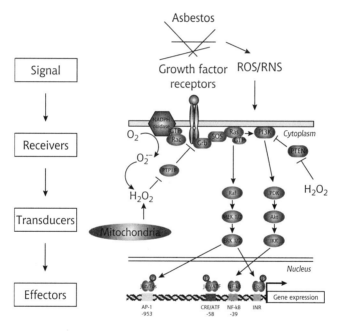

Figure 5.1 Organization of a typical cell-signaling pathway. In response to growth factors (Signal), cell surface receptors (Receivers) are activated by phosphorylation, leading to the assembly of signaling complexes at the cell membrane. These complexes activate downstream pathways that include protein kinase cascades (Transducers) leading to the activation of transcription factors (Effectors). In the instance shown here, growth factors are shown activating two classical pathways involved in cell proliferation, the SOS/Ras/Ras/ERK pathway and the PI-3K/Akt pathway. Control of each of these pathways is commonly corrupted in human cancers. Recent work shows that both of these pathways are influenced by cellular redox state, and that the production of hydrogen peroxide (H_2O_2) is required for the sustained activation, that is, necessary for the activation of gene expression and cell proliferation. H_2O_2 may be derived from NADPH oxidases at the cell surface, or from mitochondria. Shown in red are components of these pathways that regulate or be regulated by reactive oxygen species, such as the protein phosphatase PTB1B and the lipid phosphatase PTEN. See text for details.

mechanism for inactivation (eg, dephosphorylation by a phosphatase). Normally, these counteracting forces are in dynamic balance with one another, and signals impinging on the system may induce fluctuations over time scales that range from milliseconds in neurons to days in other cell types. In this sense, most cell-signaling pathways are best considered cellular rheostats rather than simple *on-off* switches.

As might be expected, disease processes are intimately linked to the corruption of cell-signaling pathways, as first understood by study of the signaling pathways that regulate cell proliferation in cancer (Hanahan and Weinberg, 2000), but now appreciated for virtually all chronic diseases. For many years, genotoxic insults have been known to alter cellular phenotypes through gene mutation. More recently appreciated is the realization that chronic environmental insults also may alter cellular phenotype through perturbation of cell-signaling pathways that regulate gene expression. Asbestos, as an inhaled particulate that persists in tissues, engenders markedly complex responses in cells and tissues over time. Here we discuss how asbestos interacts with cell-signaling pathways to modulate cell functions, including induction of proliferation and cell death, either by necrosis or by apoptosis (programmed cell death). Cell responses to asbestos are dose-related, and in many instances reflect a dependence on changes in the redox status of the cell, suggesting that asbestos interacts predominantly, albeit in complex ways, with redox-dependent signaling pathways.

ROS and RNS in Cell Signaling

ROS and RNS have several important properties that contribute to their activities as second messengers of cell signaling: they are transient in nature, diffusible within and between cells, modulate the activity of specific molecular targets, and control responses to a wide variety of extracellular and intracellular stimuli. In addition, cells have enzyme systems dedicated to the regulated production of ROS and RNS, and a variety of antioxidant defenses to limit these species to physiological levels in well-defined subcellular compartments. Depending on the chemical species, concentration and duration of exposure, ROS/RNS may alter the metabolic state of the cell, increase cell proliferation, induce cell cycle arrest, or induce cell death, either through activation of apoptotic pathways or through necrosis (lytic cell death). A number of recent reviews have addressed the role of ROS/RNS in these processes (Behrend et al., 2003; Davies, 1999; Gabbita et al., 2000; Lambeth, 2004; Sauer et al., 2001; Stone and Collins, 2002). Much effort presently is being expended on the identification of signaling proteins that are regulated by cycles of oxidation and reduction, and how imbalances in the intracellular metabolism of ROS and RNS impinge on the function of these targets. Because of considerable evidence that oxidants contribute to the bioactivity of asbestos, questions concerning the mechanisms by which asbestos acts through RNS and ROS in the pathogenesis of acute and chronic diseases are of current interest.

There are several sources of ROS and RNS in mammalian cells and tissues. Partially reduced forms of molecular oxygen in cells include superoxide anion (O_2^-), hydrogen peroxide (H_2O_2), and hydroxyl radical (OH). These may arise as (1) energy derived from carbohydrates, (2) fatty acids converted to ATP, (3) oxidative phosphorylation in mitochondria, or (4) autooxidation of quinones, flavins, and other intracellular components. Electron transfer to molecular O_2 by cytosolic enzymes may also generate intracellular ROS during normal metabolism. For example, breakdown of uric acid, amino acids, and fatty acids by oxidation generates H_2O_2 in peroxisomes. In neutrophils and professional phagocytes, the membrane bound NADPH oxidase Nox2 (or gp91[phox]) generates superoxide, which is then converted to H_2O_2 that functions as an antimicrobial agent. Other members of the Nox family of NADPH oxidases are now known to produce O_2^- as a signaling molecule in several cellular responses, most notably cell proliferation and angiogenesis (Lambeth, 2004). Since it is technically difficult to measure the production of ROS/RNS in cells, and these may be generated from multiple sources, often it is not possible to identify the source of ROS that participates in activation of cell signaling pathways, precisely.

Regulation of Cell Proliferation by ROS

In actively dividing cells, the cell cycle is controlled by the periodic expression of cyclins, unstable protein cofactors that regulate cyclin-dependent kinases (CDKs). CDK/cyclin complexes phosphorylate protein targets that control progression through G1, entry into the S phase, and mitosis (Murray, 2004). In contrast to regulation by the CDK cycle in actively proliferating cells, induction of proliferation in quiescent cells requires activation of mitogenic signaling pathways. Compelling evidence for a role for intracellular hydrogen peroxide (H_2O_2) as a second messenger in mitogenic signaling has accumulated over the past decade. For example, production of H_2O_2 is required for mitogenesis in response to the growth factors: epidermal growth factor (EGF), basic fibroblast growth factor (bFGF), platelet-derived growth factor (PDGF) and thrombospondin2 (Gabbita et al., 2000; Karin and Shaulian, 2001). In some instances, the source of H_2O_2 production in response to growth factors has been linked to Rac-dependent activation of the Nox family of NADPH oxidases (Park et al., 2004). Similar to the electron transport chain, the Nox family of membrane-bound NADPH oxidases produce O_2^-, which is rapidly converted by superoxide dismutases (SOD) to H_2O_2.

Several targets for H_2O_2 in cell proliferation in mitogenesis have been described. As shown in Figure 5.1, activation of growth factor receptors on the cell surface leads to induction of several major mitogenic pathways, including the SOS-Ras-Raf-ERK and phosphoinositol-3-kinase/Akt (PI-3K/Akt) signaling cascades. Upon binding of ligand, EGF and other similar growth factor receptors are phosphorylated on intracellular tyrosine residues, and this modification drives the recruitment and assembly of signaling proteins to the cytoplasmic face of the plasma membrane (Schlessinger, 2004). PI-3Ks act on membrane lipid phosphatidylinsitols to produce phosphatidylinositol (3,4,5) trisphosphate, which in turn recruits signaling proteins such as the serine/threonine kinase Akt to the membrane through highly specific interactions with specialized protein domains (Parsons, 2004). As shown in Figure 5.1, both the PI-3K/Akt and SOS-Ras-Raf-ERK pathways transduce signals to transcription factors that regulate expression of cyclin D1 and other genes involved in cell proliferation. Ras and other transducers provide crosstalk between these major mitogenic pathways.

Upon stimulation with growth factors, H_2O_2 produced by the activation of NADPH oxidases, mitochondria or other sources accentuates signaling through both the PI-3K/Akt and SOS-Raf-Ras-ERK pathways by the transient and reversible inactivation of phosphatases. Protein tyrosine phosphatase 1B (PTP1B), which dampens signaling by removing tyrosine residues from growth factor receptors and other signaling proteins, is transiently inactivated by H_2O_2-dependent oxidation of a cysteine residue in the enzyme's catalytic site (Lee et al., 1998). In response to EGF, inactivation of PTB1B reaches maximal levels by 10 minutes, and returns to baseline within an hour, suggesting that the transient burst of H_2O_2 production in response to mitogens lasts less than an hour. Similarly, the lipid phosphatase PTEN is transiently inactivated by oxidation in response to H_2O_2 (Lee et al.,

2002), in macrophages stimulated by lipopolysaccharide (Leslie et al., 2003) and in cells treated with peptide growth factors (Kwon et al., 2004). As for PTB1B, a cysteine residue in the active site of PTEN is reversibly inactivated by oxidation (Kwon et al., 2004). Interestingly, PI3-K activity is required for production of H_2O_2 in response to growth factors (Bae et al., 2000), most likely through activation of NADPH oxidases by the small GTPase Rac. Together these studies indicate H_2O_2 is produced in response to growth factors, accentuates mitogenic signaling through the extracellular signal-regulated kinases 1 and 2 (ERK1/2) and PI3-kinase/Akt pathways, and that one molecular target for these effects is transient and reversible oxidation of reactive site cysteines in phosphatases.

Recently it was shown that H_2O_2 induced by expression of the NADPH oxidase Nox1 up-regulates gene expression through activation of the transcription factor AP-1, with no effect on the redox state of the major thiol antioxidants, glutathione, and thioredoxin (Go et al., 2004). H_2O_2 signaling to AP-1 was mediated by activation of both the c-Jun N-terminal kinase (JNK) and ERK1/2 pathways modulated by Ras. These authors concluded, "redox signaling resulting in kinase signaling pathways is distinct from oxidative stress and is mediated by discrete, localized redox circuitry." Modification of protein thiols by cycles of oxidation and reduction is now an important area of investigation in the field of signal transduction (Forman et al., 2004; Kiley and Storz, 2004).

Cells have a variety of antioxidant defenses dedicated to the metabolism of superoxide and other forms of ROS, including SOD, catalase, and peroxiredoxins. Other systems such as thioredoxins and glutathione protect protein thiols from oxidation. Interestingly, one of these systems in mammalian cells has been adapted during evolution so that H_2O_2 may function as a signaling molecule. In bacteria, peroxiredoxins are primarily responsible for detoxification of low levels of peroxides, while catalase is reserved for protecting cells from higher levels of H_2O_2. Bacterial peroxiredoxins (Prxs) are resistant to inactivation by oxidation by H_2O_2 whereas in mammals Prxs contain a novel C-terminal protein motif that mediates inactivation of the enzyme through oxidation by its substrate (Wood et al., 2003b). It is thought that oxidative inactivation of mammalian Prxs allows H_2O_2 to reach threshold levels sufficient to oxidize cysteine residues in signaling targets such as PTB1B and PTEN, a process termed the "floodgate hypothesis" (Wood et al., 2003a). More important, recent experiments show that oxidation of Prxs is reversible, as sulfiredoxins are able to restore Prx activity once production of H_2O_2 has diminished (Budanov et al., 2004; Chang et al., 2004; Woo et al., 2003). Clearly, reversible oxidation and reduction of critical cysteine residues in phosphatases and other proteins by H_2O_2 is a component of the molecular switches that regulate signal transduction.

In a similar vein, though less well understood, RNS also participates in redox-dependent signaling. Nitric oxide (NO) is produced in high quantities by macrophages and other cells of the immune cells for the purpose of host defense, and at much lower levels in neurons and other cells types for cell signaling. NO may interact directly with cysteine residues in proteins, producing nitrosothiols, or interact chemically with ROS to produce highly reactive intermediates such as peroxynitrite. By nitrating tyrosine residues in proteins, as has been reported for the EGF receptor, peroxynitrite may then modulate signaling (van der Vliet et al., 1998). As for ROS, very low levels of RNS cooperate with low levels of growth factors to induce mitogenesis (Finkel and Holbrook, 2000).

AP-1 and Cell Cycle Progression

AP-1, the family of transcription factor complexes composed of the Jun (c-Jun, JunB, and JunD) and Fos (c-Fos, FosB, Fra1, and Fra2) families of proteins, is intimately involved in the control of proliferation, neoplastic transformation, and apoptosis (Gabbita et al., 2000; Karin and Shaulian, 2001). AP-1 is a redox-responsive transcription factor that responds in a dose-dependent manner to both growth factors and many environmental stresses, including ROS, RNS, and asbestos (Shaulian and Karin, 2001). Of interest at present is how the intensity and duration of signals emanating from specific cell-signaling pathways is interpreted by transcription factors such as AP-1 to dictate phenotypic outcomes (eg, proliferation, survival, or death).

AP-1 is regulated in part by serine/threonine protein kinases termed mitogen-activated protein kinases (MAPKs). There are three general classes of MAPKs: the extracellular signal-regulated kinases (ERK), c-Jun N-terminal kinase (JNK; also known as SAPK), and p38. MAPKs are implicated in the regulation of AP-1 in proliferation, apoptosis, and cell survival. In general, c-Jun is a target of c-jun N-terminal kinases (JNKs), and c-Fos a target of extracellular signal-regulated kinases (ERKs). Both JNK and ERK kinases are activated by oxidants, and the outcome of activation is dependent on cell type, duration of activation, and experimental conditions.

Considerable effort has been devoted to understanding the role of c-Jun and other AP-1 family members in proliferation and apoptosis. Once activated, JNK translocates into the nucleus where it phosphorylates c-Jun on serines 63 and 73 (Davis, 2000), modifications that promote transcriptional activation of gene expression. Mice lacking c-Jun do not survive embryogenesis (Johnson et al., 1993). Interestingly, mice that express a mutant form of c-Jun in which serines 63 and 73 have been replaced with alanine residues are viable and fertile, but smaller than controls (Behrens et al., 1999). These mice are resistant to certain forms of apoptotic stimuli, suggesting that JNK-dependent phosphorylation of c-Jun at serines 63 and 73 is linked to apoptosis rather than proliferation.

Of all the Jun proteins, c-Jun has the most potent activity in cooperating with activated Ras in transformation assays (Alani et al., 1991; Schutte et al., 1989a,b; Vandel et al., 1996), a result that agrees well with the observation that c-Jun $-/-$ cells have severe defects in proliferation due to a dramatic increase in the length of G1, a defect partially restored by expression of cyclin D1 (Wisdom et al., 1999). Analysis of AP-1 activity during exit from mitosis suggests that c-Jun acts as a positive effector of cyclin D1 expression, whereas JunB is a negative regulator (Bakiri et al., 2000; Chiu et al., 1989). Phosphorylation of c-Jun during entry into G1 combined with Cdc2/cyclin B-mediated destruction of JunB acts to tip the balance of AP-1 complexes toward proliferation.

In contrast to regulation of c-Jun by JNK, the Fos family of proteins are regulated by ERK1/2. Experiments in knockout mice indicate c-Fos and FosB are required for expression of cyclin D1, although it is not known if these proteins act directly through the cyclin D1 promoter (Brown et al., 1998). c-Fos is a direct target for phosphorylation by ERK1/2 (Murphy et al., 2002). During cell cycle reentry in response to serum, c-Fos is expressed, transported into the nucleus, and phosphorylated within 1 hour. Brief activation of ERK (15–30 minutes) in response to growth factors is not sufficient for proliferation due to decay of ERK signaling before c-Fos is expressed at high enough levels to promote AP-1-dependent transcription (Murphy et al., 2002). Activation of ERK for longer periods promotes phosphorylation of c-Fos on threonines (Thr) 325 and 331, modifications that promote stabilization of c-Fos, transcriptional activity, and proliferation (Monje et al., 2003; Murphy et al., 2002, 2004). These findings are of considerable import because they show that the duration of ERK signaling is linked directly to specific modifications of c-Fos that influence phenotypic outcome.

The requirement for c-Fos in cell cycle progression is transient. Once activated for transcription the protein is immediately targeted for degradation. In contrast, Fra1, which is stabilized by phosphorylation by ERK (Casalino et al., 2003), is expressed for long periods of time after cell cycle reentry (Burch et al., 2004). Fra1 appears to be an important mediator of cell proliferation through transcriptional activation of cyclin D1, and contributes to tumorigenic properties of mesothelial cells such as increased migration and invasiveness (Ramos-Nino et al., 2002, 2003). Interestingly, facets of cell adhesion and migration have also been linked recently to the generation of cellular ROS (Moldovan et al., 1999).

Apoptosis and ROS

A balance between cell proliferation and cell death governs homeostasis in many organs. At higher concentrations than those that promote proliferation, ROS can cause cell cycle arrest, or apoptosis and necrosis. These responses are often related to protracted stimulation of MAPKs or other dedicated *cell death* pathways. Interactions between these pathways may be critical to cell fate, as dysregulation of apoptosis plays an important part in human cancer (Stenner-Liewen and Reed, 2003).

Apoptosis is an ATP-dependent process of programmed cell death in response to developmental cues, metabolic imbalances, or environmental insult. Apoptosis is characterized by membrane blebbing, cell shrinkage, nuclear condensation, and DNA fragmentation. Apoptosis can be initiated by an extrinsic pathway in which external cues activate death receptor pathways or an intrinsic pathway by conditions that impair mitochondrial function. The pivotal event in the mitochondrial pathway is mitochondrial outer membrane permeabilization (MOMP), which leads to the release of cytochrome c and apoptosis-inducing factor (AIF) from the space between the inner and outer mitochondrial membranes (Green and Kroemer, 2004). Release of cytochrome c into the cytoplasm induces the formation of a protein complex termed the apoptosome, which activates downstream caspases, a family of proteases that attack a wide variety of cellular targets (Green and Kroemer, 1998). When released from mitochondria, AIF migrates into the nucleus, where it is able to initiate nuclear condensation and fragmentation, perhaps in some cases without caspase activation (Cande et al., 2002; Penninger and Kroemer, 2003). Oxygen tension, redox potential, and intracellular pH are linked to MOMP. Elevated expression of the antiapoptotic factor Bcl-2, which acts through modulation of MOMP, is found in many cancer cells that are resistant to proapoptotic signals.

The Strength and Duration of Signaling by Intracellular H_2O_2 Determines Cell Fate

As for all signaling systems involving diffusible second messengers, cells must be responsive to fluctuating levels of H_2O_2. Once a certain threshold that promotes proliferation is exceeded, oxidative modification of additional cellular targets induces cell cycle arrest or cell death, as has been reported in many models (Karin and Shaulian, 2001; Sauer et al., 2001). Thus, there is a hierarchy of cellular responses in which low levels of H_2O_2 (3–10 μm) promote proliferation, higher levels (100–150 μm) induce transient cell cycle arrest and yet higher levels (>250 μm) induce cell death (reviewed by Davies, 1999). Similarly, the duration of signaling by phospho-ERK1/2 in the nucleus in response to growth factors and other agents such as H_2O_2 has a profound effect on cell proliferation, survival, and death (reviewed by Pouyssegur et al., 2002). When added as a bolus (usually at 200–300 μm), H_2O_2 increases ERK1/2 activation in many cell types and increases cell survival (Guyton et al., 1996). Owing to the short half-life of H_2O_2, ERK1/2 activation in this instance is transient and acts in a positive fashion on cell proliferation. In situations where ROS levels are increased beyond a certain threshold (based on the status of antioxidants in the cell), ERK1/2 activation is prolonged and cells die of apoptosis or necrosis. For example, activation of ERK1/2 through the Ras/Raf pathway is required for apoptosis in response to H_2O_2 in L929 mouse fibroblasts (Lee et al., 2003).

Asbestos and Generation of ROS

The observations that various aspects of growth factors signaling, cell proliferation, senescence, and apoptosis are controlled by exogenous or endogenous sources of ROS/RNS, and that these outcomes are related to the strength and duration of dose, provides a mechanistic link to the effects of asbestos on cell-signaling pathways. There are two primary sources for the production of ROS when asbestos fibers encounter cells: (1) direct generation of ROS through surface chemistry of asbestos fibers and (2) generation of ROS by cells in response to interactions with or engulfment of fibers (Shukla et al., 2003a). As explained elsewhere in this text, there are six types of asbestos fibers with diverse chemical and physical properties. The presence and ionic state of iron appears to play a critical role in generation of ROS directly from fibers, whereas other properties of asbestos may contribute to enhanced ROS production by cells through effects on cell membranes, growth factor receptors, mitochondrial function, or other cellular processes.

A number of investigators have examined the ability of asbestos fibers to generate ROS, and these studies have implicated iron as an important parameter in the surface chemistry of various fiber types (Shukla et al., 2003a; Shukla and Mossman, 2003). The ability of asbestos to produce ROS was studied with an emphasis on production of hydroxyl radicals (OH) through reduction of O_2 to superoxide anion (O_2^-), or O_2 + e^- = O_2^- Superoxide anion is then rapidly dismutated by SOD to produce H_2O_2. In Fenton-like reactions catalyzed by asbestos, H_2O_2 + e^- = $\cdot OH$ and OH^- (Gulumian and van Wyk, 1987). The hydroxyl radical can react with other molecules such as formate to produce carboxy radicals or with lipids to produce lipid hydroperoxides. In general studies show that fibers like siderite and crocidolite that contain Fe^{2+} ions support Fenton-type reactions, with crocidolite being most active (Zalma et al., 1987). Other fiber types and iron-containing particles with Fe^{3+} ions are not active. In crocidolite asbestos ($Na_2Fe^{3+}_2Fe^{2+}_3[Si_8O_{22}](OH)_2$) iron is distributed within three crystallographic sites known as M_1, M_2, and M_3; M_4 binds alkali ions such as Na, Ca, and K. The distribution of ferric and ferrous ions among the three octahedral M_1, M_2, and M_3 sites of crocidolite varies depending on the source of the mineral, and may even vary within different areas of a single fiber. Several investigators have shown that for crocidolite, the oxidation state of iron, and its ability to be mobilized from the fiber surface, rather than the amount of iron in the crystal lattice, is important for the generation of ROS (Fenoglio et al., 2001; Ghio et al., 1992; Gulumian et al., 1993; Lund and Aust, 1990).

Chrysotile asbestos, the only member of the serpentine family, is a 1:1 layer silicate with a chemical formula of $Mg_3[SiO_5](OH)_4$. In chrysotile asbestos misalignment of layers of silicate sheets with octahedral sheets of $MgO_2(OH)_4$ cause the fiber to curl, thereby exposing Mg-hydroxide on the fiber surface. Chrysotile fibers in cylindrical layers or other spiral configurations have different physical configurations, and therefore expose different chemical groups to the environment. In contrast to crocidolite, chrysotile asbestos is not rich in iron and the surface is less effective at generating hydroxyl radicals (Gulumian and van Wyk, 1991). Comparative studies show that the ability of asbestos fibers to generate hydroxyl radicals is as follows: crocidolite > amosite > tremolite > anthophyllite > chrysotile. For all fiber types, surface chemistry is affected by the source of the mineral, mechanical, and thermal treatment of fibers, and chemical impurities, often due to contamination with other ores.

Other mechanisms for the production of ROS by asbestos require the direct interaction of asbestos with cells. One mechanism involves frustrated phagocytosis. When cells attempt to engulf long fibers, sustained production of O_2^- by oxidases in phagosomes produces an increased level of intracellular H_2O_2, which in turn may lead to a chain reaction of ·OH production by ferrous ions in the fiber (Goodglick and Kane, 1986; Hansen and Mossman, 1987). The fate of cells that attempt to engulf asbestos fibers is not well documented, but in tracheal explants fibers appear to provide foci for reactive processes that include both cell death and cell proliferation (Woodworth et al., 1983).

More important, when asbestos interacts with cells it is also capable of activating mitogenic and other signaling pathways that regulate production of H_2O_2. Usually the effects of growth factors and other stimuli that impinge on these pathways are transient in nature, and ROS production subsides, as the pathway is inactivated. As a durable particulate with unusual geometric and chemical properties, asbestos may have a unique capacity for persistent activation of signaling pathways, and thereby interfere with both the strength and duration of signals that influence phenotypic responses. Given the chemical complexity of asbestos fibers, and the observation that the surface activity of asbestos fibers may vary from fiber to fiber, or even within a single fiber, ascribing specific cellular outcomes to the generation of a single chemical species of ROS is unlikely. Rather it appears that it is the interplay between asbestos and redox-dependent signaling pathways that is important.

ROS-Dependent Effects of Asbestos on Cell-Signaling Pathways

Interaction of asbestos fibers with the cell surface activates a number of signaling cascades involving MAPKs, with the most potent effects mediated by the MAPKs ERK1/2 (Yuan et al., 2004; Zanella et al., 1996) and ERK5 (Scapoli et al., 2004). Asbestos induces increases in the second messenger diacylglycerol and stimulates protein kinase C (PKC) activity (Perderiset et al., 1991; Sesko et al., 1990), as well as rapid autophosphorylation of the epidermal growth factor receptor (EGFR) (Zanella et al., 1996). These events are linked to activation of ERK1/2 by the SOS/Ras/Raf pathway, as inhibition of EGFR tyrosine kinase activity or MEK1 blocks ERK activation in response to asbestos. Aggregation of the EGFR by long crocidolite fibers may initiate signaling cascades important for cell proliferation in disease life mesothelioma (Pache et al., 1998), for milled (non-fibrous) crocidolite is inactive in the induction of increased EGFR protein expression (Faux et al., 2000). Using transgenic mice that express a dominant-negative form of the EGFR (dnEGFR), Manning et al. (Manning et al., 2002) have shown that proliferation of bronchiolar and alveolar epithelium in response to inhalation of crocidolite requires phosphorylation of EGFR.

Activation of EGFR leads to activation of ERK1/2, which causes increased expression and activity of c-Jun and c-Fos, AP-1 DNA binding activity, and gene expression (Janssen et al., 1995; Timblin et al., 1998). Interestingly, activated ERK has been located at sites of developing fibrotic lesions in mice after 14–20 days of inhalation of chrysotile asbestos (Robledo et al., 2000). In tracheal explants, induction of PDGF-A and TGF-β gene expression by amosite asbestos is also dependent on activation of ERK (Dai and Churg, 2001).

Molecular responses to asbestos may be cell-type specific: in rat pleural mesothelial (RPM) and hamster tracheal epithelial (HTE) cells, crocidolite asbestos induces high levels of c-Jun mRNA for at least 24 hours, whereas protracted expression of c-Fos mRNA was observed in RPM, but not HTE, cells (Heintz et al., 1993; Janssen et al., 1994). In these cell types crocidolite asbestos was more active than chrysotile asbestos in the induction of both c-Jun and c-Fos mRNA. Induction of c-Fos and c-Jun proto-oncogene expression by asbestos is dependent upon redox status, for pretreatment of cells with the antioxidant N-acetyl-L-cysteine dampens induction of these genes in rat mesothelial cells (Janssen et al., 1994, 1995). In serum-stimulated mouse type II alveolar epithelial cells, the MAPK family member p38 is not activated by asbestos (Yuan et al., 2004), whereas in normal alveolar macrophages p38 is activated by asbestos (Geist et al., 2000). Cell type-specific responses to asbestos at the level of MAPK activation and proto-oncogene expression could reflect differences in antioxidant status, signal transduction pathways, cell cycle position or other factors.

Because of its central role in processes as diverse as proliferation and programmed cell death, it is often difficult to link activation of AP-1 to a specific cellular response. Nonetheless, increased expression of c-Jun in HTE cells by asbestos and H_2O_2 leads to increased cell proliferation and enhanced ability to grow in soft agar, an indication of neoplastic transformation (Timblin et al., 1995). Erionite, a potent inducer of mesothelioma in rodents and man (Mossman and Gee, 1989; Mossman et al., 1996a) also increases the expression of c-fos and c-jun mRNA in RPM cells (Janssen et al., 1995; Timblin et al., 1998). Inhalation of asbestos by rats or mice leads to dose-related increases in mRNAs encoding AP-1 family members in lung homogenates (Quinlan et al., 1994, 1995), and laser capture microscopy has shown that c-fos and c-jun mRNA expression is increased in bronchiolar cells after inhalation of asbestos (Manning et al., 2002). Experiments with transgenic mice harboring an AP-1-dependent reporter gene construct indicate that increased levels of mRNAs for AP-1 family members is accompanied by induction of AP-1-dependent gene expression (Hubbard et al., 2001). Interestingly, prolonged induction of c-Fos by asbestos appears to be linked to apoptosis, not proliferation (Zanella et al., 1999). As c-Fos is stabilized by ERK1/2, this result is in good agreement with the observation that prolonged activation of ERK1/2 is also linked to apoptosis (Yuan et al., 2004).

Together these studies indicate that activation of ERK by asbestos is manifested in increased expression of the proto-oncogenes, c-Jun, and c-Fos, as well as other AP-1 family members such as Fra1 (Ramos-Nino et al., 2002), and that these factors drive AP-1-dependent gene transcription. Aspects of these responses are cell-type specific, and the critical AP-1-dependent genes that mediate specific outcomes in response to asbestos are not yet well understood.

Asbestos, Apoptosis, and ROS

There is considerable evidence that asbestos induces apoptosis in vitro and in vivo, and that this outcome in many instances is linked to ROS. Apoptosis of alveolar type II epithelial and mesenchymal cells is an important facet of resolving airway hyperplasia in acute lung injury, but may lead to loss of barrier function, lung injury, and fibrosis if left unchecked (Kazzaz et al., 2000; Polunovsky et al., 1993; Uhal, 1997). Rats exposed to asbestos show TUNEL staining at bronchiolar-alveolar junctions' characteristic of apoptosis, but electron microscopy suggests cell lysis or necrosis is primarily responsible for bronchiolar and pulmonary epithelial cell death in these animals (Jung et al., 2000). In vitro, induction of apoptosis in human and rabbit pleural mesothelial cells is ameliorated by catalase and the iron chelator deferoxamine, implicating iron-derived ROS as a mediator (Broaddus et al., 1996). Similarly, free radical scavengers and iron chelators inhibit apoptosis of alveolar epithelial cells in response to asbestos (Aljandali et al., 2001). Antioxidants and elevated expression of mitochondrial SOD prevent cell death in response to tumor necrosis factor-α H_2O_2, and asbestos (Manna et al., 1998; Mossman et al., 1996b; Zwacka et al., 1998), again implicating ROS as intermediate in the induction of apoptosis.

Induction of cell death by asbestos appears to occur through MOMP. Asbestos reduces mitochondrial membrane potential, induces the release of cytochrome c, and activates caspase-9 in alveolar epithelial cells (Kamp et al., 2002). In contrast, inert particles such as glass beads or TiO_2 do not affect MOMP. Over-expression of the antiapoptotic factor Bcl-Xl, which counteracts MOMP, protects cells asbestos-induced losses of mitochondrial potential and subsequent DNA fragmentation. In serum-stimulated mouse, type II alveolar cells confocal microscopy shows prolonged activation of ERK1/2 in the nucleus by asbestos is associated with migration of AIF from mitochondria to the nucleus and the induction of apoptosis (Yuan et al., 2004). In contrast, cells that display ERK1/2 activation in the nucleus for less than 4 hours express cyclin D1 and go on to enter the S phase, indicating that asbestos alters the duration of ERK signaling and activation of AIF only in a subset of cells.

Although it is not yet known if these outcomes are directly linked to alterations in cellular redox status, cell autonomous effects of asbestos (ie, the decision to proliferate or die) may be mediated by mitochondrial dysfunction. Dose-dependent decreases in formazan production, an indication of mitochondrial dysfunction, increased expression of pro- and antiapoptotic genes, and increased numbers of apoptotic cells are observed in mesothelial cells exposed to asbestos (Shukla et al., 2003b). Confocal microscopy with vital dyes shows that changes in mitochondrial membrane potential under these conditions are limited to a subset of cells. Apoptosis was decreased in the presence of both an inhibitor of caspase-9 and catalase, indicating that elevated levels of H_2O_2 and activation of the intrinsic mitochondrial apoptotic pathway are involved in asbestos-induced cell death.

In summary, there is clear and convincing evidence that endogenous sources of ROS and RNS modulate gene expression and cellular phenotypes through redox-dependent signaling pathways. With the advent of new tools for identifying proteins that are regulated by cycles of oxidation and reduction, dissection of signaling pathways that respond to alterations in cellular redox status is now possible. Because the nucleus, endoplasmic reticulum, and mitochondria utilize different strategies to regulate redox status, it will be important to understand how perturbation of the redox status of one subcellular compartment influences the redox status of others. Clearly, environmental ROS/RNS interact with cellular sources of these species and thereby alter the strength, duration, and location of information flow through signaling pathways. As a durable particulate that is able to generate ROS either directly or through the perturbation of cell physiology, asbestos presents an intriguing challenge. Clearly, additional investigation of the effects of specific asbestos fibers on modulation of the intracellular levels of ROS and RNS, mitochondrial function, and the activation and subcellular distribution of redox-sensitive signaling proteins is warranted.

Importance of Cell-Signaling Events in Multistage Carcinogenesis by Asbestos

Asbestos fibers are recognized as human carcinogens by the International Agency for Research on Cancer (IARC) due to their association with increased risks of lung cancers

Multistage Carcinogenesis

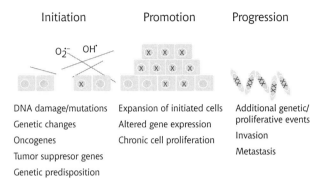

Initiation	Promotion	Progression
DNA damage/mutations	Expansion of initiated cells	Additional genetic/
Genetic changes	Altered gene expression	proliferative events
Oncogenes	Chronic cell proliferation	Invasion
Tumor suppresor genes		Metastasis
Genetic predisposition		

Figure 5.2 The multistage nature of carcinogenesis. On the basis of the experimental models and the study of human tumors, the process of carcinogenesis has been divided into several stages. During initiation, cells suffer genetic damage in critical oncogenes or tumor suppressor genes, leading to disregulation of cell growth. Inherited defects in tumor suppressor or DNA repair genes can cause a genetic predisposition to genetic changes that promote cancer formation. Through the generation of free radicals or other mechanisms, asbestos can act at this stage of tumor development, or cooperate with other carcinogens that cause mutations (eg, cigarette smoke). During promotion, cells bearing genetic defects proliferate, which may lead to changes in gene expression and altered cell phenotypes. Chronic cycles of cell injury, apoptosis and compensatory proliferation during proliferation eventually leads to genetic instability. At the latter stages of transformation, genetic instability provides the background necessary for the development of cell variants that may have the capacity to invade local tissues and metastasize to distal sites. The entire process of multistage carcinogenesis may take decades in humans.

and mesotheliomas in occupational cohorts exposed to asbestos (reviewed in Craighead and Mossman, 1982; Mossman et al., 1996a). Asbestos-induced carcinogenesis, defined as the various stages of tumor development, regardless of tissue origin, is a multistage process characterized by at least three sequential and complex phenomena: initiation, promotion, and progression. Initiation is defined as a change in genetic material, manifested by DNA damage, mutations, or other heritable changes in DNA (Figure 5.2). These genetic alterations may be rendered by increases in expression of oncogenes or decreases in expression or function of tumor suppressor genes. Genetic predisposition may play a role in the susceptibility of individuals to certain carcinogens as has been suggested for mesotheliomas found in certain regions of Turkey (Roushdy-Hammady et al., 2001).

Initiation alone does not render a cell *tumorigenic*. Additional signals in a process called "tumor promotion" are required for the expansion of the initiated cell population and subsequent genetic changes. Classically, tumor promoters have mitogenic properties that can evoke acute or chronic cell proliferation. Since a rapidly dividing cell is prone to additional genetic events that may be required for invasion and metastasis, hallmarks of *full-blown* malignant cells, a third stage of carcinogenesis, defined as *progression* has been recognized in most models of carcinogenesis.

Work from a number of laboratories suggests that asbestos may play different roles in the induction of lung cancers and mesotheliomas (Figure 5.3). For example in the development of lung cancers in asbestos workers, cigarette smoke is a major predisposing or risk factor (Mossman and Gee, 1989). Unsurprisingly, cigarette smoke contains thousands of agents, including ROS and RNS, which are known to damage DNA and

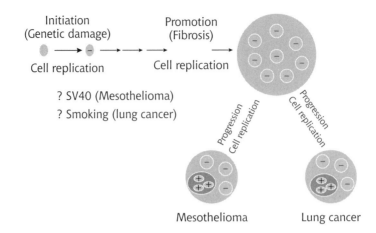

Figure 5.3 Cofactors for the induction of mesothelioma and lung cancer by asbestos. Asbestos (or other carcinogens) may cause genetic damage during the initiation phase of tumor development, leading to cell proliferation and the accumulation of cells with altered growth properties. Cofactors that contribute to uncontrolled cell growth or suppression of apoptosis, such as mutations caused by smoking or disruption of signaling pathways by SV40, may accelerate the initiation, promotion or progression phases of tumor development.

influence mitogenesis. As illustrated earlier in this chapter, ROS/RNS can be cytotoxic, cytostatic, or proliferative to cells, depending upon their concentration and the duration of exposure. Thus, ROS/RNS elaborated by asbestos may also play a role in tumor promotion, either by stimulating initial mesothelial or epithelial cell damage and subsequent compensatory hyperplasia, or by altering the cell cycle kinetics of initiated mesothelial or epithelial cells.

In contrast to lung cancers, smoking is not recognized as a risk factor in mesothelioma. In the development of this tumor type, asbestos fibers, most notably the high iron-containing amphiboles crocidolite and amosite, may initiate DNA damage in mesothelial cells, which are unusually sensitive to the cytotoxic effects of asbestos (Lechner et al., 1985) through mechanisms that involve the formation of ROS (Shukla et al., 2003a). Interestingly, mesotheliomas express high levels of thioredoxin, thioredoxin reductase and glutamate cysteine ligase (Kinnula et al., 2004), components of enzyme systems that maintain proteins in a reduced state, suggesting this cell type may be exquisitely sensitive to imbalances in ROS/RNS. The durable fibrous morphology of amphiboles also may serve as a stimulus for epithelial and mesothelial cell growth during the processes of tumor promotion in lung cancers or mesotheliomas (Woodworth et al., 1983). A dynamic interplay between cell death and cell proliferation is observed in normal mesothelial cells after exposure to crocidolite asbestos that is not observed with non-pathogenic particles or fibers (Goldberg et al., 1997).

Inactivation of the p53 and retinoblastoma (pRB) tumor suppressor proteins is a hallmark of most human malignancies. p53 is a transcription factor activated in response to oxidants, DNA damage, viral infection, and a broad array of other cellular stresses, whereas pRB is a transcriptional repressor that controls entry into the S phase. In human cells in culture, the small and large tumor antigens encoded by the DNA tumor virus SV40 (Simian virus 40) are capable of inactivating both pathways (Hanahan and Weinberg, 2000). Intriguingly, a role for SV40 T-antigen has recently been suggested in the pathogenesis of mesothelioma (Carbone et al., 2003; Carbone and Rdzanek, 2004; Klein et al., 2002). Since SV40 virus is known to replicate in human mesothelial cells, it may have multiple roles, as asbestos fibers do, in mesothelial cell carcinogenesis (Mossman and Gruenert, 2002). For example, SV40 small t-antigen activates the ERK pathway (Rundell and Parakati, 2001) and down-regulates the expression of nitric oxide synthase in human mesothelial cells (Aldieri et al., 2004). Both of these processes may favor the survival of initiated or malignant mesothelial cells. Moreover, as for other human cell types, large T-antigen may inactivate the p53 and pRB pathways, promoting survival and proliferation of cells with genetic instability.

Conclusions

Activation of ERK and other signaling pathways by asbestos, or ROS/RNS elaborated by asbestos, may be critical to elicitation of injury and proliferation in mesothelial and epithelial cells during carcinogenesis. The responses to asbestos are dose-related, and represent a dynamic balance between the induction of cell injury and cell death and promotion of cell proliferation. Chronic cell injury coupled with inflammatory responses also may promote compensatory hyperplasia over time. Because of its durability and capability to produce or modulate ROS/RNS, asbestos may have a unique ability to perturb cell-signaling pathways. For example, genetic changes resulting in the formation of unregulated and constitutively activated protein kinases are frequently observed in tumors, and increased expression of normal protein kinases have also been strongly associated with specific tumor types in man (Lawrence and Niu, 1998). Signaling through the EGFR and the erbB receptor network has been implicated in epithelial cell and mesothelial cells after acute exposures to asbestos, and these pathways may play a crucial role in both the pathogenesis and maintenance of the malignant phenotypes. This notion is supported by the observation that 40%–89% of human nonsmall cell lung tumors and approximately 60% of human mesotheliomas exhibit increased expression of EGFR (Janne et al., 2002), a state which has been linked to increases in angiogenesis and invasiveness as well as increased cell survival after chemotherapy. On the basis of the remarkable success of inhibiting specific protein kinases in several tumor types, these observations have led to chemotherapeutic strategies to inhibit EGFR function. As our understanding of the functional roles of specific signaling pathways in asbestosis and neoplastic transformation improves, and the effects of asbestos on these pathways in specific cell types are defined, it is hoped that more successful therapeutic interventions for asbestos-related diseases will emerge.

References

Alani R, Brown P, Binetruy B, et al. The transactivating domain of the c-Jun proto-oncoprotein is required for cotransformation of rat embryo cells. *Mol Cell Biol*. 1991; 11:6286–6295.
Aldieri, E, Orecchia, S, Ghigo, D, et al. Simian virus 40 infection down-regulates the expression of nitric oxide synthase in human mesothelial cells. *Cancer Res*. 2004;64:4082–4084.
Aljandali A, Pollack H, Yeldandi A, Li Y, Weitzman SA, Kamp, DW. Asbestos causes apoptosis in alveolar epithelial cells: role of iron-induced free radicals. *J Lab Clin Med*. 2001;137;330–339.
Bae YS, Sung JY, Kim OS, et al. Platelet-derived growth factor-induced H(2)O(2) production requires the activation of phosphatidylinositol 3-kinase. *J Biol Chem*. 2000;275:10527–10531.
Bakiri L, Lallemand D, Bossy-Wetzel E, Yaniv M. Cell cycle-dependent variations in c-Jun and JunB phosphorylation: a role in the control of cyclin D1 expression. *EMBO J*. 2000;19:2056–2068.

Behrend L, Henderson G, Zwacka RM. Reactive oxygen species in oncogenic transformation. *Biochem Soc Trans.* 2003;31:1441–1444.

Behrens A, Sibilia M, Wagner EF. Amino-terminal phosphorylation of c-Jun regulates stress-induced apoptosis and cellular proliferation. *Nat Genet.* 1999;21:326–329.

Broaddus VC, Yang L, Scavo LM, Ernst JD, Boylan AM. Asbestos induces apoptosis of human and rabbit pleural mesothelial cells via reactive oxygen species. *J Clin Invest.* 1996;98,2050–2059.

Brown JR, Nigh E, Lee RJ, et al. Fos family members induce cell cycle entry by activating cyclin D1. *Mol Cell Biol.* 1998;18:5609–5619.

Budanov AV, Sablina AA, Feinstein E, Koonin EV, Chumakov PM. Regeneration of peroxiredoxins by p53-regulated sestrins, homologs of bacterial AhpD. *Science.* 2004;304:596–600.

Burch PM, Yuan Z, Loonen A, Heintz NH. An extracellular signal-regulated kinase 1- and 2-dependent program of chromatin trafficking of c-Fos and Fra-1 is required for cyclin D1 expression during cell cycle reentry. *Mol Cell Biol.* 2004;24:4696–4709.

Cande C, Cohen I, Daugas E, et al. Apoptosis-inducing factor (AIF): a novel caspase-independent death effector released from mitochondria. *Biochimie.* 2002;84:215–222.

Carbone M, Pass HI, Miele L, Bocchetta M. New developments about the association of SV40 with human mesothelioma. *Oncogene.* 2003;22:5173–5180.

Carbone M, Rdzanek MA. Pathogenesis of malignant mesothelioma. *Clin Lung Cancer.* 2004;5 Suppl 2:S46–S50.

Casalino L, De Cesare D, Verde P. Accumulation of Fra-1 in ras-transformed cells depends on both transcriptional autoregulation and MEK-dependent posttranslational stabilization. *Mol Cell Biol.* 2003;23:4401–4415.

Chang TS, Jeong W, Woo HA, Lee SM, Park S, Rhee SG. Characterization of mammalian sulfiredoxin and its reactivation of hyperoxidized peroxiredoxin through reduction of cysteine sulfinic acid in the active site to cysteine. *J Biol Chem.* 2004;279:50994–51001.

Chiu R, Angel P, Karin M. Jun-B differs in its biological properties from, and is a negative regulator of, c-Jun. *Cell.* 1989;59:979–986.

Craighead JE, Mossman BT. The pathogenesis of asbestos-associated diseases. *N Engl J Med.* 1982;306:1446–1455.

Dai J, Churg, A. Relationship of fiber surface iron and active oxygen species to expression of procollagen, PDGF-A, and TGF-beta(1) in tracheal explants exposed to amosite asbestos. *Am J Respir Cell Mol Biol.* 2001;24:427–435.

Davies KJ. The broad spectrum of responses to oxidants in proliferating cells: A new paradigm for oxidative stress. *IUBMB Life.* 1999;48:41–47.

Davis RJ. Signal transduction by the JNK group of MAP kinases. *Cell.* 2000;103:239–252.

Faux SP, Houghton CE, Hubbard A, Patrick, G. Increased expression of epidermal growth factor receptor in rat pleural mesothelial cells correlates with carcinogenicity of mineral fibres. *Carcinogenesis.* 2000;21:2275–2280.

Fenoglio I, Prandi L, Tomatis M, Fubini B. Free radical generation in the toxicity of inhaled mineral particles: the role of iron speciation at the surface of asbestos and silica. *Redox Rep.* 2001;6:235–241.

Finkel T, Holbrook NJ. Oxidants, oxidative stress and the biology of ageing. *Nature.* 2000;408:239–247.

Forman HJ, Fukuto JM, Torres M. Redox signaling: thiol chemistry defines which reactive oxygen and nitrogen species can act as second messengers. *Am J Physiol Cell Physiol.* 2004;287:C246–C256.

Gabbita SP, Robinson KA, Stewart CA, Floyd RA, Hensley K. Redox regulatory mechanisms of cellular signal transduction. *Arch Biochem Biophys.* 2000;376:1–13.

Geist LJ, Powers LS, Monick MM, Hunninghake GW. Asbestos stimulation triggers differential cytokine release from human monocytes and alveolar macrophages. *Exp Lung Res.* 2000;26:41–56.

Ghio AJ, Zhang J, Piantadosi CA. Generation of hydroxyl radical by crocidolite asbestos is proportional to surface [Fe3+]. *Arch Biochem Biophys.* 1992;298:646–650.

Go YM, Gipp JJ, Mulcahy RT, Jones DP. H_2O_2-dependent activation of GCLC-ARE4 reporter occurs by mitogen-activated protein kinase pathways without oxidation of cellular glutathione or thioredoxin-1. *J Biol Chem*. 2004;279:5837–5845.

Goldberg JL, Zanella CL, Janssen YM, et al. Novel cell imaging techniques show induction of apoptosis and proliferation in mesothelial cells by asbestos. *Am J Respir Cell Mol Biol*. 1997;17:265–271.

Goodglick LA, Kane AB. Role of reactive oxygen metabolites in crocidolite asbestos toxicity to mouse macrophages. *Cancer Res*. 1986;46:5558–5566.

Green D, Kroemer, G. The central executioners of apoptosis: caspases or mitochondria? *Trends Cell Biol*. 1998;8:267–271.

Green DR, Kroemer G. The pathophysiology of mitochondrial cell death. *Science*. 2004;305: 626–629.

Gulumian M, Bhoolia DJ, Du Toit RS, et al. Activation of UICC crocidolite: the effect of conversion of some ferric ions to ferrous ions. *Environ Res*. 1993;60:193–206.

Gulumian M, van Wyk, JA. Hydroxyl radical production in the presence of fibres by a Fenton-type reaction. *Chem Biol Interact*. 1987;62:89–97.

Gulumian M, van Wyk, JA. Oxygen consumption, lipid peroxidation, and mineral fibres. In: Bown R, Hoskins J, Johnson N, eds. *Mechanisms in Fibre Carcinogenesis*. New York: Plenum Press; 1991:439–446.

Guyton KZ, Liu Y, Gorospe M, Xu Q, Holbrook NJ. Activation of mitogen-activated protein kinase by H_2O_2. Role in cell survival following oxidant injury. *J Biol Chem*. 1996;271:4138–4142.

Hanahan D, Weinberg RA. The hallmarks of cancer. *Cell*. 2000;100:57–70.

Hansen K, Mossman BT. Generation of superoxide (O_2^-) from alveolar macrophages exposed to asbestiform and nonfibrous particles. *Cancer Res*. 1987;47:1681–1686.

Heintz NH, Janssen YM, Mossman BT. Persistent induction of c-fos and c-jun expression by asbestos. *Proc Natl Acad Sci USA*. 1993;90:3299–3303.

Hubbard AK, Timblin CR, Rincon M, Mossman BT. Use of transgenic luciferase reporter mice to determine activation of transcription factors and gene expression by fibrogenic particles. *Chest*. 2001;120:24S–25S.

Janne PA, Taffaro ML, Salgia R, Johnson BE. Inhibition of epidermal growth factor receptor signaling in malignant pleural mesothelioma. *Cancer Res*. 2002;62:5242–5247.

Janssen YM, Heintz NH, Marsh JP, Borm PJ, Mossman BT. Induction of c-fos and c-jun proto-oncogenes in target cells of the lung and pleura by carcinogenic fibers. *Am J Respir Cell Mol Biol*. 1994;11:522–530.

Janssen YM, Heintz NH, Mossman BT. Induction of c-fos and c-jun proto-oncogene expression by asbestos is ameliorated by N-acetyl-L-cysteine in mesothelial cells. *Cancer Res*. 1995;55:2085–2089.

Johnson RS, van Lingen B, Papaioannou VE, Spiegelman BM. A null mutation at the c-jun locus causes embryonic lethality and retarded cell growth in culture. *Genes Dev*. 1993;7:1309–1317.

Jung M, Davis WP, Taatjes DJ, Churg A, Mossman BT. Asbestos and cigarette smoke cause increased DNA strand breaks and necrosis in bronchiolar epithelial cells in vivo. *Free Radic Biol Med*. 2000;28:1295–1299.

Kamp DW, Panduri V, Weitzman SA, Chandel N. Asbestos-induced alveolar epithelial cell apoptosis: role of mitochondrial dysfunction caused by iron-derived free radicals. *Mol Cell Biochem*. 2002;234–235:153–160.

Karin M, Shaulian E. AP-1: linking hydrogen peroxide and oxidative stress to the control of cell proliferation and death. *IUBMB Life*. 2001;52:17–24.

Kazzaz JA, Horowitz S, Xu J, et al. Differential patterns of apoptosis in resolving and nonresolving bacterial pneumonia. *Am J Respir Crit Care Med*. 2000;161:2043–2050.

Kiley PJ, Storz G. Exploiting thiol modifications. *PLoS Biol*. 2004;2:e400.

Kinnula VL, Paakko P, Soini Y. Antioxidant enzymes and redox regulating thiol proteins in malignancies of human lung. *FEBS Lett*. 2004;569:1–6.

Klein G, Powers A, Croce C. Association of SV40 with human tumors. *Oncogene*. 2002;21:1141–1149.

Kwon J, Lee SR, Yang KS, et al. Reversible oxidation and inactivation of the tumor suppressor PTEN in cells stimulated with peptide growth factors. *Proc Natl Acad Sci USA.* 2004;101:16419–16424.

Lambeth JD. NOX enzymes and the biology of reactive oxygen. *Nat Rev Immunol.* 2004;4:181–189.

Lawrence DS, Niu J. Protein kinase inhibitors: the tyrosine-specific protein kinases. *Pharmacol Ther.* 1998;77:81–114.

Lechner JF, Tokiwa T, LaVeck M, et al. Asbestos-associated chromosomal changes in human mesothelial cells. *Proc Natl Acad Sci USA.* 1985;82:3884–3888.

Lee SR, Kwon KS, Kim SR, Rhee SG. Reversible inactivation of protein-tyrosine phosphatase 1B in A431 cells stimulated with epidermal growth factor. *J Biol Chem.* 1998;273:15366–15372.

Lee SR, Yang KS, Kwon J, Lee C, Jeong W, Rhee SG. Reversible inactivation of the tumor suppressor PTEN by H_2O_2. *J Biol Chem.* 2002;277:20336–20342.

Lee YJ, Cho HN, Soh JW, et al. Oxidative stress-induced apoptosis is mediated by ERK1/2 phosphorylation. *Exp Cell Res.* 2003;291:251–266.

Leslie NR, Bennett D, Lindsay YE, Stewart H, Gray A, Downes CP. Redox regulation of PI 3-kinase signaling via inactivation of PTEN. *EMBO J.* 2003;22:5501–5510.

Lund LG, Aust AE. Iron mobilization from asbestos by chelators and ascorbic acid. *Arch Biochem Biophys.* 1990;278:61–64.

Manna SK, Zhang HJ, Yan T, Oberley LW, Aggarwal BB. Overexpression of manganese superoxide dismutase suppresses tumor necrosis factor-induced apoptosis and activation of nuclear transcription factor-kappaB and activated protein-1. *J Biol Chem.* 1998;273:13245–13254.

Manning CB, Cummins AB, Jung MW, et al. A mutant epidermal growth factor receptor targeted to lung epithelium inhibits asbestos-induced proliferation and proto-oncogene expression. *Cancer Res.* 2002;62:4169–4175.

Moldovan L, Irani K, Moldovan NI, Finkel T, Goldschmidt-Clermont, PJ. The actin cytoskeleton reorganization induced by Rac1 requires the production of superoxide. *Antioxid Redox Signal.* 1999;1:29–43.

Monje P, Marinissen MJ, Gutkind JS. Phosphorylation of the carboxyl-terminal transactivation domain of c-Fos by extracellular signal-regulated kinase mediates the transcriptional activation of AP-1 and cellular transformation induced by platelet-derived growth factor. *Mol Cell Biol.* 2003;23:7030–7043.

Mossman, BT, Gee JB. Asbestos-related diseases. *N Engl J Med.* 1989;320:1721–1730.

Mossman BT, Gruenert DC. SV40, growth factors, and mesothelioma: another piece of the puzzle. *Am J Respir Cell Mol Biol.* 2002;26:167–170.

Mossman BT, Kamp DW, Weitzman SA. Mechanisms of carcinogenesis and clinical features of asbestos-associated cancers. *Cancer Invest.* 1996a;14;466–480.

Mossman BT, Surinrut P, Brinton BT, et al. Transfection of a manganese-containing superoxide dismutase gene into hamster tracheal epithelial cells ameliorates asbestos-mediated cytotoxicity. *Free Radic Biol Med.* 1996b;21:125–131.

Murphy LO, MacKeigan JP, Blenis J. A network of immediate early gene products propagates subtle differences in mitogen-activated protein kinase signal amplitude and duration. *Mol Cell Biol.* 2004;24:144–153.

Murphy LO, Smith S, Chen RH, Fingar DC, Blenis J. Molecular interpretation of ERK signal duration by immediate early gene products. *Nat Cell Biol.* 2002;4:556–564.

Murray AW. Recycling the cell cycle: cyclins revisited. *Cell.* 2004;116:221–234.

Pache JC, Janssen YM, Walsh ES, et al. Increased epidermal growth factor-receptor protein in a human mesothelial cell line in response to long asbestos fibers. *Am J Pathol.* 1998;152:333–340.

Park HS, Lee SH, Park D, et al. Sequential activation of phosphatidylinositol 3-kinase, beta Pix, Rac1, and Nox1 in growth factor-induced production of H_2O_2. *Mol Cell Biol.* 2004;24:4384–4394.

Parsons, R. Human cancer, PTEN and the PI-3 kinase pathway. *Semin Cell Dev Biol.* 2004;15:171–176.

Penninger JM, Kroemer G. Mitochondria, AIF and caspases—rivaling for cell death execution. *Nat Cell Biol.* 2003;5:97–99.

Perderiset M, Marsh JP, Mossman BT. Activation of protein kinase C by crocidolite asbestos in hamster tracheal epithelial cells. *Carcinogenesis.* 1991;12:1499–1502.

Polunovsky VA, Chen B, Henke C, et al. Role of mesenchymal cell death in lung remodeling after injury. *J Clin Invest.* 1993;92:388–397.

Pouyssegur J, Volmat V, Lenormand, P. Fidelity and spatio-temporal control in MAP kinase (ERKs) signalling. *Biochem Pharmacol.* 2002;64, 755–763.

Quinlan TR, BeruBe KA, Marsh JP, et al. Patterns of inflammation, cell proliferation, and related gene expression in lung after inhalation of chrysotile asbestos. *Am J Pathol.* 1995;147:728–739.

Quinlan TR, Marsh JP, Janssen YM, et al. Dose-responsive increases in pulmonary fibrosis after inhalation of asbestos. *Am J Respir Crit Care Med.* 1994;150:200–206.

Ramos-Nino ME, Scapoli L, Martinelli M, Land S, Mossman BT. Microarray analysis and RNA silencing link fra-1 to cd44 and c-met expression in mesothelioma. *Cancer Res.* 2003;63:3539–3545.

Ramos-Nino ME, Timblin CR, Mossman BT. Mesothelial cell transformation requires increased AP-1 binding activity and ERK-dependent Fra-1 expression. *Cancer Res.* 2002;62:6065–6069.

Robledo RF, Buder-Hoffmann SA, Cummins, AB, Walsh ES, Taatjes DJ, Mossman BT. Increased phosphorylated extracellular signal-regulated kinase immunoreactivity associated with proliferative and morphologic lung alterations after chrysotile asbestos inhalation in mice. *Am J Pathol.* 2000;156:1307–1316.

Roushdy-Hammady I, Siegel J, Emri S, Testa JR., Carbone M. Genetic-susceptibility factor and malignant mesothelioma in the Cappadocian region of Turkey. *Lancet.* 2001;357:444–445.

Rundell K, Parakati R. The role of the SV40 ST antigen in cell growth promotion and trans-formation. *Semin Cancer Biol.* 2001;11:5–13.

Sauer H, Wartenberg M, Hescheler J. Reactive oxygen species as intracellular messengers during cell growth and differentiation. *Cell Physiol Biochem.* 2001;11:173–186.

Scapoli L, Ramos-Nino ME, Martinelli M, Mossman BT. Src-dependent ERK5 and Src/EGFR-dependent ERK1/2 activation is required for cell proliferation by asbestos. *Oncogene.* 2004;23:805–813.

Schlessinger J. Common and distinct elements in cellular signaling via EGF and FGF receptors. *Science.* 2004;306:1506–1507.

Schutte J, Minna JD, Birrer MJ. Deregulated expression of human c-jun transforms primary rat embryo cells in cooperation with an activated c-Ha-ras gene and transforms rat-1a cells as a single gene. *Proc Natl Acad Sci USA.* 1989a;86:2257–2261.

Schutte J, Viallet J, Nau M, Segal S, Fedorko J, Minna J. jun-B inhibits and c-fos stimulates the transforming and trans-activating activities of c-jun. *Cell.* 1989b;59:987–997.

Sesko A, Cabot M, Mossman B. Hydrolysis of inositol phospholipids precedes cellular proliferation in asbestos-stimulated tracheobronchial epithelial cells. *Proc Natl Acad Sci USA.* 1990;87:7385–7389.

Shaulian E, Karin M. AP-1 in cell proliferation and survival. *Oncogene.* 2001;20:2390–2400.

Shukla A, Gulumian M, Hei TK, Kamp D, Rahman Q, Mossman BT. Multiple roles of oxidants in the pathogenesis of asbestos-induced diseases. *Free Radic Biol Med.* 2003a;34:1117–1129.

Shukla A, Jung M, Stern M, et al. Asbestos induces mitochondrial DNA damage and dysfunction linked to the development of apoptosis. *Am J Physiol Lung Cell Mol Physiol.* 2003b;285:L1018–1025.

Shukla A, Mossman B. Asbestosis and asbestos-related cancers: role of reactive oxygen and nitrogen species (ROS/RNS). In: Vallyathan V, Castranova V, Shi X, eds. *Oxygen/Nitrogen Radicals: Lung Injury and Disease.* New York: Marcel Dekker; 2003:179–195.

Stenner-Liewen F, Reed J. Apoptosis and cancer: basic mechanisms and therapeutic opportunities in the postgenomic era. *Cancer Res.* 2003;63:263–268.

Stone JR, Collins T. The role of hydrogen peroxide in endothelial proliferative responses. *Endothelium.* 2002;9:231–238.

Timblin CR, Guthrie GD, Janssen YW, Walsh ES, Vacek P, Mossman BT. Patterns of c-fos and c-jun proto-oncogene expression, apoptosis, and proliferation in rat pleural mesothelial cells exposed to erionite or asbestos fibers. *Toxicol Appl Pharmacol.* 1998;151:88–97.

Timblin CR, Janssen YW, Mossman BT. Transcriptional activation of the proto-oncogene c-jun by asbestos and H_2O_2 is directly related to increased proliferation and transformation of tracheal epithelial cells. *Cancer Res.* 1995;55:2723–2726.

Uhal B D. Cell cycle kinetics in the alveolar epithelium. *Am J Physiol.* 1997;272:L1031–1045.

van der Vliet A, Hristova M, Cross CE, Eiserich JP, Goldkorn, T. (1998). Peroxynitrite induces covalent dimerization of epidermal growth factor receptors in A431 epidermoid carcinoma cells. *J Biol Chem.* 1997;273:31860–31866.

Vandel L, Montreau N, Vial E, Pfarr CM, Binetruy B, Castellazzi M. Stepwise transformation of rat embryo fibroblasts: c-Jun, JunB, or JunD can cooperate with Ras for focus formation, but a c-Jun-containing heterodimer is required for immortalization. *Mol Cell Biol.* 1996;16:1881–1888.

Wisdom R, Johnson RS, Moore C. c-Jun regulates cell cycle progression and apoptosis by distinct mechanisms. *EMBO J.* 1999;18:188–197.

Woo HA, Chae HZ, Hwang SC, et al. Reversing the inactivation of peroxiredoxins caused by cysteine sulfinic acid formation. *Science.* 2003;300:653–656.

Wood ZA, Poole, LB, Karplus PA. Peroxiredoxin evolution and the regulation of hydrogen peroxide signaling. *Science.* 2003a;300:650–653.

Wood ZA, Schroder E, Robin Harris J, Poole LB. Structure, mechanism and regulation of peroxiredoxins. *Trends Biochem Sci.* 2003b;28:32–40.

Woodworth CD, Mossman BT, Craighead JE. Induction of squamous metaplasia in organ cultures of hamster trachea by naturally occurring and synthetic fibers. *Cancer Res.* 1983;43:4906–4912.

Yuan Z, Taatjes DJ, Mossman BT, Heintz NH. The duration of nuclear extracellular signal-regulated kinase 1 and 2 signaling during cell cycle reentry distinguishes proliferation from apoptosis in response to asbestos. *Cancer Res.* 2004;64:6530–6536.

Zalma R, Bonneau L, Guignard J, Pezerat H. Production of hydroxyl radicals by iron solid compounds. *Toxicol Environ Chem.* 1987;13:171–187.

Zanella CL, Posada J, Tritton TR, Mossman BT. Asbestos causes stimulation of the extracellular signal-regulated kinase 1 mitogen-activated protein kinase cascade after phosphorylation of the epidermal growth factor receptor. *Cancer Res.* 1996;56:5334–5338.

Zanella CL, Timblin CR, Cummins A, et al. Asbestos-induced phosphorylation of epidermal growth factor receptor is linked to c-fos and apoptosis. *Am J Physiol.* 1999;277:L684–L693.

Zwacka RM, Dudus L, Epperly MW, Greenberger JS, Engelhardt JF. Redox gene therapy protects human IB-3 lung epithelial cells against ionizing radiation-induced apoptosis. *Hum Gene Ther.* 1998;9:1381–1386.

6

Benign Pleural and Parenchymal Diseases Associated with Asbestos Exposure

John E. Craighead

Introduction

Asbestosis is a disease of the 20th century. Although vague historical documentation from the distant past refers to "phythis" occurring among slaves and those involved in the trades, the etiology of these nonspecific respiratory conditions is obscure. Possibly they represented asbestosis, but disease such as silicosis (a common, recognized lung disease of antiquity), kaolinosis (due to China clay exposure), and byssinosis (caused by exposure to cotton dust), as well as a myriad of infectious processes are possible, if not likely, alternate explanations. We just do not know. In 1866, Zenker coined the term "pneumonokoniosis" to describe a condition known as hematite lung, stating "it will then be necessary to embrace under a single title all these essentially identical forms of disease...attributable to mineral dust exposure" (Meiklejohn, 1960).

As considered in Chapter 1, the first commercial chrysotile mine was opened in the Province of Québec, Canada, in the 1870s. Mining of the amphibole, crocidolite, in South Africa began shortly before the turn of the century, and shortly thereafter, this mineral was evaluated by naval shipbuilders because it is resistant to heat and fire. By the early 1900s crocidolite and chrysotile were widely used in the manufacturing of fire-resistant textiles. Workers in these early days, no doubt, sustained massive exposures, for control measures were lacking and there was little recognition of the capacity of asbestos to cause disease. However, in 1898, the British Chief Inspector of Factories and Workshops already had noted "the evil effects of asbestos dust."

Initially discovered at autopsy in the lungs of a textile worker in 1900, the ravages of asbestosis plagued workers exposed industrially in the early decades of the century (Cooke, 1924). By the end of World War I, both of the commercial amphiboles, crocidolite and amosite, and chrysotile had been widely used industrially, but in relatively modest amounts. It was not until later that the term "asbestosis" was coined, and the hallmark of the disease, the so-called curious bodies described by Cooke (1927), was recognized under the microscope. A torrent of case reports followed, for pathologists now had a definitive diagnostic marker of the disease in the form of asbestos bodies

(AB). But, because of the extended latency of asbestosis, the full impact of occupational exposure was not fully appreciated (Merewether and Price, 1930). As a result of a tragic fire aboard a passenger vessel in the late 1930s, the US Navy stipulated the incorporation of amosite into the insulation of all newly constructed vessels, a practice that continued until the 1970s. In addition to its fire-retardant properties, amosite was chosen because it was relatively light in weight and resistant to degradation by sea water. During the last half of the 20th century, unrestricted exposure to asbestos was played out in countless cases of respiratory diseases attributable to exposure. Now, asbestosis is a disappearing disease. Modern governmental regulations controlling the use of asbestos (Chapter 13) and public awareness have reduced substantially its incidence.

From a medical perspective, asbestosis can be considered either a clinical disease manifest functionally, and readily demonstrable by radiological means, or a pathological entity of variable degrees of severity, but often as scattered localized lesions in the lungs in the absence of clinically evident respiratory insufficiency. Chapter 10 addresses clinical approaches to diagnosis, and Chapter 11 provides a detailed radiological overview of its features. This chapter considers the pathogenesis and pathological features of the disease from the perspective of its epidemiology.

Asbestos Bodies

Over a century ago, in one of the earliest descriptions of what was later to be designated as an AB, Marchand (1906) noted "peculiar pigmented crystals" that were light yellow or reddish brown in lung tissue. He recorded the dimensions of these structures and demonstrated iron in the coat. As noted above, Cooke found "curious bodies" scattered in the lungs of an asbestos worker in 1927. These structures were initially designated as asbestosis (sic) bodies, a term changed to AB shortly thereafter. When similar ferritin-coated bodies were found microscopically in the absence of evidence of asbestos exposure, the term pseudo-asbestos body was coined, more commonly referred to now as a ferruginous body (Figure 6.1).

AB are now the morphologic hallmark of asbestos exposure and the key pathological criterion for the diagnosis of asbestosis in a fibrotic lung; however, the complexities of the topic verge on the enigmatic, for the AB usually are an indication of exposure to relatively long, thin fibers of amphibole (Figure 6.2), and often represent only a small proportion of the total number of asbestos fibers in the lungs. Indeed, the ratio of asbestos fibers to AB ranges from 1:1 to 3000:1. In a taxingly comprehensive analysis of the lungs of 38 patients, Murai et al. (1995) found only 17% of asbestos fibers coated to form AB with the proportion differing by mineralogical type. In this study, the vast bulk of the coated fibers were longer than 20 μm, and had a diameter of less than 0.8 μm. Roughly similar findings were reported by Churg and Warnock (1977). Clearly, amphibole cores are found in the great majority of AB that are rodlike in appearance. Some studies (Pooley and Ranson, 1986) suggest that amosite more readily forms AB than crocidolite. Only occasionally do AB develop on a chrysotile core (Figure 6.3A and 6.3B). When and if chrysotile is coated, the fibers usually are relatively long (>15 μm), thin, and curved in a complex array of configurations. In developed industrialized countries, most ferruginous bodies in the lungs of members of the general population, and in heavily exposed occupational groups, are AB; however, other types of inorganic and organic fibers, on occasion, form ferruginous bodies, sharing morphological features with AB (Churg and Warnock, 1977, 1981; Craighead et al., 1982). Structures forming on and around plate or sheet silicates such as talc, kaolin, and mica, are

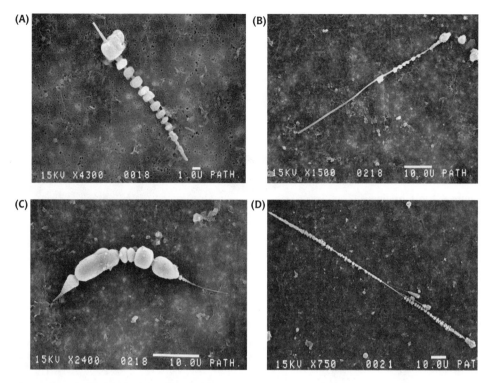

Figure 6.1 (A–D) SEM of AB developing on amphibole cores in the lung of a patient. Note the relative size of fiber and the associated body (bar).

perhaps the most commonly observed, but metal fibers, shards of silica and graphite, fibrous zeolites, fiber glass, ceramic fibers, and even fibers of wool and cotton have been described in the core of ferruginous bodies. Particles of iron such as found in the lungs of welders and steel mill workers form nonfibrous siderotic bodies (Angervall et al., 1960). Breakdown products of lung tissue, specifically, fragments of elastic fibers, can acquire an iron coat—the so-called elastosis bodies (established using a stain for elastic). Even the most experienced pathologist occasionally cannot differentiate members of this wide panoply of ferruginous bodies from true AB; thus, discrimination requires ultrastructural evaluation of the core of the body complemented by x-ray spectrometry to determine the particle's elemental composition, and selected area electron defraction to assay its crystalline features. Often, the occupational history provides meaningful insights, but it can also be misleading.

Painstaking light microscopical study complemented by iron staining of tissue sections permits the identification of an occasional AB in the lungs of unexposed members of the general public (Thompson, 1965; Utidjian et al., 1968). Such observations are increasingly rare because of the implementation of rigorous regulations limiting the use of asbestos in our modern environment. In one study from Miami, Florida, published in 1965, 26% of the lungs from routine autopsies displayed AB (Gaensler and Addington, 1969), whereas investigations in Montreal (Anjilvel and Thurlbeck, 1966) documented AB in 2% of routine autopsies. Three percent of autopsies in London yielded AB (Gibbs, A, unpublished). Examination of digests of lung demonstrates AB in a sizable proportion of the population. In a study by Churg and Warnock (1977), 12% of a large group

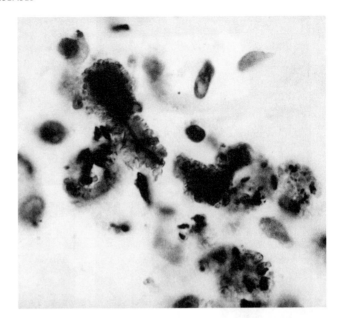

Figure 6.2 A ferruginous body with a carbon-black fibrous core. This graphite body superficially resembles an AB but the AB cores are colorless. Note the carbonaceous granules in the alveolar macrophages.

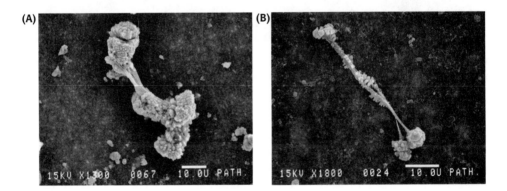

Figure 6.3 SEM of AB developing on a long, thick fiber core of chrysotile. (A) Note the fibrils are focally splaying out. The bar measures 10 μm in another chrysotile AB (B).

of urban dwellers had more than 100 AB/gram of wet lung tissue. In a second study, these investigators found an average of 2000 AB/gram of dry lung, whereas Roggli et al. (2004) demonstrated fewer than 20 AB/gram of wet lung tissue in an unexposed control population. These findings emphasize the influences of various technical approaches on the results of assays (Chapter 12) as well as differences between various control populations. Unfortunately, standardized techniques for evaluating tissue samples have not been generally accepted by workers in the field and samples for comparative interlaboratory quality control exercises unfortunately are not generally available (Davis et al., 1986).

Digests of hilar and mediastinal lymph nodes (Gloyne, 1933; Godwin and Jagatic, 1968; Roggli and Benning, 1990) from heavily exposed patients also demonstrate AB and uncoated fibers when examined by electron microscopy. Laboratory contamination of tissue samples during preparation is an ever-present concern and must be prevented. Nonetheless, asbestos has been found to be widely distributed in tissues throughout the body, presumably transported by lymphatics (Sebastien, 1977). This assumption is based on the demonstration of uncoated amphibole and chrysotile fibers at the confluence of lymphatic vessels (so-called black spots) on the visceral and parietal pleural surfaces of the lung (Boutin et al., 1996), in digests of abdominal tissues (Dodson et al., 1985) and in the urine of asbestos workers (Cook and Olson, 1979). It is not known whether the AB in these organs form locally or represent the transport of AB intact to lymph nodes, and tissues outside the thoracic cavity. In an exhaustive autopsy study, Auerbach et al. (1980) found AB in histological sections of several major abdominal organs.

As indicated above, fiber length and diameter are key factors influencing AB development (Pooley, 1972). Perhaps exogenous and endogenous iron concentrations in the lung tissue are important. The ferrintin-protein coats of AB are applied by phagocytic macrophages. Several macrophages appear to act in concert to fully envelope a long fiber, but a "zipper-like" action by a single macrophage migrating over the surface of a fiber is also a possibility (Morgan and Holmes, 1985; Suzuki and Churg, 1969). The durability of the fiber appears to be a key consideration. The rapid dissolution of chrysotile in vivo is thought to account for its infrequent presence in the core of AB. But, it should be noted that chrysotile fibers have a net-positive ionic charge in contrast to the near-neutral charge of amphibole fibers. Host factors may also play a role. For unknown reasons, AB develop readily in the lungs of experimentally exposed guinea pigs, but rarely in the tissues of rats, mice, and hamsters. Whereas newly introduced "bare" asbestos fibers prompt acute inflammation in lung tissue, the AB usually is not accompanied by acute inflammatory cells and foreign body giant cells rarely are seen (with the exception of the tissue response to the blunt fibers of anthophyllite, Craighead et al., 1982). This observation has lead to the prevailing but unproven notion that AB are biologically inert and lack pathogenic importance (McLemore et al., 1981).

Asbestosis

Classically, clinical asbestosis in its advanced form is a diffuse fibrotic pulmonary disease, more prominent in the lower lobes than in the upper lobes, often, but not invariably, associated with diffuse pleural fibrosis or typical parietal pleural plaques (PP), or both, and less commonly, diffuse bilateral thickening of the visceral pleura (Figures 6.4, 6.5, and 6.6). The fibrosis is particularly prominent in subpleural lung tissues where extensive retraction of the scarred parenchyma at the periphery of the lung tends to result in pseudo-cyst formation, a feature known as "honeycombing." This lesion should be differentiated from the peripheral blebs and bullae of emphysema, particularly the paraseptal form of this disease process. Elsewhere, septal and interstitial fibrosis are prominent features often accompanied by large numbers of AB lodged in both the fibrotic scars and the air spaces. Digests of the lungs usually demonstrate thousands of AB and countless uncoated fibers of variable lengths (Table 6.1). Quantitation of the numbers of fibers in the lung tissue is relative, for the amounts demonstrated in lung digests reflect the technical approach and equipment used by the investigator (Chapter 12).

Asbestosis usually has a clinical latency of 5–15 years or more, although subclinical disease can often be evident pathologically much earlier. The elapsed time between the initial exposure and the appearance of clinical disease is dependent upon mineralogical type as well as both the duration and intensity of exposure (Table 6.2). In the pathfinding studies of heavily exposed textile workers by Dreessen et al. (1938), 27% of the mill workers developed clinical asbestosis after exposure for only 5–9 years. In the 1930s, no industrial setting was more hazardous than the textile factory. But, studies of amosite miners in South Africa suggest that asbestosis gradually develops in a

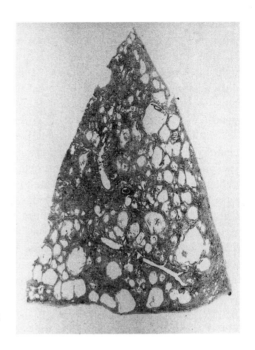

Figure 6.4 Asbestosis involving lower lung zones. Honeycombing is evident in areas with extensive scarring.

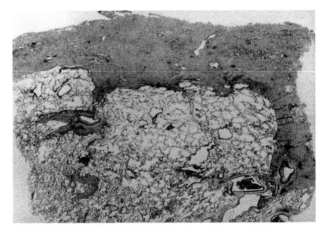

Figure 6.5 Diffuse pleural fibrosis extending into the septum. Note the absence of lung parenchymal fibrosis (asbestosis).

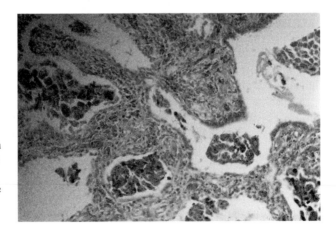

Figure 6.6 Wedge of lower lobe showing advanced diffuse fibrosis (Grade 4) with extensive honeycombing. The lesion superficially resembles emphysema but the spaces are formed by the retraction of fibrous tissue.

Table 6.1 Asbestos Fiber Dry Lung Content ($f \times 10^6$ g Wet Lung) of Amosite Factory Workers by Grade of Pulmonary Fibrosis*

Grade	Amosite		Chrysotile		Cases Studied
	Mean	SD	Mean	SD	
0.0	3.9	4.2	3.4	4.2	3
0.5	5.1	5.6	3	4	5
1.0	321.3	343.6	24.8	27.4	4
1.5	469.9	821.5	4.7	8.6	6
2.0	671.5	510.6	9.6	11.4	3
2.5	1656.6	2342.3	.0	.0	2
3.0	194.7	175.2	26.6	16.8	4
4.0	1916.3	2693.1	19.2	41.1	11

* From Gibbs et al. (1994).

Table 6.2 Asbestosis in Textile Industry*

Years Employed	Clinical Asbestosis			
	Number Examined	Number	Group Incidence %	Average Age
0–4	89	0	—	—
5–9	141	36	26	36
10–14	84	27	32	40
15–19	28	15	54	43
20+	21	17	81	53
Totals	363	95	26	41

* From Merewether and Price (1930).

substantial proportion of workers exposed to amosite after extended latency periods, that is, decades (H. Sluis-Cremer, 1981, personal communication). It appears the amosite-associated asbestosis is progressive even without continued environmental exposure, ultimately affecting the majority of the members of an exposed population of workers.

In the initial two-thirds of this century, asbestosis was often a debilitating and occasionally fatal disease. Its prevalence and severity is no longer a compelling public health problem. Stringent regulations invoked in developed countries worldwide have had their desired effect (Chapter 13). Thus, the classical description of the overt, severe disease described above is largely of historical interest. Now the pathologist and clinician are challenged to diagnose a disease of only microscopical proportions that is often localized and results in minimal symptomatology and little if any disability. In this limited form of the disease, the distribution can be sufficiently spotty and sparse that multiple tissue sections of lung must be reviewed microscopically by the pathologist to locate diagnostic histopathological changes. Rarely are these localized lesions evident radiologically, and symptoms attributable to asbestos disease are either not present or are obscured by underlying chronic obstructive pulmonary disease consequent to smoking. Customarily, pleural plaques (PP) and bilateral pleural fibrosis are evident, providing a hint of the possible existence of underlying asbestosis.

In the absence of contemporary exposure, the localized disease is characterized microscopically by peribronchiolar fibrosis and bland, stellate, microscopic scars predominantly

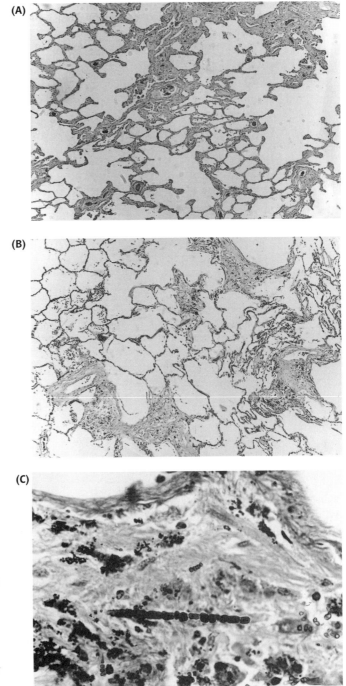

Figure 6.7 Scattered
foci of interstitial fibrosis
(A) often displaying a
stellate configuration
adjacent to blood vessels
and bronchioles (B).
Grade 2 asbestosis. Note
the AB embedded in scar
tissue (C).

located in perivascular and peribronchial sites (Figure 6.7A and 6.7B). To a variable extent, interstitial fibrosis is found in the nearby parenchyma. AB are embedded in the fibrotic tissue or are found in air spaces, usually with a predilection for the respiratory bronchioles. Fiber burden analyses of lungs in these cases show increased concentrations of AB and uncoated fibers, but substantially fewer than in the classical form of the debilitating disease.

In systematic studies of cases of asbestosis evaluated by fiber burden analysis, the median AB count was 3.7×10^5 per gram of dry lung; in 95% of cases the AB content was 1.7×10^4 per gram of dry lung tissue (Roggli et al., 1992). In 95% of the cases, the AB content was 1.7×10^3 or greater. Comparative data for normal controls and patients with idiopathic pulmonary fibrosis are illustrated in Figure 6.8. The results of a fiber burden analysis of the lungs of amosite factory workers correlated with a quantitative assessment of the severity of asbestosis are summarized in Table 6.1 (Gibbs et al., 1991).

As discussed in more detail below, the initial lesions of asbestosis are confined to the respiratory bronchioles. A report by a committee sponsored by the National Institute of Occupational Safety and Health (NIOSH) (Craighead et al., 1982) stated that the "minimal features of the disease are the demonstration of discrete foci of fibrosis in the walls of respiratory bronchioles associated with accumulations of AB." In practice, this has been interpreted to imply two or more AB in more than one anatomical acinar unit of the lungs. The report further states "the demonstration of AB in the absence of fibrosis is insufficient evidence to justify the diagnosis [of asbestosis]...." More recently, the so-called Helsinki criteria were published by an unofficial group of interested pathologists and scientists (Henderson et al., 1997). They tendered a similar definition of asbestosis "diffuse interstitial fibrosis in well inflated lung tissue remote from a lung cancer or other mass lesion, plus the presence of either two or more AB in tissue with a section area of 1 cm²." A definitive diagnosis of asbestosis cannot be made pathologically in cases that show the characteristic distribution of fibrosis in the absence of AB, even in a patient with a history of exposure. This latter point is of particular significance because

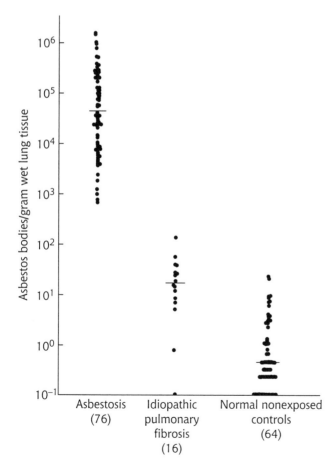

Figure 6.8 Relative numbers of AB in lung samples from an unexposed control population and patients with idiopathic pulmonary fibrosis in comparison with patients having pathological asbestosis. Note log scale. Number of subjects in brackets. (Roggli et al., 1992; published with permission).

fibrosis of the walls of the respiratory bronchioles (with or without evidence of inflammation) is a common denominator for injuries due to different types of toxic inhalant injuries to the lungs, the most common of which is cigarette smoke (Adesina et al., 1991; Hogg et al., 2004) (Figure 6.9). Thus, bronchiolar wall fibrosis is a nonspecific change that can only be attributed to asbestos exposure when AB are present in the lumina or in the fibrotic wall of the respiratory bronchioles. As the disease process progresses, fibrosis of the membranous bronchioles and alveolar ducts is observed. Finally, it is a generalized process and increasing numbers of fibers and AB are found in digests of the scarred lung tissue. A classification schema for quantitating the extent and severity of asbestosis is outlined in Appendix 6.1.

A particularly contentious point centers on the question: How many AB must be found microscopically in the presence of pulmonary fibrosis to warrant the diagnosis of asbestosis? Churg (1983) expressed the view that the presence of a single AB in a fibrotic lung is a sufficient basis for the histological diagnosis. This is an unduly liberal criterion. Contrariwise, it has been suggested that >50% of the bronchioles are involved in Grade I asbestosis. As noted above, nonspecific pulmonary fibrosis in smokers is commonly found in persons of advanced age with emphysema. And, as noted above, an occasional AB can often be demonstrated in the lungs of average citizens. Moreover, the pathophysiological distortion of the lungs in emphysematous pulmonary disease tends to enhance the retention of asbestos fibers and the elimination of dust is impeded by cigarette smoking. The attendees at the Helsinki meeting (Henderson et al., 1997) suggested that a fiber analysis yielding "asbestos fibers that fall into the range recorded by the same laboratory" could serve as a surrogate basis for a "histologic" diagnosis of asbestosis. Unfortunately, there is no scientific basis for this claim, but the lack of evidence does not exclude this possibility. Environmental scientists futilely continue to search for quantitative tools to describe the severity of fibrotic disease in the lung.

Although asbestosis is classically considered a diffuse parenchymal disease, exposures of the magnitude and duration required to cause the fibrotic reaction has profound effects on the tracheal and bronchial mucosa. In human lung tissue obtained either by biopsy or autopsy, hyperplasia of the epithelial cells lining the respiratory tract and either mucinous or squamous metaplasia (or both) are often observed in the bronchial epithelium (McGavran and Brody, 1989). These changes are mimicked in vitro when organ cultures of the bronchial mucosa are experimentally exposed to asbestos (Mossman et al., 1980, 1982) (Figure 6.10). Dramatic molecular and metabolic events occur in these epithelial cells, the details of which are considered in Chapter 8. Similar morphological changes and biochemical events are found in the bronchial tissue of smokers. Combustion

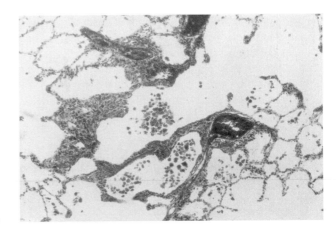

Figure 6.9 Respiratory bronchiole in the lung of a 22-year-old smoker dying traumatically. There was no occupational history of exposure to "toxic" inhalants.

(A)

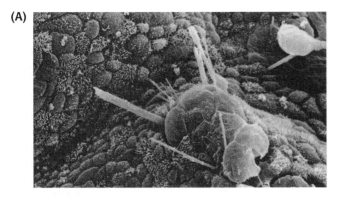

(B) Intercellular
movement
of fiber

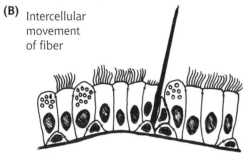

Stimulation of
squamous
metaplasia

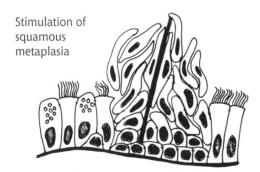

Figure 6.10 SEM demonstrating the interaction of crocidolite with epithelium of hamster trachea in organ culture (A). The fibers are enveloped by the mucosa after which squamous metaplasia evolves (B). Seen here is the early stage of this process. Some observers have misinterpreted these illustrations to suggest that fibers penetrate (like an arrow) epithelial cells. Sequential ultrastructural studies show this is not the case.

products of tobacco and asbestos may act in concert to predispose or accentuate the pathologic process (McFadden et al., 1986), and most probably, malignant transformation of the bronchial mucosa among asbestos workers who smoke. Studies using organ cultures of hamster trachea have demonstrated the interaction of the asbestos-exposed mucosa with polycyclic aromatic hydrocarbons, resulting in the induction of carcinomas in vitro (Craighead and Mossman, 1979).

Churg has championed the notion that small-airway disease, that is, the alveolitis and respiratory bronchiolar fibrosis resulting from asbestos exposure, is not the disease asbestosis (Churg et al., 1985). As these authors note, morphological changes in distal airways often occur in the absence of diffuse interstitial fibrosis. Nonsmokers exposed occupationally to asbestos display a physiological degree of air flow obstruction (Begin et al., 1983a, 1987; Cohen et al., 1984; Chapter 10). This may be a distinction without clinical relevance. The physiological alterations attributed to obstructive lung disease in smokers appear to be compounded by long-term exposure to asbestos, just as the typical radiological lesions, that is, the small, irregular shadow of asbestosis in chest x-rays are more apparent in those who smoke (Eidelman et al., 1990).

Pathogenesis

Observations on animals experimentally exposed to asbestos, complemented by detailed studies of humans, have provided insights into the cellular and molecular events that contribute to the development of pulmonary fibrosis in the asbestos worker. The intensity of the exposure, as well as the mineral type and fiber length, prove to be key considerations influencing events deep in the lungs. The threshold dosage required to produce disease (both clinically and histopathologically) remains undefined, although it is substantially lower for amphiboles than chrysotile, and relates directly to the relative proportion of long fibers (>5 μm in length) inhaled. A recent report by a committee appointed by the US Environmental Protection Agency (EPA) concluded that fibers less than 5 μm in length are not pathogenic. It should be recalled that industrial grades of asbestos are comprised of a heterogenous collection of fibers of differing lengths and breadth, the majority of which are <5 μm in length. Longer fibers are usually quite limited in crude mill products, but of these, the occasional fiber can be 10 or 20 μm (or more) in length. In the past, asbestos was sieved in the mill to produce grades that differed in mean length. Relatively long fibers were the most valuable and used in textile manufacturing whereas the "cheap," short fiber preparations were often incorporated into building materials such as cement and joint compounds.

Host factors remain undefined, although, as already noted, smoking has an effect on the lung's capacity to clear fibers and appears to accentuate the pathological changes observed in the lungs of persons with asbestosis (Weiss, 1984). Students of this disease are impressed by the variability in the extent of pulmonary parenchymal disease developing among workers seemingly exposed to comparable amounts of asbestos (Wagner, 1978). Becklake has suggested that persons with a mesomorphic body configuration are more likely to develop asbestosis, but support for this interesting concept is lacking. Begin and Sebastien (1989) documented variability in response among outbred sheep experimentally exposed to chrysotile. In view of the recognized differences among humans in their capacity to mobilize an inflammatory response, and form scar tissue, it would not be surprising to learn that some of us are more prone to develop asbestosis than others. Unfortunately, clinical or experimental evidence to support this hypothesis, at present, is limited.

As noted above, the anatomic site where events initially play out after exposure is the respiratory bronchiole, a location where the velocity of air flow is nil, and inhaled fibers tend to deposit passively. Experimental studies have shown that the depth of penetration of asbestos in the lungs is inversely proportional to fiber diameter, not to length (Chapter 12). Thus, the rigid and thin fibers of amphiboles more readily find their way deep into the lungs, regardless of length, than do the pliable fibers and bundles of chrysotile. The initial actor on the stage is the pulmonary alveolar macrophage called forth by chemotactic cytokines generated locally. Epithelial cells of the bronchiolar lumina appear to play a role in events by elaborating oxygen free radicals, products that damage tissues directly and alter molecular signaling. A sentinel and scavenger cell, the alveolar macrophage (Figure 6.11) elaborates chemotactic products that provoke an acute inflammatory response, calling forth polymorphonuclear leukocytes, also armed with the capacity to generate oxidants and proteases. This reaction mediates both local injury that may be followed by scarring, depending on the severity of the exposure, and the capacity of the tissues to generate antioxidants and antiproteases that have the potential to neutralize the adverse effects of the inflammatory cell products. These early events have been characterized as alveolitis, a picture demonstrated in the lungs of experimentally exposed animals. The events at the local level correlate with the finding of inflammatory cells and cytokines in bronchoalveolar lavage specimens from persons exposed to asbestos (see below; Figure 6.12).

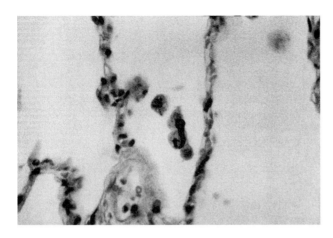

Figure 6.11 AB in alveolar macrophages in the lungs of a patient with no pathological evidence of asbestosis.

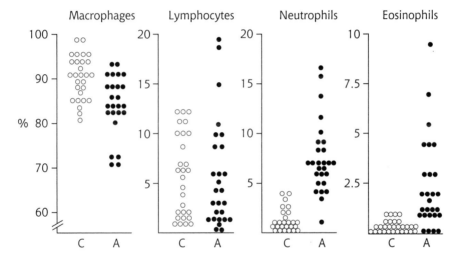

Figure 6.12 Proportions of macrophages, lymphocytes, neutrophils, and eosinophils in bronchoalveolar lavage samples from 29 nonasbestos-exposed control subjects (C) and 27 individuals with pulmonary asbestosis (A). (Robinson et al., 1986; published with permission.)

The events that transpire thereafter depend upon the lungs' capacity to inactivate the pathogenic products of the inflammatory cells, specifically the antioxidants and antiproteases. If the oxidants entering the pulmonary acinus on a single occasion exceed this threshold, acute injury to the structural components of the lung occurs, and fibrosis may develop in its wake (Figure 6.13). Clearly, a single insult would not result in clinical or microscopically evident, chronic lung disease. Rather, asbestosis is manifest as a physiological important fibrotic disease process when and if repeated, that is, day after day, exposures gradually result in scarring of the parenchyma throughout the lungs (Figure 6.14). This then is a cumulative pathological process that evolves in the heavily exposed worker over a period of years until it ultimately becomes symptomatic (Figure 6.15). Because it obviously is impossible to quantitate fiber concentrations in the individual anatomical units of the lung, as these events unfold, and because the majority of inhaled fibers are eliminated in the upper reaches of the respiratory tract, the exposure level required to produce asbestosis is not known. These uncertainties account for our

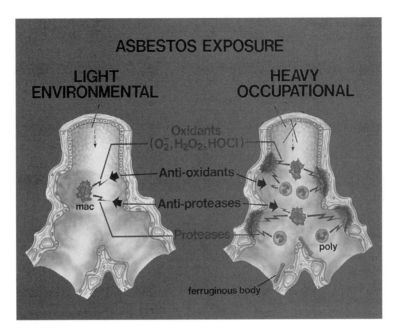

Figure 6.13 Hypothetic interaction of asbestos with airways mucosa, resulting in the elaboration of oxidants and proteases. Naturally occurring inhibitors of these agents neutralize their effect, unless the tissue is "overwhelmed" by a "toxic" amount of asbestos. Tissue injury and repair follow.

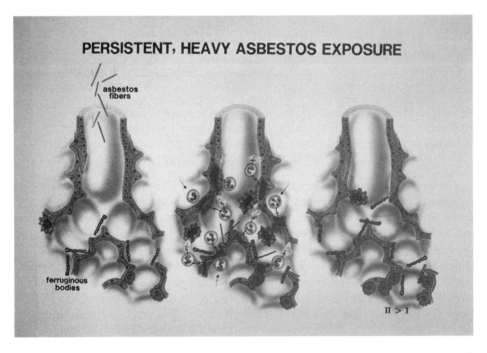

Figure 6.14 Daily inhalation of asbestos in high concentrations repeatedly damages the mucosa of the bronchial tree ultimately resulting in injuries and irreversible cumulative scarring of airways.

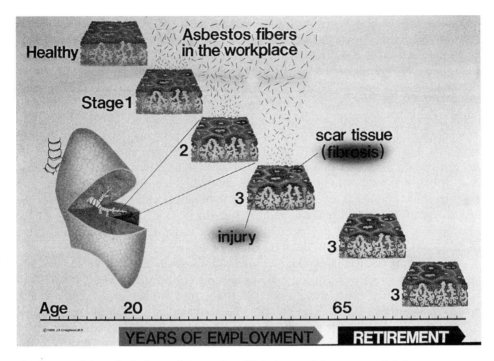

Figure 6.15 A hypothetical cumulative series of injuries result from repeated daily exposures
to amounts of asbestos that exceed threshold over extended periods of time (usually >10 years).
The residual accumulation of superimposed scars is the clinical and pathological disease process,
asbestosis.

inability to define reliable thresholds for exposure in the workplace, and understandably
are a basis for the conservative posture of regulatory agencies. Moreover, based on
these considerations, it is our view that the commonly employed terminology, that is,
fiber years, is only a term of convenience, for it inadequately characterizes the intensity
of exposure required to produce the disease asbestosis. For example, an exposure to
2 f/mL for 30 years (ie, 60 f/mL-yrs) is not the pathological equivalent of an exposure
to 6 f/mL for 10 years. In quantitative assessments, fiber mineralogical type is a critical
consideration. Commercial amphiboles are roughly three- to fourfold more pathogenic
than chrysotile.

   With this overview as background, we now turn to a consideration of the cellular and
biochemical events that have been demonstrated to occur in the lung after exposure.

   Numerous attempts have been undertaken to assay the products elaborated by the
inflammatory and epithelial cells exposed to asbestos in vitro, and in experimental animal
models. Unfortunately, these laboratory investigations, by their nature, are artificial, and
the dosages to which cells in culture are exposed, generally exceed realistic comparisons
to events in the lung of the exposed worker. As noted above, the initial accumulation of
macrophages in the distal airways after inhalation of asbestos is followed by an influx of
polymorphonuclear leukocytes (Spurzem et al., 1987; Warheit et al., 1984). Though the
mechanisms by which these macrophages are attracted to sites of asbestos deposition are
complex, Kagan et al. (1983) and Warheit et al. (1985, 1986) detected activated complement in the bronchoalveolar washings of chrysotile-exposed animals. An inhibitor of
these components of complement reduced or eliminated the inflammatory response in
vivo. On the basis of the studies of Garcia et al. (1989), migration of polymorphonuclear

leukocytes to sites of asbestos deposition may be mediated by leukotrienes. Oxidants appear to have a similar chemotactic effect. It is uncertain how inflammatory mediators interact at the local level in the human lung (Bonner et al., 2002; Cummins et al., 2003; Hayes et al., 1990; Kanazawa et al., 1970; Lounsbury et al., 2002; Thomas et al., 1994).

Abundant experimental evidence documents the elaboration of oxidants by macrophages and polymorphonuclear leukocytes in vitro, implying that similar events occur in the intact lung after exposure (Quinlan et al., 1994; Schapira et al., 1994; Chapter 5). The interface of scavenger cells with an "indigestible" inorganic fiber results in macrophage activation and the elaboration of digestive (proteolytic) enzymes (Kamp et al., 1993). Evidence to support this contention is based on the elegant studies of Mossman et al. (1990) who inhibited inflammation and pulmonary scarring in the lungs of mice experimentally exposed to asbestos by the long-term intravascular administration of the antioxidants, superoxide dismutase, and catalase. In these studies, the activity of the enzymes was facilitated and prolonged by binding the enzymes to polyethylene glycol, a chemical that prolongs the half-life of the inhibitor in vivo.

An interacting cascade of cytokines and growth factors is essential for the development of pulmonary fibrosis. Among these factors, *tumor necrosis factor alpha* (TNF-α) is a major catalyst (Dubois et al., 1989; Liu et al., 1998; Walker et al., 1995). *Tumor growth factor alpha* (TGF-α) also proves to be an important inducer of mesenchymal cell proliferation and seems to promote fibrogenic activity. A related growth factor, *tumor growth factor beta* (TGF-β), stimulates the deposition of extracellular matrix, a fundamental component of the scarring process, and *platelet-derived growth factor* (PDGF) is a highly effective mitogen for mesenchymal cells (Brody, 1993; Lasky et al., 1995). Based on these and many other in vitro studies, one presumes that similar events occur in the human lung, although the concentrations of the mediators in situ, and the timing, at present, has not been documented.

Asbestos inhaled deep into the lungs initially interacts with epithelial cells of the bronchioles (Brody, 1986, 1993), triggering the elaboration of cytokines and growth factors. Interstitial mesenchymal cells appear to be involved; ultrastructural studies have demonstrated interlinking anatomic bonds between stromal cells of the pulmonary interstitium and epithelial cells lining the airways, suggesting communication, but if and how these cells interact is currently unknown. Of interest is the elaboration of early response oncogenes in epithelial cells exposed to asbestos fibers (Timblin et al., 2001, 2002). These mediators of cell proliferation might well initiate the deposition of fibrous tissue at the local level.

Progression of Asbestosis

The thesis presented in this chapter thus far argues that clinical asbestosis is a diffuse fibrotic disease process resulting from cumulative, superimposed injuries to the lung parenchyma that ultimately evolves into debilitating lung disease over a period of years. This concept is based on the notion that injury ceases when exposure terminates. It allows for individual variability in the luxuriance of the inflammatory response and the subsequent cellular and molecular events that result in both local tissue injury and repair, as discussed above. Nonetheless, many clinicians and the writer are convinced, based on clinical evidence, that the clinical disease process progresses after exposure ceases in some, but not all, long-term survivors with asbestosis (Becklake et al., 1979; Britton et al., 1977; Goff and Gaensler, 1972; Jones et al., 1989; Liddell et al., 1977; Rossiter et al., 1980; Souranta et al., 1982; Viallat et al., 1983). This conclusion is based on systematic studies of serial chest x-rays of patients, and to a more limited extent, serial physiological monitoring. If so, one must ask what pathogenic mechanisms are involved, and what artifacts may distort the clinical evidence? The first fragmentary body of evidence argues that when progression can be documented, it usually occurs in those with moderately severe radiological disease. But exceptions occur. The writer has documented the initial appearance and progression of x-ray changes in a heavily exposed insulator, several years after exposure ceased. Goff and Gaensler (1972) described another such patient, a woman with an intense exposure to crocidolite for only a 9-month period. In systematic studies of Australian crocidolite miners, short-term (median duration, 4 months) exposure resulted in progressive pulmonary fibrosis after a latency period, a process that then continued to progress through retirement for periods as long as three decades (Cookson et al., 1986). Similar observations have been reported by Rubino et al. (1979) in chrysotile-exposed miners, and by Sluis-Cremer (1981, personal communication) among amosite miners. The likelihood that asbestosis will progress appears to correlate with cumulative exposure.

Some have suggested that the physical presence of asbestos in the lung interstitium serves as an "irritant," triggering a subtle chronic inflammatory response. Fragmentary evidence suggests that amphibole exposure is more likely to lead to progressive disease because of its biopersistence. Others have argued that the progression of disease has an immunological basis, but the evidence supporting such conjecture is limited. Noteworthy are the experimental studies conducted in sheep by Begin and colleagues that document but do not explain progression (1983b).

One could argue that smoking, with the resulting emphysema and fibrosis, contributes to the progression of radiological changes in the asbestotic patient. For example, Souranta and associates (1982) showed that 50% of smokers had demonstrable evidence of progression of asbestosis radiologically, whereas only 25% of nonsmokers exhibited similar long-term changes. It is now well recognized that smoking accentuates the small, irregular shadows that are the radiological hallmark of the disease. The gradual loss of lung function that accompanies aging and obesity, or the superimposition of cardiovascular disease might explain progressive physiologic deterioration in some patients (Niewoehner and Kleinerman, 1974). Other possibilities abound. For example, idiopathic pulmonary fibrosis could account for the appearance of diffuse pulmonary disease in some patients. Clearly, a biological explanation is lacking for the clinically documented progression of the pulmonary fibrotic changes resulting from asbestos exposure.

Cytology of Sputum and Bronchoalveolar Lavaged (BAL) Fluid

Cytological evaluation of respiratory tract washings and sputum is an underutilized but a potentially useful means for assessing exposure to asbestos and the possible existence of asbestosis. This work can best be conducted by a cytopathologist collaborating with a pulmonologist skilled in BAL. As might be expected, staining of specimens to demonstrate the iron coat of the AB increases the sensitivity of the assessment (Wheeler et al., 1988).

Begin et al. (1983b) documented a pulmonary inflammatory response after experimental exposure of sheep to chrysotile asbestos and, Robinson et al. (1986) conducted similar studies using BAL of crocidolite- and chrysotile-exposed workers. Unfortunately, the value of this latter investigation, with regard to appraising the cellular events in the lungs after exposure to asbestos, was compromised by the confounding influence of concomitant cigarette smoking (Rebuck and Braude, 1983). But overall, the evidence indicated that patients with asbestosis display increases in the absolute numbers of neutrophils and eosinophils in lavage fluids recovered from deep in the lung. As shown in

Figure 6.12, and in a report by Wallace et al. (1989), the relative numbers of lymphocytes also tend to be higher in asbestos-exposed workers, although there are no striking alterations in lymphocyte subsets. Unfortunately, systematic, sequential clinical studies have not yet documented the populations of inflammatory cells in lung washings at various stages in the development and progression of asbestos pulmonary disease, in the absence of smoking.

In a detailed cytopathologic evaluation of more than 500 asbestos workers, 84% of whom smoked, Greenberg et al. (1976a,b) diagnosed squamous metaplasia in 42%, moderate atypia of bronchial epithelial cells in 8%, and severe atypia in 2%. The number of AB in the specimens did not correlate with the cytological changes (Farley et al., 1977). It appears that sputum cytology has little or no value in assessing possible preneoplastic changes *attributable to asbestos* in the epithelium of the bronchial tree of heavy smokers (Greenberg et al., 1976c).

Comprehensive cytological evaluations of sputum samples have demonstrated AB in the majority of specimens from active asbestos workers. The presence of AB in the sputum correlates with the length of occupational exposure (Farley et al., 1977). In a study correlating the results of fiber burden analysis of lung tissue with the presence of AB in the sputum, Roggli et al. (1980) related the lung content of asbestos to the proportion of sputum specimens displaying AB. Sebastien et al. (1988) found that the presence of a single AB per milliliter of BAL fluid corresponded with a concentration of 1×10^3 AB/gram in the digest of the lung parenchyma. When a careful microscopical search is conducted, AB can be found in the sputum of an occasional patient lacking a history of exposure.

The sensitivity of BAL as a means for documenting asbestos exposure has been explored in several studies (De Vuyst et al., 1982; Roggli et al., 1986; Schwartz et al., 1991; Sebastien et al., 1988; Teschler et al., 1994; Wheeler et al., 1988). In the work of De Vuyst et al. (1982), patients with known heavy and prolonged exposure had AB in BAL with concentrations as high as 4.2×10^4 per mL of fluid. Among those with suspected exposure, more than 90% were positive, whereas only 12% of controls had AB in BAL fluids, and the concentrations of AB were relatively low. Interestingly enough, 70% of patients with mesotheliomas had a positive lavage. Teschler et al. (1993) systematically evaluated the number of AB in lavage fluid from the various lobes of the right lung. They found the concentrations in the lower lobe lavage to be more than twofold higher than in specimens from the upper lung lobes. This finding, of course, correlates with the well-recognized tendency for asbestosis to appear initially in the lower lobes of the lungs.

Enthusiastic acceptance of BAL analysis as a measure of exposure is compromised by studies of BAL fluid from 9 of 31 sarcoidosis patients that demonstrated AB by electron microscopy. In addition, two of five cases of idiopathic pulmonary fibrosis proved positive (Roggli et al., 1986). Finally, in an analysis by Schwartz et al. (1991), it was concluded that "BAL is a reproducible bioassay of exposure but appear to have little utility in most clinical settings." However, as this brief review clearly shows, BAL assays conducted by experienced clinicians and cytologists can often provide valuable information when evaluated in the context of all the available clinical evidence. This is particularly the case when and if semiquantitative assessments for AB in the specimen are done.

Benign Pleural Disease

In 1943, Siegal et al. discovered pleural calcification in chest x-rays of 6.3% of talc miners and millers in northern New York. The cause of these changes was unknown, although contamination of the talc with other inorganic particulates was a consideration.

Twelve years later, bilateral pleural thickening was detected in 5% of asbestos workers (Jacob and Bohlig, 1955). Shortly thereafter, Frost and coworkers (1956) noted pleural calcifications in workers exposed to asbestos. Several additional surveys documented a similar association, although a causative link was not established (Meurman, 1968). In 1960, Kiviluoto described pleural calcification in residents of various regions of Finland who had no known occupational exposure to asbestos.

On the basis of the observation of Selikoff and his associates (1965), it soon was generally accepted that the pleural lesions were an important concomitant feature of pulmonary asbestosis. At the time, they coined the term "pleural asbestosis," a designation accepted by some, and rejected by most others, to date. It was later found that not all of those with radiological evidence of circumscribed plaques in North America had documented asbestos exposure (Churg, 1982) and nonasbestiform fibers in the form of erionite, a naturally occurring fibrous zeolite in Turkey (Baris et al., 1987; Chapter 3), and man-made ceramic fibers (Lockey et al., 1996) were found to cause pleural calcification.

The pathogenic mechanism by which durable fibrous material of certain dimensions results in pleural disease has been the subject of considerable speculation and some incisive research (Britton, 1982; Herbert, 1986; Hillerdal, 1980; Schwartz, 1991). Several components of the puzzle have now been established. It has been found that asbestos relocates from the lung parenchyma to the visceral pleura by at least two mechanisms. First, it transmigrates from the air spaces across anatomical boundaries to the pleura (Morgan et al., 1977) and second, it is transported to the pleura by lymphatics originating in the lung parenchyma and passes through a network of interconnecting lymphatic vessels located in the pleural connective tissue. A portion ultimately deposits at confluences of these channels in the form of the so-called black spots (the black appearance is attributable to the concomitant deposition of carbon) (Boutin et al., 1996; Mitchev et al., 2002; Figure 6.16). Fibers also enter major lymphatic channels coursing through the lung septae to be transported to lymph nodes in the hilum and mediastinum (Roggli and Benning, 1990). Interestingly enough, after the intravenous inoculation of asbestos, the mineral can be found in low concentrations in washings of the pleural cavity (Sebastien et al., 1977). Studies of pleural effusion fluid in humans have demonstrated the presence of a small number of asbestos fibers, and analyses of the circumscribed plaques that develop in the parietal pleura have yielded an occasional particle of asbestos.

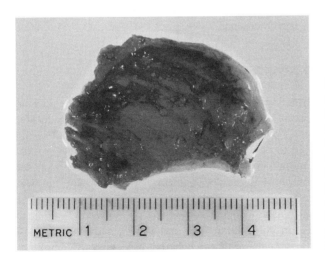

Figure 6.16 Experimental demonstration of crocidolite (blue asbestos) accumulation in the lymphatics of parietal pleura of a rat in which asbestos suspension was introduced into the pleural cavity. The publication of Boutin et al. (1996) illustrates a similar feature on the human visceral pleura. Analyses demonstrate amphiboles in these sites.

Benign Pleural Effusion

In 1962, Eisenstadt described benign, spontaneously occurring effusions in the pleural cavities of two refinery workers. Ten years later, a report by Gaensler and Kaplan (1971) considered the etiology of the pleural effusions detected in 91 hospitalized patients, 12 of whom had a history of consequential long-term exposure to asbestos (Miller et al., 1983). It was concluded that the effusions in approximately 13% of this study group could be attributed to asbestos exposure. In a later publication, these workers (Epler et al., 1982) showed that the prevalence of effusions in a population of asbestos workers was dosage dependent; 7% of those with "severe exposure" exhibited effusions (an incidence of 9 per 1000 persons/years), whereas only 0.2% of those with "peripheral," that is, relatively light exposures, had effusions. In the studies of Hillerdal and Ozesmi (1987), the left chest was affected more often than the right; they claimed that the mean latency period was some 30 years from time of first exposure with a range of 1–58 years! In contrast, Robinson and Musk (1981) found a mean latency period of 16 years in crocodilite-exposed patients. Effusions persist for variable periods of time, but on the average, the duration proves to be approximately 4 months. In the majority of cases, effusions failed to reoccur. Since many effusions are asymptomatic and thus, go unrecognized by the patient and his physician, the quantitative information cited above must be qualified (Epler et al., 1982; Smyrnios et al., 1990).

The pathogenesis of the asbestos-association effusion is obscure, but there is no evidence to suggest that it reflects a cause and effect relationship to the accumulation of asbestos fibers or AB in the visceral or parietal pleura or in the pleural cavity. However, correlative studies comparing the microscopical features of the visceral and parietal pleura with the pleural exudate have not been carried out thus far. Hillerdal and Ozesmi (1987) found the exudate in thoracentesis specimens from patients with effusions was hemorrhagic in about half their cases. In about a third or more, the number of eosinophils in the exudates was elevated, the remaining cells being polymorphonuclear leukocytes and lymphocytes. The finding of eosinophils in the exudates, as shown in several studies, suggests that immunologic events are responsible. Others have suggested that the exudate on the pleura reflects alveolitis in the subjacent lung. It appears unlikely these questions will be resolved by further clinical investigation. Animal models of asbestos-related pleural effusions have not been developed, although direct inoculation of asbestos into the pleural cavity provokes an acute inflammatory reaction (Shore et al., 1983). There is no evidence to indicate that the effusions are a prognostic indicator of a predisposition to neoplasia, specifically, mesothelioma.

Diffuse Pleural Thickening

In 1973, Navratil and Dobias termed the pleural lesions associated with asbestosis as either "hyalinosis simplex," that is, an asymptomatic pleural plaque customarily located on the parietal pleura or "hyalinosis complicata." The latter lesion was defined as diffuse fibrosis of the pleura, believed to be a progressive process often resulting in functional restrictive impairment of pulmonary function (Figure 6.7C). They hypothesized that pleural effusions cause or contribute to the development of the lesion, an unproven concept that continues to be in vogue.

Visceral pleural changes occur in asbestos-exposed workers (1) as the sole radiological evidence of past exposure; (2) in conjunction with parietal PP, and the much less common, visceral PP; and (3) as associated with parenchymal asbestosis (Solomon and

Webster, 1976). Diffuse pleural thickening (DPT) has been defined radiologically as "a smooth, noninterrupted pleural density extending over at least one-fourth of the chest wall with or without costophrenic angle obliteration" (McCloud et al., 1985).

All too often, the radiologic picture overlaps the appearance of confluent plaques on the parietal pleura (see below), with both lesions displaying variable degrees of calcification. Histologically, the DPT exhibits a nonspecific proliferation of vascularized connective tissue anointed with varying numbers of lymphocytes and macrophages. Fibrin and an inflammatory cell exudate often are layered on the pleural surfaces. In some cases, the rind of connective tissue obliterates the pleural space, but in many, it can be readily stripped from the underlying pulmonary parenchyma by the surgeon, so-called decortication. Visceral DPT, on occasion, displays the hyalinized, "waxy" appearance observed in typical parietal PP microscopically. Indeed, in some cases, fibrosis of the visceral pleura is sufficiently circumscribed to yield the gross "ivory" appearance of a plaque (Gibbs et al., 1991). One wonders whether or not hyalinized DPT may represent the end-stage of the resolution of the fibrin envelope that so often adheres to an inflamed pleura. AB are not a feature of the lesion. The nonspecific, thin, fibrous adhesions commonly present in the pleural cavity of adults are not a marker of asbestos exposure.

In a survey of more than 1.3×10^3 asbestos-exposed workmen using traditional chest x-rays, McCloud et al. (1985) detected circumscribed PP in 16.5% of patients, and DPT in 13.5%. They concluded that almost a third of the lesions were the residue of a benign pleural effusion, whereas confluent plaques accounted for about 25% of the radiological change. By serial monitoring crocidolite miners in Western Australia, de Klerk et al. (1989) noted that "minor pleural thickening frequently progressed...but a thickness greater than 5 μm was uncommon." The total cumulative exposure to crocidolite directly correlated with the onset of DPT between 5 and 15 years after initial exposure. Subsequently, there was no evidence of progression of the lesion 15 years and longer after the onset of the changes in the pleura. In a further study of many of these same subjects, the proportion with unilateral and bilateral costophrenic angle blunting (approximately 15%) was equivalent to the number of cases of DPT (Hillerdal and Musk, 1990).

On occasion, fibrosis of the mediastinal surface of the lung involves the pericardium, resulting in a "shaggy" appearance radiologically. Pericardial effusions and a constrictive fibrous pericarditis have been described in association with asbestosis, but this is, no doubt, a rare complication (Davies et al., 1991; Trosini-Desert et al., 2003). More often, it reflects contiguous spread of a malignant process.

Those assembled in Helsinki opined in 1997 "low exposure...may induce pleural plaques.... In contrast, for diffuse pleural fibrosis, higher exposure levels may be required. And, bilateral diffuse pleural fibrosis is often associated with moderate or heavy exposure, as seen in the cases with asbestosis..." (Henderson et al., 1997). Smith et al. (2003) have taken issue with this conclusion. In a comprehensive study of shipyard employees, the age of the workers and latency period for the development of DPT and PP were comparable, and no significant differences in the severity of the exposure could be documented.

Rounded Atelectasis (Blesovsky's Syndrome [1966])

This uncommon, generally asymptomatic, localized lung lesion is of considerable clinical importance because it readily simulates radiologically a bronchogenic carcinoma in the periphery of the lung (Menzies and Fraser, 1987) (Chapters 7 and 11). Rounded Atelectasis (RA) is often a complication of progressive, severe, visceral pleural disease but it may represent a change secondary to pleural effusion or both. Development of the lesion is often associated with scarring that radiates from the pleura into the pulmonary parenchyma, the so-called "crow's foot" lesion (Franzblau and Selikoff, 1988; Hillerdal, 1989; Menzies and Fraser, 1987; Schneider et al., 1980; Stark, 1982; Solomon et al., 1979). RA has no specific prognostic significance and is not an indication of underlying parenchymal asbestosis.

Pleural Plaques

These unique, asbestos-associated lesions have distinctive radiological features (Chapter 11) and a characteristic gross and microscopical appearance (Figures 6.17 and 6.18). As noted above, PP also develop in persons exposed environmentally to nonasbestiform fibrous mineral such as Turkish erionite (Baris et al., 1987), talc in New York State (Siegal et al., 1943), and ceramic fibers (Lockey et al., 1996). On rare occasions, they also develop spontaneously in the general urban and rural residents of North America, and in members of the rural populations of Central Europe in the absence of occupational asbestos exposure. Throughout rural Finland, the prevalence is high (Kiviluoto, 1960; Meurman, 1966, 1968), but to an undocumented extent, they have been noted radiologically in residents of Bulgaria (Zolov et al., 1967), Slovenia (Hromek, 1962), and Bohemia (Marsova, 1964). An abundance of epidemiological evidence associates PP with occupational exposure to amosite, anthophyllite, crocidolite, and fibrous tremolite/actinolite). It is doubtful that chrysotile, in the absence of a tremolite, induces the lesion. Although a substantial proportion of long-term Canadian miners and millers of chrysotile ore display PP in routine chest x-rays, automotive mechanics, drywallers, and chrysotile textile workers have not been shown to develop PP as a result of their employment. To the extent these workers are exposed to chrysotile, the fibers are usually short, that is, $<5 \mu m$.

Studies that focus on the epidemiology of PP are compromised by the insensitivity of the traditional chest x-ray as a tool for detecting the lesion. Moreover, interobserver variability

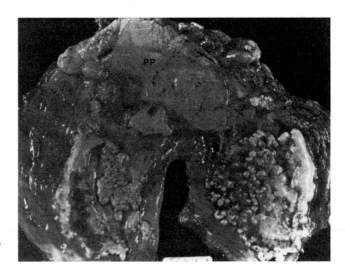

Figure 6.17 Pleural surface of diaphragm and parietal pericardium (PP) of man with history of occupational exposure to asbestos. The disklike configuration and nodularity are typical of these lesions. Isolated plaques are often located on the domes of the diaphragms, the only evidence of past exposure to asbestos.

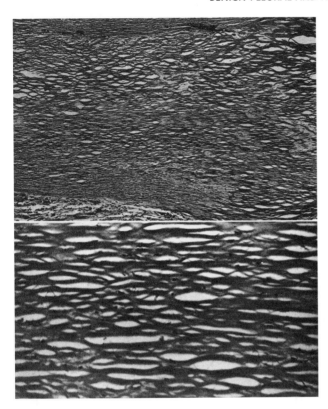

Figure 6.18 Microscopic features of typical pleural plaques. Note "basket-weave" arrangement of collagen bundles and relative acellularity of tissue. These lesions usually are not vascularized. (Published with permission from Craighead et al. 1982.)

in interpretation compromises the reproducibility of results. High-resolution computer axial tomography is the current technology of choice, but for reasons of expense and convenience, the approach has yet to be used in surveys of large populations. Systematic postmortem studies similarly have not been carried out, although it is generally accepted that autopsies often reveal PP that are not detected by the most modern radiological approaches (Robinson, 1972). The quantitative data concerned with the relationship of exposure to PP formation is based on fiber burden analyses of the lungs (Chapter 12). Lung burdens of asbestos are substantially lower in persons with PP than in those with asbestosis, although, of course, PP occur commonly in the chest of heavily exposed patients, particularly those with asbestosis (Kishimoto et al., 1989; Sison et al., 1989).

A substantial body of clinical evidence indicates that PP demonstrable in traditional chest x-rays have a minimum latency period of roughly 15 years. With the passage of time, the lesions tend to calcify and thus, as the worker ages, PP are increasingly obvious in x-rays.

Figure 6.19 depicts the writer's concept of the mechanism whereby PP develop in the parietal pleura of the chest. It is based on the assumption that amphibole asbestos transmigrates into and through the visceral pleura (Sebastien, 1977) to accumulate in and around the orifices of the stomata of the parietal pleural lymphatics (Wang, 1975). This is a dynamic process since approximately 25% of the body's plasma volume passes through the pleural cavities and is filtered through the stomata each day (Stewart and Burgen, 1958). Accordingly, enormous volumes of fluid are cleared on a continuous basis. Fibers at the orifices of the stomata are believed to initiate an inflammatory response, ultimately leading to the deposition of fibrous tissue in the network of the fibrin deposited at the sites of inflammation (Shore et al., 1983). In this regard, it is noteworthy that Von Recklinghausen (1863) described "whirlpools forming in certain sites on the

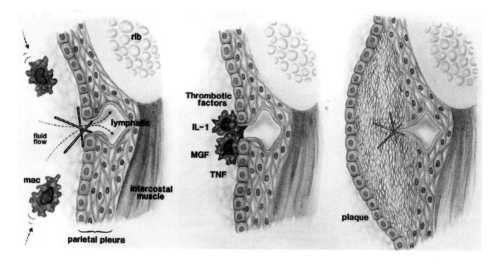

Figure 6.19 Hypothetical mechanism of plaque formation in parietal pleura. Asbestos fiber suspended in the fluid of the pleural cavity is drawn to stomata of the pericostal lymphatics where it initiates an inflammatory response mediated by cytokines. Fibrous tissue then proliferates in relatively circumscribed site. The mechanistic basis for the distinctive, relatively acellular character of the PP is unknown.

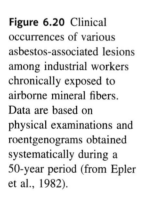

Figure 6.20 Clinical occurrences of various asbestos-associated lesions among industrial workers chronically exposed to airborne mineral fibers. Data are based on physical examinations and roentgenograms obtained systematically during a 50-year period (from Epler et al., 1982).

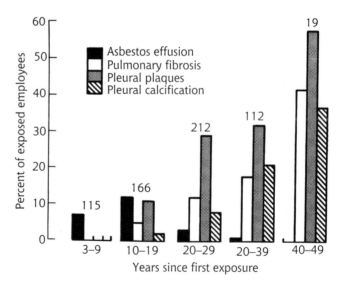

abdominal diaphragm surface" where particles enter the lymphatics. An experimental animal model of PP formation has yet to be developed.

Weiss et al. (1981), Hillerdal (1978), and Hedenberg et al. (1979) in radiological studies conducted in the United States and Sweden, found PP in a statistically greater number of asbestos-exposed workers who smoked. The pathogenic basis for this finding is obscure, although one could speculate that smokers retain more asbestos fibers in the chest than nonsmokers. The number of shipyard workers developing asbestosis and the various pleural markers of amphibole asbestos are shown in Figure 6.20 (Epler et al., 1982).

As discussed in greater detail in Chapter 7, PP are not a risk factor for the development of bronchogenic carcinoma, although there is not universal agreement on this matter (Edge, 1979; Harber et al., 1987; Hillerdal and Henderson, 1997; Hughes and Weill, 1991; Kiviluoto et al., 1979; Thringer, 1980; Wain et al., 1984).

Appendix: Pathologic Grading of Asbestosis

In 1965, the Working Group on Asbestos and Cancer of the International Union Against Cancer (UICC) recommended a classification schema for asbestosis that was based on both an assessment of the severity of fibrosis and the extent of the changes in the lung as a whole. Shortly thereafter, Hinson et al. (1973) proposed a grading protocol based on gross and microscopic criteria that could be applied to pulmonary fibrosis in general, and to asbestosis specifically. This grading system has not been applied systematically in large-scale studies.

Grading protocols for the radiologic assessment of the pneumoconioses are at an advanced stage of development (Chapter 11). Groups of radiologists working largely under the auspices of the UICC and the International Labor Organization (ILO) proposed protocols that were generally accepted and have been applied in numerous epidemiologic studies. The UICC/ILO grading system was developed with silicosis and coal workers' pneumoconiosis in mind, and was not as applicable to asbestosis as might be desired. Because of this problem, the standard UICC and ILO approach was amalgamated into the UICC/ILO 1971 system used universally for all pneumoconioses, including asbestosis. A version updated in 1980 is now used.

The histologic grading system is a modification and extension of the protocol of Hinson et al. (1973) although it is based exclusively on microscopic criteria. It presupposes systematic study of the lung tissue at the time of autopsy and requires representative sampling of the lungs. Although perfusion fixation of the lungs obtained at autopsy would be highly desirable, the schema is applicable to lung tissue obtained under less-than-ideal conditions of fixation (ie, without perfusion). It also can be used in the evaluation of lung biopsy material, accepting the limitations of the sample. Under this circumstance, evaluation of the pathologic material might appropriately be carried out in conjunction with radiologic studies to assess the distribution of disease. Use of the grading schema makes it possible for the diagnostic pathologist to communicate with other medical professionals regarding the severity of the disease.

Grading of Asbestosis

The grading system (Figure 6A.1) is intended only for the semiquantitative estimation of the degree of asbestosis, and not as an aid to diagnosis. Therefore, the diagnosis of asbestosis should be established before grading is attempted. Because fibrosis of the peribronchiolar and interstitial tissues is the key lesion in asbestosis, this grading system is based solely on the evaluation of fibrosis. The numbers of AB, macrophages, and inflammatory cells within the tissues and changes in the epithelium are not considered, even though the presence of AB in the lungs is the hallmark of the diagnosis.

Each histologic slide is evaluated from two perspectives. Initially, the severity of the lesion either in or surrounding the bronchioles is assessed and the numeric score recorded. Then, the proportion of the bronchioles in the sections that have any degree of involvement is evaluated (not just the proportion involved to the most severe degree). This grade, which represents the extent of the disease, is recorded as a letter score.

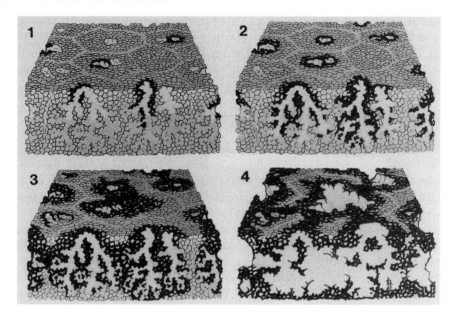

Figure 6A.1 Stages in the development of asbestosis. Initially, the lesions develop in the walls of the respiratory bronchioles (stage 1). As the lesion progresses, bridging occurs between individual respiratory units, and the alveolar walls are involved (stages 2 and 3). With the progression of the disease, more respiratory units are involved. Destruction of the parenchyma by the contraction of scars occurs in stage 4. The "honeycomb" lung, which is characteristic of advanced disease, results from the contraction of fibrotic scars.

To establish an overall grade for a tissue section, the distribution letter score is converted to a number and multiplied by the lesion score. To characterize the disease of a patient, the products of the scores of all the slides are added and the sum divided by the number of slides examined. This average indicates the degree of disease.

Asbestosis Grading Schema

Severity

Lesions associated with individual respiratory bronchioles are evaluated. The grade is based on the most severe lesion in the slide, not a visual average of the changes found in the various individual respiratory units, as follows:

Grade 0: No fibrosis is associated with bronchioles.

Grade 1: Fibrosis involves wall of at least one respiratory bronchiole with or without extension into the septa of the immediately adjacent layer of alveoli; no fibrosis is present in more distant alveoli.

Grade 2: Fibrosis appears as in grade 1, plus involvement of alveolar ducts or two or more layers of adjacent alveoli; there still must be a zone of nonfibrotic alveolar septa between adjacent bronchioles.

Grade 3: Fibrosis appears as in grade 2, but the coalescence of fibrotic change such that all alveoli between at least two adjacent bronchioles have thickened, fibrotic septa; some alveoli may be obliterated completely.

Grade 4: Fibrosis appears as in grade 3, but with the formation of new spaces of a size larger than alveoli, ranging up to as much as 1 cm; this lesion has been termed *honeycombing*. Spaces may or may not be lined by epithelium.

Table 6A.1 Asbestos Grading Schema*

Score		1	2	3	4	6	8 and 9	12
Grades from products								
Magnitude of increase	...	2×	1.5×	1.3×	1.5×	1.5×	1.3×
	1+	2+	3+	4+	5+	6+	7+
Straight grades								
Magnitude of increase	...	2×	1.5×	1.3×	1.25×	1.2×	1.1×

* Published with permission from Craighead et al. (1982).

Extent

The proportion of the respiratory bronchioles involved by the disease process is assessed. The grades pertain to the relative numbers of bronchioles in the slide involved by *any degree* of fibrosis—not just the numbers involved to the maximum degree as recorded under severity—as follows:

Grade A (1): Only occasional bronchioles are involved—most show no lesion.
Grade B (2): More than occasional involvement is seen, but less than half of all bronchioles are involved.
Grade C (3): More than half of all bronchioles are involved.

Multiplication of the scores for severity and extent requires explanation because it might be argued that a product score is inappropriate. For example, a product score of 4 obtained on a tissue with grade 4 severity with an extent score of A has implications with regard to disease that differ from a tissue with grade 2 severity and grade B extent. Although theoretically the validity of this argument cannot be refuted, the severity and extent of the lesions are found to vary independently, but seem to be interdependent. Thus, severe lesions are usually found when disease is widespread in the tissue.

The second concept, which argues for the multiplication of the severity and extent scores, relates to the range of possible scores that result (Table 6A.1). Thus, the products of grades (1 × 1, 1 × 2, 2 × 3, etc.) produce a series of eight possible scores (1, 2, 3, 4, 6, 8, 9, and 12).

References

Adesina AM, Vallyathan NV, McQuillen EN, Weaver DO, Craighead JE. Bronchiolar inflammation and fibrosis associated with smoking: a morphological cross-sectional population analysis. *Am Rev Respir Dis.* 1991;143:144–149.

Angervall H, Hansson G, Rockert H. Pulmonary siderosis in electrical worker. A note on pathological appearances. *Acta Pathol Microbiol Scand.* 1960;49:373–392.

Anjilvel L, Thurlbeck WM. Incidence of asbestos bodies in lungs at random necropsies in Montreal. *Canad M A J.* 1966;95:1179–1182.

Auerbach O, Conston AS, Garfinkel L, Parks VR, Kaslow HD, Hammond EC. Presence of asbestos bodies in organs other than the lung. *Chest.* 1980;77:133–137.

Baris I, Simonato L, Artvinti M, et al. Epidemiological and environmental evidence of the health effects of exposure to erionite fibres: a four year study in the Cappadocian region of Turkey. *Int J Cancer.* 1987;39:10–17.

Becklake MR, Liddell FDK, Manfreda J, McDonald JC. Radiological changes after withdrawal from asbestos exposure. *Br J Ind Med.* 1979;36:23–28.

Begin R, Sebastien P. Excessive accumulation of asbestos fibre in the bronchoalveolar space may be a marker of individual susceptibility to developing asbestosis: experimental evidence. *Br J Ind Med.* 1989;46(12):853–855.

Begin R, Boileau R, Peloquin S. Asbestos exposure, cigarette smoking, and airflow limitation in long-term Canadian chrysotile miners and millers. *Am J Ind Med.* 1987;11:55–66.

Begin R, Cantin A, Berthiaume Y, Biolaeu R, Peloquin S, Masse S. Airway function in lifetime-nonsmoking older asbestos workers. *Am J Med.* 1983a;75:631–638.

Begin R, Rola-Pleszczynski M, Masse S, Nadeau D, Drapeau G. Assessment of progression of asbestosis in the sheep model by bronchoalveolar lavage and pulmonary function tests. *Thorax.* 1983b;38:449–457.

Blesovsky A. The folded lung. *Br J Dis Chest.* 1966;60:19–22.

Bonner JC, Rice AB, Ingram JL, et al. Susceptibility of cyclooxygenase-2-deficient mice to pulmonary fibrogenesis. *Am J Pathol.* 2002;161:459–470.

Boutin C, Dumortier P, Rey F, Viallat JR, De Vuyst P. Black spots concentrate oncogenic asbestos fibers in the parietal pleura. Thoracoscopic and mineralogic study. *Am J Respir Crit Care Med.* 1996;153:444–449.

Britton MG, Hughes DTD, Wever AMJ. Serial pulmonary function tests in patients with asbestosis. *Thorax.* 1977;32:45–52.

Britton MG. Asbestos pleural disease. *Br J Dis Chest.* 1982;76:1–10.

Brody AR. Asbestos-induced lung disease. *Environ Health Perspect.* 1993;100:21–30.

Brody AR. Pulmonary cell interactions with asbestos fibers in vivo and in vitro. *Chest.* 1986;89(3 Suppl):155S-159S.

Churg A. Asbestos fibers and pleural plaques in a general autopsy population. *Am J Pathol.* 1982;109:88–96.

Churg A. Current issues in the pathologic and mineralogic diagnosis of asbestos-induced disease. *Chest.* 1983;84:275–280.

Churg A, Warnock ML. Analysis of the cores of ferruginous (asbestos) bodies from the general population. I. Patients with and without lung cancer. *Lab Invest.* 1977;37:280–286.

Churg AM, Warnock ML. Asbestos and other ferruginous bodies: their formation and clinical significance. *Am J Pathol.* 1981;102:447–456.

Churg A, Wright JL, Wiggs B, Pare PD, Lazar N. Small airways disease and mineral dust exposure. Prevalence, structure, and function. *Am Rev Respir Dis.* 1985;131:139–143.

Cohen BM, Adasczik A, Cohen EM. Small airways changes in workers exposed to asbestos. *Respiration.* 1984;45:296–302.

Cook PM, Olson GF. Ingested mineral fibers: elimination in human urine. *Science.* 1979; 204:195–198.

Cooke WE. Fibrosis of lungs due to inhalation of asbestos dust. *Br Med J.* 1924;2:147.

Cooke WE. Pulmonary asbestosis. *Br Med J.* 1927;2:1024.

Cookson W, de Klerk N, Musk AW, Glancy JJ, Armstron B, Hobbs M. The natural history of asbestosis in former crocidolite workers in Wittenoom Gorge. *Am Rev Respir Dis.* 1986;133:994–998.

Craighead JE, Abraham JL, Churg A, et al. The pathology of asbestos-associated diseases of the lungs and pleural cavities: diagnostic criteria and proposed grading schema. Report of the Pneumoconiosis Committee of the College of American Pathologists and the National Institute for Occupational Safety and Health. *Arch Pathol Lab Med.* 1982;106:544–596.

Craighead JE, Mossman BT. Carcinoma induction by 3-methylcholanthrene in hamster tracheal tissue implanted in syngeneic animals. *Prog Exp Tumor Res.* 1979;24:48–60.

Cummins AB, Palmer C, Mossman BT, Taatjes DJ. Persistent localization of activated extra-cellular signal-regulated kinases (ERK1/2) is epithelial cell-specific in an inhalation model of asbestosis. *Am J Pathol.* 2003;162:713–720.

Davies D, Andrews MI, Jones JS. Asbestos induced pericardial effusion and constrictive pericarditis. *Thorax.* 1991;46:429–432.

Davis JMG, Glyseth B, Morgan A. Assessment of mineral fibres from human lung tissue. *Thorax.* 1986;41:167–175.

de Klerk NH, Cookson WO, Musk AW, Armstrong BK, Glancy JJ. Natural history of pleural thickening after exposure to crocidolite. *Br J Ind Med.* 1989;46:461–467.

De Vuyst P, Jedwab J, Dumortier P, et al. Asbestos bodies in bronchoalveolar lavage. *Am Rev Respir Dis.* 1982;126:972–976.

Dodson RF, O'Sullivan MF, Corn CJ, Williams MG Jr, Hurst GA. Ferruginous body formation on a nonasbestos mineral. *Arch Pathol Lab Med.* 1985;109:849–852.

Dreessen WC, Dallavalle JM, Edwards TI, Miller JW, Savers RR. *A study of asbestosis in the asbestos textile industry.* Washington, DC: US Treasury Department Public Health Service. Public Health Bulletin No 241; 1938.

Dubois CM, Bissonnette E, Rola-Pleszczynski M. Asbestos fibers and silica particles stimulate rat alveolar macrophages to release tumor necrosis factor. Autoregulatory role of leukotriene B$_4$. *Am Rev Respir Dis.* 1989;139:1257–1264.

Edge JR. Incidence of bronchial carcinoma in shipyard workers with pleural plaques. *Ann NY Acad Sci.* 1979;330:289–294.

Eidelman D, Saetta MP, Ghezzo H, et al. Cellularity of the alveolar walls in smokers and its relation to alveolar destruction. Functional implications. *Am Rev Respir Dis.* 1990;141:1547–1552.

Eisenstadt HB. Pleural asbestosis. *Am Practitioner.* 1962;13:573–578.

Epler GR, McCloud TC, Gaensler EA. Prevalence and incidence of benign asbestos pleural effusion in a working population. *JAMA.* 1982;247:617–622.

Farley ML, Greenberg SD, Shuford EH Jr, Hurst GA, Spivey CG, Christianson CS. Ferruginous bodies in sputa of former asbestos workers. *Acta Cytologica.* 1977;21:693–700.

Franzblau A, Selikoff IJ. Asbestos-associated rounded atelectasis in a cohort of insulation workers. [Abstract] *VIIth International Pneumonoconiosis Conference.* August 23–26, 1988, Pittsburgh, PA.

Frost J, Georg J, Moller PF. Asbestosis with pleural calcification among insulation workers. *Danis Med Bull.* 1956;3:202–204.

Gaensler EA, Addington WW. Asbestos or ferruginous bodies. *N Engl J Med.* 1969;280:488–92.

Gaensler EA, Kaplan AI. Asbestos pleural effusion. *Ann Int Med.* 1971;74:178–191.

Garcia JGN, Griffith DE, Cohen AB, Callahan KS. Alveolar macrophages from patients with asbestos exposure release increased levels of leukotriene B$_4$. *Am Rev Respir Dis.* 1989;139:1494–1501.

Gibbs AR, Gardner MJ, Pooley FD, Griffiths DM, Blight B, Wagner JC. Fiber levels and disease in workers from a factory predominantly using amosite. *Environ Health Perspect.* 1994;102(Suppl 5):261–263.

Gibbs AR, Stephens M, Griffiths DM, Blight BJ, Pooley FD. Fibre distribution in the lungs and pleura of subjects with asbestos related diffuse pleural fibrosis. *Br J Ind Med.* 1991;48:762–770.

Gloyne SR. The morbid anatomy and histology of asbestosis. *Tubercle.* 1933;14:550–558.

Godwin MC, Jagatic G. Asbestos and mesothelioma. *JAMA.* 1968;204:1009.

Goff AM, Gaensler EA. Asbestosis following brief exposure in cigarette filter manufacture. *Respiration.* 1972;29:83–93.

Greenberg SD, Hurst GA, Christianson SC, Matlage WJ, Hurst IJ, Mabry LC. Pulmonary cytopathology of former asbestos workers. Report of the first year. *Am J Clin Pathol.* 1976a;66:815–822.

Greenberg SD, Hurst GA, Matlage WT, Christianson CS, Hurst IJ, Mabry LC. Sputum cytopathological findings in former asbestos workers. *Texas Medicine.* 1976b;72:39–43.

Greenberg SD, Hurst GA, Matlage WT, Miller JM, Hurst IJ, Mabry LC. Occupational carcinogenesis. High-risk industrial groups: identification, education, and surveillance. Tyler Asbestos Workers Program. *Ann NY Acad Sci.* 1976c;271:353–364.

Harber P, Mohsenifar Z, Oren A, Lew M. Pleural plaques and asbestos-associated malignancy. *J Occup Med.* 1987;29:641–644.

Hayes AA, Venaille TJ, Rose AH, Musk AW, Robinson BWS. Asbestos-induced release of a human alveolar macrophage-derived neutrophil chemotactic factor. *Exp Lung Res.* 1990;16:121–130.

Hedenberg L, Hermansson L, Liden MA, Thuringer G. Directed health survey of workers exposed to asbestos. Lakartidningen 78:4151–4152, 1978 (Abstract in International Cancer Research Data Bank Cancergram on Environmental and Occupational Carcinogenesis, Series CK02, No 4, April 1979:6, National Cancer Institute).

Henderson DW, Rantanen J, Barnhartt S, et al. Asbestos, asbestosis, and cancer: the Helsinki criteria for diagnosis and attribution. *Scand J Work Environ Health.* 1997;23:311–316.

Herbert A. Pathogenesis of pleurisy, pleural fibrosis, and mesothelial proliferation. *Thorax.* 1986;41:176–189.

Hillerdal G. Pleural plaques in a health survey material. *Scand J Respir Dis.* 1978;59:257–263.

Hillerdal G. The pathogenesis of pleural plaques and pulmonary asbestosis: possibilities and impossibilities. *Eur J Respir Dis.* 1980;61:129–138.

Hillerdal G. Rounded atelectasis: clinical experience with 74 patients. *Chest.* 1989;95:836–841.

Hillerdal G, Henderson DW. Asbestos, asbestosis, pleural plaques and lung cancer. *Scand J Work Environ Health.* 1997;23:93–103.

Hillerdal G, Musk AW. Pleural lesions in crocidolite workers from Western Australia. *Br J Ind Med.* 1990;47:782–783.

Hillerdal G, Ozesmi M. Benign asbestos pleural effusion: 73 exudates in 60 patients. *Eur J Respir Dis.* 1987;71:113–121.

Hogg JC, Chu F, Utokaparch S, et al. The nature of small-airway obstruction in chronic obstructive pulmonary disease. *N Engl J Med.* 2004;350:2645–2653.

Hromek J. Hromadny vyskyt caracteristickych pleuralnich zmen u obyvatelstva zapadni easti byaleho kraje Jihlava. *Rozhledy Tuberk.* 1962;22:405–414.

Hughes JM, Weill H. Asbestosis as a precursor of asbestos related lung cancer: results of a prospective mortality study. *Br J Ind Med.* 1991;48:229–233.

Jacob B, Bohlig H. Die rontgenologische Komplikationen der Lungenasbestose. *Fortschr Roentgenstr.* 1955;83:515–525.

Jones RN, Diem JE, Hughes JM, Hammad YY, Glindmeyer HW, Weill H. Progression of asbestos effects: a prospective longitudinal study of chest radiographs and lung function. *Br J Ind Med.* 1989;46:97–105.

Kagan E, Oghiso Y, Hartmann D-P. Enhanced release of a chemoattractant for alveolar macrophages after asbestos inhalation. *Am Rev Respir Dis.* 1983;128:680–687.

Kamp DW, Dunne M, Dykewicz MS, Sbalchiero JS, Weitzman SA, Dunn MM. Asbestos-induced injury to cultured human pulmonary epithelial-like cells: role of neutrophil elastase. *J Leukocyte Biol.* 1993;54:73–80.

Kanazawa K, Birbeck MS, Carter RL, Roe FJ. Migration of asbestos fibers from subcutaneous injection sites in mice. *Br J Cancer.* 1970;24:96–106.

Kishimoto T, Ono T, Okada K, Ito H. Relationship between number of asbestos bodies in autopsy lung and pleural plaques on chest x-ray film. *Chest.* 1989;95:549–552.

Kiviluoto R, Meurman LO, Hakama M. Pleural plaques and neoplasia in Finland. *Ann NY Acad Sci.* 1979;330:31–33.

Kiviluoto R. Pleural calcification as a roentgenologic sign of non-occupational endemic anthophyllite-asbestosis. *Acta Radiol Suppl.* 1960;194:1–67.

Lasky JA, Coin PG, Lindroos PM, Ostrowski LE, Brody AR, Bonner JC. Chrysotile asbestos stimulates platelet-derived growth factor-AA production by rat lung fibroblasts in vitro: evidence for an autocrine loop. *Am J Respir Cell Mol Biol.* 1995;12:162–170.

Liddell D, Eyssen G, Thomas D, MacDonald C. Radiological changes over twenty years in relation to chrysotile exposure in Québec. In: Walton WH, ed. *Inhaled Particles IV.* Oxford, England: Pergamon Press; 1977:799–812.

Liu J-Y, Brass DM, Hoyle GW, Brody AR. TNF-α receptor knockout mice are protected from the fibroproliferative effects of inhaled asbestos fibers. *Am J Pathol.* 1998;153:1839–1847.

Lockey J, Lemasters G, Rice C, et al. Refractory ceramic fiber exposure and pleural plaques. *Am J Respir Crit Care Med.* 1996;154:1405–1410.

Lounsbury KM, Stern M, Taatjes D, Jaken S, Mossman BT. Increased localization and substrate activation of protein kinase Cδ in lung epithelial cells following exposure to asbestos. *Am J Pathol.* 2002;160:1991–2000.

Marchand F. Über eigentümliche Pigmentkristalle in den Lungen. Verhandl. d. Deutsch. path. *Gesellsch.* 1906;10:223–228.

Marsova D. Beitrag zur Xtiologie der Pleuraverkalkungen. *Z Turberk.* 1964;121:329–334.

McCloud TC, Woods BO, Carrington CB, Epler GR, Gaensler EA. Diffuse pleural thickening in an asbestos-exposed population: prevalence and causes. *Am J Roentgenol.* 1985;144:9–18.

McFadden D, Wright JL, Wiggs B, Churg A. Smoking inhibits asbestos clearance. *Am Rev Respir Dis.* 1986;133:372–374.

McGavran PD, Brody AR. Chrysotile asbestos inhalation induces tritiated thymidine incorporation by epithelial cells of distal bronchioles. *Am J Respir Cell Mol Biol.* 1989;1:231–235.

McLemore TL, Roggli V, Marshall MV, Lawrence EC, Greenberg SD, Stevens PM. Comparison of phagocytosis of uncoated versus coated asbestos fibers by cultured human pulmonary alveolar macrophages. *Chest.* 1981;80(1 Suppl):39–42.

Meiklejohn A. The origin of the term "pneumonokoniosis." *Br J Ind Med.* 1960;17:155–160.

Menzies R, Fraser R. Round atelectasis: pathologic and pathogenetic features. *Am J Surg Pathol.* 1987;11:674–681.

Merewether ERA, Price GW. Report on effects of asbestos dust on the lungs and dust suppression in the asbestos industry; Her Majesty's Stationery Office, London; 1930.

Meurman L. Asbestos bodies and pleural plaques in a Finnish series of autopsy cases. *Acta Pathol Microbiol Scand.*; Munksgaard, Kopenhagen (Suppl 181), 1966.

Meurman LO. Pleural fibrocalcific plaques and asbestos exposure. *Environ Res.* 1968;2:30–46.

Miller A, Teirstein AS, Selikoff IJ. Ventilatory failure due to asbestos pleurisy. *Am J Med.* 1983;75:911–919.

Mitchev K, Dumortier P, De Vuyst P. "Black spots" and hyaline pleural plaques on the parietal pleura of 150 urban necropsy cases. *Am J Surg Pathol.* 2002;26:1198–1206.

Morgan A, Evans JC, Holmes A. Deposition and clearance of inhaled fibrous minerals in the rat: studies using radioactive tracer techniques. In: Walton WH, ed. *Inhaled Particles IV,* Oxford: Pergamon Press; 1977:259–274.

Morgan A, Holmes A. The enigmatic asbestos body: its formation and significance in asbestos-related disease. *Environ Res.* 1985;38:283–292.

Mossman BT, Adler KB, Craighead JE. Cytotoxic and proliferative changes in tracheal organ and cell cultures after exposure to mineral dusts. In: Brown RC ed. *The In Vitro Effects of Mineral Dusts.* London: Academic Press; 1980:241.

Mossman BT, Adler KB, Jean L, Craighead JE. Mechanisms of hypersecretion in rodent tracheal explants after exposure to chrysotile asbestos. Studies using lectins. *Chest.* 1982; 81S:23S–24S.

Mossman BT, Marsh JP, Sesko A, et al. Inhibition of lung injury, inflammation, and interstitial pulmonary fibrosis by polyethylene glycol-conjugated catalase in a rapid inhalation model of asbestosis. *Am Rev Respir Dis.* 1990;141:1266–1271.

Murai Y, Kitagawa, M, Kiraoka T. Asbestos body formation in the human lung: distinctions, by type and size. *Arch Environ Health.* 1995;50:19–25.

Navratil M, Dobias J. Development of pleural hyalinosis in long-term studies of persons exposed to asbestos dust. *Environ Res.* 1973;6:455–472.

Niewoehner DE, Kleinerman J. Morphologic basis of pulmonary resistance in the human lung and effects of aging. *J Appl Physiol.* 1974;36:412–418.

Pooley FD. Asbestos bodies, their formation, composition and character. *Environ Res.* 1972;5:363–379.

Pooley FD, Ranson DL. Comparison of the results of asbestos fibre dust counts in lung tissue obtained by analytical electron microscopy and light microscopy. *J Clin Pathol.* 1986;39:313–317.

Quinlan TR, Marsh JP, Janssen YMW, Borm PA, Mossman BT. Oxygen radicals and asbestos-mediated disease. *Environ Health Perspect.* 1994;102(Suppl 10):107–110.

Rebuck AS, Braude AC. Bronchoalveolar lavage in asbestosis. *Arch Intern Med.* 1983;143:950–952.

Robinson JJ. Pleural plaques and splenic capsular sclerosis in adult male autopsies. *Arch Pathol.* 1972;93:118–122.

Robinson BW, Musk AW. Benign asbestos pleural effusion: diagnosis and course. *Thorax.* 1981;36:896–900.

Robinson BWS, Rose AH, James A, Whitaker D, Musk AW. Alveolitis of pulmonary asbesto-sis. Bronchoalveolar lavage studies in crocidolite- and chrysotile-exposed individuals. *Chest.* 1986;90:396–402.

Roggli VL, Benning TL. Asbestos bodies in pulmonary hilar lymph nodes. *Modern Pathol.* 1990;3:513–517.

Roggli VL, Greenberg SD, McLarty J, et al. Comparison of sputum and lung asbestos body counts in former asbestos workers. *Am Rev Respir Dis.* 1980;122:941–945.

Roggli VL, Greenberg SD, Pratt PC. *Pathology of Asbestos-Associated Disease.* Boston, MA: Little Brown & Co.; 1992.

Roggli VL, Oury TD, Sporn TA. *Pathology of Asbestos Associated Diseases*, 2nd ed. New York: Springer; 2004.

Roggli VL, Piantadosi CA, Bell DY. Asbestos bodies in bronchoalveolar lavage fluid. A study of 20 asbestos-exposed individuals and comparison to patients with other chronic intersti-tial lung diseases. *Acta Cytologica.* 1986;30:470–476.

Rossiter CE, Heath JR, Harries PG. Royal naval dockyards asbestosis research project: nine year follow-up study of men exposed to asbestos in Devonport Dockyard. *J Royal Soc Med.* 1980;73:337–344.

Rubino GF, Newhouse M, Murray R, Scansetti G, Piolatto G, Aresini G. Radiological changes after cessation of exposure among chrysotile asbestos miners in Italy. *Ann NY Acad Sci.* 1979;330:157–161.

Schapira RM, Ghio AJ, Effros RM, Morrisey J, Dawson CA, Hacker AD. Hydroxyl radicals are formed in the rat lung after asbestos instillation in vivo. *Am J Respir Cell Mol Biol.* 1994;10:573–579.

Schneider HJ, Felson B, Gonzalez LL. Rounded atelectasis. *Am J Roentgenol.* 1980;134:225–232.

Schwartz DA. New developments in asbestos-induced pleural disease. *Chest.* 1991;99:191–198.

Schwartz DA, Galvin JR, Burmeister LF, et al. The clinical utility and reliability of asbestos bodies in bronchoalveolar fluid. *Am Rev Respir Dis.* 1991;144:684–688.

Sebastien P, Armstrong B, Monchaux G, Bignon J. Asbestos bodies in bronchoalveolar lavage fluid and in lung parenchyma. *Am Rev Respir Dis.* 1988;137:75–78.

Sebastien P, Fondimare A, Bignon J, Morchaux G, Desbordes J, Bonnaud G. Topographic dis-tribution of asbestos fibers on human lung in relation to occupational and non-occupational exposure. In: Walton WA, ed. *Inhaled Particles IV.* Oxford: Pergamon Press; 1977:435–444.

Selikoff IJ. The occurrence of pleural calcification among asbestos insulation workers. *Ann NY Acad Sci.* 1965;132:351–367.

Shore BL, Daughaday CC, Spilberg I. Benign asbestos pleurisy in the rabbit. A model for the study of pathogenesis. *Am Rev Respir Dis.* 1983;128:481–485.

Siegal W, Smith AR, Greenburg L. The dust hazard in tremolite talc mining. *Am J Roent-genol Radium Therapy Nucl Med.* 1943;49:11–29.

Sison RF, Hruban RH, Moore GW, Kuhlman JE, Wheeler PS, Hutchins GM. Pulmonary disease associated with pleural "asbestos" plaques. *Chest.* 1989;95:831–835.

Smith KA, Sykes LJ, McGavin CR. Diffuse pleural fibrosis—an unreliable indicator of heavy asbestos exposure? *Scand J Work Environ Health.* 2003;29:60–63.

Smyrnios NA, Jederlinic PJ, Irwin RS. Pleural effusion in an asymptomatic patient. Spectrum and frequency of causes and management considerations. *Chest.* 1990;97:192–196.

Solomon A, Webster I. The visceral pleura in asbestosis. *Environ Res.* 1976;11:128–134.

Solomon A, Irwig LM, Sluis-Cremer GK, Thomas RG, Du Toit RS. Thickening of pulmo-nary interlobar fissures: exposure-response relationship in crocidolite and amosite miners. *Br J Ind Med.* 1979;36:195–198.

Souranta H, Huuskonen MS, Zitting A, Juntunen J. Radiographic progression of asbestosis. *Am J Ind Med.* 1982;3:67–74.

Spurzem JR, Saltini C, Rom W, Winchester RJ, Crystal RG. Mechanisms of macrophage accu-mulation in the lungs of asbestos-exposed subjects. *Am Rev Respir Dis.* 1987;136:276–280.

Stark P. Round atelectasis: another pulmonary pseudotumor. *Am Rev Respir Dis.* 1982;125:248–250.

Stewart PB, Burgen AS. The turn-over of fluid in the dog's pleural cavity. *J Lab Clin Med.* 1958;52:212–230.

Suzuki Y, Churg J. Structure and development of the asbestos body. *Am J Pathol.* 1969;55:79–107.

Teschler H, Friedrichs KH, Hoheisel GB, et al. Asbestos fibers in bronchoalveolar lavage and lung tissue of former asbestos workers. *Am J Respir Crit Care Med.* 1994;149:641–645.

Teschler H, Konietzko N, Schoenfeld B, Ramin C, Schraps T, Costabel U. Distribution of asbestos bodies in the human lung as determined by bronchoalveolar lavage. *Am Rev Respir Dis.* 1993;147:1211–1215.

Thomas G, Ando T, Verma K, Kagan E. Asbestos fibers and interferon-γ up-regulate nitric oxide production in rat alveolar macrophages. *Am J Respir Cell Mol Biol.* 1994;11:707–715.

Thompson JG. Asbestos and urban dweller. *Ann New York Acad Sci.* 1965;132:196–214.

Thringer G. Are pleural plaques a predictor for carcinoma of the lung? *Eur J Repsir Dis.* 1980;61(Suppl. 107):109–110.

Timblin C, Robledo R, Rincon M, Cummins A, Pfeiffer L, Mossman B. Transgenic mouse models to determine the role of epidermal growth factor receptor in epithelial cell proliferation, apoptosis, and asbestosis. *Chest.* 2001;120:22S–24S.

Timblin CR, Shukla A, Berlanger I, BeruBe KA, Churg A, Mossman BT. Ultrafine airborne particles cause increases in protooncogene expression and proliferation in alveolar epithelial cells. *Toxicol Appl Pharmacol.* 2002;179:98–104.

Trosini-Desert V, Chambellan A, Germaud P, Chailleux E. Constrictive pericarditis due to asbestos exposure. *Rev Mal Respir.* 2003;20:622–627.

Utidjian MD, Gross P, deTreville RTP. Ferruginous bodies in human lungs: prevalence at random autopsies. *Arch Environ Health.* 1968;17:327–333.

Viallat JR, Boutin C, Pietri JF, Fondarai J. Late progression of radiographic changes in Canari chrysotile mine and mill exworkers. *Arch Environ Health.* 1983;38:54–58.

Von Recklinghausen F. Zur Fettresorportion. *Wirchow's Arch Pathol Anat.* 1863;26:172–208.

Wagner JC. *Susceptibility to the asbestos-related disease.* In: *Proceedings of Asbestos Symposium, Johannesburg, 1977.* Glen HW, ed. Randburg, South Africa: National Institute for Metallurgy; 1978:109–113.

Wain SL, Roggli VL, Foster WL Jr. Parietal pleural plaques, asbestos bodies, and neoplasia. A clinical, pathologic, and roentgenographic correlation of 25 consecutive cases. *Chest.* 1984;86:707–713.

Walker C, Everitt J, Ferriola PC, Stewart W, Mangum J, Bermudez E. Autocrine growth stimulation by transforming growth factor α in asbestos-transformed rat mesothelial cells. *Cancer Res.* 1995;55:530–536.

Wallace JM, Oishi JS, Barbers RG, Batra P, Aberle DR. Bronchoalveolar lavage cell and lymphocyte phenotype profiles in healthy asbestos-exposed shipyard workers. *Am Rev Respir Dis.* 1989;139:33–38.

Wang NS. The preformed stomas connecting the pleural cavity and the lymphatics in the parietal pleura. *Am Rev Respir Dis.* 1975;111:12–20.

Warheit DB, Chang LY, Hill LH, Hook GER, Crapo JD, Brody AR. Pulmonary macrophage accumulation and asbestos-induced lesions at sites of fiber deposition. *Am Rev Respir Dis.* 1984;129:301–310.

Warheit DB, George G, Hill LH, Snyderman R, Brody AR. Inhaled asbestos activates a complement-dependent chemoattractant for macrophages. *Lab Invest.* 1985;52:505–514.

Warheit DB, Hill LH, George G, Brody AR. Time course of chemotactic factor generation and the corresponding macrophage response to asbestos inhalation. *Am Rev Respir Dis.* 1986;134:128–133.

Weiss W. Cigarette smoke, asbestos, and small irregular opacities. *Am Rev Respir Dis.* 1984;130:293–301.

Weiss W, Levin R, Goodman L. Pleural plaques and cigarette smoking in asbestos workers. *J Occup Med.* 1981;23:427–430.

Wheeler TM, Johnson EH, Coughlin D, Greenberg SD. The sensitivity of detection of asbestos bodies in sputa and bronchial washings. *Acta Cytologica.* 1988;32:647–650.

Zolov Chr, Bourilkov T, Babadjov L. Pleural asbestosis in agricultural workers. *Environ Res.* 1967;1:287–292.

7

Lung Cancer Associated with Asbestos Exposure

Richard Attanoos

Introduction

Lung cancer (LC) is a major cause of death worldwide and accounts for approximately 12% of all cancer deaths. Among men, LC is the most common cancer in developed countries where age-adjusted incidence rates exceed $1 \times 10^2/1 \times 10^5$ population. Among women, the incidence is lower, approximately $30/1 \times 10^5$ population. LC carries a poor prognosis (Parkin et al., 1997, 1999). The mortality rates are generally 85%–90% and more than half the patients die within 1 year of diagnosis. It is estimated that between 80% and 90% of LC in men are etiologically related to tobacco, whereas the number of smokers' cancer is lower in women. Overall, asbestos-exposed subjects are at increased risk of LC and there is now sound evidence that a synergistic interaction between asbestos and tobacco smoke exists, further increasing the risk, under circumstances discussed in detail below.

In this chapter, the history of asbestos-related LC is reviewed together with the prevailing theories of lung carcinogenesis in asbestos-exposed subjects. The synergism between tobacco smoke and asbestos, clinical, pathological, and mineralogical evidence for ascription of LC to asbestos exposure is assessed together with a review of the recent consensus document, the so-called "Helsinki criteria."

Historical Perspective

The association between LC and tobacco smoking was established in the 1950s and the relative LC risk was related to the pattern, intensity, and duration of smoking and the tar content of the cigarettes. Moreover, relative LC risk was found to decrease after smoking cessation (Doll and Hill, 1952, 1964).

The earliest documentation of LC in asbestos workers dates to the 1930s (Chapter 1). However, the reality of the association of LC and asbestosis was not appreciated until 1949 after publication in the United Kingdom of the first systematic inquiry recorded in the Annual Report of the Chief Inspector of Factories (Merewether, 1949). LC was reported in 13.2% of 235 male deaths complicated by asbestosis, compared to 1.2% of almost 7×10^3 deaths due to silicosis. In 1951, Gloyne published a survey of more than 1.2×10^3 industrial postmortem examinations, noting LC in more than 14%. In 1955, two key publications provided irrefutable evidence of the association between LC and asbestos exposure. The first was a case-controlled study by Breslow (1955) using case material from California hospitals, and the second by Doll (1955). This latter publication was a retrospective cohort mortality study of workers in a textile factory located in Rochdale, United Kingdom.

Asbestos-Related LC: Mechanistic Considerations

Despite considerable epidemiological and clinical study and both animal modeling and in vitro molecular research, fundamental issues remain unresolved. These include

- Asbestos-related LC cannot be distinguished from LC of other causes on clinical or pathological grounds. There exist no recognized specific anatomical, histological, molecular, or genetic features that relate the causation to asbestos.
- The mechanisms of asbestos-related lung carcinogenesis are incompletely understood. This has importance with respect to LC attribution. Legal arguments center on whether LC risk is only elevated in persons with coexistent asbestosis, or whether LC risk relates to cumulative asbestos exposure (in the absence of asbestosis).
- Epidemiological studies performed in asbestos-exposed workers identify a complex interrelationship between LC risk, cumulative asbestos exposure (dose-response), asbestos fiber type, and features of the industrial workplace. All published studies have inherent flaws and purported conclusions should be closely scrutinized (Chapter 4). Prospective cohort mortality studies in which asbestos exposures in workers are well defined are valuable for addressing questions of causation but exceedingly difficult to design and carry out. Case-referent and postmortem studies are often criticized because of bias in the selection of cases and controls, but can take into account factors that are difficult to anticipate prospectively.

Estimates of LC risk in various epidemiological studies have focused on asbestos exposure measurements in the workplace and correlate dose with clinical response (LC and/or asbestosis). Dust measurements for various asbestos-exposed cohorts are recorded in numerous publications. However, reliable data of asbestos exposure in the workplace is difficult to obtain (Ayer et al., 1965) for reasons considered in detail in Chapter 4. Sampling of workplace air was rarely sampled for asbestos in epidemiological studies before the 1940s.

Underestimates of exposure in epidemiological cohorts results in an overestimation of LC risk. As discussed in Chapter 4, studies that compare results generated from different sampling methods often incorporate measurement conversion factors. In reality, few published epidemiological studies employ reliable information on work history and actual exposure measurements, even when dose-response assessments are crudely estimated. Table 7.1 summarizes dose-response data for a number of relatively robust epidemiological cohorts. Importantly, there exist few reliable data correlating workplace environmental exposure levels with the respirable fraction of asbestos (ie, asbestos inhaled, deposited, and retained) within lung tissue. Therefore, the significance of workplace environmental exposure levels recorded in the literature remain questionable as it is only the respirable fraction of the cumulative asbestos dosage that has pathogenetic significance. The prudent investigator is obliged to address the strengths and shortcomings of the environmental sampling utilized in a study.

Leaving aside the practical difficulties that exist in assimilating the asbestos exposure data, estimates of LC risk are also problematic because of the long latent period between

Table 7.1 Relative Risk (RR) for Lung Cancer in Selected Studies

Study	Cohort*	RR
Acheson et al. (1982)	Chrysotile textile 125	0.8
Peto (1985)	Manufacturers 100	1
Dement et al. (1983a,b)	Chrysotile textile 25	4
Dement et al. (1994)	Manufacturers 33	3
Nicholson et al. (1979)	Chrysotile miners 667	0.15
McDonald et al. (1983)	Miners 2500	0.04
Henderson and Enterline (1979)	Cement manufacture 100	1
Weill (1994)	Cement workers 50	2
Nicholson et al. (1981)	US Insulation manufacture 23	4.3
McDonald et al. (1984)	Friction products 2000	0.05
Berry (1994)	Chrysotile 1600	0.06
Sluis-Cremer and Bezuidenhout (1989)	Crocidolite mining 19	5.2
de Klerk et al. (1989)	Crocidolite miners 100	1

* f/mL-year resulting in twofold increase in lung cancer.

initial asbestos exposure and response, that is, LC. (This usually exceeds 20 years with no recognized upper limit.) The confounding effect of increases in the prevalence of smoking in cohorts of tobacco smokers is an additional problem. A review of published epidemiological studies led Browne (1986) to conclude that LC risk was not increased until a cumulative asbestos exposure of 25–100 f/mL-yrs. The report of the Ontario Royal Commission (Dupre et al., 1984) indicated that this level of exposure was sufficient to produce asbestosis. Without good basis, the figure of 25 f/mL-yrs has been considered a level of exposure necessary to increase LC risk twofold. This criterion was accepted in the consensus document—so-called Helsinki criteria (1977)—and interestingly, by some courts in the United States.

A linear increase in cancer risk is evident at high levels of asbestos exposure but at lower levels of cumulative exposure. A less than linear response is often observed. However, epidemiological studies are not well suited for determining risk when dosage approaches threshold. To date, a threshold for the carcinogenic effect of asbestos has not been demonstrated in human or animal studies.

Table 7.1 illustrates the differences between LC risk (ie, dose-response coefficient) in various epidemiological studies and highlights the importance of the type of asbestos

work (process) together with fiber type. In a meta-analysis of 17 epidemiological studies, Hodgson and Darnton (2000) acknowledged that it was difficult to establish a clear
view of the quantified risk of LC. The mean risk for all amphibole cohorts was 4.8% per
f/mL-yr (95% CI = 3.9–5.8). For pure chrysotile cohorts a value of 0.5 % per f/mL-yr
exposure is regarded as the upper limit for LC (ie, 200 f/mL-yrs for LC risk doubling).
For "commercial" chrysotile mining the estimate of 0.06% per f/mL-yr exposure reflects a
LC doubling risk at 1600 f/mL-yrs. The mean estimate for cohorts of workers exposed to
a mixture of asbestos fiber types is 0.32% per f/mL-yr exposure with an upper estimate of
0.5% per f/mL-yr exposure constituting a value of 300 f/mL-yrs for a doubling LC risk.

LC risk differs with fiber type; consistently higher rates have been found in occupational cohorts exposed to amphiboles in comparison to chrysotile. In a review of
epidemiological data by Hodgson and Darnton (2000), the risk differential between
chrysotile and the two commercial amphiboles (amosite and crocidolite) was estimated
to be between 1:10 and 1:50. The difference in carcinogenic potency has been attributed without scientific verification to fiber surface properties (intrinsic redox potential),
geophysical chemical factors, and biopersistence. As noted elsewhere in this book, fiber
burden analysis undertaken after death (often many years after exposure) is not a robust
indicator of prior chrysotile asbestos exposure due to the mineral's relatively low biopersistence. Thus, work histories serve as the most reliable means of assessing exposure,
despite the shortcomings inherent in retrospectively gathered exposure information.

It is well established that LC risk in asbestos workers varies with industrial process—being relatively high in insulators, intermediate in textile workers, and low in
friction product workers and asbestos-cement manufacturers. In simple terms, this can
be attributed to different workplace conditions and industrial processes. Most probably,
however, it reflects the difference in the total inhaled, deposited, and retained asbestos
as well as asbestos fiber type and fiber size. The proportional mortality ratio (PMR) for
LC in different cohorts of asbestos workers is shown in Table 7.2. The data from these

**Table 7.2 Proportional Mortality Ratios (PMR) for Lung
Cancer in Selected Studies by Asbestos Type**

Study	Cohort	PMR
Acheson et al. (1984)	Factory Amosite	6.6
Levin et al. (1998)	Factory Amosite	7.4
Acheson et al. (1982)	Gas mask workers Chrysotile	1.4
McDonald et al. (1983)	Textile factory Chrysotile	0
McDonald et al. (1984)	Friction products Chrysotile	1.9
Thomas et al. (1982)	Cement factory Chrysotile	0
Gardner et al. (1986)	Cement factory Chrysotile	0
Dement et al. (1994)	Textile factory Chrysotile	6.75

studies cannot be evaluated comparatively because standardization for variables was not done.

Recently, a number of case-control studies have been published and for completeness, they merit inclusion. In a German population-based, matched case-control study involving more than 800 male LC cases and a comparable number of controls (Pohlabeln et al., 2002), exposure was computed as lifelong working hours. A panel of experts estimated the cumulative exposure on a time:intensity scale. Applying the two-phase paradigm, the odds ratio (OR) for LC associated with exposure of 25 f/mL-yrs was 1.94 and the excess was statistically significant.

A Swedish population-based case-referent study investigated the LC risk associated with occupational exposure. It focused on dose-response relationships and the interaction with tobacco smoking (Gustavsson et al., 2002). Cases of LC among males aged 40–75 years were identified during a 5-year period. LC risk increased almost linearly with cumulative dose of asbestos. The risk at a cumulative dose of 4 f/mL-yrs was 1.9 (95% CI = 1.3–2.7). In this study, the effects of asbestos exposure and smoking were considered to be between additive and multiplicative.

LC, Tobacco Smoke, and Asbestos

The risk of LC in asbestos-exposed nonsmokers can only be assessed using very large cohorts. The inaccuracies of classifying persons as current smokers, that is, smokers and nonsmokers, together with the impact of passive smoking among workers all potentially inflate the risk of LC in bona fide lifelong nonsmokers. In an analysis of almost 1.78×10^5 insulation workers, the LC risk was increased by fivefold in nonsmokers who were exposed to asbestos for 20 or more years, compared with nonsmoking control subjects. However, the results were based on only four cases and therefore, there exists the potential for substantial statistical variation in this figure (Table 7.3). More recently, Liddell (2001) noted that nonsmokers have a relative risk (RR) of LC due to asbestos exposure that is about twice as high as the RR for smokers. The absolute risk of LC is, of course, substantially less in nonsmokers than in smokers. In practice, lung tumors are rare among asbestos-exposed subjects who are lifelong nonsmokers.

Data from studies of various occupational groups are consistent with a multiplicative model whereby both asbestos and smoking are independently capable of causing LC and act

Table 7.3 Synergistic Interaction between Tobacco Smoking, Asbestos Exposure, and Lung Cancer Risk*

Asbestos Exposure Ratio	Smoking	Mortality
No	No	1
Yes	No	5.2[†]
No	Yes	10.9
Yes	Yes	53.2

* From Selikoff and Hammond, 1979.

[†] At face value the lung cancer risk appears approximately fivefold increased in occupationally exposed nonsmokers as compared with nonsmokers in the control reference population (nonasbestos-exposed). However, the results are based on only four cases and therefore, there exists substantial statistical variation in this figure. In fact, the actual mortality ratio is not known but probably lies greater than 1.00 and may be a little higher than 12.00.

synergistically when exposure to both occurs. This model is consistent with the multistage theory of carcinogenesis whereby cancer occurs as a result of a sequence of genetic changes that release the normal cell from regulatory mechanisms (Saracci, 1977).

It was previously believed that long-term smoking cessation results in normalization of LC risk. However, recently published data (Halpern et al., 1993) shows that while smoking cessation is beneficial at any age, risk reduction is far less than complete. (For example, smoking cessation for 50 years results in a 5% excess LC risk in persons aged 75–80 years.)

Considerable controversy exists as to whether asbestos per se or asbestosis predisposes one to LC. Opinions are divided into three groups:

1. *Fibrosis/cancer hypothesis.* The risk of LC is only increased when asbestosis is present.
2. *Fiber burden hypothesis.* The risk of LC is increased only when exposure is sufficient to produce asbestosis, even in the absence of radiologically and pathologically demonstrable asbestosis.
3. Any asbestos exposure increases the risk of LC.

Fibrosis/Cancer Hypothesis

As noted above, numerous studies have shown that LC risk is increased in persons with clinical asbestosis. Proponents of the fibrosis/cancer hypothesis are of the opinion that it is only in the presence of asbestos-induced lung fibrosis that LC risk is materially increased. They argue that

- Severe interstitial lung fibrosis unrelated to asbestos exposure is associated with increased risk of LC.
- Epidemiological studies have established a link between asbestosis and LC and not asbestos exposure per se.
- In inhalation studies, LC only develops in animals with asbestosis.

Studies Supporting Fibrosis/Cancer Hypothesis

Numerous studies supporting the fibrosis hypothesis can be identified in the literature. Prospective and retrospective epidemiological cohort studies and clinical case-referent studies support this thesis.

In published cohorts, when clinical asbestosis is present, the incidence of LC is high, ranging between 30% and 50% of deaths (Berry, 1981; Coutts et al., 1987). The Annual Report of the Chief Inspectors of Factories on Industrial Health for 1958 demonstrates an association between asbestosis and LC. In a series of 365 deaths in which postmortem examination confirmed asbestosis, almost 18% (65 cases) had concomitant LC. The LC mortality of factory workers in East London for the period 1933–1980 was reported by Newhouse et al. (1985). Ninety percent of LC patients had associated asbestosis.

In 1955, Doll published a retrospective cohort mortality study of asbestos textile workers. LC was found to be a specific industrial hazard for those who had worked with asbestos for at least 20 years. The average risk for employees with 20 or more years of exposure was approximately ten times that experienced by the general population. An increased LC standardized mortality ratio (SMR) was detected only in men with asbestosis.

In the North American insulation workers cohort mortality study there were 544 recorded deaths from LC (Suzuki and Selikoff, 1986). The study cohort included only four cancers in nonsmokers. In a subcohort where nonneoplastic tissue was available for assessment, all but one case had histological evidence of fibrosis; in 90.7% it was either moderate or severe. In a related occupational cohort, Kipen et al. (1987) studied a series of 450 deaths from LC among North American asbestos insulation workers. Lung tissue for histological analysis was available in only 138 and asbestosis was demonstrated in every case. The study has been criticized for use of nonstandardized pathology criteria for the diagnosis of asbestosis. Some asbestosis cases were diagnosed on the basis of pleural/subpleural changes (rather than lung parenchymal fibrosis) and some cases had no demonstrable asbestos bodies (AB). For example, fibrosis of the subpleural connective tissue was considered to be asbestosis. Critics have highlighted the lack of a control group.

In 1989, Sluis-Cremer and Bezuidenhout reported a necropsy series of almost 400 amphibole asbestos miners in South Africa. Of the 35 persons who died of LC, 24 had asbestosis, and the remaining 11 were smokers. The LC SMR increased by almost six-fold in the presence of moderate to severe asbestosis, but not in those without lung parenchymal disease. Smoking, age, and the severity of the fibrosis correlated with LC risk; adjusting for asbestosis and proportional mortality was not increased in persons without asbestosis. This study is particularly important as the quality of the occupational history and clinical records were outstanding. Moreover, a pathological confirmation of diagnoses was undertaken. Critics of this study suggest that there was selection bias (only 37% of the workforce were studied), and the use of a nonstandardized pathological terminology with respect to the diagnosis of asbestosis. In addition, it was acknowledged that applicants for compensation had been selected for study (Rudd, 1990). (This may have introduced bias by overrepresenting cases with asbestosis.)

In 1991, Hughes and Weill reported a prospective mortality study of 839 workers from two asbestos-cement manufacturing plants. In 1969, 154 deaths had occurred and 29 were due to LC (all cigarette smokers). Workers without radiological evidence of lung fibrosis did not experience a raised LC risk. The SMR increased (fourfold) only in those with radiological detectable irregular lung opacities (ie, radiological evidence of asbestosis with a UICC/ILO score of greater than 1/0). The authors concluded that lung fibrosis (ie, asbestosis) was a necessary precursor for asbestos-induced LC. This study represented the first prospective cohort mortality study among asbestos-exposed workers. Unfortunately, it had low statistical power (Rudd, 1987). In workers without small opacities followed for at least 20 years from first exposure, LC developed in 10, whereas 9.5 cases were expected. Since 95% CI on the case would be 0.51–1.94, the study did not have the statistical power to exclude an almost twofold risk of LC in those without radiological evidence of asbestosis.

Weiss (1999) undertook a meta-analysis of 38 published cohort studies hypothesizing that excesses in LC occur among workers who developed asbestosis. Asbestosis proved to be a much better predictor of excess LC risk than asbestos exposure data.

LC risk is known to be increased in persons with diffuse interstitial fibrosis irrespective of causation with a RR ranging between 2X and 14X (Turner-Warwick et al., 1980). In the study of Nagai et al. (1992), LC occurred in 11% of nonsmokers and 38% of smokers with idiopathic pulmonary fibrosis. This paper links the synergistic effect of tobacco smoking with fibrosis in the absence of asbestos exposure.

Davis and Cowie (1990) reviewed the literature on asbestosis in rats exposed to asbestos in the laboratory. Cancer was associated with the fibrosing process and overall, the incidence paralleled the degree of fibrosis. These studies have been criticized because exposure levels and the route of administration of asbestos to the animals were not comparable to the human experience. Clearly, extrapolation between exposures in animals and comparisons to human disease are problematic.

Fiber Burden Hypothesis

Proponents of the fiber burden hypothesis maintain that it is the cumulative asbestos exposure to asbestos that increases the risk of LC. Thus, the incidence of cancer is increased only when exposure is sufficient to produce asbestosis even in the absence of clinical and/or pathological evidence of lung disease. They justify this position based upon the following considerations:

- In vitro studies indicate that asbestos can induce transformation in cells along a dose gradient (low for mesothelium, intermediate for bronchial epithelial cells, and highest for fibroblasts). Hypothetically, this infers that carcinogenicity and fibrogenicity represent separate processes.
- LC risk correlates with increased fiber burdens in the lung independent of fibrosis and smoking.

A number of epidemiological (mainly case-control design) studies have been published in which results suggest that LC risk is elevated without radiographic evidence of asbestosis.

Martischnig et al. (1977) evaluated 200 cases of LC (without clinical or radiological evidence of asbestosis) and an equal number of control subjects. Exposure was documented in 29% LC subjects and 14% controls, yielding an OR of 2.35 (95% CI = 1.39–3.97). The study has been criticized based on control selection, occupational history retrieval, and the lack of a pathological assessment of asbestosis.

A case-control study by Wilkinson et al. (1995) yielded similar results. The authors reviewed 271 LC patients and 678 control subjects. The OR was 2.03 in subjects with fibrosis and radiological opacities of greater than 1/0 compared with 1.56 in subjects displaying no radiological evidence of lung fibrosis. The authors concluded that LC risk was increased in some persons without radiological evidence of asbestosis. This study warrants a number of criticisms (Jones et al., 1996) that are summarized below: (1) the control group included a number of subjects with histories of dust exposures, thus confounding the radiological interpretation; (2) authors ignored the patients' own assessment of asbestos exposure and based it on a job classification questionnaire; (3) furthermore, occupations listed in the "probable and possible" exposure categories included many with inadequate evidence of asbestos-related LC and exposure to other minerals such as silica that might have resulted in radiological opacities; (4) combining the "definite and probable" categories produced an excess OR of 1.49 (95% CI = 1.09–2.04) but the "definite" category alone only produced an OR of less than 1.00. In both categories, the OR for less than 10 years' exposure was much higher than the OR for 10 years or more exposure (ie, an inverse dose-response). The OR for those with 10 or more years' exposure was not significantly greater than 1.0 in all subjects or in men aged 40 or older. Furthermore, while the authors imply that the study supports the view that asbestos (not asbestosis) increases the risk of LC, histological asbestosis not detected by x-rays may have been present in the lungs of the exposed subjects. Accordingly, the results in no way contradict the view that fibrosis in a subcohort of persons accounts for the increased risk of LC.

A radiographic study of asbestos-cement workers in Ontario (Finkelstein, 1997) demonstrated a significant increase in LC mortality in subjects lacking evidence of asbestosis. Among 123 subjects without asbestosis at least 20 years after first exposure, there were 12 LC deaths compared with 2.17 expected, giving an SMR of 5.53 (95% CI = 2.86–9.66) compared to 9.96 among the 20 LC with asbestosis. Among 128 subjects without asbestosis at least 25 years after first exposure, there were nine LC deaths compared with 1.55 expected, giving an SMR of 5.81 (95% CI = 2.66–11.0). The study did not identify a dose-response relation between the risk of LC and tobacco smoking. This suggests serious selection bias within the cohort.

De Vos Irvine et al. (1993) carried out an analysis of all men with LC in the west of Scotland diagnosed between 1975 and 1984. The incidence of malignant mesotheliomas (MM) was considered a proxy for asbestos exposure and mortality from chronic bronchitis was used as a proxy for past smoking. The relation between LC and asbestos exposure, after allowing for the effect of smoking, was calculated by a weighted stepwise multiple linear regression. The study showed that an estimated 5.7% (95% CI = 2.3–9.1%) of all LC (a total of 1081 cases) were asbestos-related. Given the small number of recorded cases of asbestosis in the study, it is probably not a prerequisite for the development of asbestos-related LC. This study provided no documentation of the presence or absence of asbestosis in the study groups. And, the surrogate markers are nonspecific.

Recently, epidemiological evidence pertinent to this issue was critically reviewed (Hessel et al., 2005). After an assessment of nine key publications, the authors conclude that results are not definitive.

With respect to mineralogical analysis, proponents of the fiber burden hypothesis draw support from the publications discussed below. Anttila et al. (1993) analyzed asbestos fiber burdens in relation to lobe of origin of the cancer in 90 consecutive patients. The location of the tumor did not correlate with fibrosis, smoking, or the number of fibers less than 3 μm in length. The authors suggested that asbestos causes an excess of tumors in the lower lobe at relatively low exposure levels independent of pulmonary fibrosis. However, the study is subject to bias as subjects with diffuse interstitial fibrosis and LC would have been precluded from undergoing surgical resection on the basis of lung function tests. In this way, the study selects cases with little or no fibrosis and with a lower fiber burden. In a related publication claiming similar conclusions (Karjalainen et al., 1993), cases with radiological evidence of fibrosis were found to have lower lobe LC. Moreover, almost all cases with fibrosis had the highest asbestos fiber burdens invalidating the association between asbestos exposure alone and lower lobe tumors among persons without asbestosis. The confounding effects of tobacco smoking could not be adjusted adequately as nonsmokers had lower asbestos fiber burdens in comparison to smokers.

Karjalainen et al. (1994) investigated the asbestos-associated risk of LC according to histological type of cancer, lobe of origin, fiber burdens, and types of amphibole fibers. Fiber counts were performed on the lungs of surgically treated male LC patients, and autopsy cases among men serving as referents. The risk of LC was increased according to the pulmonary concentration of asbestos fibers. For fiber counts between 1 and 4.9×10^6/g (dry lung) the OR was 1.7 (95% CI = 0.9–3.2) and for counts of 5×10^6 or more, the OR was 5.3 (95% CI = 1.9–14.8). When seven cases of asbestosis were excluded, the OR for counts between 1 and 4.9×10^6/g was 1.5 (95% CI = 0.8–2.9) and for 5×10^6 or more 2.8 (95% CI = 0.9–8.7). Critics have suggested that the excess risk was accounted for by the cases with asbestosis. Proponents of the paper have countered this argument. They stress that the results still indicate that the trend was similar after excluding the asbestosis cases. The wide CI were simply a reflection of the low statistical power of the study. Regardless, the results of fiber burden analyses has been given substantial weight with respect to asbestos attribution in LC cases by the quorum of participants in the formulation of the Consensus document—Helsinki criteria—as discussed below.

Helsinki Criteria

In 1997, a workshop attended by invited participants from eight countries convened to review the recent research data pertaining to clinical criteria for causality and to establish guidelines for diagnosing asbestos-related disease—The Helsinki criteria (Consensus Report, 1997). The meeting discussants concluded that the presence of asbestosis is not required for attribution of LC to asbestos. Instead, they focused on the cumulative asbestos exposure as assessed clinically by estimation of cumulative exposure, or pathologically by measurement of the asbestos content of lung tissue samples. They proposed that any of the following criteria are sufficient for attribution of a causal role to asbestos for LC, provided there is a minimum 10-year interval from first exposure to onset of the cancer:

- The presence of asbestosis diagnosed clinically, radiologically (including by high-resolution CT scan), or histologically.
- Estimated cumulative exposure of 25 f/mL-yrs (or more), the presumptive threshold level for the development of asbestosis from mixed fiber exposure.
- A count of around $5-15 \times 10^3$ AB per gram of dry lung tissue.
- A count of $>2 \times 10^6$ or more amphibole asbestos fibers 5 μm or longer per gram of dry lung tissue.
- A count of $>5 \times 10^6$ or more amphibole asbestos fibers 1 μm or longer per gram of dry lung tissue.
- A fiber count in the range associated with asbestosis carried out in the same laboratory.
- An occupational history of 1 year of heavy exposure to asbestos (eg, manufacture of asbestos products, asbestos spraying, insulation work with asbestos materials) or 5–10 years of moderate exposure (eg, construction or shipbuilding).
- Because of rapid clearance of chrysotile, occupational histories are probably a better indicator of LC risk from chrysotile than fiber analysis.

Helsinki Criteria—Critique

Attribution of disease due to asbestos exposure has long been the subject of debate. The workshop participants proposed rules for attributing LC to asbestos exposure. Alas, the issue now seems to have greater importance in litigation, than in science. Meeting participants constituted a small, self-selected group of interested parties with potential diverse opinions not necessarily represented in the final published report. This is unfortunate because the gathering reviewed considerable data, identified and clarified a number of diagnostic problems, and highlighted a conceptual medicolegal argument, that is, necessity to demonstrate a doubling of the RR for LC attribution purposes. However, in many of the most contentious areas, sound scientific evidence proved to be lacking. As a consequence, the criteria are easily challenged. Thus, the conclusions are in no way robust, valid, or specific. In essence, the conclusions represent a position statement generated by a select group of researchers who do not necessarily reflect the views of the scientific community as a whole.

- That LC should be attributed to asbestos, when asbestosis can be diagnosed either clinically, radiologically, or histologically, is not particularly contentious. In general, medical opinion is united in accepting that LC risk is elevated when there is concomitant asbestosis. However, due to the difficulties of diagnosing bona fide cases of minimal grade 1 asbestosis there is little or no data assessing whether, in these cases, LC risk is indeed increased. And, there has been no systematic evaluation of this issue using pathological criteria for the diagnosis of asbestosis. The problems associated with the diagnosis of minimal asbestosis are protean and are discussed in Chapter 6.

- Estimated cumulative exposures of 25 f/mL-yrs or more constitutes sufficient exposure to double the risk for LC. It represents a threshold level for the development of asbestosis resulting from mixed fiber exposure. Obviously, assessment of exposure data retrospectively is difficult, if not impossible. A number of specific comments merit discussion. At 25 f/mL-yrs, only a minority of asbestos-exposed workers develop radiologically detectable asbestosis, a small percentage of whom will subsequently develop LC. When asbestosis becomes radiologically detectable, only 33% LC are attributable to asbestos constituting a relative risk of 1.5. The published percentage increase in relative LC risk is between 0.5%–4% for each f/mL-yr of exposure. Without explanation, the upper limit of 4% (constituting a doubling of LC risk at 25 f/mL-yrs) was accepted by the Committee. If the lower figure of 0.5% had been taken, a doubling of LC risk would require 200 f/mL-yrs. Good scientific method suggests that the median figure for percentage increase in RR of LC per year of exposure might have been more reasonably incorporated. In the published report, only two identifiable points of reference were cited. The first refers to a German report from an insurance group claiming that a dose exceeding 25 f/mL-yrs has been estimated to cause a twofold risk of LC (Tossavainen, 1997). De Vuyst reviewed "Guidelines for the attribution of LC to asbestos" and states that "relative risk is roughly doubled in cohorts exposed to mixed fibers (amphiboles + chrysotile) at a cumulative exposure of 25 f/cc-yrs." These statements are not substantiated by references in the peer-reviewed publications. A further problem is that the workshop participants accepted 25 f/mL-yr exposure as a basis for doubling the LC risk, irrespective of asbestos fiber type and size distribution, factors known to be of great significance in LC pathogenicity. Recently, a German group attempted to correlate fiber-years exposure with pulmonary asbestos burden and asbestosis and seriously questioned the validity of the 25 f/mL-yr cumulative asbestos exposure parameter as a criterion for medicolegal purposes.

- Workplace cumulative exposure estimates are a surrogate for asbestos deposition and retention. The major factors influencing deposition are (1) the number of fibers in the breathing zone, (2) fiber dispersal (clumped fibers are too large to be deposited), and (3) fiber size distribution. Surveys of airborne measurements do not take these factors into account.

- The third proposed criterion is the significance of work history. As suggested in the report, an occupational history of 1 year of heavy exposure to asbestos (ie, manufacture of asbestos products, asbestos spraying, insulation work with asbestos materials) or 5–10 years of moderate exposure (ie, construction or shipbuilding) is considered sufficient exposure to elevate LC risk twofold. The German Accident Insurance Institution, with a database of more than 2.7×10^4 workplace measurements was used as a basis for translating work place history into a meaningful assessment of cumulative asbestos exposure. While this system aids a disability claimant, there is an unfortunate introduction of bias. Exposure data generated in this way is not comparable with information from epidemiological studies when the mean or median (50th percentile) value is used to calculate time weighted average exposure.

- Anecdotal estimates of exposure are fraught with difficulties because an individual's assessment is subject to (1) poor recall of work place conditions decades prior to the development of the LC, (2) a lack of knowledge as to what was in the work place "dust" to which he or she was exposed. Some problems can be overcome by a structured questionnaire and expert knowledge of the industrial situations where the individual worked. However, in many cases, particularly in those with multiple employments, or in employment where no airborne measurements exist, there remain many uncertainties as to relative amounts of asbestos exposure that took place. The terms light, moderate, and heavy exposure are very subjective terms and mean little outside particular industries.
- The final attribution criteria relates to fiber burden analysis of lung. The European Respiratory Society Working Group has formulated guidelines for minalogical analysis (De Vuyst et al., 1998). It should be emphasized that the evidence base for the Helsinki consensus viewpoint, that is, there is a twofold increase in LC risk when either 2 million amphibole fibers (more than 5 μm) or 5×10^6 amphibole fibers (more than 1 μm in length) per gram of dry lung tissue, appears to be based on the results of a single case-control study undertaken in a Finnish population. Karjalainen et al. (1994) examined the lung fiber burden in surgically treated male LC patients and compared fiber burden levels in a large number of control cases. Odds ratios of LC in cancer cases and autopsy controls were assessed and correlated with fiber burden. As noted above, due to the small study size, the results had low statistical power. Nonetheless, the study formed the basis of mineralogical attribution criteria for LC.
- The Helsinki report also suggests that LC can be attributed to asbestos when the lung fiber burden falls "within the range recorded for asbestosis in that laboratory," that is, lung fiber burden should be assigned a similar significance to cases of asbestosis.

Pathobiology and Pathogenesis

The mechanism of asbestos-induced carcinogenesis is not known. While a number of postulated tissue events have been suggested, a Consensus Report by the International Agency for Research against Cancer (IARC; Kane et al., 1996) concluded that there were many weaknesses and gaps in current theories. Moreover, mechanisms may differ depending upon dose.

After inhalation, fibers deposit within the respiratory tract, at an anatomical site determined by fiber diameter and length. As discussed in Chapter 2, the depth of penetration is inversely proportional to fiber diameter. Thus, long, thin fibers may lodge deep in the parenchyma and either intercept respiratory bronchiolar bifurcations or reach alveolar sacs. An important factor in asbestos pathogenicity relates to the durability of the asbestos in the tissue.

One proposed sequence of tissue events has been postulated to account for the development of asbestos-induced fibrosis and LC (Meldrum, 1996; Mossman et al., 1996). Following asbestos fiber deposition, there is an acute inflammatory cellular response and within the resultant inflammatory milieu various cytokines, growth factors, proteases, and free radicals are elaborated that induce a chronic cellular proliferative state. Chronic cellular proliferation thereby occurs in parallel with the development of alveolar wall interstitial widening, and fibrosis, that is, epithelial cell and fibroblastic proliferation coexist. Chronic tissue proliferative states increase DNA copy errors and thereby result in clastogenic effects and the initiation of carcinogenesis. According to this postulated sequence of events, asbestos exposures that are insufficient to elicit a chronic inflammatory reaction and cellular proliferative state would not result in an increased risk of LC. This model suggests a threshold for LC comparable to levels that induce asbestosis. This pathogenetic model is often advocated by the proponents of the Fibrosis/cancer hypothesis and is supported by the weight of evidence generated from epidemiological data.

Critics of this postulated mechanism of asbestos-mediated lung carcinogenesis claim that, leaving aside epidemiological studies, the question of biological plausibility arises. The fibrosis of asbestosis develops in the alveoli and small airways whereas most LC arise in the major bronchi, remote from the fibrosis. Therefore, it is difficult to understand how fibrosis at one site in the lung can be a necessary precursor of malignant transformation at a distant site (Abraham, 1994).

An alternative sequence of events is based on the notion that asbestos fibers are directly genotoxic. In vitro studies have shown that asbestos causes DNA strand breaks (Libbus et al., 1989; Rom et al., 1991), and has genotoxic effects in cells by the induction of chromosomal aberrations, thus, initiating the carcinogenic process. Asbestos may also directly induce cellular proliferation by two mechanisms—activation of proto-oncogenes that encode transcription factors and, by the inactivation of tumor suppressor genes. In concert, there no doubt is a cascade of genetic events resulting in DNA synthesis and bronchial epithelial cell proliferation. Asbestos fibers phagocytosed by alveolar macrophages may induce free oxygen radicals. Short fibers generate fewer active oxygen species than do long, thin fibers (reflecting fiber surface area). Crocidolite, with its high iron content, has a higher intrinsic redox potential than does chrysotile (Chapter 5).

Recently, molecular studies have been published that attempt to identify markers of asbestos-mediated LC based on the premise that asbestos exposure increases k-ras codon 12 mutations in adenocarcinomas of the lung (Nelson et al., 1999).

Tobacco contains a complex mixture of initiators and promoters of carcinogenesis. In vitro studies have demonstrated that asbestos (crocidolite) and tobacco act synergistically by increasing DNA strand breakage (Rom et al., 1991).

A pathogenic construct consistent with the notion that prolonged heavy asbestos exposure predisposes to cancer centers on the biologic changes that occur in the bronchial epithelium attributed to both smoking and asbestos exposure. The occurrence of squamous metaplasia in the bronchial epithelium consequent to smoking has long been recognized. The observation that asbestos similarly induces metaplasia based on observations on the lung in autopsy cases of asbestosis (Figure 7.1) and the initiation of these changes by introducing asbestos onto the epithelial surface of tracheal organ cultures in vitro (Mossman and Craighead, 1979; Figure 7.1). The process of squamous metaplasia is associated with increased mitotic activity and cell turnover as fibers are taken up from the epithelial surface (Mossman and Craighead, 1978, 1979). Under these circumstances, one might anticipate the intracellular molecular events outlined in detail in Chapter 5 would transpire in bronchial stem cells. Under this presumptive set of circumstances, one could envision that asbestos would serve (1) as a promoter to facilitate the mutagenic actions of the carcinogens in tobacco smoke, or (2) as a vehicle for transport of carcinogens on the fiber surface to actively dividing cells in the metaplastic epithelium. Uptake of tobacco smoke carcinogens thus would be facilitated.

(A)

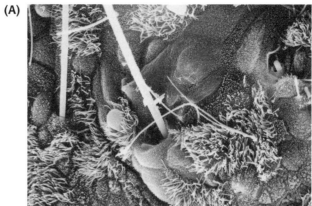

(B)

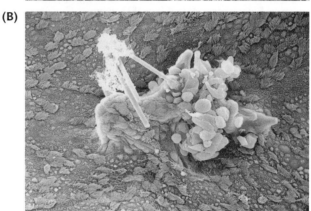

Figure 7.1 (A) Initial interaction of chrysotile and crocidolite fibers with the hamster tracheal mucosa in organ culture as illustrated by scanning electron microscopy. Note the uptake of the fibers by the mucosal epithelial cells. (B) Early squamous metaplasia in response to crocidolite, a change that is commonly noted in the human lung in asbestosis. These alterations are accompanied by dramatic molecular and biochemical events in the cells that are believed to increase susceptibility to tobacco carcinogens (Craighead and Mossman, 1979).

Asbestos-Related LC: Clinical Observation

Several studies have recorded a predominance of lower lobe carcinomas in asbestos-exposed subjects with an approximate upper lobe to lower lobe ratio of 1:2 (Kannerstein and Churg, 1972; Whitwell et al., 1974). The reverse lobar distribution had been claimed in LC in tobacco smokers. However, recent studies show no major differences in the proportion of peripheral versus central, and upper lobe versus lower lobe cancers in patients who are asbestos exposed.

Uncommonly, peripheral LC grow subjacent to and through the serosa to be manifest clinically as diffuse pleural-based masses mimicking MM. Such lung carcinomas have been referred to as "pseudomesotheliomatous carcinomas." All major histological types of LC display this unusual gross appearance, although adenocarcinomas most commonly display this pattern. Apart from bronchogenic carcinoma, a variety of primary pleural-based sarcomas and histogenetically diverse metastatic neoplasms (carcinoma, melanoma, primitive neuroectodermal tumors, non-Hodgkin's lymphoma) may exhibit this feature. There is no evidence to suggest that asbestos contributes to the development of these pleural lesions.

Pleural plaques are not a risk factor for bronchogenic carcinoma (Edelman, 1990; Hughes and Weill, 1991; Kiviluoto et al., 1979; Partanen et al., 1992; Wain et al., 1984; Weiss, 1993), although some observers have argued to the contrary. As might be expected, plaques commonly occur in those who ultimately develop MM, but there is no evidence to suggest that they predispose one to the development of the neoplasm. Whereas plaques are exceedingly common in the rural Finnish population, mesotheliomas are not increased in prevalence.

References

Abraham JL. Asbestos inhalation, not asbestosis, causes lung cancer. *Am J Ind Med*. 1994;26:839–842.

Acheson ED, Gardner MJ, Pippard EC, Grime LP. Mortality of two groups of women who manufactured gas masks from chrysotile and crocidolite asbestos: a 40 year follow-up. *Br J Ind Med*. 1982;39:344–348.

Acheson ED, Gardner MJ. Asbestos: the control limit for asbestos. UK Health and Safety Commission HMSO; 1983.

Acheson ED, Gardner MJ, Winter PD, Bennett C. Cancer in a factory using amosite asbestos. *Int J Epidemiol*. 1984;13:3–10.

Anttila S, Karjalainen A, Taikina-aho O, Kyyronen P, Vainio H. Lung cancer in the lower lobe is associated with pulmonary asbestos fiber count and fiber size. *Environ Health Perspect*. 1993;101:166–170.

Ayer HE, Lynch JR, Fanney JH. A comparison of impinger and membrane filter techniques for evaluating air samples in asbestos plants. *Ann NY Acad Sci*. 1965;132:274–287.

Berry G. Mortality and cancer incidence of workers exposed to chrysotile asbestos in the friction products industry. *Ann Occup Hyg*. 1994;38:539–546.

Berry G . Mortality of workers certified by pneumoconiosis medical panels as having asbestosis. *Br J Ind Med*. 1981;38:130–137.

Breslow L . Industrial aspects of bronchiogenic neoplasms. *Dis Chest*. 1955;28:421–430.

Browne K. Is asbestos or asbestosis the cause of the increased risk of lung cancer in asbestos workers? *Br J Ind Med*. 1986;43:145–149.

Coutts II, Gilson JC, Kerr IH, Parkes WR, Turner-Warwick M. Mortality in cases of asbestosis diagnosed by a pneumoconiosis medical panel. *Thorax*. 1987;42:111–116.

Davis JM, Cowie HA. The relationship between fibrosis and cancer in experimental animals exposed to asbestos and other fibers. *Environ Health Perspect*. 1990;88:305–309.

de Klerk NH, Armstrong BK, Musk AW, Hobbs MS. Cancer mortality in relation to measures of occupational exposure to crocidolite at Wittenoom Gorge in Western Australia. *Br J Ind Med*. 1989;6:529–536.

Dement JM, Harris RL Jr, Symons MJ, Shy CM. Exposures and mortality among chrysotile asbestos workers. Part 1: exposure estimates. *Am J Ind Med*. 1983a;4:399–419.

Dement JM, Harris RL Jr, Symons MJ, Shy CM. Exposures and mortality among chrysotile asbestos workers. Part II: mortality. *Am J Ind Med*. 1983b;4:421–433.

Dement JM, Brown DP, Okun A. Follow-up study of chrysotile asbestos textile workers: cohort mortality and case-control analyses. *Am J Ind Med*. 1994;26:431–447.

De Vos Irvine H, Lamont DW, Hole DJ, Gillis CR. Asbestos and lung cancer in Glasgow and the west of Scotland. *Br Med J*. 1993;306:1503–1506.

De Vuyst P, Karjalainen A, Dumortier P, et al. Guidelines for mineral fibre analyses in biological samples: report of the ERS Working Group, European Respiratory Society. *Eur Respir J*. 1998;11:1416–1426.

Doll R. Mortality from lung cancer in asbestos workers. *Br J Ind Med*. 1955;12:81–86.

Doll R, Hill AB. A study of the aetiology of carcinoma of the lung. *Br Med J*. 1952;2:1271–1286.

Doll R, Hill AB. Mortality in relation to smoking: ten years' observations of British Doctors. *Br Med J*. 1964;5395:1399–1410.

Dupre JS, Mustard JS, Uffen RJ. Report of the Royal Commission on Matters of Health and Safety arising from the use of asbestos in Ontario. Ontario Ministry of the Attorney General, Ontario. 1984:281.

Edelman DA. Does asbestosis increase the risk of lung cancer? *Int Arch Occup Environ Health.* 1990;62:345–349.

Finkelstein MM. Radiographic asbestosis is not a prerequisite for asbestos-associated lung cancer in Ontario asbestos cement workers. *Am J Ind Med.* 1997;32:341–348.

Gardner MJ, Winter PD, Pannett B, Powell CA. Follow-up study of workers manufacturing chrysotile asbestos cement products. *Br J Ind Med.* 1986;43:726–732.

Gloyne SR. Pneumoconiosis. A histological survey of necropsy material in 1205 cases. *Lancet.* 1951;1:810–814.

Gustavsson P, Nyberg F, Pershagen G, Scheele P, Jakobsson R, Plato N. Low-dose exposure to asbestos and lung cancer: dose-response relations and interaction with smoking in a population-based case-referent study in Stockholm, Sweden. *Am J Epidemiol.* 2002;155:1016–1022.

Halpern MT, Gillespie BW, Warner KE. Patterns of absolute risk of lung cancer mortality in former smokers. *J Natl Cancer Inst.* 1993;85:457–464.

Hammond EC, Selikoff IJ, Seidman H. Asbestos exposure, cigarette smoking and death rates. *Ann NY Acad Sci.* 1979;330:473–490.

Henderson VL, Enterline PE. Asbestos exposure: factors associated with excess cancer and respiratory disease mortality. *Ann NY Acad Sci.* 1979;330:117–126.

Hessel PA, Gamble JF, McDonald JC. Asbestos, asbestosis, and lung cancer: a critical assessment of the epidemiological evidence. *Thorax.* 2005;60:433–436.

Hodgson JT, Darnton A. The quantitative risks of mesothelioma and lung cancer in relation to asbestos exposure. *Ann Occup Hyg.* 2000;44:565–601.

Hughes JM, Weill H. Asbestosis as a precursor of asbestos related lung cancer: results of a prospective mortality study. *Br J Ind Med.* 1991;48:229–233.

Jones RN, Hughes JM, Weill H. Asbestos exposure, asbestosis, and asbestos-attributable lung cancer. *Thorax.* 1996;51(Supp 2):S9–S15.

Kannerstein M, Churg J. Pathology of carcinoma of the lung associated with asbestos exposure. *Cancer.* 1972;30:14–21.

Karjalainen A, Anttila S, Heikkila L, Kyyronen P, Vainio H. Lobe of origin of lung cancer among asbestos-exposed patients with or without diffuse interstitial fibrosis. *Scand J Work Environ Health.* 1993;19:102–107.

Karjalainen A, Anttila S, Vanhala E, Vainio H. Asbestos exposure and the risk of lung cancer in a general urban population. *Scand J Work Environ Health.* 1994;20:243–50.

Kane AB, Boffetta P, Saracci R, et al. Mechanisms of fiber carcinogenesis. IARC Scientific Publications 140 Lyon, 1996.

Kipen HM, Lilis R, Suzuki Y, Valciukas JA, Selikoff IJ. Pulmonary fibrosis in asbestos insulation workers with lung cancer: a radiological and histopathological evaluation. *Br J Ind Med.* 1987;44:96–100.

Levin JL, McLarty JW, Hurst GA, Smith AN, Frank AL. Tyler asbestos workers: mortality experience in a cohort exposed to amosite. *Occup Environ Med.* 1998;55:155–160.

Libbus BL, Illenye SA, Craighead JE. Induction of DNA strand breaks in cultured rat embryo cells by crocidolite asbestos as assessed by nick translation. *Cancer Res.* 1989;49:5713–5718.

Liddell FD. The interaction of asbestos and smoking in lung cancer. *Ann Occup Hyg.* 2001;45:341–356.

Martischnig KM, Newell DJ, Barnsley WC, Cowan WK, Feinmann EL, Oliver E. Unsuspected exposure to asbestos and bronchogenic carcinoma. *Br Med J.* 1977;1:746–749.

McDonald AD, Fry JS, Woolley AJ, McDonald JC. Dust exposure and mortality in an American chrysotile asbestos friction products plant. *Br J Ind Med.* 1984;41:151–157.

McDonald AD, Fry JS, Woolley AJ, McDonald J. Dust exposure and mortality in an American chrysotile textile plant. *Br J Ind Med.* 1983;40:361–367.

Meldrum M. Review of Fiber Toxicology 1996; p13–14 and 42–47. HMSO: Health and Safety Executive ISBN 0 7176 1205 8, 1996.

Merewether ERA. Asbestosis and carcinoma of the lung. In: Annual Report on the Chief Inspector of Factories for the year 1947. London: HMSO Stationery Office; 1949.

Mossman BT, Craighead JE. Induction of neoplasms in hamster tracheal grafts with 3-methylcholanthrene coated Lycra fibers. *Cancer Res.* 1978;38:3717–3722.

Mossman BT, Craighead JE. Use of hamster tracheal organ cultures for assessing the cocarcinogenic effects of inorganic particulates on the respiratory epithelium. *Prog Exp Tumor Res.* 1979;24:37–47.

Mossman BT, Kamp DW, Weitzman SA. Mechanisms of carcinogenesis and clinical features of asbestos-associated cancers. *Cancer Invest.* 1996;14:466–480.

Nagai A, Chiyotani A, Nakadate T, Konno K. Lung cancer in patients with idiopathic pulmonary fibrosis. *Tohoku J Exp Med.* 1992;167:231–237.

Nelson HH, Christiani DC, Wiencke JK, Mark EJ, Wain JC, Kelsey KT. k-ras mutation and occupational asbestos exposure in lung adenocarcinoma: asbestos related cancer without asbestosis. *Cancer Res.* 1999;59:4570–4573.

Newhouse ML, Berry G, Wagner JC. Mortality of factory workers in East London 1933–1980. *Br J Ind Med.* 1985;42:4–11.

Nicholson WJ, Selikoff IJ, Seidman H, Lilis R, Formby P. Long-term mortality experience of chrysotile miners and millers in Thetford Mines, Québec. *Ann NY Acad Sci.* 1979;330:11–21.

Parkin DM, Pisani P, Ferlay J. Estimates of the worldwide incidence of 25 major cancers in 1990. *Int J Cancer.* 1999;80:827–841.

Parkin DM, Whelan SL, Ferlay, et al. (eds.) In: *Cancer in Five Continents*, Vol. VII. International Agency for Research on Cancer (IARC) Scientific Publication No. 143, Lyon: IARC; 1997.

Partanen T, Nurminen M, Zitting A, Koskinen H, Wiikeri M, Ahlman K. Localized pleural plaques and lung cancer. *Am J Ind Med.* 1992;22:185–192.

Peto J. Relationship of mortality to measures of environmental asbestos pollution in an asbestos textile factory. *Ann Occup Hyg.* 1985;29:305–355.

Pohlabeln H, Wild P, Schill W, et al. Asbestos fibre years and lung cancer: a two phase case-control study with expert exposure assessment. *Occup Environ Med.* 2002;59:410–414.

Roggli VL, Vollmer RT, Greenberg SD, McGavran MH, Spjut HJ, Yesner R. Lung cancer heterogeneity: a blinded and randomized study of 100 consecutive cases. *Hum Pathol.* 1985;16:569–579.

Rom WN, Travis WD, Brody AR. Cellular and molecular basis of the asbestos related diseases. *Am Rev Respir Dis.* 1991;143:408–422.

Rudd RM. Pulmonary asbestosis in asbestos insulation workers with lung cancer (letter). *Br J Ind Med.* 1987;44:428–429.

Rudd RM. Relation between asbestosis and bronchial cancer in amphibole asbestos miners. *Br J Ind Med.* 1990;47:215–216.

Saracci R. Asbestos and lung cancer: an analysis of the epidemiological evidence on the asbestos-smoking interaction. *Int J Cancer.* 1977;20:323–331.

Selikoff IJ and Hammond EC. Asbestos and smoking. *JAMA.* 1979;242:458–459.

Sluis-Cremer GK, Bezuidenhout BN. Relation between asbestosis and bronchial cancer in amphibole asbestos miners. *Br J Ind Med.* 1989;46:537–540.

Suzuki Y, Selikoff IJ. Pathology of lung cancer among asbestos insulation workers. *Fed Proc.* 1986;45:744A.

Thomas HF, Benjamin IT, Elwood PC, Dweetnam PM. Further follow-up study of workers from an asbestos cement factory. *Br J Ind Med.* 1982;39:273–276.

Tossavainen A. *Asbestos, asbestosis and cancer, Exposure Criteria for Clinical Diagnosis, in Asbestos, Asbestosis and Cancer,* Proceedings of an International Expert Meeting, Research Report 14, 8–27, 1997.

Turner-Warwick M, Burrows B, Johnson A. Cryptogenic fibrosing alveolitis—clinical features and their influence on survival. *Thorax.* 1980;35:171–180.

Wain SL, Roggli VL, Foster WL Jr. Parietal pleural plaques, asbestos bodies, and neoplasia. A clinical, pathologic, and roentgenographic correlation of 25 consecutive cases. *Chest.* 1984;86:707–713.

Weill H. Biological effects: asbestos-cement manufacturing. *Ann Occup Hyg.* 1994;38:533–538.

Weiss W. Asbestos-related pleural plaques and lung cancer. *Chest.* 1993;103:1854–1859.

Weiss W. Asbestosis: a marker for the increased risk of lung cancer among workers exposed to asbestos. *Chest.* 1999;115:536–549.

Whitwell F, Newhouse ML, Bennett DR. A study of the histological cell types of lung cancer in workers suffering from asbestosis in the United Kingdom. *Br J Ind Med.* 1974;31:298–303.

Wilkinson P, Hansell DM, Janssens J, et al. Is lung cancer associated with asbestos exposure when there are no small opacities on the chest radiograph? *Lancet.* 1995;345:1074–1078.

8

Malignant Diseases of the Pleura, Peritoneum, and Other Serosal Surfaces

Allen R. Gibbs and John E. Craighead

Introduction

This chapter focuses on malignant mesothelioma (MM) and other mesothelial lesions and conditions that mimic MM. Formerly a rare tumor, MM is now, alongside lung cancer, the most important occupational cancer among industrial populations worldwide. MM is, with rare exceptions, a diffuse tumor that arises in the serosal surfaces of the pleura, peritoneum, pericardium, ovary, and tunica vaginalis of the testis. The most frequent location is the pleura (>90%) followed by the peritoneum (6%–10%); the other sites are rare (Jones et al., 1995; Roggli, 1981). As a result of serosal effusion and diffuse serosal thickening by tumor, patients with pleural tumors typically present with chest pain and shortness of breath and abdominal pain with distension in the peritoneal cases (Chapter 10).

MM of the pleura is more common in males than females because of its strong association with occupational asbestos exposure. In several countries, including Australia, United Kingdom, and France (Banaei et al., 2000; Health and Safety Executive, 2001; Leigh et al., 2002), the annual incidence is steadily increasing but in many developed countries, including the United States, Holland, and Sweden, it seems to have reached a plateau (Chapter 16; Hemminki and Li, 2003; Price and Ware, 2004; Segura et al., 2003). The disease is strongly associated with past use of commercial amphibole asbestos (Chapter 4) and for most industrialized countries, the incidence is in the range of 14–30 cases per million per year for persons >15 years of age (Banaei et al., 2000; Health and Safety Executive, 2001; Peto et al., 1999; Tossavainen and Takahashi, 2000). Australia has the highest incidence of any country due mainly to the mining and use of crocidolite in the past; in 1997, the rate was 50.6 per million per year for males >20 years and 9.0 for females (Leigh et al., 2002). In South Africa, a recent updated study of the birth cohort mortality in and around Prieska Northern Cape Province (where crocidolite was mined from 1893 to the 1960s) the rates for males and females were respectively, 366 and 172 per million person/years (Kielkowski et al., 2000). Nonoccupational environmental exposures have occurred in these countries and elsewhere worldwide (Chapters 3 and 4).

Prognosis and Treatment

As discussed in detail in Chapter 14, treatment is not curative, although there is increasing interest in extrapleural pneumonectomy that, in combination with chemotherapy and radio-therapy, has effectively lengthened survival periods in patients with limited disease. Indeed, a few long-term survivals have been achieved. However, for patients with pleural MM, the median survival is between 4 and 18 months after diagnosis, and it is the rare patient who lives longer than 3 years (Curran et al., 1998; Edwards et al., 2000; Herndon et al., 1998; Ruffie et al., 1989; Steele, 2002). The epithelioid type shows a slightly better median sur-vival (a few months) than the sarcomatoid type. The morphologic variants are not thought to differ except for the desmoplastic form that customarily pursues an aggressive course. Peritoneal MM is usually widespread in the abdomen by the time of diagnosis and survival time is shorter on average than with pleural MM. Median survivals range from 4 to 12 months (Antman et al., 1983b; Moertel, 1972; Sugarbaker et al., 2002). Adverse prognostic factors include an advanced stage of disease, and age at the time of presentation, as well as a "poor" physical status of the patient (Rusch and Venkatraman, 1999).

Etiology

Although a strong link between MM and amphibole asbestos exposure is established, not all cases are etiologically related to asbestos. In the adult male population, 20%–40% of MM are idiopathic, and in women in the United States, the incidence of spontaneous idiopathic MM exceeds 50%.

Asbestos

The link between asbestos exposure and MM was reported in 1960 among residents exposed to crocidolite asbestos in the mining areas of the Northern and North Western Cape Province of South Africa (Wagner et al., 1960). The first medically documented case occurred in 1956 when a Bantu man came to necropsy with a clinical diagnosis of tuberculosis (Wagner, 1991). The pathologist, Dr Christopher Wagner, was amazed to discover an unusual gelatinous tumor that filled the thoracic cavity, and was further surprised by finding asbestos bodies in the lung parenchyma. This prompted him to con-tact Dr CA Sleggs, superintendent at a regional tuberculosis hospital, who noted that in his experience, a proportion of patients with clinically diagnosed tuberculosis did not respond to chemotherapy and died. Interestingly enough, they resided in the Northern Cape Province where the blue asbestos mines were located west of Kimberly. It was promptly established that some of these cases were, in fact, MM. Since then, countless papers in the medical and scientific literature have reported MM in patients exposed to asbestos under a variety of circumstances, including occupational (Acheson et al., 1982; Edwards et al., 1996; Howel et al., 1999; Jones et al., 1996; McDonald and McDonald, 1980), domestic (paraoccupational) (Gibbs et al., 1990; Newhouse and Thompson, 1965), and environmental circumstances (Coplu et al., 1996; Chapter 4). In subjects heavily exposed to amphibole asbestos early in their working life more than 1 in 10 will die from MM, for example, insulators and shipyard workers, but in those exposed to lesser amounts, mortality rates are substantially lower. The proportion of MM linked to expo-sure varies among countries, regions within countries and with gender, and appears to relate mainly to the commercial use of amphibole asbestos. As noted above, in the United

States where women rarely are exposed to amphibole asbestos, the overall incidence is low and the majority of cases are idiopathic. The incidence of asbestos-related MM in the United Kingdom is higher.

There is a marked difference in pathogenicity between the various fibers (Gibbs, 1990; Hodgson and Darnton, 2000; Chapter 4). Mesotheliomas occur rarely among persons exclusively exposed to "chrysotile" and it is currently believed that "pure" chrysotile does not cause the neoplasm (Berman and Crump, 2004). Although a number of cases of MM have been associated with presumptive "chrysotile only" exposure, fiber burden studies of the lungs usually demonstrate commercial and sometimes noncommercial amphibole asbestos fibers (Chapter 12).

In the late 1950s and early 1960s, Wagner visited hospitals in the vicinity of amosite and chrysotile mines in South Africa (Wagner, 1991) but failed to find cases of MM despite the fact that the three major commercial types had been mined commercially in South Africa for at least 30 years. Therefore, even at that time, there appeared to be a marked difference between crocidolite and the other types of commercial asbestos in the apparent causation of MM. This continues to be the pattern in South Africa; recently published papers indicate that there is still a high MM rate among crocidolite miners, a much lower rate in amosite miners; cases have not been identified among chrysotile miners (Kielkowski et al., 2000; Rees et al., 1999a,b). The absence of MM in the chryostile cohort is readily explained by the exceedingly low concentrations of tremolite demonstrable in the finished milled products (Rees et al., 2001). Studies of World War II gas mask assemblers described a high rate of MM in women who worked with crocidolite filters but a virtual absence among those using chrysotile filters (Acheson et al., 1982; Jones et al., 1996). Studies of asbestos cement plant workers have related MM risk to commercial amphibole, not chrysotile, exposure (Gardner et al., 1986; Hughes et al., 1987; Thomas et al., 1982). Several cohort and case-control studies of friction product manufacturing workers and mechanics who handled products containing chrysotile have consistently failed to show an elevated risk for developing MM (Goodman et al., 2004; Newhouse and Sullivan, 1989; Paustenbach et al., 2004), as discussed in detail in Chapter 4.

The noncommercial forms of amphibole are an important cause of MM because they are a contaminant of chrysotile asbestos in many (but not all) deposits in the Province of Québec (McDonald et al., 1997), vermiculite ores in Libby, Montana (McDonald et al., 2002), and occur as natural deposits in a number of countries (Coplu et al., 1996; Luce et al., 2000; Sakellariou et al., 1996; Chapter 4). The Québec mining experience initially led to the notion that exposure to chrysotile could cause MM, although infrequently, but it was not until much later that the significance of a relatively small amount of tremolite in the ore was appreciated (McDonald et al., 1980; Pooley, 1976). However, chrysotile significantly "contaminated" with tremolite appears to be uncommon in manufactured products in the developed countries and is responsible for very few MM.

There is now a consensus that exposure to commercial amphibole asbestos, crocidolite and amosite, is highly hazardous, whereas chrysotile rarely, if ever, causes MM (Berman and Crump, 2004; Gibbs, 1990; Hodgson and Darnton, 2000; Mossman et al., 1990). In a recent meta-analysis of asbestos-exposed cohorts, Hodgson and Darnton (2000) calculated the theoretical ratio of MM potency: chrysotile 1; amosite 100; crocidolite 500. (It should be realized that these investigators did not allow for tremolite "contamination" of chrysotile and that the ratio applies to chrysotile containing tremolite in the Québec mining cohort and not to mineralogically "pure" chrysotile; McDonald and McDonald, 1997.) Another analysis commissioned by the United States Environmental Protection Agency (EPA) calculated a 1000-fold difference in MM carcinogenicity between commercial amphibole and chrysotile asbestos (Berman and Crump, 2004). Clearly, exposures to crocidolite and amosite are etiologically responsible for the majority of MM occurring in developed countries.

Latency (usually considered to be the time period measured from first exposure to diagnosis or death), is long for asbestos-induced MM. A review by Lanphear and Buncher (1992) of 1690 cases of MM reported a median latency of 32 years; in 99%, it was longer than 15 years, and in 96%, it was more than 20 years. Another case series published in 1997 gave a range of 15–67 with a mean of 41 years (Yates et al., 1997). Reports of MM resulting from exposure to asbestos commencing at birth documented a minimal latency of more than 20 years, with an average of about 50 years (Coplu et al., 1996; Sakellariou et al., 1996). The risk of MM developing after asbestos exposure has been estimated to increase exponentially in proportion to the third or fourth power of time. Therefore, as the intensity of exposure decreases, one expects the duration of latency to increase (Peto et al., 1982). However, even with very heavy exposures to commercial amphibole asbestos such as those in insulators and asbestos product workers in the past, the average latency remains at more than 30 years and a number of cases arising in the 1990s and 2000s can be linked to World War II exposures.

MM of the peritoneum generally results from relatively heavy exposures to commercial amphibole asbestos and there is a much higher prevalence of pleural plaques (PP) and asbestosis than with pleural MM (Browne and Smither, 1983). However, a lower proportion of peritoneal cases are linked to asbestos (Brenner et al., 1981; Spirtas et al., 1994) in both men and women; one of us (JEC) has assembled a series comprised of young men with peritoneal MM who have no history of asbestos exposure.

Although the data is limited, the link between pericardial and gonadal MM and asbestos exposures appears to be less strong than with the pleural and peritoneal types.

Other Mineral Fibers

Erionite

Erionite is not an asbestos mineral but a fibrous zeolite. It shows a striking physical resemblance to crocidolite, but has different chemical and crystallographic properties. It is a durable fiber that persists in lung tissues for many years. Exposure is associated with the development of MM in residents of the Cappadocian region of Southern Turkey who are exposed lifelong in dwellings carved out of the igneous tuff of the region (Selcuk et al., 1992). Both experimental and human studies suggest that erionite has a greater MM-producing capacity than crocidolite. This work supports the notion that the surface properties of the fiber are important since the two types of fiber have similar physical dimensions, but erionite fibers possess a greater surface area (Coffin et al., 1989). The latency of erionite-induced MM appears to be similar to that for amphibole asbestos.

Organic Fibers

Organic fiber exposure has been postulated to be a cause of MM. Tumor has been reported to occur in sugar cane workers who presumably inhaled crystalline silica fibers of plant origin (Newman, 1986). However, there has not been any recent confirmatory information published on this topic.

Man-Made Mineral Fibers

The majority of man-made mineral fibers appear to have short biopersistence and an increased risk of MM has not been noted in persons exposed to these fibers. Occasional cases described among workers in this industry have been found to be associated with exposure to asbestos. One of the authors (AG) observed a MM in a glass fiber worker but elevated levels of commercial amphibole asbestos were identified in the lungs, indicating the need to exclude confounding factors (Gold, 1967; McDonald and McDonald, 1980). Refractory ceramic fibers are the exception since these particles have a much greater biopersistence; inhalation studies in rats have yielded a high rate of MM (McConnell et al., 1995; Miller et al., 1991). As noted in Chapter 6, exposure to ceramic fibers has been associated with the development of PP, but a conclusive link has not been established between MM and exposure (Brown et al., 2005; Lockey et al., 1996; Rodelsperger, 1995). Refractory ceramic fibers have been identified in the lung tissues of a small number of cases of MM but in association with commercial amphibole asbestos (Roggli et al., 2004).

Therapeutic Irradiation

MM of the pleura and peritoneum has been reported in humans after therapeutic irradiation and thorium dioxide (thorotrast) administration. The latency period ranges from 7 to 50 years with a mean of 21 years (Anderson et al., 1985; Babcock et al., 1976; Cavazza et al., 1996; Gilks et al., 1988; Maurer and Egloff, 1975; Shannon et al., 1995; Stey et al., 1995; Stock et al., 1979). MM associated with irradiation is usually described in persons undergoing treatment for Wilms' tumor (Anderson et al., 1985; Austin et al., 1986), Hodgkin's disease and other malignant lymphomas (Lerman et al., 1991; List et al., 1985; Valagussa et al., 1986) metastatic testicular seminoma and teratomas, and breast carcinoma (Antman et al., 1983a; Bokemeyer and Schmoll, 1993; Neugut et al., 1997; Shannon et al., 1995; Stock et al., 1979). The risk is extremely low since a review of 2.5×10^5 women with breast carcinoma and 1.4×10^4 patients with Hodgkins' lymphoma (in whom 24.8% and 50.6%, respectively, received radiation treatment) revealed no increase incidence of MM compared to controls (Neugut et al., 1997). One of us (AG) has consulted on a case of pleural MM that developed several decades after aggressive radiation treatment to the mediastinum for metastatic lymph node involvement by a testicular teratoma. There was no history of asbestos exposure and mineral fiber analysis of the lung showed background levels of asbestos. A fiber burden analysis has been reported in only one additional case; again, the asbestos concentration did not exceed background (Austin et al., 1986). One of us (JEC) has documented MM in three older women with breast cancer whose malignant pleural disease was localized to the radiation field, and we (JEC) have recently seen two cases of pelvic MM developing in women treated in the past for cervical squamous carcinoma with intravaginal radioactive cesium. Animal studies also demonstrate the development of MM after irradiation (Sanders and Jackson, 1972).

Viruses

A viral etiology was suggested several decades ago when MM was described in chicken associated with avian leukosis virus infection (Chabot et al., 1970; Peterson et al., 1984). An interest in the possible viral etiology was rekindled again in the 1990s when Simian virus 40-like molecular sequences were described in MM tissue by workers in several different laboratories. Subsequently, a number of additional reports confirmed this finding (Jasani et al., 2001), but some investigators could not repeat the results (Manfredi et al., 2005). Recently, it was suggested that the observation was an artifact due to plasmid contamination by the assay reagents (Lopez-Rios et al., 2004).

The occurrence of Simian virus 40 infections within the human population appears to be mainly linked with contamination of poliovirus vaccines used between 1955 and 1963

(Sweet and Hilleman, 1960). As an oncogenic virus, it produces MM when introduced into the pleural cavity of hamsters. The biological plausibility for Simian virus 40 being either a cause or a cofactor with asbestos, in inducing MM, is indicated by several additional types of laboratory experiments. SV40 is capable of transforming human cells in vitro. It also appears to act synergistically with asbestos in inducing malignant transformation of human mesothelial cells (Bocchetta et al., 2000; Cicala et al., 2004). By inhibiting apoptosis, the infection could provide cells with sufficient time in the replicative cycle to accumulate genetic alterations. Its activity appears to be related both to the viral large T antigen (T-ag) and small T antigen (t-Ag) that inactivate the supressor genes, p53 and pRb, enhancing activity of telomerase, ERKs, and AP-1 (Mossman and Gruenert, 2002). Recently, the virus was also shown to stimulate the release of vascular endothelial growth factor from human mesothelial cells, a factor critical in angiogenesis in some experimental systems (Cacciotti et al., 2002).

Epidemiological support for the viral hypothesis is lacking since data from a small number of studies are inconclusive (Dang-Tan et al., 2004). However, the results of the epidemiological investigations are problematic since there are, as of yet, no good screening methods for determining active or past exposure. And, it is not known which individuals received the virus-contaminated vaccines and the Simian virus 40 exposure dosage. Therefore, one cannot readily compare nonexposed controls with exposed. A new generation of molecular epidemiological studies will be necessary to pursue this avenue of research.

Chronic Inflammation

Occasional cases of MM have been described associated with prolonged chronic inflammation of serosal membranes. Examples include chronic empyema, chronic peritonitis (Hillerdal and Berg, 1985; Riddell et al., 1981), and the intrapleural implantation of leucite spheres for treatment of pulmonary tuberculosis (Roviaro et al., 1982). The tumor develops spontaneously in an occasional patient with Familial Mediterranean fever, a heritable disease characterized by chronic and recurrent episodes of serosal inflammation (Livneh et al., 1999).

Genetic Factors

Familial clusters of MM have been described, although they are comparatively rare; they suggest a strong genetic influence at least in some cases (Bianchi et al., 1993; Dawson et al., 1992; Musti et al., 2002; Roushdy-Hammady et al., 2001). The majority, but not all, have been linked with exposure of multiple family members to asbestos or erionite, the Turkish fibrous zeolite. In addition, multigenerational studies have shown an increased incidence of cancer in first-degree relatives (Heineman et al., 1996; Roushdy-Hammady et al., 2001).

Limited molecular studies suggest various factors may play a role in individual susceptibility. For example genetic polymorphisms in the coding genes for phase II proteins, such as GST and NAT, which deactivate carcinogens, might be important in individual susceptibility (Hirvonen et al., 1995; Puntoni et al., 2003). A study of chromosomal damage in the peripheral blood lymphocytes using the cytokinesis-block micronucleus assay showed an increased frequency of micronuclei in MM patients as compared to healthy controls, patients with lung cancer, and those with benign respiratory disease. These observations suggest that genetic factors may predispose one to MM development (Bolognesi et al., 2002).

Experimental studies in mice support the notion that genetic factors contribute to the development of MM. Intragastric administration of 3-methylcholanthrene induces peritoneal MM in variable numbers of inbred mice of different strains (Rice et al., 1989). And, our studies (Craighead et al., 1993) of mice inoculated intraperitoneally with crocidolite again show difference in the susceptibility of different murine strains. The durations of latency also differed among the mouse strains studied.

Others

Exposures to nickel, beryllium, and fiberglass have been postulated to be a cause of MM but these claims remain to be confirmed. Epidemiological surveys of fiberglass workers have provided no evidence to suggest that occupational exposure causes MM.

Idiopathic

It has been estimated that about 20%–40% of MM occurring in the United States today are idiopathic and appear to develop spontaneously despite an intensive search for the cause. In the United Kingdom a higher proportion of cases are amphibole asbestos-associated. Pathologists recognized spontaneously developing MM long before the commercial exploitation of asbestos; the first idiopathic lesion was diagnosed in the mid-1800s (Craighead, 1987; Wagner 1870). There is evidence for a background rate of MM and this has been estimated at about 1–8 cases per million per year (Price and Ware, 2004; see Chapter 16). Support for this conclusion comes from several sources: (1) the constancy of risk over time for MM in females in the United States (Price and Ware, 2004); (2) cases of MM in which there is no history of exposure to asbestos, and lung asbestos fiber burdens are not elevated (Gibbs et al., 1989; Roggli et al., 2002); (3) the spontaneous occurrence of MM in children and adolescents (Fraire et al., 1988).

Ascertainment of cases is high in the United States because of the availability and widespread use of diagnostic reagents by pathologists, and the intense pursuit of "new" cases for litigation (Chapter 15).

Pathological Features

Gross Features

MM arising in the peritoneal cavity more often presents as massive ascites and less often as tumor masses palpable on external examination. At surgery and autopsy, tumor nodules are usually scattered diffusely over the serosal surfaces and mesenteries. To a variable extent, the tumor encompasses the small and large intestines and invests the liver and spleen. The omentum is usually involved forming a solid "cake-like" mass. On occasion, MM presents as an umbilical mass or as a mass in the spermatic cord simulating a hernia or a primary neoplastic lesion arising at that site. Customarily, the tumor does not invade the peritoneal organs but the masses often result in bowel obstruction.

Occasional cases of peritoneal MM present as inflammatory lesions without being evident gross tumor. These lesions are often manifest clinically as acute appendicitis, acute cholecystitis, or as an incarcerated umbilical hernia (Kerrigan et al., 2003). Even more rare is the formation of intestinal intraluminal polyps resulting from intramucosal spread of peritoneal MM (Mayall and Gibbs, 1991).

Pleural MM usually presents clinically as an effusion that inexorably reoccurs despite repeated thorocentesis. On internal examination tumor nodules are scattered over the parietal and visceral pleural surfaces and in the major fissures (Figure 8.1, see the color insert). As the lesion progresses, the lung is encompassed and invaded by neoplastic tissue that often extends into the chest wall leading to unremitting pain, and into the pericardial cavity, occasionally resulting in constrictive heart failure. Intrapulmonary lesions can be massive and simulate a primary LC, grossly and radiologically (Figure 8.2, see the color insert).

As noted above, primary tumors arising in the tunica vaginalis often simulate inguinal hernias. They can either spread into the peritoneal cavity, or involve the testis and subcutaneous tissues of the penis with associated lymphadenitis.

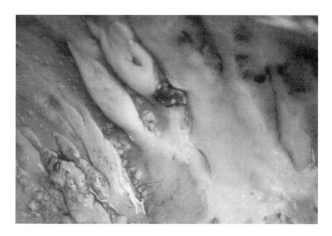

Figure 8.1 Parietal pleura of asbestos worker showing deposits of mesothelioma (tan), plaques (ivory), and chest wall adipose (yellow).

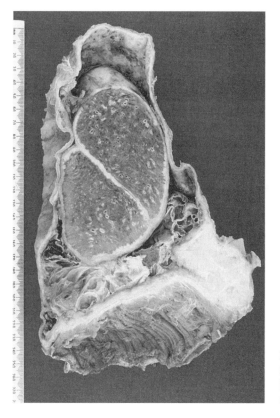

Figure 8.2 Diffuse MM encompassing the lung and extension along the interlobar fissure. Note the involvement of the diaphragm.

Often, tumors of the pleura grow through the diaphragm and spread into the peritoneum where the distribution of lesions simulates a primary peritoneal MM. Similarly, peritoneal MM, on occasion, spread into the chest cavity. In rare cases, one is uncertain where the tumor actually originated. Metastatic spread usually occurs late in the disease. The opposite lung is the most common site for a pleural MM. Accumulations of tumor in the posterior "gutters" of the chest cavity and retroperitoneal space can lead to vertebral involvement and occasional neurological complaints as the tumor invades the spinal canal and the cord. Distant metastasis to such organs as the brain occur, but rarely. It has been estimated that about one percent of pleural MM find their way to the central nervous system.

Rarely, MM presents as a localized lesion with a pedunculated or sessile pleural attachment (Allen et al., 2005; Crotty et al., 1994). About half of the cases survive for longer than 2 years from the time of diagnosis, suggesting a more protracted clinical course than with diffuse disease. These localized lesions must be differentiated from the fibrous tumor of the pleura, described below.

The typical macroscopic growth pattern of MM can also be simulated by other tumors. The term "pseudomesotheliomatous tumor" is applied to these lesions (Harwood et al., 1976). The most common nonmesotheliomatous cancer to display this growth pattern is adenocarcinoma developing at the periphery of the lung (Koss et al., 1998), but a wide variety of neoplasms result in this gross appearance on occasion including primary pleural sarcomas, malignant lymphomas, thymic epithelial tumors, and metastatic carcinomas (Attanoos et al., 2002b; Attanoos and Gibbs, 2003; Lin et al., 1996; Mayall and Gibbs, 1992; Moran et al., 1992). In a recent study, almost 90% of the pleural tumors mimicking MM were primary lung carcinomas, of which 70% were adenocarcinomas. The remaining cancers of the pleura arose outside the chest cavity (Attanoos and Gibbs, 2003).

Synchronous carcinomas have been found in 1.8% of 500 MM examined at autopsy (Attanoos et al., 2003b ; Mayall and Gibbs, 1992). This can result in misdiagnosis usually because of misinterpretation of conflicting immunohistochemical results. Recently, one of us (JEC) discovered a bronchogenic keratinizing squamous carcinoma arising among massive accumulations of metastatic MM in the lung parenchyma of a long-term survivor.

Light Microscopy

The World Health Organization (WHO) classifies MM into (1) epithelioid; (2) sarcomatoid, which includes desmoplastic as a subtype; and (3) biphasic. However, within these general types are found a number of distinctive histologic patterns, which at present have no clinical significance but are important considerations for the diagnostic histopathologist. MM occasionally are composed of cells that are difficult to classify as either epithelioid or sarcomatoid for they resemble transitional carcinoma.

Epithelioid MM are comprised of cells that typically are low columnar or cuboidal in shape with a relatively clear nucleoplasm often displaying a prominent nucleolus. They frequently form tubulopapillary (Figure 8.3, see the color insert) and adenomatoid (Figure 8.4, see the color insert) structures surrounded by variable amounts of connective tissue. The tumors often form solid sheets of polygonal cells, either mimicking large cell undifferentiated lung carcinomas, or pleomorphic carcinomas in which are found large bizarre tumor giant cells (Figure 8.5, see the color insert). Other phenotypes include (1) deciduoid (Figure 8.6, see the color insert), (2) small dark round cell, (3) clear cell (Figure 8.7, see the color insert), (4) lipid rich, and (5) hepatoid (Figure 8.8, see the color insert);

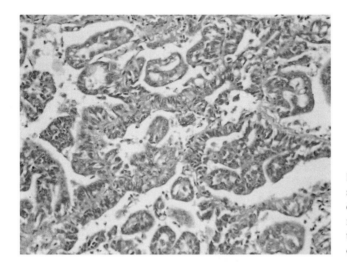

Figure 8.3 Epithelioid MM showing tubulopapillary differentiation. Note the minimal pleomorphism of tumor cells and the absence of mitotic figures.

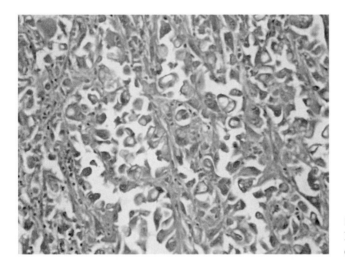

Figure 8.4 Epithelioid MM showing adenomatoid differentiation.

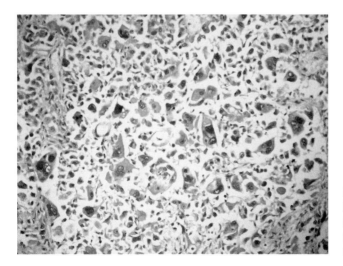

Figure 8.5 Epithelioid MM showing marked pleomorphism with tumor giant cells. Note the lack of stroma.

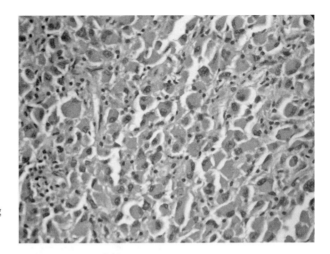

Figure 8.6 Epithelioid MM comprised of cells resembling the decidua in the pregnant uterus.

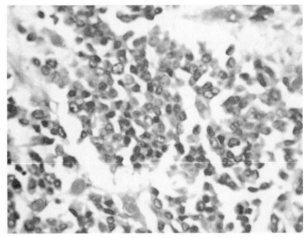

Figure 8.7 Epithelioid MM exhibiting small tumor cells with relatively high nuclear:cytoplastmic ratios.

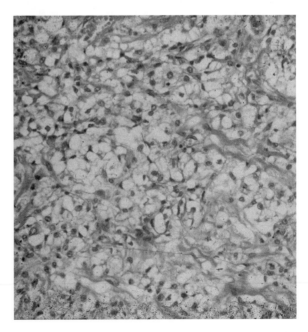

Figure 8.8 Epithelioid MM displaying a prominent clear cell pattern.

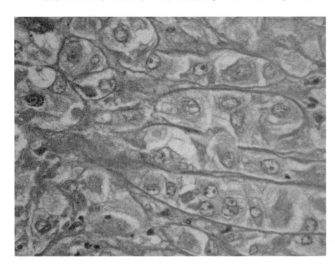

Figure 8.9 Epithelioid MM showing trabecular arrangement simulating hepatoma.

some of these forms are not infrequently seen as a minor component, but rarely do they predominate (Figure 8.9, see the color insert). The amount of stroma varies in quality and quantity; it may be sparse or copious, myxoid or fibrous. This feature affects the gross consistency of the lesion. Occasionally, an epithelioid MM can be desmoplastic with more than 50% of the tumor being composed of bland appearing fibrous tissue. Frequently, a tumor represents a montage of histological types, with differing features at various topographical locations.

Sarcomatoid MM exhibit a variety of patterns often intermixed with one another; the most frequently occurring lesion displays sheets and bundles of spindle cells resembling fibrosarcoma intermixed with tumor giant cells, at times resembling a malignant fibrous histiocytoma (Figure 8.10, see the color insert). On occasion, the cytoplasm of the spindle cells may be highly eosinophilic, resembling smooth muscle cells and sometimes rhabdomyoblastic-like. A small proportion of MM show cartilaginous, osteoid, and bone formation (Figure 8.11, see the color insert). Overall, the connective tissue in sarcomatoid MM often exhibits a hyaline cast and is whorled and complex. The desmoplastic variant of MM provides one of the most challenging diagnostic problems in pathology with regard to distinguishing the neoplasm from fibrous pleuritis (Figures 8.12 and 8.13, see the color insert). To comply with the WHO definition, 50% or more of the tumor should be desmoplastic and characterized by dense, bland appearing fibrous tissue. Mangano et al. (1998) proposed the following criteria for diagnosis: the presence of (1) frank sarcomatoid foci; (2) bland necrosis; (3) invasion of adipose, skeletal muscle, or lung; and (4) metastasis. These criteria appear robust. The lymphohistiocytoid variant is rare, exhibiting a pattern that resembles malignant lymphoma (Figure 8.14, see the color insert). It is composed of histiocytoid-like mesothelial cells set in a "sea" of lymphocytes and plasma cells.

Biphasic MMs are composed of a combination of any of the epithelioid and any of the sarcomatoid patterns, but to comply with the WHO definition, each component should comprise at least 10% of the tumor (Figure 8.15, see the color insert). Sometimes it is difficult to decide whether or not there is a true sarcomatoid component or prominent stromal reaction in an epithelioid MM. Interobserver reproducibility in this situation is poor, but differences in assessments are of little clinical importance unless correct diagnosis is jeopardized. Therefore, one should not place inordinate reliance on published figures indicating the proportions of the various histological types of MM. And, as noted above, topographical differences in histological features commonly occur in the tumor of individual cases.

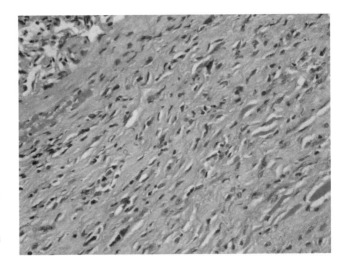

Figure 8.10 Sarcomatoid MM. The illustration demonstrates atypical spindle cells, dispersed in dense connective tissue.

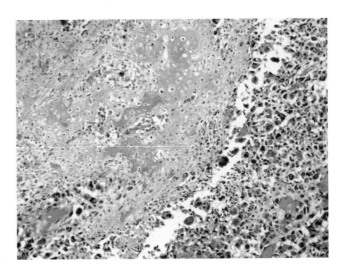

Figure 8.11 Sarcomatoid MM showing malignant spindle cells stroma with calcification and ossification.

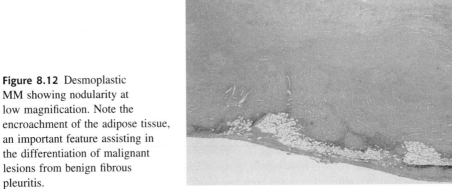

Figure 8.12 Desmoplastic MM showing nodularity at low magnification. Note the encroachment of the adipose tissue, an important feature assisting in the differentiation of malignant lesions from benign fibrous pleuritis.

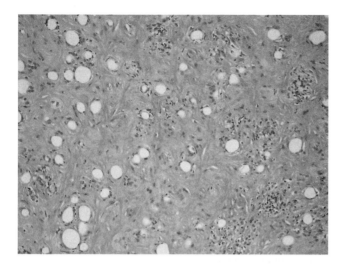

Figure 8.13 Desmoplastic MM showing extensive infiltration of adipose by relatively bland connective tissue.

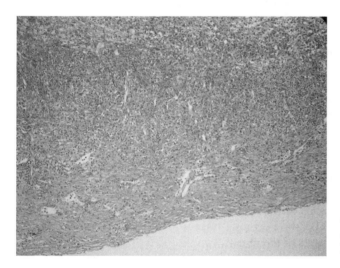

Figure 8.14 Lymphohistio-cytoid MM. Note cellularity superficially suggesting a lymphoma.

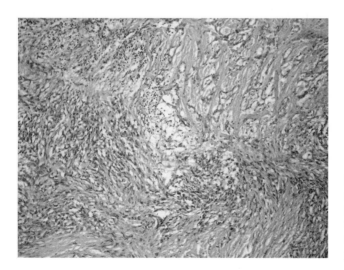

Figure 8.15 Biphasic MM revealing malignant spindle cells and foci of tubular epithelioid tumor cells arranged in cords and pseudoglands.

On light microscopy, the typical patterns of spread within the lung are direct subpleural and lymphangitic but occasionally one sees an intraalveolar growth pattern which in sarcomatoid MM mimics epithelioid haemangioendothelioma and in epithelioid MM suggests desquamative interstital pneumonia. A lepidic growth pattern may be seen, which mimics bronchioloalveolar carcinoma (Nind et al., 2003).

Sussman and Rosai (1990) reported six cases of metastatic MM initially presenting as isolated cervical, mediastinal, and inguinal lymphadenopathy. They emphasized the importance of immunohistochemistry and electron microscopy as adjuvants to diagnosis as discussed in detail below.

Histo- and Immunohistochemistry

Formerly, histochemical stains utilizing the periodic acid Schiff (PAS) reaction to demonstrate neutral mucin after diastase (to eliminate glycogen from the tissue) and alcian blue staining at low pH to demonstrate hyaluronic acid were the main adjuncts to the diagnosis of the epithelioid MM. In these procedures, diastase or amylase digestion was carried out to establish the specificity of the PAS reaction for acid mucopolysaccharides.

MM produce extracellular hyaluronic acid, an acid mucin, that is stained by alcian blue at pH 2.5; if the tissue is pretreated with hyaluronidase, the staining is reduced, and the material is an acid micropolysaccharide, probably hyaluronic acid. However, there are several drawbacks to this procedure: (1) the loss of the acid mucin during routine processing of tissue in aqueous fixatives, (2) the poor enzymatic specificity of the hyaluronidase, and (3) interpretive difficulties attributable to mucopolysaccharides in the stromal connective tissue.

The demonstration of neutral mucin in the form of vacuoles (not granular) within tumor cells or glandular lumina by PAS after diastase pretreatment is strongly suggestive of adenocarcinoma as opposed to MM. However, a negative result is unhelpful since about 50% of pulmonary adneocarcinomas fail to produce neutral mucin, and on rare occasions, epithelioid MM stain positively by PAS after diastase digestion. And, hyaluronidase resistant alcian blue positivity is sometimes demonstrable due to the presence of crystalline hyaluronic acid or peptidoglycans in tissues (Cook et al., 2000; Hammar et al., 1996). In these cases, diagnosis rests on the typical gross, light microscopic, and ultrastructural features of the tumor.

Immunohistochemistry has become the main adjunct to light microscopy for the diagnosis of MM. The immunohistochemical panel should be tailored to the diagnostic problem at hand. When the differential is between epithelioid MM and adenocarcinoma, the most common issue in practice, a combination of two or more mesothelial with two or more epithelial markers is most useful, the choice to a large extent depending on the experience of the pathologist (Table 8.1). The most useful mesothelial markers are cytokeratins, calretinin (nuclear staining) (Figure 8.16, see the color insert), thrombomodulin and epithelial membrane antigen (EMA) (membranous type staining). Wilms' tumor susceptibility gene-1 is less specific and sensitive for mesothelial cells. Some investigators recommend the use of N-cadherin (Peralta-Soler et al., 1995). D2–40, a recently described monoclonal antibody is a marker of the lymphatic endothelium, but it appears promising as a mesothelial marker (Chu et al., 2005). *HBME-1* and mesothelin (Figure 8.17, see the color insert) are relatively nonspecific markers. There is some variation in the sensitivity of the various mesothelial markers with histological pattern—calretinin reactivity is prominent in tubulopapillary, adenomatoid (solid and pleomorphic areas) MM—whereas thrombomodulin exhibits the highest sensitivity in small cell areas (Attanoos et al., 2001).

The most useful epithelial markers in our experience are the carcinoembryonic antigen (CEA) monoclonal antibody, CD15, Ber EP4, MOC 31 and thyroid transcription

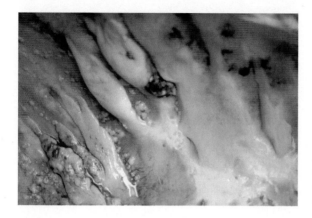

Figure 8.1 Parietal pleura of asbestos worker showing deposits of mesothelioma (tan), plaques (ivory), and chest wall adipose (yellow).

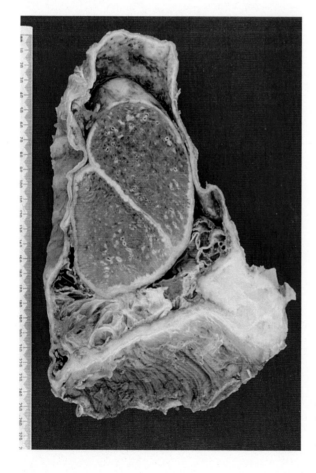

Figure 8.2 Diffuse MM encompassing the lung and extension along the interlobar fissure. Note the involvement of the diaphragm.

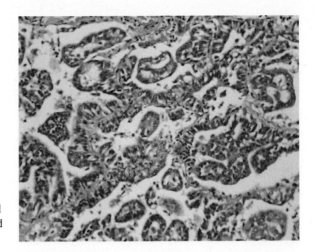

Figure 8.3 Epithelioid MM showing tubulopapillary differentiation. Note the minimal pleomorphism of tumor cells and the absence of mitotic figures.

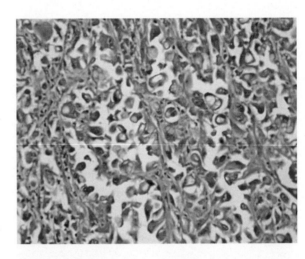

Figure 8.4 Epithelioid MM showing adenomatoid differentiation.

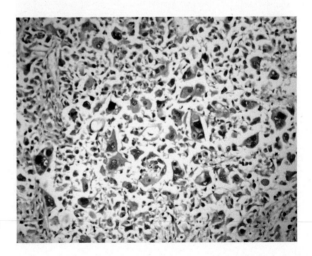

Figure 8.5 Epithelioid MM showing marked pleomorphism with tumor giant cells. Note the lack of stroma.

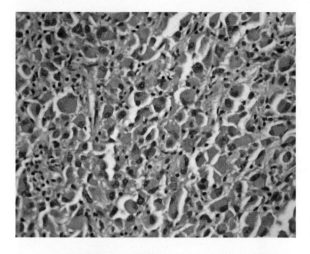

Figure 8.6 Epithelioid MM comprised of cells resembling the decidua in the pregnant uterus.

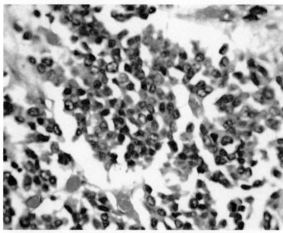

Figure 8.7 Epithelioid MM exhibiting small tumor cells with relatively high nuclear:cytoplasmic ratios.

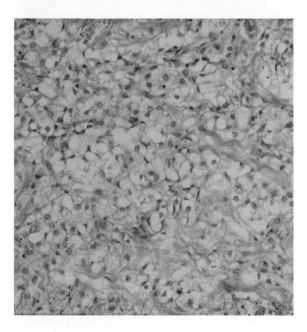

Figure 8.8 Epithelioid MM displaying a prominent clear cell pattern.

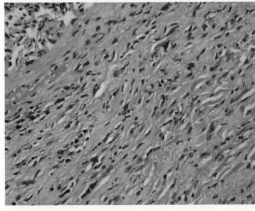

Figure 8.9 Epithelioid MM showing trabecular arrangement simulating hepatoma.

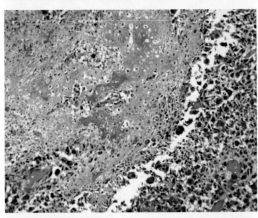

Figure 8.10 Sarcomatoid MM. The illustration demonstrates atypical spindle cells, dispersed in dense connective tissue.

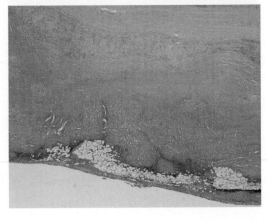

Figure 8.11 Sarcomatoid MM showing malignant spindle cells stroma with calcification and ossification.

Figure 8.12 Desmoplastic MM showing nodularity at low magnification. Note the encroachment of the adipose, an important feature assisting in the differentiation of malignant lesions from benign fibrous pleuritis.

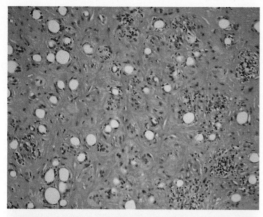

Figure 8.13 Desmoplastic MM showing extensive infiltration of adipose by relatively bland connective tissue.

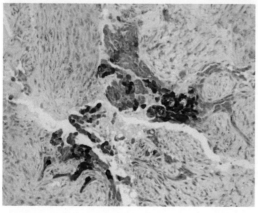

Figure 8.14 Lymphohistiocytoid MM. Note cellularity superficially suggesting a lymphoma.

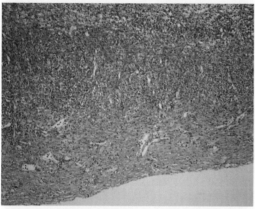

Figure 8.15 Biphasic MM revealing malignant spindle cells and foci of tubular epithelioid tumor cells arranged in cords and pseudoglands.

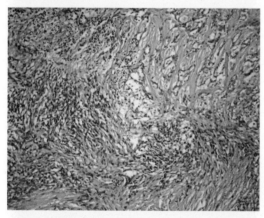

Figure 8.16 Epithelioid MM demonstrating by immunochemistry strong nuclear and cytoplasmic reactivity with calretinin antibody.

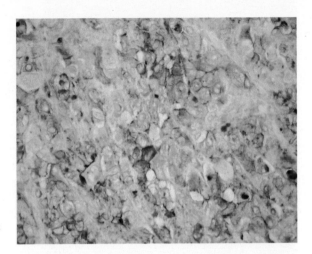

Figure 8.17 Epithelioid MM showing strong cytoplasmic immunopositivity for mesothelin antibody.

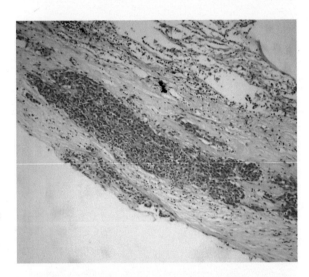

Figure 8.18 A pleural biopsy showing atypical mesothelial cell proliferations but no definite invasion of surrounding reactive connective tissue. Note lung in upper right corner.

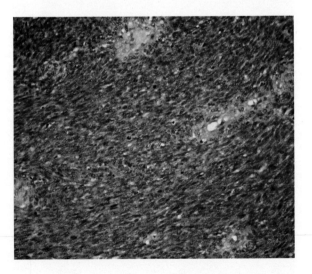

Figure 8.19 Synovial sarcoma showing fascicles of dense "blue" staining spindle cells. It is not possible to differentiate this tumor definitively from a sarcomatous MM.

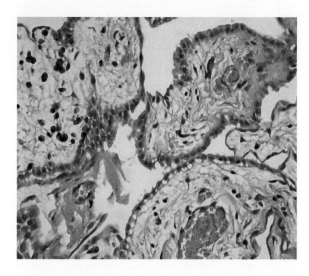

Figure 8.20 A well-differentiated papillary mesothelioma showing well-formed papillae with fibrous cores that are lined by relatively bland mesothelial cells. There is no evidence of stromal invasion.

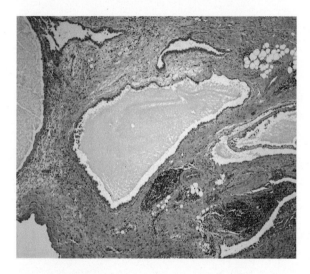

Figure 8.21 A benign multicystic MM from the peritoneal cavity.

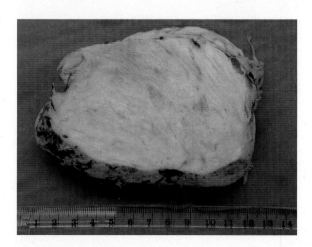

Figure 8.22 A benign solitary fibrous tumor with a gray/cream solid fibrous cut surface that arose in the visceral pleura of the lung.

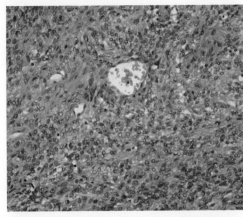

Figure 8.23 A benign solitary fibrous tumor showing relatively bland spindle cells displaying "patternless" features.

Figure 8.24 A solitary fibrous tumor showing hypercellular areas of spindle cells with mitoses indicating a malignant potential.

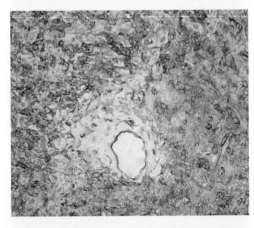

Figure 8.25 A solitary fibrous tumor of the pleura showing immunopositivity for CD34 antibody.

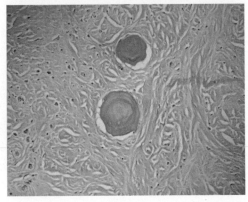

Figure 8.26 A calcifying fibrous pseudotumor showing a hyalinized stroma with lamellar (psammoma) calcified bodies.

Table 8.1 Routine Immunohistochemical Panel for Differentiating Epithelioid MM from Pulmonary Adenocarcinoma

Mesothelial Markers	Epithelial Markers
Cytokeratin 5 and 6	CEA
Calretinin	CD15
Thrombomodulin	Ber EP4
WT-1	MOC31
EMA (membranous)	TTF-1
N-cadherin	E-cadherin
D2-40	B72.3

It is recommended that a laboratory should concentrate on two or three of each group for regular use in diagnosis.

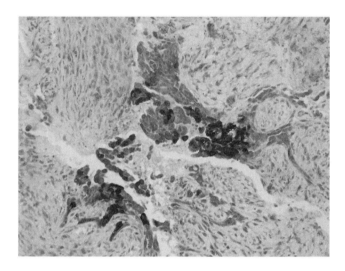

Figure 8.16 Epithelioid MM demonstrating by immunochemistry strong nuclear and cytoplasmic reactivity with calretinin antibody.

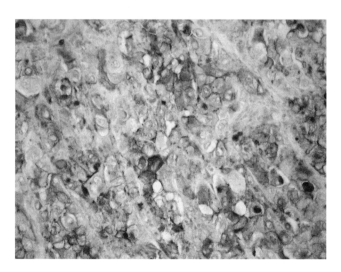

Figure 8.17 Epithelioid MM showing strong cytoplasmic immunopositivity for mesothelin antibody.

Table 8.2 Routine Immunohistochemical Panel for Differentiating Sarcomatoid MM from Primary and Metastatic Sarcomas Located within the Pleura

AE1/AE3, CAM5.2, MNF 116
Calretinin
Cytokeratin 5/6
CD31
CD34

factor 1 (TTF-1). Others have also recommended BG-8, B72.3, and E-cadherin (Leers et al., 1998; Ordonez, 2003; Peralta-Soler et al., 1995). The immunohistochemistry panel will require amendment when the differential diagnosis includes tumors other than pulmonary adenocarcinomas. Cytokeratin 5/6 is frequently positive in squamous cell and genitourinary carcinomas and thus, is not a useful procedure.

When the diagnostic question relates to a spindle cell lesion we use a panel composed of cytokeratin (AE1/AE3 and MNF116), calretinin, CD31, and CD34 antibody (Table 8.2). The latter procedures are useful for the diagnosis of intraserosal malignant vascular tumors.

The use of immunohistochemical markers for differentiating malignant from reactive mesothelial lesions is fraught with difficulty although some investigators find p53 and EMA positivity with a membrane pattern of reactivity a useful predictor of malignancy, and desmin positivity in epithelioid lesions is predictive of benignancy (Attanoos et al., 2003a).

An awareness of artifactual tinctorial reactions is important in avoiding misdiagnosis. In addition, hyaluronic acid rich MM may produce aberrant immunophenotypes including false immunoreactivity with a number of epithelial markers, in particular CEA and CD15 (Robb, 1989). These reactions can usually be abolished by hyaluronidase treatment of tissue sections prior to immunohistochemistry.

Electron Microscopy

Immunohistochemistry has largely replaced ultrastructural examination of suspected MM for diagnostic purposes. Epithelioid MM typically show abundant parallel arrays of intermediate filaments, long, wavy surface microvilli, and prominent accumulations of intracytoplasmic glycogen (Oury et al., 1998; Plate 8.1). However, these features tend to be lost as MM becomes less differentiated (Dardick et al., 1987). In contrast, adenocarcinomas usually display short, straight, blunt, and fuzzy microvilli. Microvilli are observed on the abluminal surface of MM cells that directly contact the underlying connective tissue, whereas this feature is not observed in adenocarcinomas (Dewar et al., 1987). Microvilli are generally retained in formalin-fixed, paraffin-embedded tissue; thus, electron microscopy can be useful in examining epithelial lesions when the immunochemical phenotype is ambiguous. Sarcomatoid MM typically display nondescript ultrastructural features being composed of spindle-shaped cells with elongated nuclei resembling tumor cells of fibrosarcoma. Microvilli are not present. Occasionally, epithelioid differentiation is observed in sarcomatous MM.

Cytopathology

The majority of MM present clinically with effusions either in the chest or abdominal cavities. Aspirates of these fluids can be utilized for cytodiagnosis. Pathologists differ with regard to their enthusiasm for tendering a definitive diagnosis of MM based on cytopathology. Assuming satisfactory technical procedures, the sensitivity ranges from a few percent to more than 90%, but it improves with the expertise and experience of the cytopathologist. False-positive cytological diagnoses of malignancy are uncommon. However, confusion between MM and adenocarcinoma are more frequent, although this error is declining with the use of immunohistochemistry. Whenever possible, pathologists should prepare adequate material for establishing the immunochemical phenotype of a specimen.

The laboratory should receive all the fluid aspirated from a patient. Centrifuged deposits are used for direct smears and the preparation of cell blocks. The latter should be fixed appropriately for light microscopic and ultrastructural examination. Immunohistochemical procedures can be performed on either cell block sections or smears.

Positive diagnoses can usually only be made on the epithelioid or biphasic forms of MM since the sarcomatoid type rarely releases diagnostic cells into the fluid (Plate 8.2A). Evaluation is a two-stage process requiring answers to the following questions: (1) Is it malignant? (2) Is it mesothelial? However, a firm diagnosis should not be made in the absence of good clinical and radiological information. There are a number of features helpful in distinguishing MM from adenocarcinoma and benign reactive mesothelial proliferations. Those that suggest malignancy are (1) nuclear irregularity, (2) hyperchromasia and nuclear enlargement, and (3) clusters of atypical cells. Features that suggest a mesothelial phenotype include (1) aggregates of cells having a "knobby" contour, (2) pseudoacini lined by cuboidal cells, (3) solid connective tissue cores, (4) optically dense cytoplasm (in PAP stains dense green and in MGG basophilia), (5) brush-like borders related to surface microvilli, (6) cell-to-cell apposition and cell engulfment, (7) a peripheral arrangement of small vacuoles, and sometimes, (8) a large solitary vacuole. A stepwise logistic regression analysis of 24 cytological features investigating the separation of MM, adenocarcinoma, and benign mesothelial proliferations revealed five variables that were the most useful in distinguishing MM from adenocarcinoma (Stevens et al., 1992). These are (1) true papillary aggregates, (2) multinucleation with atypicalities, (3) cell-to-cell apposition favoring MM, (4) acinus-like structures, and (5) balloon-like vacuolation characteristic of adenocarcinoma. Four variables were selected to distinguish MM from benign mesothelial proliferations: (1) nuclear pleomorphism, (2) macronucleoli, (3) cell-to-cell engulfment indicating malignancy, and (4) monolayer cell clusters indicating benign prolilferations. Probably the most characteristic feature of MM is numerous aggregates of cells displaying macronucleoli and prominent cell engulfment. Cellular aggregates are not a reliable criterion of malignancy since they can occur in association with benign proliferations (Spriggs and Jerome, 1979).

Fine needle aspiration cytology can be utilized in suspected MM cases presenting without effusions. However, this technique is unlikely to be fruitful in evaluating sarcomatoid MM. In these cases, core needle biopsies can be useful.

Biomarkers

As noted above, hyaluronic acid is commonly found in epithelial MM by histochemistry, although technical considerations detract from the utility of histological approaches to identify the material in cells and tissues. Assays of pleural fluid and blood serum have demonstrated elevated concentrations of glycosaminoglycans including hyaluronic acid in patients with MM although the specificity of the findings is occasionally in doubt (Dahl et al., 1989; Meyer and Chaffee, 1939; Roboz et al., 1985; Waxler et al., 1979). Unfortunately, clinical surveys using modern chemical and immunohistochemical tests have not been reported and this potentially sensitive tool for early diagnosis and monitoring clinical progression of the malignancy has yet to be exploited.

Recently, Pass et al. (2005) reported that the glycoprotein, osteopontin, might prove to be a sensitive indicator for monitoring MM progression. The utility of this serum assay remains to be explored in routine diagnostic studies. Similarly, Robinson et al. (2003) associated increased serum concentrations of a glycoprotein, mesothelin, with MM.

Differential Diagnosis of Malignant Mesothelioma

Reactive versus Malignant Lesions

The diagnostic problems can be divided broadly into two categories: (1) reactive versus MM and (2) MM versus other malignant tumors.

Is an epithelioid mesothelial proliferation reactive or malignant? Cytological features often used in other sites to determine the likelihood of malignancy (such as pleomorphism, prominent nucleoli, and increased mitotic rate) are not always helpful in evaluating benign mesothelial lesions (Galateau-Salle et al., 2005). Reactive lesions can take the form of florid proliferations usually forming sheets of cells and lacking papillae, although occasional papillae and gland-like structures are often seen. Necrosis in the absence of inflammation favors malignancy, although MM display necrosis infrequently or to only a limited extent. Invasion of stroma indicates malignancy, although this feature may be difficult to evaluate in thickened, inflamed serosal membranes where cells are entrapped (Figure 8.18, see the color insert). Reverse "zonation," where the cellular proliferation is greater in the deeper areas of the pleura away from the surface, suggests malignancy. Convincing infiltration of either adipose or chest wall muscle indicates malignancy. Features suggesting benignancy include an overall sparsity of glandular structures, linearity of cells and glandular structures parallel to the serosal surface, and a sudden "cut off" of mesothelial cells at a relatively shallow depth from the surface (Galateau-Salle et al., 2005). Immunohistochemical markers can be helpful in differential diagnosis. Strong membrane staining of cells for EMA and positive nuclear staining for p53 suggest malignancy whereas positive desmin staining suggests a reactive process (Attanoos et al., 2003a).

Another diagnostic problem is the differentiation of reactive fibrosis from a desmoplastic/sarcomatoid MM. Benign spindle cell reactions, usually termed either fibrous or organizing

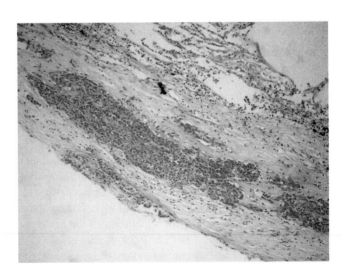

Figure 8.18 A pleural biopsy showing atypical mesothelial cell proliferations but no definite invasion of surrounding reactive connective tissue. Note lung in upper right corner.

pleurisy or pleuritis are an ever-present concern. Reactive proliferations usually show zonation, the process being most cellular in proximity to the surface and less so in the deeper layers. Features which point to malignancy include lack of (1) zonation, (2) nodularity, (3) frankly sarcomatoid areas, (4) foci of bland necrosis, (5) invasion of adipose tissue, skeletal muscle, or lung, and (6) distant metastases (Churg et al., 2000; Mangano et al., 1998). Immunohistochemistry is of limited help. Broad spectrum cytokeratin stains are useful in fibrous lesions because they show the orientation of the spindle cells better than conventional stains and they can highlight infiltration of structures such as adipose. The mere presence of cytokeratin positive cells are not diagnostic of malignancy because they are often present in reactive fibrosis (reflecting mesothelial elements), although in the latter lesions, one observes a mixture of cells only some of which contain cytokeratin.

Epithelioid Malignant Mesothelioma

Distinguishing between an epithelioid MM and a pulmonary adenocarcinoma is the most frequent diagnostic problem confronted by the histopathologist. Immunohistochemical panel (Table 8.1) will establish the diagnosis, except in rare cases, but electron microscopy may be useful on occasion as discussed above. Extrapulmonary carcinomas not infrequently metastasize to the pleura. The diagnostic immunohistochemical panel might then require modification. For example, when the differential diagnosis of a small cell is the problem, additional immunohistochemical markers may be required such as the lymphoid cell markers, CD56 and CD45, thus excluding either small cell carcinoma or malignant lymphoma. Particularly difficult is the identification of either a metastatic renal cell carcinoma or a serous papillary tumor of ovarian origin from a MM since these epithelial tumors exhibit similar immunohistochemical phenotypes. Calretinin, cytokeratin 5/6 and Ber EP4 reactivity appear to be the most useful discriminant markers (Ordonez, 1998; Osborn et al., 2002). CD10, initially believed to be a marker for renal cell carcinoma, has now been found not to be useful (Ordonez, 2004). Primary thymic epithelial tumors occasionally arise in, or spread into, the pleura (Moran et al., 1992). They express cytokeratin 5 and 6 and thrombomodulin within the epithelial cells, and calretinin within the cells of the stroma as well as a lobulated architecture and organoid features. Aberrant expression of CD20 and the presence of immature lymphocytes (CD1a, CD2, CD99, and TdT immunopositive) indicate the correct diagnosis (Attanoos et al., 2002a).

Sarcomatoid Malignant Mesothelioma

There are a number of sarcomas that arise within the serosa and form diffuse masses that mimic sarcomatoid MM. These lesions include synovial sarcoma (SS), malignant vascular tumors, primitive neuroendocrine tumors (PNET)/Ewings sarcoma, desmoplastic round cell tumors, and malignant solitary fibrous tumors (Attanoos et al., 2003; Aubry et al., 2001; Lin et al., 1996; Praet et al., 2002).

Immunopositivity for cytokeratin is useful in separating sarcomatoid MM from fibrosarcoma and leiomyosarcoma although occasionally cells in the latter tumor can display positive reactivity. These neoplasms in the lungs are usually either consequent to direct extension from the chest wall, or reflect hematogenous metastases. Therefore, knowledge of the gross appearances and distribution of the tumor elsewhere in the body is helpful.

Synovial sarcoma is a so-called "blue" celled tumor (Figure 8.19, see the color insert). It displays long, interweaving fascicles, frequently in a hemangiopericytomatous pattern and hyaline fibrosis. These features should alert the pathologist to the possible diagnosis. Immunohistochemical diagnostic differentiation is problematic because the tumor is also

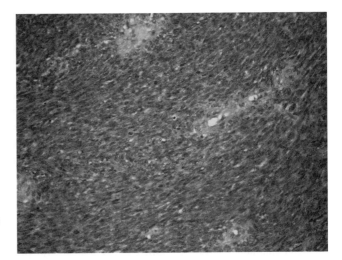

Figure 8.19 Synovial sarcoma showing fascicles of dense "blue" staining spindle cells. It is not possible to differentiate this tumor definitively from a sarcomatous MM.

cytokeratin and calretinin positive (Miettinen et al., 2001). Synovial sarcomas frequently express Bcl-2 in contrast to epithelioid MM which are negative. Molecular identification of the specific SYT/SSX translocation in tumor DNA is occasionally necessary. Malignant vascular tumors can mimic both epithelioid and sarcomatoid MM. They may show cytokeratin immunopositivity. CD31, CD34, and factor 8 reactivity are useful for identifying these tumors (Attanoos et al., 2000; Lin et al., 1996).

Primitive neuroectodermal tumors (PNET) (formerly known as Ewing's sarcoma and Askin tumors when arising in the chest) typically occur as large localized masses involving the pleura and chest wall, usually in children and young adults. Histologically, they display sheets of discohesive small, round, dark tumor cells commonly accompanied by areas of necrosis and rosette-like structures. These lesions can be misdiagnosed as small cell MM. Glycogen may be seen in the cytoplasm utilizing the PAS reaction with and without diastase digestion. Immunohistochemistry characteristically is positive for MIC2 and negative for cytokeratin. However, focal reactivity for cytokeratin, chromogranin, and synaptophysin can be seen. These lesions show a characteristic DNA translocation: t(11; 22)(q24; q12) although this finding is not consistently specific (Thorner et al., 1996).

Desmoplastic round cell tumor is a malignant lesion composed of nests of small, round cells with sparse cytoplasm set in either a dense fibrous or cellular spindle cell stroma. This tumor most frequently occurs in adolescents and young adults in whom it usually presents in the abdomen or pelvis (although rare cases have been reported in the pleura, thorax, and paratesticular region) (Cummings et al., 1997; Parkash et al., 1995). They are typically immunoreactive for cytokeratin and desmin, often with a "dot-like" cytoplasmic pattern and demonstrable Wilms' tumor antigen. These lesions characteristically have the translocation t(11; 22)(p13; q12; Liu et al., 2000).

Malignant solitary fibrous tumors of the pleura (see below) can mimic sarcomatoid MM histologically. Characteristically, they are localized rather than diffuse and are frequently CD34 immunopositive. However, when malignant, they often lose their CD34 immunoreactivity. In contrast to MM, they are cytokeratin negative. Identification of benign appearing areas typical of solitary fibrous tumor can be helpful in diagnosis. Unfortunately, the term benign mesothelioma has been used in the past when referring to these lesions. There is no biological relationship of the solitary fibrous tumor to MM.

Malignant Mesothelioma of other Serosal Sites

Peritoneum

Peritoneal MM is less common than pleural MM and there is no evidence to indicate that exposure to chrysotile, even when contaminated by tremolite, causes peritoneal MM (Doll and Peto, 1986). The age distribution of pleural and peritoneal MM are similar, but there is less male preponderance. The ratio of peritoneal to pleural MM in asbestos-exposed cohorts increases as the exposure to commercial amphiboles increases (Browne and Smither, 1983). A study of more than 1.6×10^6 deaths in men in England and Wales from 1979 to 1990 identified 2.8×10^3 cancers of the pleura and 362 cancers of the peritoneum (ratio 8:1; Coggon et al., 1995; Table 8.3). Striking occupational differences in the proportional mortality rate (PMR) for pleural and peritoneal cancers were found in this comparison. Construction workers, including asbestos laggers, had the highest mortality rate due to peritoneal cancer but only a slight increase in mortality for pleural cancers. Several occupations with increased mortality for pleural cancers showed a deficit of peritoneal cancers, for example, sheet metal workers, upholsterers, carpenters, and electricians, a probable indication of a lesser degree of exposure. In early studies, peritoneal MM were frequently associated with asbestosis. The study of Coggon et al. (1995) showed that PMRs for asbestosis were more closely related to peritoneal than pleural

Table 8.3 PMR for Pleural and Peritoneal Cancers in Men in the United Kingdom According to Job Category*

Occupation	No of Cases Pleura	No of Cases Peritoneal	Ratio Peritoneal/ Pleura
Construction workers	160	990	6.2
Smiths and forgemen	133	561	4.2
Vehicle body builders	649	877	1.4
Construction managers	240	349	1.4
Plasterers	207	265	1.3
Sheet metal workers	186	235	1.3
Machine tool operators	116	136	1.2
Chemical workers	144	146	1.0
Boiler operators	240	171	0.7
Carpenters	167	102	0.6
Builders and handymen	166	98	0.6
Plumbers and gas fitters	450	283	0.6
Production fitters	208	103	0.5
Professional engineers	162	46	0.3
Architects and surveyors	160	58	0.3
Electrical engineers	227	58	0.2
Electricians	349	83	0.2
Metal plate workers	709	78	0.1
Welders	247	33	0.13
Upholsterers	366	0	—
Electrical plant operators	301	0	—
Chemical engineers and scientists	274	0	—
Preparatory fiber processors	139	0	—

* From Coggon et al. (1995).

cancer. The exposure response relations for MM were nonlinear, with the risk of pleural MM rising more steeply at lower levels of exposure, but less steeply at high exposures. With heavy exposures, the risk of peritoneal MM and asbestosis increased much more than the risk for developing pleural MM.

Overall, attributable risk of MM due to asbestos exposure was lower for the peritoneum (58%) than the pleura (88%) in men in the United States (Spirtas et al., 1994). Cases of peritoneal MM in men are documented when there is no recognized amphibole asbestos exposure (Brenner et al., 1981; Craighead, unpublished).

Pericardium

About 150 cases of primary pericardial MM have been described in the literature. These lesions must be distinguished from pleural MM that have spread to the pericardium (which is not uncommon) (Thomason et al., 1994; Vigneswaran and Stefanacci, 2000). Morphologically, they appear similar to their pleural counterpart. Some cases have been associated with asbestos exposure. Pericardial MM has a poor prognosis but rarely are they localized and may be surgically resected with long-term survival. Grossly, the tumors involve the parietal and visceral pericardium diffusely to encase and invade the heart. Therefore, they usually present with pericardial effusions and/or mediastinal masses. Consequently, these tumors can result in arrythmias, congestive heart failure, pericardial constriction, and tamponade.

Gonads

Very rarely MM arise in the tunica vaginalis of the testis and in the testicular and ovarian parenchyma (Attanoos and Gibbs, 2000; Clement et al., 1996; Jones et al., 1995). In a recent study of almost 1.2×10^5 MM cases collected from the MM Registry of the United Kingdom Health and Safety Executive over a 24-year period, primary MM of the tunica vaginalis and ovary comprised 0.09% and 0.03% of all cases, respectively (Attanoos and Gibbs, 2000). The age of these lesions at presentation is similar to pleural and peritoneal MM and they present as mass lesions and associated effusions (hydrocele or ascites). Knowledge of the natural history and etiology of these lesions is limited because of their rarity and poor documentation. Only 50% (or less) appear to be associated with exposure to commercial amphibole asbestos and the clinical course is more favorable than the pleural and peritoneal MM.

Hernial Sacs

Occasionally, florid mesothelial hyperplasia is found in inguinal hernia sacs presumably because of the architectural disorganization and repeated episodes of inflammation. Entrapment of mesothelial cells can occur which is highly suggestive of invasion microscopically. Therefore, circumspection should be exercised before a diagnosis of MM is made in tissues from these sites. On rare occasions, MM arise within hernial sacs (Kerrigan et al., 2003), but a peritoneal lesion that spread into the hernia must be excluded.

Other Mesothelial Lesions

Well-Differentiated Papillary Mesothelioma

It is important to recognize this rare tumor because it does not behave like a conventional MM and is not associated with exposure to asbestos (Figure 8.20, see the color

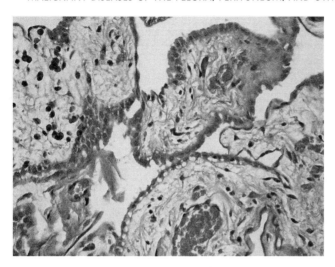

Figure 8.20 A well-differentiated papillary mesothelioma showing well-formed papillae with fibrous cores that are lined by relatively bland mesothelial cells. There is no evidence of stromal invasion.

insert). It is encountered most frequently in the peritoneum of women in the third and fourth decades incidentally during surgical treatment for other conditions (Daya and McCaughey, 1990; Goepel, 1981; Hoekman et al., 1996). Rarely, well-differentiated papillary mesotheliomas have been described in the pleura, pericardium, and tunica vaginalis (Barbera and Rubino, 1957; Butnor et al., 2001; Galateau-Salle et al., 2004; Sane and Roggli, 1995) in men. In most patients, the tumors behave in a benign or indolent fashion and remissions occur commonly. Although long-term survival is well documented, occasional cases with a more aggressive course have been reported and progression to a conventional MM has been described (Foyle et al., 1981; Goepel, 1981) although these lesions could have contained an unrecognized invasive component. Thus, tumors should be adequately sampled before a definitive diagnosis is tendered.

Grossly the nodular lesions of well-differentiated papillary mesotheliomas are gray-white and usually less than 2 cm in maximum dimension. Microscopically, there is little or no invasion of the tissue underlying the implants. The diagnosis is accomplished by light microscopy; the lesions characteristically display a uniform, well-defined, complex papillary structure lined by a single layer of bland cuboidal or columnar mesothelial cells with subnuclear vacuolation. Mitoses are either rare or absent. The tumors can be distinguished from conventional epithelial MM by the lack of (1) a diffuse growth pattern and invasion of adjacent structures and (2) cytological atypia and cellular stratification. The prominent uniform papillary architecture is invariably evident. The lining cells of the papillae exhibit the typical mesothelial cell immunohistochemical phenotypes.

Multicystic Mesothelioma (Cystic Mesothelioma and Peritoneal Inclusion Cysts)

These tumors are comparatively rare and occur most frequently in the peritoneum (Katsube et al., 1982; Ross et al., 1989; Weiss and Tavassolli, 1988) and very rarely in the pleura (Ball et al., 1990; Figure 8.21, see the color insert). Multicystic mesotheliomas are not associated with asbestos exposure. The majority are benign but some reoccur after surgery and rarely has death followed. Frequent coexistent conditions are endometriosis and pelvic inflammatory disease. Grossly, these lesions form single or multiple thin-walled cysts containing gelatinous fluid. Microscopically, the cysts are multilocular and lined by a single layer of cuboidal or flattened mesothelial cells without evidence of invasion. They are distinguished from diffuse MM by their localized nature and lack of histological complexity.

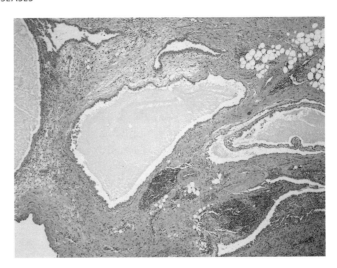

Figure 8.21 A benign multicystic MM from the peritoneal cavity.

Adenomatoid Tumors

These benign lesions are usually discovered incidentally in the genital organs of men (epididymis and spermatic cord) and women (fallopian tube and uterus) (Taxy et al., 1974). Rarely is the tumor found in the omentum, mesentery, and pleura (Craig and Hart, 1979; Kaplan et al., 1996; Young et al., 1991).

The lesions are minute (<5 mm in greatest dimension) and microscopically show glandular spaces and papillae lined by large mesothelial cells and solid sheets with intra-cytoplasmic vacuoles. Immunohistochemistry and electron microscopy establish their mesothelial origin. Cytological atypia is absent. They can be mistaken for MM with adenomatoid features since the tumors appear infiltrative microscopically.

Solitary Fibrous Tumor

Solitary fibrous tumor is now the preferred term for this tumor that has also been called pleural fibroma and localized fibrous mesothelioma in the past (Travis et al., 2004) (Figures 8.22–8.25, see the color insert). It is thought to develop from the submesothe-lial fibrous connective tissue. There is no recognized association with asbestos exposure. The majority behave in a benign fashion but, on rare occasions, metastasize. Under these circumstances, the diagnosis must be questioned. Solitary fibrous tumors are often detected incidentally by the radiologist but sizable lesions may present with shortness of breath, chest pain, general malaise, and other poorly defined general thoracic symptoms. Occasionally, the tumor is associated with hypoglycemia or clubbing of fingers. Solitary fibrous tumors can occur at almost any age, but they are most frequently discovered in individuals of more than 40 years of age. It has no sex predilection.

Grossly, they typically arise from the visceral pleura and are well defined, solid, gray, firm lesions that occasionally show cystic change, calcification, or foci of necrosis. Rarely do they develop in the mediastinum, lung, and other soft tissue sites. These solitary lesions vary in size from about 1 cm to more than 30 cm in maximum dimension. Rarely are they multiple. They may be pedunculated or push into the lung parenchyma and they may arise from an interlobar fissure.

Microscopically, solitary fibrous tumors display a variegated appearance with spindle cell areas of low and relatively high cellularity, arranged haphazardly ("patternless"), in

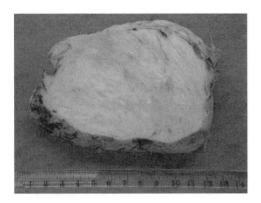

Figure 8.22 A benign solitary fibrous tumor with a gray/cream solid fibrous cut surface that arose in the visceral pleura of the lung.

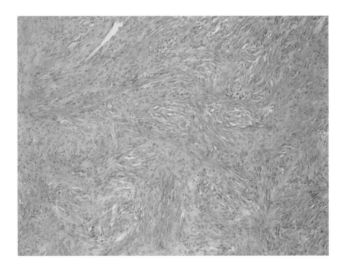

Figure 8.23 A benign solitary fibrous tumor showing relatively bland spindle cells displaying "patternless" features.

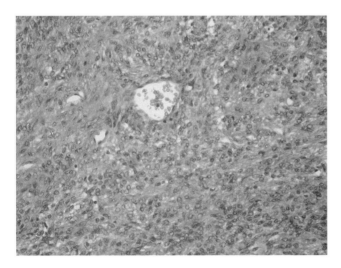

Figure 8.24 A solitary fibrous tumor showing hypercellular areas of spindle cells with mitoses indicating a malignant potential.

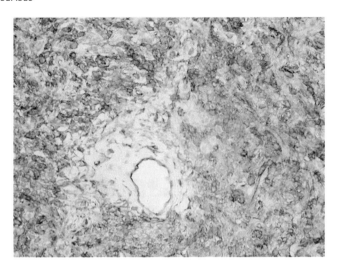

Figure 8.25 A solitary fibrous tumor of the pleura showing immunopositivity for CD34 antibody.

a pericytic fashion around hyalinized blood vessels or in a storiform pattern. Features that suggest a more aggressive behavior include greater cellularity, an infiltrative growth pattern, and high mitotic activity (>4 mitoses per 10 high power fields). These lesions are designated malignant solitary fibrous tumors. However, on occasion, solitary fibrous tumors with relatively bland histolological features behave aggressively with invasion of thoracic structures (Brunnemann et al., 1999;).

Immunostains are positive for CD34 (>90%), CD99 (>90%), Bcl-2 (>80%) and negative for cytokeratin, EMA, desmin, S100, and CD31. The malignant forms usually do not express CD34 and Bcl-2. The differential diagnosis with sarcomatoid MM is discussed above.

Analysis of lung tissue from patients with fibrous tumor of the pleura have not revealed increased concentrations of asbestos attributable to occupational exposure. A few cases of solitary fibrous tumor developing after therapeutic irradiation of the lung have been reported.

Calcifying Fibrous Pseudotumor of the Pleura

This is a rare, relatively acellular, fibrous lesion that simulates a fibrous plaque (of the type associated with asbestos exposure) and arises in the visceral pleura (Pinkard et al., 1996; Figure 8.26, see the color insert). It is characterized by psammoma-like foci of calcification. It tends to occur in young adults and is usually discovered incidentally on chest radiographs. The lesions are often multiple but confined to the pleura without invasion of the lung. It is not associated with asbestos exposure.

Pathogenesis

Tumors exhibiting features similar but not identical to sarcomatoid and epitheloid MM in humans are readily produced in rats by the intrapleural and intraperitoneal introduction of massive amounts of asbestos, various man-made fibers, some talcs, and aluminum fibers (Plate 8.3). Aerosol exposure has failed to consistently cause MM in animals and results are compromised by the background occurrence of MM in certain aging

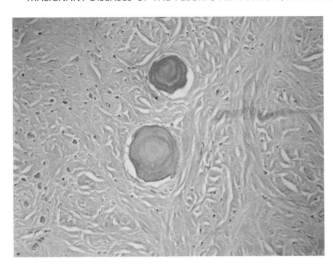

Figure 8.26 A calcifying fibrous pseudotumor showing a hyalinized stroma with lamellar (psammoma) calcified bodies.

rat strains. A vast literature on the subject has accumulated, initially triggered by the pathfinding studies of Stanton and his associates (1977). Ideally, animal studies would provide a useful laboratory tool for the screening of potential or suspect carcinogenic agents. Unfortunately, this goal has not been realized since fibrous materials such as chrysotile and fiberglass that have little or no MM-producing capacity in humans readily induce MM in rodents. The surface area of the foreign material as reflected in its diameter and length is critical rather than a particle's chemical or crystallographic characteristics. Thus, animal models of MM caused by asbestos and other minerals may be comparable to foreign body carcinogenesis, a popular research topic in years past (Bischoff and Bryson, 1964; Brand, 1975).

The research observations of Stanton were prophetic with regard to fiber dimension for he and his associates (1977) hypothesized that fibers in the neighborhood of 8 μm in length and less than 0.25 μm in breadth would be carcinogenic in humans, whereas shorter and blunter fibers had little or no MM-producing capacity. This has proven to be the case in man. Similarly, Davis et al. (1989) showed that though chrysotile was pathogenic in animals, the material failed to produce tumors when the fibers were destroyed by ball milling. Interestingly enough, brake shoe dust is not pathogenic in animals (Chapter 3).

Epidemiological studies in populations of industrial workers have shown a dose-response relationship between cumulative exposure to amphibole asbestos and the rate of MM. Only massive amounts of foreign material are carcinogenic in rats, even when injected as a bolus into a body cavity.

The pathogenicity of asbestos is linked to the physical and chemical properties of the fiber, specifically its (1) dimensions, (2) geometry, (3) chemical composition, (4) surface properties, and (5) durability (biopersistence). These features vary with fiber type but an important difference between chrysotile and the amphiboles is the much shorter duration of biopersistence of the former in the lung; the half-life of chrysotile is measured in terms of days or weeks whereas amphiboles are retained in the lungs for decades, if not a lifetime (Bernstein et al., 2003, 2004, 2005; Churg, 1994; Churg and Vedal, 1994; de Klerk et al., 1996). This feature is a critical determinant of disease.

As noted above, the efficiency of fiber deposition within the lung is largely dependent on diameter and density with fiber length being of lesser importance (Jones, 2004; Lippman, 1990). Mineral fibers with diameters 1 μm or less in diameter show the optimum deposition efficiency. The depth of penetration of the fibers is inversely proportional to the fiber diameter, not its length as discussed in more detail in Chapter 2. Inhaled fibers preferentially accumulate at the junctions of terminal bronchioles and alveolar ducts but after a few months the pattern of distribution changes with translocation and accumulation of fibers subpleurally (Morgan et al., 1977). The mucociliary escalator system clears fibers deposited in the airway. Clearance of fibers that have deposited in the alveoli is accomplished through the lymphatics and by macrophage-mediated phagocytosis. These mechanisms are less efficient when the fibers are relatively long and become negligible when fibers are 16 μm or greater in length. Abundant experimental and epidemiological evidence indicates that short fibers (5 μm or less in length) are unlikely to result in MM, at least in part due to their relatively rapid clearance (Agency for Toxic Substances and Disease Registry, 2003).

Surface properties are determined by the mechanical and thermal evolution of the fibers, by chemical treatment and by the presence of impurities. Differences between fiber types influence their capacity to generate various chemical species of radicals (reactive oxygen and nitrogen species) that potentially result in DNA damage of mesothelial cells (Shukla et al., 2003a). For example, the ionic iron in amphiboles serves as a catalyst facilitating the generation of radicals (Chapter 5).

The importance of asbestos fiber translocation to the pleura is unclear since changes in the mesothelium can result indirectly from responses to fibers deposited in the alveolar regions of the lung in close proximity to the subpleural membrane (Adamson et al., 1993; Coin et al., 1992). However, both amphibole and chrysotile fibers translocate to the pleura. Using thoracoscopic biopsy samples, Boutin et al. (1996) demonstrated "commercial" amphibole fibers within the parietal pleura, the particles concentrating at the confluence of lymphatics where carbon particles also accumulated ("black spots"). At these "black spots" the concentrations of amphiboles were high in asbestos-exposed subjects substantially exceeding the number of chrysotile fibers. Outside the "black spots" the concentration of fibers was low. More than 20% of the fibers were >5 μm in length and all the relatively "long" fibers were amphibole. It has been postulated that fibers also reach the pleura by direct mechanical translocation through the tissue (Oberdorster, 1994), rather than by the route of the lymphatics.

The long latency of MM suggests, but does not prove, that multistep carcinogenesis is involved. Presumably, multiple cumulative genetic alterations are required to convert a normal mesothelial cell to a malignant one. Cytogenetic abnormalities and genomic imbalances have been found in MM but these features may follow, not precede, neoplastic transformation. Many of these alterations are incompatible with cell survival, but the likelihood of a cell becoming malignant presumably is increased if mutations accumulate prior to apoptosis. As discussed in Chapter 5, asbestos can act directly and indirectly on cells through the generation of reactive oxygen and nitrogen species as well as growth factors. The complex cellular events that lead to MM alters the balance between apoptosis and proliferation (Goldberg et al., 1997).

As discussed above, the surface reactivity and oxidant inducing potential of the fiber is linked to the bioavailability of iron at its surface, which could either come from the amphibole fiber or an endogenous accumulation of iron in the lungs. These reactions depend on both the content of iron and the oxidation state of the iron; the ability of various types of asbestos fibers to generate oxidants is as follows: crocidolite > amosite > tremolite > anthophyllite > chrysotile (Gulumian and van Wyck, 1991). Persistence of asbestos fibers in the lung is associated with continual redox cycling of iron and depletion of antioxidant defenses such as ascorbate and GSH (Fubini and Mollo, 1995). It can be modified by surfactants, proteins, or immunoglobulins present in the lung tissue (Kane,

2003). Asbestos-induced DNA damage is dependent on the intracellular concentrations of redox-active iron as well as glutathione depletion (Ault and Eveleigh, 1999). Mitochondrial DNA is more susceptible to oxidative damage than nuclear DNA and the former may be an important target of asbestos (Shukla et al., 2003a). Asbestos also modifies lipids in cell membranes resulting in alterations in their structure and function.

In vitro experiments have shown interference with normal chromosomal segregation by asbestos fibers resulting in aneuploidy and extensive numerical and structural chromosomal abnormalities. DNA damage to mesothelial and pulmonary epithelial cells includes altered DNA bases, single strand breaks, chromosomal damage, and sister chromatid changes. Loss of a copy of chromosome 22 is one of the most frequent changes seen in human MM but alterations to chromosomes 1, 3, 4, 5, 6, 7, 9, 11, 13, 14, 15, 18, 19, and 20 are relatively frequent. More than 10 clonal chromosomal abnormalities have been observed in MM, usually in combination. It is, of course, unknown which, if any, of these structural chromosomal changes occurs after malignant transformation; they could represent chromosomal instability in proliferating tumor cells.

Signaling pathways initiated at the external cell surface or within the cytoplasm regulate transactivation of transcription factors and gene expression that affect proliferation, apoptosis, cell survival, and production of cytokines (Sandhu et al., 2000; Shukla et al., 2003b). These events are described in detail in Chapter 5.

Abnormal expression of several oncogenes and growth factors has been found in in vitro experimental studies. These include PDGF, TGF-α, TGF-β, IGF-1, IL-1α, IL-1β, G-CSF, GM-CSF, MCP-1, LIF, TNFα, IL-6, and IL-8. What role, if any, these factors play in transformation and the subsequent growth of the neoplasm in humans is unknown.

Tumor suppressor gene protein products alter the balance between cell proliferation and apoptosis, favoring the latter. Those that appear to be important in MM include P16INK4, P53, and NF2. There is in vitro and in vivo evidence of homozygous deletion and methylation of P16 in MM; inactivation of P16 (together with P14 ARF (another tumor suppressor gene present at the same 9p21 locus), influence RB and P53 dependent growth regulatory pathways. These events could alter G1 arrest by the mesothelial cell thereby favoring cell division over apoptosis. Mutations of P53 are rarely identified in MM but immunohistochemistry shows frequent accumulation of P53 antigen in tumor cells, an indication of dysfunction. NF2 is located on chromosome 22 and mutations have been identified in about 40% of MM. It encodes a protein (schwannin or merlin) that connects the cytoskeleton to the plasma membrane. NF2 mutation is thought to be involved with progression rather than initiation of MM.

In conclusion, the hypothetical sequence of events in the pathogenesis of MM involves fiber-induced generation of reactive oxygen and nitrogen radicals, directly or indirectly, resulting in DNA damage and the elaboration of multiple growth factors that stimulate receptor tyrosine kinases and downstream signaling cascades. In turn, transcription factors are activated and the gene expression necessary for cell proliferation is induced (Chapter 5). Based on in vitro observations, some investigators have suggested that malignant transformation results from a physical interaction of asbestos fibers with the mitotic spindle but the evidence supporting this concept is limited (Ault et al., 1995).

References

Acheson ED, Gardner MJ, Pippard EC, Grime LP. Mortality of two groups of women who manufactured gas masks from chrysotile and crocidolite asbestos: a 40-year follow-up. *Br J Ind Med.* 1982;39:344–348.

Adamson IY, Balowska J, Bowden DH. Mesothelial proliferation after instillation of long or short asbestos fibers into mouse lung. *Am J Pathol.* 1993;142:1209–1216.

Agency for Toxic Substances and Diseases Registry. Report of the expert panel on health effects of asbestos and synthetic vitreous fibers: the influence of fiber length. 2003; U.S. Department of Health and Human Services.

Allen TC, Cagle PT, Churg AM, et al. Localized malignant mesothelioma. *Am J Surg Pathol.* 2005;29:866–873.

Roggli VL, Sharma A. Analysis of tissue mineral fiber content. In: Roggli VL, Oury TD, Sporn TA, eds. *Pathology of Asbestos-Associated Diseases*, 2nd ed. New York: Springer; 2004; 309–354.

Anderson KA, Hurley WC, Hurley BT, Ohrt DW. Malignant pleural mesothelioma following radiotherapy in a 16-year old boy. *Cancer.* 1985;56:273–276.

Antman KH, Corson JM, Li FP, et al. Malignant mesothelioma following radiation exposure. *J Clin Oncol.* 1983a;1:695–700.

Antman KH, Pomfret EA, Ainser J, MacIntyre J, Osteen RT, Greenberger JS. Peritoneal mesothelioma: natural history and response to chemotherapy. *J Clin Oncol.* 1983b;1:386–391.

Attanoos RL, Gibbs AR. Primary malignant gonadal mesotheliomas and asbestos. *Histopathol.* 2000;37:150–159.

Attanoos RL, Gibbs AR. 'Pseudomesotheliomatous' carcinomas of the pleura: a 10-year analysis of cases from the environmental lung disease research group, Cardiff. *Histopathol.* 2003;43:444–452.

Attanoos RL, Galateau-Salle F, Gibbs AR, Muller S, Ghandour F, Dojcinov SD. Primary thymic epithelial tumors of the pleura mimicking malignant mesothelioma. *Histopathol.* 2002a;4:42–49.

Attanoos RL, Griffin A, Gibbs AR. The use of immunohistochemistry in distinguishing reactive from neoplastic mesothelium. A novel use for desmin and comparative evaluation with epithelial membrane antigen, p53, platelet-derived growth factor-receptor, p-glycoprotein and Bcl-2. *Histopathol.* 2003a;43:231–238.

Attanoos RL, Suvarna SK, Rhead E, et al. Malignant vascular tumors of the pleura in 'asbestos' workers and endothelial differentiation in malignant mesothelioma. *Thorax.* 2000;55:860–863.

Attanoos RL, Thomas DH, Gibbs AR. Synchronous diffuse malignant mesothelioma and carcinomas in asbestos exposed individuals. *Histopathol.* 2003b;43:387–392.

Attanoos RL, Webb R, Dojcinov SD, Gibbs AR. Malignant epithelioid mesothelioma: antimesothelial marker expression correlates with histological pattern. *Histopathol.* 2001;39:584–588.

Attanoos RL, Webb R, Djocinov SD, Gibbs AR. Value of mesothelial and epithelial antibodies in distinguishing diffuse peritoneal mesothelioma in females from serous papillary carcinoma of the ovary and peritoneum. *Histopathol.* 2002b;40:237–244.

Aubry M-C, Bridge JA, Wickert R, Tazelaar HD. Primary monophasic synovial sarcoma of the pleura: five cases confirmed by the presence of SYT-SSX fusion transcript. *Am J Surg Pathol.* 2001;25:776–781.

Ault JG, Cole RW, Jensen CG, Jensen LC, Bachert LA, Rieder CL. Behavior of crocidolite asbestos during mitosis in living vertebrate lung epithelial cells. *Cancer Res.* 1995;55:792–798.

Aust A, Eveleigh J. Mechanisms of DNA oxidation. *Exp Biol Med.* 1999;222:246–252.

Austin MB, Fechner RE, Roggli VL. Pleural malignant mesothelioma following Wilms' tumor. *Am J Clin Pathol.* 1986;86:227–230.

Babcock TL, Powell DH, Bothwell RS. Radiation induced peritoneal mesothelioma. *J Surg Oncol.* 1976;8:369–372.

Ball NJ, Urbanski SJ, Green FH, Kieser T. Pleural multicystic mesothelial proliferation. The so-called Multicystic mesothelioma. *Am J Surg Pathol.* 1990;14:375–378.

Banaei A, Auvert B, Goldberg M, Gueguen A, Luce D, Goldberg S. Future trends in mortality of French men from mesothelioma. *Occup Environ Med.* 2000;57:488–494.

Barbera V, Rubino M. Papillary Mesothelioma of the tunica vaginalis. *Cancer.* 1957;10:183–189.

Berman DW, Crump KS. Final draft: technical support document for a protocol to assess asbestos-related risk. Washington, DC: EPA; 2004.

Bernstein DM, Chevalier J, Smith P. Comparison of Calidria chrysotile asbestos to pure tremolite: inhalation biopersistence and histopathology following short-term exposure. *Inhal Toxicol.* 2003;15:1387–1419.

Bernstein DM, Chevalier J, Smith P. Comparison of Calidria chrysotile asbestos to pure tremolite: final results of the inhalation biopersistence and histopathology examination following short-term exposure. *Inhal Toxicol.* 2005;17:427–449.

Bernstein DM, Rogers R, Smith P. The biopersistence of Brazilian chrysotile asbestos following inhalation. *Inhal Toxicol.* 2004;16:745–761.

Bianchi C, Brollo A, Zuch C. Asbestos-related familial mesothelioma. *Eur J Cancer Prev.* 1993;2:247–250.

Bischoff F, Bryson G. Carcinogenesis through solid state surfaces. *Prog Exp Tumor Res.* 1964;5:85–133.

Bocchetta MI, Di Resta A, Powers R, et al. Human mesothelial cells are unusually susceptible to simian virus 40 mediated transformation and asbestos cocarcinogenicity. *Proc Natl Acad Sci USA.* 2000;97:10214–10219.

Bokemeyer C, Schmoll HJ. Secondary neoplasms following treatment of malignant germ cell tumors. *J Clin Oncol.* 1993;11:1703–1709.

Bolognesi C, Filiberti R, Neri M, et al. High frequency of micronuclei in peripheral blood lymphocytes as index of susceptibility to pleural malignant mesothelioma. *Cancer Res.* 2002;62:5418–5419.

Boutin C, Dumortier P, Rey F, Viallat JR, DeVuyst P. Black spots concentrate oncogenic asbestos fibers in the parietal pleura. *Am J Respir Crit Care Med.* 1996;153:444–449.

Brand KG. Foreign body induced sarcomas. In: Becker FF ed. *Cancer—A Comprehensive Treatise. Etiology: Chemical and Physical Carcinogenesis*, New York: Plenum Press; 1975: 485.

Brenner J, Sordillo PP, Magill GB, Golbey RB. Malignant peritoneal mesothelioma. *Am J Gastroenterol.* 1981;75:311–313.

Brown RC, Bellmann B, Muhle H, Davis JM, Maxim LD. Survey of the biological effects of refractory ceramic fibers: overload and its possible consequences. *Ann Occup Hyg.* 2005;49:295–307.

Browne K, Smither WJ. Asbestos-related mesothelioma: factors discriminating between pleural and peritoneal sites. *Br J Ind Med.* 1983;40:145–152.

Brunnemann RB, Ro JY, Ordonez NG, Mooney J, El-Naggar AK, Ayala AG. Extrapleural solitary fibrous tumor: a clinicopathologic study of 24 cases. *Mod Pathol.* 1999;12:1034–1042.

Butnor K, Sporn TA, Hammar SP, Roggli VL. Well-differentiated papillary mesothelioma. *Am J Surg Pathol.* 2001;25:1304–1309.

Cacciotti P, Strizzi L, Vianale G, et al. The presence of simian virus 40 sequences in mesothelioma and mesothelial cells is associated with high levels of vascular endothelial growth factor. *Am J Respir Cell Mol Biol.* 2002;26:189–193.

Cavazza A, Travis LB, Travis WD, et al. Post-irradiation malignant mesothelioma. *Cancer.* 1996;77:1379–1385.

Chabot JF, Beard D, Langlois AJ, Beard JW. Mesotheliomas of peritoneum, epicardium and pericardium induced by strain MC29 avian leukosis virus. *Cancer Res.* 1970;30:1287–1308.

Chu AY, Litzky LA, Pasha TL, Acs G, Zhang PJ. Utility of D2–40, a novel mesothelial marker, in the diagnosis of malignant mesothelioma. *Mod Pathol.* 2005;18:105–110.

Churg A. Deposition and clearance of chrysotile asbestos. *Ann Occup Hyg.* 1994;38:625–633.

Churg A, Colby TV, Cagle P, et al. The separation of benign and malignant mesothelial cell proliferations. *Am J Surg Pathol.* 2000;24:1183–1200.

Churg A, Vedal S. Fiber burden and patterns of asbestos-related disease in workers with heavy mixed amosite and chrysotile exposure. *Am J Respir Crit Care Med.* 1994;150:663–669.

Cicala C, Pompetti F, Carbone M. SV40 induces mesothelioma in hamsters. *Am J Pathol.* 2004;142:1524–1533.

Clement PB, Young RH, Scully RE. Malignant mesotheliomas presenting as ovarian masses. *Am J Surg Pathol.* 1996;20:1067–1080.

Coffin DL, Peters SE, Palekar LD, Stahel EP. A study of the biological activity of erionite in relation to its chemical and structural characteristics. In: Wehner AP, ed. *Biological Interactions of Inhaled Mineral Fibers and Cigarette Smoke*, Columbus: Batelle Memorial Institution; 1989: 313–323.

Coggon D, Inskip H, Winter P, Pannett B. Differences in occupational mortality from pleural cancer, peritoneal cancer and asbestosis. *Occup Environ Med.* 1995;52:775–777.

Coin PG, Roggli VL, Brody A. Deposition, clearance, and translocation of chrysotile asbestos from peripheral and central regions of rat lung. *Env Res.* 1992;58:97–116.

Cook DS, Attanoos R.L, Jalloh SS, Gibbs AR. 'Mucin positive' epithelial mesothelioma of the peritoneum: an unusual diagnostic pitfall. *Histopathol.* 2000;17:33–36.

Coplu L, Dumortier P, Demir AU, et al. An epidemiological study in an Anatolian village in Turkey environmentally exposed to tremolite asbestos. *J Environ Pathol Toxicol Oncol.* 1996;15:177–182.

Craig JR, Hart WR. Extragenital adenomatoid tumor. *Cancer.* 1979;64:1336–1346.

Craighead JE. Current pathogenetic concepts of diffuse malignant mesothelioma. *Human Path.* 1987;18:544–557.

Craighead JE, Richards SA, Calore JD, Fan D, Weaver DL. Genetic factors influence malignant mesothelioma development in mice. *Eur Respir Rev.* 1993;3:1259–1260.

Crotty TB, Myers JL, Katzenstein AL, Tazelaar HD, Swensen SJ, Churg A. Localized malignant mesothelioma: a clinicopathologic and flow cytometric study. *Am J Surg Pathol.* 1994;18:357–363.

Cummings OW, Ulbright TM, Young RH, Del Tos AP, Fletcher CD, Hull MT. Desmoplastic small round cell tumors of the paratesticular region. A report of six cases. *Am J Surg Pathol.* 1997;21:219–225.

Curran D, Sahmoud T, Therasse P, van Meerbeeck J, Postmus PE, Giaccone G. Prognostic factors in patients with pleural mesotheliomas: the European Organization for Research and Treatment of Cancer experience. *J Clin Oncol.* 1998;16:145–152.

Dahl IM, Solheim ØP, Erikstein B, Müller E. A longitudinal study of the hyaluronan level in the serum of patients with malignant mesothelioma under treatment. Hyaluronan as an indicator of progressive disease. *Cancer.* 1989;64:68–73.

Dang-Tan T, Mahmud SM, Puntoni R, Franco EL. Polio vaccines, Simian Virus 40, and human cancer: the epidemiologic evidence for a causal association. *Oncogene.* 2004;23:6535–6540.

Dardick I, Jabi M, McCaughey WT, Deodhare S, van Nostrand AW, Srigley JR. Diffuse epithelial mesothelioma: a review of the ultrastructural spectrum. *Ultrastruct Pathol.* 1987;11:503–533.

Davis JMG. Mineral fibre carcinogenesis: experimental data relating to the importance of fibre types, size, deposition, dissolution and migration. In: Bignon J, Peto J, Saracci R, eds. *Mineral Fibresin the Non-occupational Environmet*, Lyon, France: IARC Scientific Publication; 1989:90:33–45.

Dawson A, Gibbs A, Browne K, Pooley F, Griffiths M. Familial mesotheliomas: details of 17 cases with histopathologic findings and mineral analysis. *Cancer.* 1992;70:1183–1187.

Daya D, McCaughey WT. Well-differentiated papillary mesothelioma of the peritoneum. A clinicopathologic study of 22 cases. *Cancer.* 1990;65:292–296.

de Klerk NH, Musk AW, Williams V, Filion PR, Whitaker D, Shilkin KB. Comparison of measures of exposure to asbestos in former crocidolite workers from Wittenoom Gorge, W. Australia. *Am J Ind Med.* 1996;30:579–587.

Dewar A, Valente M, Ring NP, Corrin B. Pleural mesothelioma of epithelial type and pulmonary adenocarcinoma: an ultrastructural and cytochemical comparison. *J Pathol.* 1987;152:309–316.

Doll R, Peto J. Asbestos. Effects on Health of Exposure to Asbestos. 1986. London, Her Majesty's Stationery Office.

Edwards JG, Abrams KR, Leverment JN, Spyt TJ, Waller DA, O'Byrne KJ. Prognostic factors for malignant mesothelioma in 142 patients: validation of CALGB and EORTC prognostic scoring systems. *Thorax*. 2000;55:731–735.

Edward AT, Whitaker D, Browne K, Pooley FD, Gibbs AR. Mesothelioma in a community in the north of England. *Occup Environ Med*. 1996;53:547–552.

Foyle A, Al-Jabi M, McCaughey WT. Papillary peritoneal tumors in women. *Am J Surg Pathol*. 1981;5:241–249.

Fraire AE, Cooper S, Greenberg SD, Buffler P, Langston C. Mesothelioma of childhood. *Cancer*. 1988;62:838–847.

Fubini B, Mollo L, Giamello E. Free radical generation at the solid/liquid interface in iron containing minerals. *Free Rad Res*. 1995;23:593–614.

Galateau-Salle F, Brambilla E, Cagle P, et al. Pathology of malignant mesothelioma: an update prepared by the International Mesothelioma Panel. Galateau-Salle F. 2005. London: Springer-Verlag.

Galateau-Salle F, Vignaud JM, Burke L, et al. Mesopath Group: Well-differentiated papillary mesotheliomas of the pleura: a series of 24 cases. *Am J Surg Pathol*. 2004;28:534–540.

Gardner MJ, Winter PD, Pannett B, Powell CA. Follow-up study of workers manufacturing chrysotile asbestos cement products. *Br J Ind Med*. 1986;43:726–732.

Gibbs AR. Role of asbestos and other fibres in the development of diffuse malignant mesothelioma. *Thorax*. 1990;45:649–654.

Gibbs AR, Griffiths DM, Pooley FD, Jones JS. Comparison of fibre types and size distributions in lung tissues of paraoccupational and occupational cases of malignant mesothelioma. *Br J Ind Med*. 1990;47:621–626.

Gibbs AR, Jones JS, Pooley FD, Griffiths DM, Wagner JC. Non-occupational malignant mesotheliomas. *IARC Sci Publ*. 1989;90: 219–228.

Gilks B, Hegedus C, Freeman H, Fratkin I, Churg A. Malignant peritoneal mesothelioma after remote abdominal radiation. *Cancer*. 1988;61:2019–2021.

Goepel JR. Benign papillary mesothelioma of peritoneum: a histological, histochemical and ultrastructural study of six cases. *Histopathol*. 1981;5:21–30.

Gold C. A primary mesothelioma involving the rectovaginal septum and associated with beryllium. *J Pathol Bacteriol*. 1967;93:435–442.

Goldberg JL, Zanella CL, Janssen YM, et al. Novel cell imaging techniques show induction of apotosis and proliferation in mesothelial cells by asbestos. *Am J Respir Cell Mol Biol*. 1997;17:265–271.

Goodman M, Teta MJ, Hessel PA, et al. Mesothelioma and lung cancer among motor vehicle mechanics: a meta-analysis. *Ann Occup Hyg*. 2004;48:309–326.

Gulumian M, van Wyck J. Oxygen consumption, lipid peroxidation and mineral fibers. In: Brown R, Hoskins J, Johnson N, eds. *Mechanisms in Fiber Carcinogenesis*, New York: Plenum Press; 1991:439–446.

Hammar SP, Bockus DE, Remington FL, Rohrbach KA. Mucin-positive epithelial mesotheliomas: a histochemical, immunohistochemical, and ulltrastrucural comparison with mucin-producing pulmonary adenocarcinomas. *Ultrastruct Pathol*. 1996;20:293–325.

Harwood TR, Gracey DR, Yokoo H. Pseudomesotheliomatous carcinoma of the lung. A variant of peripheral lung cancer. *Am J Clin Pathol*. 1976;65:159–167.

Health and Safety Executive. Health and safety statistics 2000/01. 2001. London, HSE Books.

Heineman EF, Bernstein L, Stark AD, Spirtas R. Mesothelioma, asbestos, and reported history of cancer in first-degree relatives. *Cancer*. 1996;77:549–554.

Hemminki K, Li X. Mesothelioma incidence seems to have leveled off in Sweden. *Int J Cancer*. 2003;103:145–146.

Herndon JE, Green MR, Chahinian AP, Corson JM, Suzuki Y, Vogelzang NJ. Factors predictive of survival among 337 patients with mesothelioma treated between 1984 and 1994 by the Cancer and Leukemia group B. *Chest*. 1998;113:723–731.

Hillerdal G, Berg J. Malignant mesothelioma secondary to chronic inflammation and old scars. Two new cases and review of the literature. *Cancer.* 1985;55:1968–1972.

Hirvonen A, Pelin K, Tammilehto L, Karjalainen A, Mattson K, Linnainmaa K. Inherited GSTM1 and NAT2 defects as concurrent risk modifiers in asbestos-related human malignant mesothelioma. *Cancer Res.* 1995;55:2981–2983.

Hodgson JT, Darnton A. The quantitative risks of mesothelioma and lung cancer in relation to asbestos exposure. *Ann Occup Hyg.* 2000;44:565–601.

Hoekman K, Tognon G, Risse EK, Bloemsma CA, Vermorken JB. Well-differentiated papillary mesothelioma of the peritoneum: a separate entity. *Eur J Cancer.* 1996;32A:255–258.

Howel D, Gibbs A, Arblaster L, et al. Mineral fibre analysis and routes of exposure to asbestos in the development of mesothelioma in an English region. *Occup Environ Med.* 1999;56:51–58.

Hughes JM, Weill H, Hammad YY. Mortality of workers employed in two asbestos cement manufacturing plants. *Br J Ind Med.* 1987;44:161–174.

Jasani B, Cristaudo A, Emri SA, et al. Association of SV40 with human tumors. *Semin Cancer Biol.* 2001;11:49–61.

Jones AD. Respirable industrial fibres: deposition, clearance and dissolution in animal models. *Ann Occup Hyg.* 2004;37:211–216.

Jones JS, Gibbs AR, McDonald JC, Pooley FD. Mesothelioma following exposure to crocidolite (blue) asbestos. A fifty year follow-up study. Antypas G, Proceedings, 2nd International Congress on Lung Cancer. 1996: 407–411. Italy, Monzuzzi Editore.

Jones MA, Young RH, Scully RE. Malignant mesothelioma of the tunica vaginalis. A clinicopathologic analysis of 11 cases with review of the literature. *Am J Surg Pathol.* 1995;19:815–825.

Kane AB. Asbestos bodies: clues to the mechanism of asbestos toxicity? *Hum Pathol* 2003;34:735–736.

Kaplan MA, Tazelaar HD, Hayashi T, Schoer KR, Travis WD. Adenomatoid tumors of the pleura. *Am J Surg Pathol.* 1996;20:1219–1223.

Katsube Y, Mukai K, Silverberg SG. Cystic mesothelioma of the peritoneum: a report of five cases and review of the literature. *Cancer.* 1982;50:1615–1622.

Kerrigan SA, Cagle P, Churg A. Malignant mesothelioma of the peritoneum presenting as an inflammatory lesion. A report of four cases. *Am J Surg Pathol.* 2003;27:248–253.

Kielkowski D, Nelson G, Rees D. Risk of mesothelioma from exposure to crocidolite asbestos: a 1995 update of a South African mortality study. *Occup Environ Med.* 2000;57:563–567.

Koss MN, Fleming M, Przygodzki RM, Sherrod A, Travis W, Hocholzer L. Adenocarcinoma simulating mesothelioma. A clinicopathologic and immunohistochemical study of 29 cases. *Ann Diagn Pathol.* 1998;2:93–102.

Lanphear BP, Buncher CR. Latent period for malignant mesothelioma of occupational origin. *J Occup Med.* 1992;34:718–721.

Leers MP, Aarts MM, Theunissen PH. E-cadherin and calretinin: a useful combination of immunochemical markers for differentiation between mesothelioma and metastatic adenocarcinoma. *Histopathol.* 1998;32:209–216.

Leigh J, Davidson P, Hendrie L, Berry D. Malignant mesothelioma in Australia, 1945–2000. *Am J Ind Med.* 2002;41:188–201.

Lerman Y, Learman Y, Schachter P, Herceg E, Lieberman Y, Yellin A. Radiation associated malignant pleural mesothelioma. *Thorax.* 1991;46:463–464.

Lin BT, Colby T, Gown AM, et al. Malignant vascular tumor of the serous membranes mimicking mesothelioma. A report of 14 cases. *Am J Surg Pathol.* 1996;20:1431–1439.

Lippmann M. Effects of fiber characteristics on lung deposition, retention and disease. *Environ Health Perspect.* 1990;88:311–317.

List AF, Doll DC, Greco FA. Lung cancer in Hodgkin's disease: association with previous radiotherapy. *J Clin Oncol.* 1985;3:215–221.

Liu J, Nau MM, Yeh JC, Allegra CJ, Chu E, Wright JJ. Molecular heterogeneity and function of EWS-WT1 fusion transcripts in desmoplastic small round cell tumors. *Clin Cancer Res.* 2000;6:3522–3529.

Livneh A, Langevitz P, Pras M. Pulmonary associations in familial Mediterranean fever. *Curr Opin Pulm Med.* 1999;5:326–331.

Lockey J, Lemasters G, Rice C, et al. Refractory ceramic fiber and pleural plaques. *Am J Respir Crit Care Med.* 1996;154:1405–1410.

Lopez-Rios F, Illei PB, Rusch V, Ladanyi M. Evidence against a role for SV40 infection in human mesotheliomas and high risk of false-positive PCR results owing to presence of SV40 sequences in common laboratory plasmids. *Lancet.* 2004;364:1157–1166.

Luce D, Bugel I, Goldberg P, et al. Environmental exposure to tremolite and respiratory cancer in New Caledonia:a case control study. *Am J Epidemiol.* 2000;151:259–265.

Manfredi JJ, Dong J, Liu WJ, et al. Evidence against a role for SV40 in human mesothe-lioma. *Cancer Res.* 2005;65:2602–2609.

Mangano WE, Cagle PT, Churg A, Vollmer RT, Roggli VL. The diagnosis of desmoplastic malignant mesothelioma and its distinction from fibrous pleurisy: a histologic and immu-nohistochemical analysis of 31 cases including p53 immunostaining. *Am J Clin Pathol.* 1998;110:191–199.

Maurer R, Egloff B. Malignant peritoneal mesothelioma after cholangiography with thorotrast. *Cancer.* 1975;36:1381–1385.

Mayall FG, Gibbs AR. Malignant peritoneal mesothelioma giving rise to multiple intestinal polyps. *Histopathology.* 1991;18:480–482.

Mayall FG, Gibbs AR. 'Pleural' and pulmonary carcinosarcomas. *J Pathol.* 1992;167:305–311.

McConnell EE, Mast RW, Hesterberg TW, et al. Chronic inhalation toxicity of a kaolin-based refractory ceramic fiber in Syrian golden hamsters. *Inhalation Toxicol.* 1995;7:503–532.

McDonald AD, McDonald JC. Malignant mesothelioma in North America. *Cancer.* 1980;46:1650–1656.

McDonald AD, Case BW, Churg A, et al. Mesothelioma in Quebec chrysotile miners and millers: epidemiology and aetiology. *Ann Occup Hyg.* 1997;41:707–719.

McDonald JC, McDonald AD. Chrysotile, tremolite and carcinogenicity. *Ann Occup Hyg.* 1997;41:699–705.

McDonald JC, Harris J, Armstrong B. Cohort Mortality study of vermiculite miners exposed to fibrous tremolite. *Ann Occup Hyg.* 2002;46(Suppl. 1):93–94.

McDonald JC, Liddell FD, Gibbs GW, Eyssen GE, McDonald AD. Dust exposure and mor-tality in chrysotile mining, 1910–75. *Br J Ind Med.* 1980;37:11–24.

Meyer K, Chaffee E. Hyaluronic acid in pleural fluid associated with malignant tumor involv-ing pleura and peritoneum. *Proc Soc Exp Biol.* 1939;42:797–800.

Miettinen M, Limon J, Niezabitowski A, Lasota J. Calretinin and other mesothelioma mark-ers in synovial sarcoma: analysis of antigenic similarities and differences with malignant mesothelioma. *Am J Surg Pathol.* 2001;25:610–617.

Miller WC, Hesterberg TW, Hamilton RD. Oncogenicity study of refractory ceramic fibers (RCF) in hamsters. MTC Report 092518. 1991:1–69. Littleton, Colorado, Mountain technol-ogy Center.

Moertel C. Peritoneal mesothelioma. *Gastroenterology.* 1972;63:346–350.

Moran CA, Travis WD, Rosado-de-Christenson M, Koss MN, Rosai J. Thymomas presenting as pleural tumors. Report of eight cases. *Am J Surg Pathol.* 1992;16:138–144.

Morgan A, Evans JC, Holmes A. Deposition and clearance of inhaled fibrous materials in the rat. Studies using radioactive tracer techniques. In: Walton WH, McGovern B. *Inhaled Particles IV*, New York: Pergamon Press; 1977: 259–274.

Mossman B, Gruenert DC. SV40, growth factors, and mesothelioma: another piece of the puzzle. *Am J Respir Cell Mol Biol.* 2002;26:167–170.

Mossman BT, Bignon J, Corn M, Seaton A, Gee JB. Asbestos: scientific developments and implications for public policy. *Science.* 1990;247:294–301.

Musti M, Cavone D, Aalto Y, Scattone A, Serio G, Knuutila S. A cluster of familial malignant mesothelioma with del(9p) as the sole chromosomal anomaly. *Cancer Genet Cytogenet.* 2002;138:73–76.

Neugut AI, Ahsan H, Antman K. Incidence of malignant pleural mesothelioma after thoracic radiotherapy. *Cancer.* 1997;80:948–950.

Newhouse ML, Sullivan KR. A mortality study of workers manufacturing friction materials: 1941–86. *Br J Ind Med.* 1989;46:176–179.

Newhouse ML, Thompson H. Mesothelioma of pleura and peritoneum following exposure to asbestos in the London area. *Br J Ind Med.* 1965;22:261–269.

Newman RH. Fine biogenic silica fibres in sugar cane: a possible hazard. *Ann Occup Hyg.* 1986;30:365–370.

Nind NR, Attanoos RL, Gibbs AR. Unusual intraparenchymal growth patterns of malignant pleural mesothelioma. *Histopathology.* 2003;42:150–155.

Oberdorster G. Macrophage-associated responses to chrysotile. *Ann Occup Hyg.* 1994;38:601–615, 421–422.

Ordonez N. The immunohistochemical diagnosis of mesothelioma: a comparative study of epithelioid mesothelioma and lung adenocarcinoma. *Am J Surg Pathol.* 2003;27:1031–1051.

Ordonez NG. Role of immunohistochemistry in distinguishing epithelial peritoneal mesotheliomas from peritoneal and ovarian serous carcinomas. *Am J Surg Pathol.* 1998;22:1203–1214.

Ordonez NG. The diagnostic utility of immunohistochemistry in distinguishing between mesothelioma and renal cell carcinoma: a comparative study. *Hum Pathol.* 2004;35:697–710.

Osborn M, Pelling N, Walker MM, Fisher C, Nicholson AG. The value of 'mesothelioma-associated' antibodies in distinguishing between metastatic renal cell carcinomas and mesotheliomas. *Histopathology.* 2002;41:301–307.

Oury TD, Hammar SP, Roggli V. Ultrastructural features of diffuse malignant mesotheliomas. *Hum Pathol.* 1998;29:1382–1392.

Parkash V, Gerald WL, Parma A, Miettinen M, Rosai J. Desmoplastic small round cell tumor of the pleura. *Am J Surg Pathol.* 1995;19:659–665.

Pass HI, Lott D, Lonardo F, et al. Asbestos exposure, pleural mesothelioma, and serum osteopontin levels. *N Engl J Med.* 2005;353:1564–1573.

Paustenbach DJ, Finley BL, Lu ET, Brorby GP, Sheehan PJ. Environmental and occupational health hazards associated with the presence of asbestos in brake linings and pads (1900 to present): a "state of the art" review. *J Toxicol Environ Health B Crit Rev.* 2004;7:25–80.

Peralta-Soler A, Knudsen KA, Jaurand MC, et al. The differential expression of N-cadherin and E-cadherin distinguishes pleural mesotheliomas from lung adenocarcinomas. *Hum Pathol.* 1995;26:1363–1369.

Peterson JT Jr, Greenberg SD, Buffler PA. Non-asbestos related malignant mesothelioma. A review. *Cancer.* 1984;54:951–960.

Peto J, Decarli A, La Vecchia C, Levi F, Negri E. The European mesothelioma epidemic. *Br J Cancer.* 1999;79:666–672.

Peto J, Seidman H, Selikoff IJ. Mesothelioma mortality in asbestos workers: implications for models of carcinogensis and risk assessment. *Br J Cancer.* 1982;45:124–135.

Pinkard NB, Wilson RW, Lawless N, et al. Calcifying fibrous pseudotumor of pleura. A report of three cases of a newly described entity involving the pleura. *Am J Clin Pathol.* 1996;105:189–194.

Pooley FD. An examination of the fibrous mineral content of asbestos lung tissue from the Canadian chrysotile mining industry. *Env Res.* 1976;12:281–298.

Praet M, Forsyth R, Dhaene K, et al. Synovial sarcoma of the pleura: report of four cases. *Histopathology.* 2002;41(Suppl. 2):147–149.

Price B, Ware A. Mesothelioma trends in the United States. An update based on surveillance, epidemiology, and end results program data for 1973 through 2003. *Am J Epidemiol.* 2004;159:107–112.

Puntoni R, Filiberti R, Cerrano PG, Neri M, Andreatta R, Bonassi S. Implementation of a molecular epidemiology approach to human pleural malignant mesothelioma. *Mutat Res.* 2003;544.385–396.

Rees D, Goodman K, Fourie E, et al. Asbestos Exposure and mesothelioma in South Africa. *South African Medical J.* 1999a;89:627–634.

Rees D, Myers JE, Goodman K, et al. Case-control study of mesothelioma in South Africa. *Am J Ind Med.* 1999b;35:213–222.

Rees D, Phillips JI, Garton E, Pooley FD. Asbestos lung fiber concentration in South African chrysotile mine workers. *Ann Occup Hyg.* 2001;45:473–477.

Rice JM, Kovatch RM, Anderson LM. Intraperitoneal mesotheliomas induced in mice by a polycyclic aromatic hydrocarbon. *J Toxicol Environ Health.* 1989;27:1530–1560.

Riddell RH, Goodman MJ, Moossa AR. Peritoneal malignant mesothelioma in a patient with recurrent peritonitis. *Cancer.* 1981;48:134–139.

Robb JA. Mesothelioma vs. adenocarcinoma: false-positive CEA and Leu-M1 staining due to hyaluronic acid. *Hum Pathol.* 1989;20:400.

Robinson BW, Creaney J, Lake R, et al. Mesothelin-family proteins and diagnosis of mesothelioma. *Lancet.* 2003;362:1612–1616.

Roboz J, Greaves J, Silides D, Chahinian AP, Holland JF. Hyaluronic acid content of effusions as a diagnostic aid for malignant mesothelioma. *Cancer Res.* 1985;45:1850–1854.

Rodelsperger K, Woitowitz HJ. Airborne fibre concentrations and lung burden compared to the tumour response in rats and humans exposed to asbestos. *Ann Occup Hyg.* 1995;39:715–725.

Roggli VL. Pericardial mesothelioma after exposure to asbestos. *N Engl J Med.* 1981;304:1045.

Roogli VL. Asbestos bodies and nonasbestos ferruginous bodies. In: Roggli VL, Oury TD, Sprin TA, eds., *Pathology of Asbestos-Associated Diseases.* 2nd ed. New York: Springer 2004; 34–70.

Roggli VL, Sharma A, Butnor KJ, Sporn T, Vollmer RT. Malignant mesothelioma and occupational exposure to asbestos: a clinicopathologic correlation of 1445 cases. *Ultrastruct Pathol.* 2002;26:55–65.

Ross MJ, Welch WR, Scully RE. Multilocular peritoneal inclusion cysts (so-called cystic mesotheliomas). *Cancer.* 1989;64:1336–1346.

Roushdy-Hammady I, Siegel J, Emri S, Testa JR, Carbone M. Genetic-susceptibility factor and malignant mesothelioma in the Cappadocian region of Turkey. *Lancet.* 2001;357:444–445.

Roviaro GC, Sartori F, Calabro F, Varoli F. The association of pleural mesothelioma and tuberculosis. *Am Rev Respir Dis.* 1982;126:569–571.

Ruffie P, Feld R, Minkin S, et al. Diffuse malignant mesothelioma of the pleura in Ontario and Quebec: a retrospective study of 332 patients. *J Clin Oncol.* 1989;7:1157–1168.

Rusch VW, Venkatraman ES. Important prognosis factors in patients with malignant pleura mesothelioma, managed surgically. *Ann Thorac Surg.* 1999;68:1799–1804.

Sakellariou K, Malamou-Mitsi V, Haritou A, et al. Malignant pleural mesothelioma from nonoccupational exposure asbestos exposure in Metsovo (northwest Greece): slow end of an epidemic? *Eur Respir J.* 1996;9:1206–1210.

Sanders CL, Jackson TA. Induction of mesotheliomas and sarcomas from "hot spots" of 239 PuO 2 activity. *Health Phys.* 1972;22:755–859.

Sandhu H, Dehnen W, Roller M, Abel J, Unfried K. mRNA expression patterns in different stages of asbestos-induced carcinogenesis in rats. *Carcinogenesis.* 2000;21:1023–1029.

Sane AC, Roggli VL. Curative resection of a well-differentiated papillary mesothelioma of the pericardium. *Arch Pathol Lab Med.* 1995;119:266–267.

Segura O, Burdorf A, Looman C. Update of predictions of mortality from pleural mesothelioma in the Netherlands. *Occup Environ Med.* 2003;60:50–55.

Selcuk ZT, Coplu L, Emri S, Kalyoncu AF, Sahin AA, Baris YI. Malignant pleural mesothelioma due to environmental mineral fiber exposure in Turkey: an analysis of 135 cases. *Chest.* 1992;102:790–796.

Shannon VR, Nesbitt JC, Libshitz HI. Malignant pleural mesothelioma after radiation therapy for breast cancer. A report of two additional patients. *Cancer.* 1995;76:437–441.

Shukla A, Gulumian M, Hei TK, Kamp D, Rahman Q, Mossman BT. Multiple roles of oxidants in the pathogenesis of asbestos induced diseases. *Free Radic Biol Med.* 2003a;34:1117–1129.

Shukla A, Ramos-Nino M, Mossman B. Cell signaling and transcription factor activation by asbestos in lung injury and disease. *Int J Biochem Cell Biol.* 2003b;35:1198–1209.

Spirtas R, Heineman EF, Bernstein L, et al. Malignant mesothelioma: attributable risk of asbestos exposure. *Occup Environ Med.* 1994;51:804–811.

Spriggs AI, Jerrome DW. Benign mesothelial proliferation with collagen formation in pericardial fluid. *Acta Cytol.* 1979;23:428–430.

Stanton MF, Laynard M, Tegeris A, Miller E, May M, Kent E. Carcinogenicity of fibrous glass: pleural response in the rat in relation to fiber dimension. *J Natl Cancer Inst.* 1977;58:587–603.

Steele JP. Prognostic factors in mesothelioma. *Semin Oncol.* 2002;29:36–40.

Stevens NW, Leong AS, Fazzalari NL, Dowling KD, Henderson DW. Cytopathology of malignant mesothelioma: a stepwise logistic regression analysis. *Diagn Cytopathol.* 1992;8:333–341.

Stey C, Landolt-Weber U, Vetter W, Sauter C, Marincek B. Malignant peritoneal mesothelioma after Thorotrast exposure. *Am J Clin Oncol.* 1995;18:313–317.

Stock RJ, Fu YS, Carter JR. Malignant peritoneal mesothelioma following radiotherapy for seminoma of the testis. *Cancer.* 1979;44:914–919.

Sugarbaker PH, Acherman YI, Gonzalez-Moreno S, et al. Diagnosis and treatment of peritoneal mesothelioma: the Washington Cancer Institute experience. *Semin Oncol.* 2002;29:51–61.

Sussman J, Rosai J. Lymph node metastasis as the initial manifestation of malignant mesothelioma. Report of six cases. *Am J Surg Pathol.* 1990;14:819–828.

Sweet BH, Hilleman MR. The vacuolating virus, S.V. 40. *Proc Soc Exp Biol Med.* 1960;105:420–427.

Taxy JB, Battifora H, Oyasu R. Adenomatoid tumors: a light microscopic, histochemical and ultrastructural study. *Cancer.* 1974;34:306–316.

Thomas HF, Benjamin IT, Elwood PC, Sweetnam PM. Further follow-up study of workers from an asbestos cement factory. *Br J Ind Med.* 1982;39:273–276.

Thomason R, Schlegel W, Lucca M, Cummings S, Lee S. Primary malingant mesothelioma of the pericardium. Case report and literature review. *Tex Heart Inst J.* 1994;21:170–174.

Thorner P, Squire J, Chilton-MacNeil S, et al. Is the EWS/FLI-1 fusion transcript specific for Ewings sarcoma and peripheral primitive neuroectodermal tumor? A report of four cases showing this transcript in a wider range of tumor types. *Am J Pathol.* 1996;148:1125–1138.

Tossavainen A, Takahashi K. Epidemiological trends for asbestos related cancers. People and Work Research Reports 36, Helsinki: Finnish Institute of Occupational Health; 2000:26–30.

Travis WD, Brambilla E, Muller-Hermelink HK, Harris CC. *Tumors of the Lung, Pleura, Thymus and Heart. World Health Organization Classification of Tumors. Pathology & Genetics*, Lyon, France: IARC Press; 2004.

Valagussa P, Santoro A, Fossati-Bellani F, Fanfi A, Bonadonna G. Second acute leukemia and other malignancies following treatment for Hodgkin's disease. *J Clin Oncol.* 1986;4:830–837.

Vigneswaran WT, Stefanacci PR. Pericardial mesothelioma. *Curr Treat Options Oncol.* 2000;1:299–302.

Wagner E. Das tuberkelahnliche lymphadenom. *Arch d Heilkunde.* 1870;11:497–526.

Wagner JC. The discovery of the association between blue asbestos and mesotheliomas and the aftermath. *Br J Ind Med.* 1991;48:399–403.

Wagner JC, Sleggs CA, Marchand P. Diffuse pleural mesothelioma and asbestos exposure in the North Western Cape Province. *Br J Ind Med.* 1960;17:260–271.

Waxler B, Eisenstein R, Battifora H. Electrophoresis of tissue glycosaminoglycans as an aid in the diagnosis of mesotheliomas. *Cancer.* 1979;44:221–227.

Weiss SW, Tavassolli FA. Multicystic mesothelioma: an analysis of pathological findings and biological behaviour in 37 cases. *Am J Surg Pathol.* 1988;12:737–746.

Yates D, Corrin B, Stidolph P, Browne K. Malignant mesothelioma in south East England: clinicopathological experience of 272 cases. *Thorax.* 1997;52:507–512.

Young RH, Silva EG, Scully RE. Ovarian and juxtaovarian adenomatoid tumors: a report of six cases. *Int J Gynecol Pathol.* 1991;10:364–371.

9

Nonthoracic Cancers Possibly Resulting from Asbestos Exposure

John E. Craighead

Introduction

Studies of asbestos workers in the 1970s and 1980s in both Europe and North America suggested on the basis of preliminary epidemiological evidence that cancer in several major organ systems, other than the lungs and pleura, might result from exposure to asbestos. Unfortunately, many of these early investigations were poorly controlled and both socioeconomic and lifestyle information such as diet, tobacco use, and alcoholic beverage abuse were not available for consideration. Nonetheless, evidence gradually accumulated in the medical literature implicating asbestos as a carcinogen or cocarcinogen in many organ systems, even though the relative risks (RR) were usually of a low order. The demonstration of asbestos bodies (AB) and fibers in various tissues by pathologists further served to support the conclusion that asbestos exposure could result in systemic neoplastic disease (Auerbach et al., 1980; Huang et al., 1988; Kanazawa, 1970; Sebastien et al., 1980).

On the basis of these incomplete observations, concerns found their way into governmental regulations and medical review articles, too often in the form of realities, and then into litigation as the foundation for personal injury suits. A flurry of epidemiological and experimental studies followed in an effort to shed further light on the issues and to elucidate the possible pathobiological mechanisms involved. During the past two decades, considerable new information has accumulated and the fear that asbestos causes multisystem malignant disease has quelled. This chapter summarizes the available information with respect to the organ systems most often implicated.

In 1965, Sir Bradford Hill published a list of incisive questions that in his opinion medical scientists should address before considering whether or not an exposure to an extraneous substance in our environment has the capacity to cause a specific disease. Hill's criteria are now widely accepted as a basis for determining cause and effect relationships. As the information considered in detail below illustrates, associations can occasionally be found in epidemiological studies, but the key question remains how and when can causation be established in an imperfect world when the seemingly obvious may not be the answer to the riddle. The demanding considerations of Hill summarized and briefly discussed below are of paramount importance in evaluating the various cancers considered in this chapter.

1. *Strength*: The strength of an association can only be established on the basis of a statistical analysis of the results of appropriately designed and conducted epidemiological investigations. Hill emphasized that "no formal tests of significance can answer ... questions." Such tests can, and should, remind us of the effects that the play of chance can create and they will instruct us in the likely magnitude of the (hypothesized) effects. Beyond that, they, that is, statistical analyses, contribute nothing to the "proof" of (a) hypothesis.

2. *Consistency*: To paraphrase Hill, one must ask—has the observed association been repeatedly found by different scientists in various locations and populations, as well as under different circumstances and time frames?

3. *Specificity*: "If ... an association is limited to specific workers and to particular sites and types of disease, and there is no association between the work and other modes of dying, then clearly that is a strong argument in favor of causation." In more recent years, statisticians have turned to multivariate analyses to exclude confounding factors that commonly influence the health of members of a study group. For example, smoking, alcoholic beverage abuse, and familial patterns of disease inheritance.

4. *Temporality*: What is the temporal relationship of the hypothesized association? Which is the cart and which the horse? This question is particularly relevant with diseases of slow development. For example, does a particular diet lead to disease or do the early stages of the disease lead to peculiar dietary habits?

5. *Biological Gradient*: "if the association is one that reveals a ... dose-response curve, then we should look ... carefully for such evidence."

6. *Plausibility*: This concept depends on the biological knowledge of the day. Hill advises caution before dismissing a concept of pathogenesis. It is too early to be shortsighted. The association we observe may be one new to science or medicine and we must not dismiss it too lightheartedly as just too odd. As Sherlock Holmes advised Dr Watson, "when you have eliminated the impossible, whatever remains, *however improbable*, must be the truth."

7. *Coherence*: "A cause and effect interpretation of ... data should not seriously conflict with the generally known facts of the natural history and biology of the disease."

8. *Experiment*: "Occasionally it is possible to appeal to experimental, or semiexperimental, evidence. For example, because of an observed association some preventive action is taken. Does it in fact prevent? The dust in the workshop is reduced, lubricating oils are changed, persons stop smoking cigarettes. Is the frequency of the associated events affected? Here the strongest support for the causation hypotheses may be revealed."

9. *Analogy*: "A search of the medical literature often yields surprising but obscure analogies relevant to our understanding of disease. Just as we must be cautious not to exclude evidence based on the questionable plausibility of a hypothesis, so we can learn much by identifying analogous and insightful biological occurrence of an unrelated nature."

Oral and Nasopharyngeal Carcinoma

Perhaps no anatomical region where cancer commonly occurs is more difficult to define, and delineate structurally from adjacent topographical areas (Forastiere et al., 2001). For the purpose of categorization, disease is generally assigned a site of origin on the

Table 9.1 Upper Respiratory and Digestive Tract Associated Cancers by Anatomical Site*

Site	Rates/1×10^5 Person-Years	
	Males	Females
Oropharynx	2.1	1.1
Nasopharynx	1.8	1.4
Pyriform sinus	2.3	1.7
Hypophrarynx	2.1	1.5

* US National Cancer Institute: Surveillance, Epidemiology and End Results (SEER) data for 1975–1998.

basis of the *International Classification of Causes of Disease*, but the potential exists for errors. Thus, inaccuracies of classification, no doubt, often occur. For these reasons, epidemiological studies based on crude mortality data invariably are compromised by potential inaccuracies. More refined incidence estimations of cancer origin by anatomical site have been published in the National Cancer Institute Surveillance, Epidemiology, and End Results (SEER) reports, summarized in Table 9.1.

Oral and nasopharyngeal cancers display dramatic geographic and regional differences in prevalence, and the incidence also relates to the patient's sex. Worldwide, these diseases are often associated with tobacco and alcoholic beverage abuse (Craighead, 1995; Nam et al., 1992; Talamini et al., 1998) but geographic difference in incidence might be related in part to nutritional and dietary factors (McLaughlin et al., 1988). The role of viruses in the causation of malignant lesions in the oropharynx is also a subject of contemporary consideration. Papillomaviruses have now been implicated in the causation of some squamous carcinomas of the mouth, including the tongue, and nasopharyngeal carcinomas are strongly associated with Epstein-Barr virus infections in certain regions of the Orient (Craighead, 1999; Mork et al., 2001; Van Houten et al., 2001).

Selikoff et al. (1979) reported a RR of 2.1 for cancer of the oropharynx on a best estimate appraisal of disease in members of a large cohort of asbestos insulation workers. A study from South Africa (Botha et al., 1986) compared the incidence of cancer of the lips, oral cavity, and pharynx in males residing in a crocidolite mining region, with persons living elsewhere in that country. They found a Standardized Mortality Ratio (SMR) of 2.24 for white males, and 2.72 for "colored" males. In these studies no effort was made to address the issues of smoking and alcoholic beverage abuse. In contrast negative results were obtained in systematic epidemiological investigations by Mancuso and Coulter (1963), Puntoni et al. (1979), Blot et al. (1979), Enterline et al. (1987), and Cantor et al. (1986), unfortunately all mortality studies. Several other negative studies have not been cited here either because of the limited size of their study group, or the lack of anatomical detail regarding the original location of the lesions. Since many of the neoplasms in the oropharynx are localized and cured by treatment, morbidity data would prove more valuable for a critical evaluation of risk factors. Reports analyzing the incidence of nonfatal premalignant and malignant diseases in relation to asbestos exposure have not been published.

Laryngeal Carcinoma

Cancer of the larynx is a relatively uncommon disease comprising about 1% of human malignancies. It predominantly occurs in males in the later decades of life (Brownson and Chang, 1987; Burch et al., 1981; Elwood et al., 1984; Herity et al., 1982; Luce et al., 1988; Muscat and Wynder, 1992; Rothman et al., 1980; Williams and Horm, 1977). Cancer of the larynx is usually of the squamous cell type and is readily diagnosed with a high degree of specificity by both the clinician and the pathologist. Early disease is readily amenable to treatment; thus, retrospective mortality studies using death certificate data are an unsuitable means of evaluating disease occurrence.

Numerous epidemiological studies and reviews in the literature have documented the strong association of laryngeal carcinoma with cigarette smoking (Tuyns et al., 1988). The disease also occurs in those who use cigars and pipes, but the incidence is substantially lower. The relative prevalence of the disease increases in relation to the intensity of cigarette use. Few cases have been reported in those who do not smoke. Alcoholic beverage abuse is a risk factor, but the association is relatively weak.

Is laryngeal carcinoma causatively associated with asbestos exposure? It should be emphasized at the outset that investigations designed to address this question are difficult to conduct because of the low incidence of the disease and the difficulty documenting exposure. Invariably, the confounding influences of cigarette and alcohol use must be considered. Rarely is adequate information available, yet changes in the cigarette consumption patterns of a study population could have dramatic effects on the occurrence of laryngeal carcinoma.

The possible association of laryngeal carcinoma with asbestos exposure has been examined in several case-control studies published in the last several decades. Investigations of this type are no better than the care with which they are designed and conducted. Retrospective inquiries are fraught with hazard since patients may be reluctant to implicate themselves for such known health abuses as smoking and alcohol use. Furthermore, recollections and documentation of asbestos exposure and particularly, the duration and intensity of such an exposure, is subject to question. This was pointed out in a paper by Stell and McGill (1973) when they stated: "it was often necessary to ask leading questions about exposure to asbestos." In the studies reported, there is a consistent problem with regard to controlling for alcohol and cigarette abuse. This problem proved to be a deficiency in the publication authored by Shettigara and Morgan (1975). Hillerdal and Lindholm (1980) attempted to associate asbestos exposure with laryngeal carcinoma by considering radiologically detected pleural plaques in patient and control groups as a measure of exposure, ignoring the questions of cigarette and alcohol abuse. The diagnosis of pleural plaques by radiologic means is imprecise and, in certain regions of Scandinavia, where the study was carried out, pleural plaques often occur in the general population in the absence of occupational asbestos exposure (Chapter 6). In a paper by Burch et al. (1981), the following conclusion was reached: "the RR for males exposed to asbestos after the effects of cigarette smoking were controlled was 2.3, and the effect seemed restricted to cigarette smokers." Findings in the literature implicating asbestos were based on small numbers of cases and controls and consequently were subject to large sampling errors.

In a paper by Rothman et al. (1980), it was concluded that "there seems to be little question that asbestos is a risk factor, probably a strong risk factor in most populations. ... Lack of sufficient data and uncontrolled confounding effects of smoking, however, preclude any precise determination of increased risk attributable to asbestos." These authors also state that "few of the occupational studies ... cited here were able to control adequately for tobacco use, but it is evident from the figures ... that small differences in tobacco use could account for substantial differences in risk." Rothman's survey of published reports is deficient in that it only cites a few case-control studies, but fails to note a number of published reports that do not support their conclusions (Blot et al., 1980; Brown et al., 1988;

Flanders et al., 1984; Hinds et al., 1979; Newhouse et al., 1980; Olsen and Sabroe, 1984; Parnes, 1990; Rubino et al., 1979; Thomas et al., 1982; Tsai et al., 1996; Zagraniski et al., 1986). Moreover, Rothman et al. (1980) recalculated his data in an attempt to overcome the problems of matching controls with patients by age and smoking background. This reduces the number of individuals included in the analysis substantially, and thus broadened the confidence limits. After considering the methodological problems confounding attempts to assess relationships between asbestos and laryngeal cancer, it is hardly surprising that RR estimates range from 1.4 to 13 in various studies.

In a case-control study by Hinds et al. (1979), it was noted that neither asbestos exposure nor exposure to other toxic substances were found to increase significant risk. The work was undertaken in the Puget Sound area of Washington, where an increased incidence of malignant mesothelioma (MM) had been noted among "blue collar" workers, presumably due to shipyard employment. It is noteworthy that this study tended to have more nonsmokers and light smokers in the control group than in the case group. This imbalance presumably would increase the likelihood that an asbestos effect would be demonstrated if synergism played a role. It was not! In a study of shipyard workers in coastal Virginia (Blot et al., 1980), "no overall excess of laryngeal cancer associated with shipbuilding was found." In contrast, Puntoni et al. (1979) calculated an elevated RR (1.96) among Genoa, Italy shipyard workers. Newhouse et al. (1980) studied the etiology of carcinoma of the larynx in patients hospitalized in Great Britain. Those in the group with laryngeal carcinomas comprised a larger number of smokers than controls, yet no association was found between asbestos exposure and the occurrence of the disease.

Two cohort investigations have been carried out in an effort to compare the prevalence of laryngeal carcinoma in asbestos workers with members of the general population. These studies are deficient inasmuch as the prevalence of cigarette and alcohol abuse in the control and the exposed populations of workers cannot be assessed and compared accurately. Indeed, it is likely that the use of tobacco products would be greater in the workers than in a control population drawn from all strata of society. A study by McDonald et al. (1980) in Québec, Canada, which included almost 1.1×10^4 men working in the asbestos industry, failed to demonstrate an excess of deaths due to laryngeal cancer.

Analyses by pathologists have demonstrated asbestos fibers and AB in a wide variety of organs in the absence of disease (Auerbach et al., 1980). It is not surprising, therefore, that studies in which laryngeal tissue is digested in lye and examined microscopically have yielded a few AB. When AB were found, "no dysplastic epithelial changes were present in the mucosa." (Roggli et al., 1980). In a study by Hirsh et al. (1979), asbestos fibers in small numbers were found by electron microscopy in the laryngeal tissue of two men believed to have asbestosis and pleural plaques. Both were smokers. One had a laryngeal polyp and the second, laryngeal carcinoma. This work was not controlled by carrying out parallel analyses on tissue from those without laryngeal diseases. This study, then, provides no definitive information.

A review by Chan and Gee (1988) states that "Available epidemiological evidence does not support a causal association between asbestos and laryngeal cancer." Another review article by Edelman (1989) concludes that "based on data from 13 cohort and 8 case-control studies … neither case-control nor cohort studies have established an increased risk of laryngeal cancer for asbestos workers." And, an editorial by Liddell (1990) concludes: "thus, it is my opinion that the evidence of a link between exposure to asbestos and laryngeal carcinoma definitely fails to satisfy the criteria for causation set by Bradford Hill."

A meta-analysis by Goodman et al. (1999) yielded an overall SMR of 157 (95% confidence limits 95–245) but failed to demonstrate an apparent dosage effect. This study displayed a number of inconsistencies not the least of which was an inability to control for smoking. A meta-analysis by Smith et al. (1990) documented modest elevations in SMR in four of seven cohorts, but broad confidence limits for the data shed doubt on the validity of conclusions.

In summary, tobacco smoking is clearly the only established risk factor in the patho-genesis of laryngeal carcinoma. Accordingly, it is not surprising that populations of so-called "blue collar" workers experience more laryngeal carcinoma than members of the general public inasmuch as tobacco abuse occurs more commonly in this category of worker. On the basis of their occupational activities, these individuals would be expected to allege an exposure to asbestos more frequently than members of the general popula-tion. However, they also report a higher prevalence of exposure to other foreign materials in the workplace, including nonasbestos dusts and toxic chemicals. For example, in one report, the following substances were listed as suspect etiological agents: mustard gas, nickel, soot, tars and minerals, pesticides, naphthalene, leather, wood dust, and ball bear-ings. With the possible exception of tars and soot, these materials are not recognized risk factors for laryngeal cancer. The currently published data fails to provide a compelling basis for concluding that asbestos exposure is a risk factor for laryngeal carcinoma. It is not surprising that AB and fibers in small numbers have been demonstrated in laryngeal tissue of some patients, given the role of the larynx as a portal to the respiratory tract. Clearly, the presence of AB in this tissue does not serve as a basis for implicating asbes-tos in the etiology of laryngeal cancer.

Esophageal Cancer

In the general population, the lifetime risk of esophageal cancer is 0.8% for men and 0.3% for women. Cancer develops throughout the extent of the esophagus from the oral pharynx to the cardia of the stomach (Ries et al., 2002), but the morphological types and the pathogenic features differ by anatomical region. Squamous carcinoma customarily occurs in the proximal and middle esophagus; it has a strong association with tobacco and alcohol abuse (Gao et al., 1994; Yu et al., 1988). In contrast, most neoplasms in the lower esophagus are adenocarcinomas. In this segment, particularly in the distal esophagus and the adjacent cardia of the stomach, the lesions often develop in the wake of Barrett's esophagitis, often accompanied by hiatus hernia and gastric regurgitation, the so-called gastroesophageal reflux disorder (GERD; Chow et al., 1995; Garewal and Sampliner, 1989; Spechler and Goyal, 1986). In this condition, there is an association with dietary indiscretions and smoking (Wu et al., 2001). The adenocarcinomas arise in the glandular epithelium of the distal esophagus usually developing after a pro-tracted history of GERD and chronic esophagitis (Brown et al., 1994; Chow et al., 1995; Gammon et al., 1997; Jankowski et al., 1999; Lagergren et al., 1999). Currently, for unknown reasons, adenocarcinomas of the distal esophagus are increasingly prevalent in middle-aged men and women, more so in Whites than in African Americans (Blot, 1994; Enzinger and Mayer, 2003).

Extensive epidemiological studies have been carried out on workers in a number of dif-ferent industries where asbestos exposure has occurred in an effort to determine whether or not asbestos contributes to carcinoma development in the esophagus (Puntoni et al., 1979; Rubino et al., 1979). Some early studies provided positive suggestive results, but these investigations, unfortunately, were not well controlled (Newhouse et al., 1985). In addition, dietary, smoking, and alcohol histories were not obtained. For example, Selikoff cited a RR of 2.5 based on both the investigator's evaluation of the clinical evidence and death certificate data from a 1.78×10^4 cohort of insulation workers (Selikoff et al., 1979). But, these observations are of limited value and do not provide definitive evidence. When more carefully designed epidemiologic investigations were carried out, no increase in prevalence of esophageal tumors was found among occupationally exposed workers (Enterline et al., 1987; Zoloth and Michaels, 1985). Thus, the evidence thus far, including a recent meta-analysis by Goodman et al. (1999), fails to demonstrate an epidemiological association between exposure and the development of esophageal cancer.

Studies have also been carried out in several sites in the United States in an effort to determine whether or not an increased concentration of asbestos in potable water results in the development of cancer of the digestive tract (Marsh, 1983; Sigurdson et al., 1981). These investigations have failed to demonstrate an increased prevalence of esophageal cancer in persons residing in areas where water concentrations of chrysotile and amphibole asbestos are believed to be excessively high, in comparison to North American overall.

Numerous experimental studies have been conducted in an attempt to demonstrate the development of cancers of the digestive tract in animals fed massive amounts of asbestos in their food during the course of their lifetime (Condie, 1983). Postmortem examinations have failed to demonstrate the occurrence of digestive tract cancers that can be attributed to asbestos.

Gastric Carcinoma

A considerable body of information has accumulated on the natural history of gastric carcinomas worldwide, particularly since these cancers were a significant cause of mortality among men in generations past (Graham 1975; Haenszel and Correa, 1975). In more recent years, the number of new cases of gastric carcinoma in developed countries has decreased substantially; in the United States; the incidence has declined by about 75% since 1930.

Epidemiological studies provide insights into the factors that may influence the development of these cancers but the etiology is uncertain in most cases. There are a number of possible etiologies to consider. First, gastric carcinoma is not one disease but several different morphologic and biological entities occurring in different anatomic regions of the stomach. Accordingly, the occurrence of these various cancers may be influenced by different environmental and heritable influences. For example, atrophic gastritis and the associated adenocarcinoma occur in persons with pernicious anemia, whereas nutritional factors may play an etiological role in cancer developing in various localized regions of the world. In some foreign populations, overcooked food and smoked meat products have been associated with an increased prevalence of gastric carcinomas and in some instances, chemicals have been implicated, but proof of a causative relationship is lacking. Of particular note is the unusually high prevalence of gastric carcinoma in Japan, China, Chile, Costa Rica, Iceland, and Finland. In these countries, the disease is two to three times more common than in North America and Western Europe.

It is noteworthy that both in developed and developing countries, the male:female ratios are comparable and there is no consistent gradient in risk between urban and rural populations. The disease process seems to occur more frequently in persons of lower socioeconomic classes and "blue collar" workers (Englund, 1981; Wu-Williams et al., 1990). Nonasbestos miners, fishermen, and agriculture workers have an unusually high prevalence in a few studies. Genetic factors most probably contribute to the development of at least some gastric cancers (Lindor et al., 2005).

In recent years, *Helicobacter pylori*, infection of the gastric mucosa, has been associated with the development of ulcerative disease and cancer in the upper digestive tract of humans. The mechanism(s) accounting for the carcinogenesis of *H pyloris* in the stomach remains to be determined (Blaser, 1999; Nogueira et al., 2001).

Studies by Selikoff and his associates (1964, 1968, 1979; Doll and Peto, 1987) suggested that insulation workers were at increased risk for developing gastric carcinoma. Unfortunately, this work was not carefully controlled for dietary factors (Weisburger and Raineri, 1975), alcoholic beverage consumption (Gammon et al., 1997; Hoey et al., 1981), and tobacco use (Zhang et al., 1997). A few additional studies (Enterline et al., 1987; Kang et al., 1997) tended to yield data consistent with the conclusion of Selikoff, but more recent investigations have consistently failed to demonstrate an epidemiological relationship between gastric carcinoma and exposure to asbestos. Further, a dose-response relationship has not been demonstrated. A review of 45 published studies by Morgan et al. (1985) and an additional literature review by Edelman (1988) failed to demonstrate an association of gastric carcinomas with asbestos exposure. The work of Hodgson and Jones (1986) documented mortality of more than 3.1×10^4 male asbestos workers in the United Kingdom. No excess of digestive tract cancer was found in this investigation. An unpublished evaluation by Weiss of 17 cohort studies (Tables 9.2 and 9.3) and a recent meta-analysis by Goodman et al. (1999) also failed to demonstrate an association. Assorted additional studies of diverse occupational groups support this conclusion (Acheson et al., 1984; Berry and Newhouse, 1983; Clemmesen and Hjalgrim-Jensen, 1981; Coggon et al., 1990; Gardner et al., 1986; Hughes et al., 1987; McDonald et al., 1984; Ohlson et al., 1984; Peto et al., 1985; Puntoni et al., 1979; Rubino et al., 1979; Sanden and Jarvholm, 1987; Seidman et al., 1986).

Different approaches to this question have been explored. More specifically, epidemiological studies have been carried out to determine whether the asbestos content of potable water in various communities is associated with an increased prevalence with gastric carcinoma. These investigations have not demonstrated an increase in prevalence

Table 9.2 Gastric Cancer Risk in Cohorts of Asbestos Workers

Ref. No.	Author/Year	No. in Cohort	Type of Work	Gastric Cancer		
				Obs. No.	Exp. No.	O/E
1	Clemmesen and Hjalgrim-Jensen/1981	5686	Asbestos cement factory	14	9.7	1.44
2	Acheson et al./1984	5969	Amosite factory	7	7.5	0.94
3	Ohlson et al./1984	3297	Railroad maintenance	41	71.6	0.57*
4	Peto et al./1985	3211	Textile factory	29	29.0	1.00
5	Hilt et al./1985	287	Chemical plant	3	4.3	0.70
6	Seidman et al./1986	820	Amosite factory	11	5.8	1.90
7	Gardner et al./1986	2167	Chrysotile asbestos-cement factory	15	13.7	1.09
8	Hughes et al./1987	6931	Asbestos-cement factory	22	19.5	1.13
Total		28,368		142	161.1	0.88

* $p < .05$.

Table 9.3 Gastric Cancer Risk in Cross-sectional Cohorts of Asbestos Workers*

				Gastric Cancer		
Ref. No.	*Author/Year*	*No. in Cohort*	*Type of Work*	*Obs. No.*	*Exp. No.*	*O/E*
9	Mancuso and Coulter/1963	1266	Factory	2	1.7	1.18
10	Selikoff et al./1979	632	Insulators— New York/	19	5.4	3.52[†]
		17,800	New Jersey Insulators—US/ Canadian	18	14.2	1.26
11	Puntoni et al./1979	2190	Shipyard	38	28.0	1.36
12	Englund et al./1980	18,421	Plumbers	35	25.1	1.39
		1699	Insulators	8	5.3	1.50
13	Hodgson and Jones/1986	15,999[‡]	All workers in England and Wales	27	26.9	1.00
14	Enterline et al./1987	1074	Factory production and maintenance	20	11.9	1.80[†]
15	Sanden and Jarvholm/1987	3787	Shipyard	3	3.4	0.88
Total		62,968		170	121.9	1.39[†]

* Unpublished summaries kindly provided by William Weiss, MD.
[†] $p < .05$.
[‡] Number obtained from RD Jones, personal communication, October 13, 1986; representing all workers first employed before 1969.

of gastric cancer in communities where the asbestos content of the water is exceedingly high (Marsh, 1983). Experimental investigations have been carried out in several animal species to determine whether or not cancer can be induced in the digestive tract by the feeding of enormous amounts of asbestos. These studies have also proved to be negative (Condie, 1983), or lacked consistent results (Kogan et al., 1987).

In summary, the medical literature documents a number of factors that seem to influence the occurrences of gastric carcinoma. Overall, the observations reported in epidemiological studies are inconsistent with the notion that asbestos contributes to the development of this disease process. And, experimental studies have proven negative.

Colorectal Carcinoma

Colorectal cancer is the second most common malignancy of older men, and the fourth among women of advancing age. Because of its frequent occurrence, the subject of its causation has been the basis for considerable research during the last several decades. Epidemiological studies demonstrate a strong association of colorectal cancer with dietary influences, particularly, the consumption of large amounts of animal fat and red meat, and a relatively fiber-free diet (Ghadirian et al., 1997; La Vecchia et al., 1988; Slattery et al., 1988; Willett et al., 1990). Some investigations have also found a possible association with smoking and alcoholic beverage consumption (Giovannucci et al., 1994a,b; Hilt et al., 1985; Lieberman et al., 2003; Newcomb et al., 1995; Nyrén et al., 1996; Wu and Henderson, 1995). Individuals with colorectal cancer commonly have a strong family history of this disease, and recent studies have documented an autosomal dominant mode of inheritance of a predisposition to colorectal cancer, particularly disease occurring at a relatively young age (Bonelli et al., 1988; Fuchs et al., 1994; Sondergaard et al., 1991). In addition, there are several uncommon, but increasingly well-defined genetic syndromes that predispose one to cancer. Among those that claim an African heritage, there is a 50% greater likelihood of developing colorectal cancer than among Caucasians (Haggitt and Reid, 1986). From these clinical and epidemiological observations, one can conclude that the etiology of colorectal cancer is multifactorial, although the precise mode by which these influences may interact, remains to be defined (Burt et al., 1985; Young and Wolf, 1988).

Detailed studies of the molecular biology and cytogenetics of colorectal cancer indicate that the tumor cells acquire a series of mutational and chromosomal changes that influence the development of the disease. This is reflected in the loss of certain genes and the overexpression of others, ultimately resulting in neoplastic change. It appears that in some cancers, there may be a cumulative influence of several different genetic factors in the development of the tumor.

Can asbestos influence the development of colorectal cancer either as a causative or as a contributory factor? As discussed below, the experimental and epidemiological evidence strongly argues against such a thesis.

From an epidemiological perspective, more than 25 different evaluations of occupationally exposed populations have been carried out to explore this question. These studies have been analyzed in reviews (Demers et al., 1994; Edelman, 1988; Garabrant et al., 1992; Morgan et al., 1985; Weiss, 1995). The latter report evaluates both cohort and case-control studies and considers the estimated intensity of exposure in the analysis. A dosage gradient was not found (Table 9.4).

A meta-analysis by Frumkin and Berlin (1988) suggested that there existed an association of carcinoma of the colorectal tissue with asbestos exposure, but this analysis, in our view, was imperfect because it was based on the notion that the prevalence of lung cancer in a study population is a surrogate for exposure. Rather, the analysis of Frumkin and Berlin can be interpreted to argue for an association of cancer of the colon and rectum with cigarette smoking, a possibility that has not been established, as of yet.

A meta-analysis by Homa et al. (1994) suggested that "exposure to amphibole asbestos may be associated with colorectal cancer, but the findings may reflect an artifact ...." An additional recent meta-analysis by Goodman et al. (1999) in which 69 individual cohorts were evaluated, yielded an SMR of 89, a finding that is compellingly negative.

In a death certificate survey conducted in more than half of the United States, Kang et al. (1997) found a small but significant elevation in the proportional mortality ratio among mechanical, electrical, and electronic engineers, but not in occupations where heavy exposures to asbestos might be expected to occur, such as among insulation workers and plumbers.

Table 9.4 SMR for Lung and Colorectal Cancer by Estimated Exposure Intensity*

| | | Dosage | | |
		Low	Medium	High
Lung carcinoma	SMR	1.03	1.24	1.67
	95% CL	0.9–1.2	1–1.5	1.5–1.9
Colorectal carcinoma	SMR	0.63	0.84	0.64
	95% CL	0.5–0.8	0.6–1.1	0.6–1.2

* Adapted from Demers et al. (1994).

Epidemiological studies have also been conducted to evaluate the association of carcinoma of colorectal tissue with environmental exposure to asbestos in potable water supplies. The US Environmental Protection Agency (EPA) has shown that most Americans are exposed to particulates of asbestos in the water, but almost invariably; these particulates are short (<5 μm) fibers of chrysotile. However, in a study conducted among residents of Duluth, Minnesota that derives its potable water from Lake Superior where the concentrations of amphibole asbestos in the water ranged from 1 to 30 million fibers/L, there was no increase in the occurrence of gastrointestinal neoplasms (Sigurdson et al., 1981). In the six communities studied intensively, the prevalence of colorectal carcinoma was not increased in proportion to the relative amounts of asbestos in the drinking water (Kanarek et al., 1980; Levy et al., 1976; Marsh, 1983). This enormous body of data fails to provide compelling evidence that asbestos in drinking water is a contributory factor in the development of cancer of the colon and rectum.

Debate on this issue continues. Studies by de la Provôte et al. (2002) recently suggested a link of asbestos with lower gastrointestinal tumors, and a paper by Jakobsson et al. (1994) records data indicating that right colon malignant lesions are associated with exposure to asbestos-cement dust, but again, the increase in the risk of disease proved to be minimal.

Attempts to identify occupational groups at high risk for colorectal cancer have been carried out by Berg and Howell (1975) and Spiegelman and Wegman (1985). An association of the neoplasm with specific high-risk groups was not found.

Ingested asbestos transmigrates through the colonic mucosa and is transported through the body by lymphatics in rats administered massive doses of chrysotile and amosite asbestos per os (Westlake et al., 1965). In the studies conducted by Sebastien et al. (1980), fibers were detected at relatively high concentrations in the thoracic duct lymph of experimental animals for 16 hours after ingestion of asbestos. Most fibers were short (ie, <5 μm), although a few of the crocidolite fibers recovered were relatively long, and one measured 41 μm in length! Bolton et al. (1982) were unable to reproduce these findings. However, experimental work in animals has shown that the feeding of asbestos to animals does not contribute to the development of cancer in the lower digestive tract (Condie, 1983; Cunningham et al., 1977; Donham et al., 1980; McConnell et al., 1983a,b; Truhaut and Chouroulinkov, 1989). These observations further argue against the notion that occupational exposure to asbestos contributes to the development of colorectal cancer.

AB and fibers have been found in digests of the colonic tissue of asbestos workers who had carcinoma of the colon, but not in the tissues of unexposed persons with the same tumor (Ehrlich et al., 1985, 1991). No information was provided documenting the presence or absence of AB and asbestos fibers in colorectal tissues of asbestos workers without cancer. In some of the positive cases reported by Ehrlich et al. (1985, 1991), large numbers of short fibers (ie, <5 μm) of chrysotile were found in the colonic tissue. Unfortunately, the report did not provide sufficient information to allow one to rule out contamination of the specimen during collection or processing, an ever-present concern.

Using light microscopy, Rosen et al. (1974), failed to find "typical" AB in digests of the colon of 19 patients with carcinoma of the colon. They reported the presence of small numbers of "atypical" bodies and some ferruginous bodies in some of these cases. In a study of this type the investigator is obliged to carefully discriminate between "true" AB and artifacts.

Recently, Dodson et al. (2000) documented the presence of asbestos fibers in mesenteric and omental tissues of noncancer patients. Again, the ever-present potential problems of contamination of the specimens was not excluded. The mechanisms of transport of asbestos to these tissues is unclear and has not been investigated experimentally.

Pancreatic Carcinoma

Roughly 3% of cancers in the United States develop in nonendocrine pancreatic tissue. Because of the organ's subtle location in the retroperitoneal space, and the tendency for this cancer to become symptomatic only after it has become inoperable, the mortality rate is high. The disease almost invariably is an adenocarcinoma that tends to occur in the fifth and sixth decades of life and affects males more often than females. Attempts to establish an etiology based on epidemiological studies have failed, although cigarette smoking is a possible causative or contributory factor. The risk tends to increase in relationship to tobacco consumption, and appears to be reduced after cessation. But the evidence is by no means compelling. Selikoff and his associates (1980) found no increase in risk among heavy smokers who were asbestos factory workers and insulators. Chemicals of several different formulations induce pancreatic carcinoma in laboratory animals, but asbestos has not been shown to be carcinogenic experimentally.

On the basis of the study of Selikoff and Seidman (1981) and a subsequent national survey of disease in insulators, the question arose, does asbestos have a causative or contributory role in pancreatic cancer? Surveys of workers in refineries and petrochemical plants (Tsai et al., 1996), textile factory (Brown et al., 1994; Dement, 1994), railroad shops (Ohlson et al., 1984), an insulation factory (Acheson et al., 1984) and shipyards (Puntoni et al., 1979) have failed to demonstrate an association (Table 9.5). And, a recent meta-analysis by Goodman et al. (1999) came to a similar conclusion. In the absence of compelling epidemiological evidence, one is obliged to conclude that asbestos is not a risk factor for pancreatic carcinoma.

Renal Cell Carcinoma

The etiology and pathogenesis of the commonly occurring renal cell carcinoma of the kidney is obscure, but exposure to cigarette smoke, drugs such as Phenacetin, petrochemical effluents, and heavy metals, including lead and calcium, have been implicated as possible causes (Brownson, 1988; McLaughlin et al., 1984).

In 1979, Selikoff and his associates noted an apparent increase in the prevalence of renal cell carcinoma among North American insulation workers. Studies by Enterline (1987), Puntoni and coworkers (1979), and Maclure (1987) demonstrated a similar increase in risk for asbestos workers. Unfortunately, the Enterline (1987) and Puntoni et al. (1979) investigations failed to consider the prevalence of tobacco use. In addition, the tumors of the renal parenchyma (renal cell carcinoma) were not differentiated in the analysis from transitional cell carcinomas that develop in the renal pelvis. Both of these

Table 9.5 Results of Epidemiological Studies Examining the Possible Association of Asbestos Exposure with Pancreatic Carcinoma

	SMR	RR
Selikoff et al. (1980)	—	1.8
Acheson et al. (1984)	96	—
Putino et al. (1979)	—	<1
Ohlson et al. (1984)	111	—
Dement et al. (1994)	128	—
Tsai et al. (1996)	84	—

malignant lesions are epidemiologically associated with cigarette smoking, and a dosage effect has been documented for the cancers of the urinary drainage system (Hartge et al., 1987; La Vecchia et al., 1990). Thus, the variables of asbestos exposure and tobacco use, accompanied by inattention to considerations of tumor type and latency period, have compromised analyses.

Evaluations of renal parenchymal tissue from nonoccupationally exposed persons at autopsy (Huang et al., 1988) have yielded asbestos fibers and a microscopical survey (Auerbach et al., 1980) documented AB in histologic sections. Rats administered asbestos by lavage similarly had demonstrable asbestos in the renal parenchyma (Patel-Mandlik and Millette, 1983). In a single obscure publication by Gibel et al., 1976, several rats fed high concentrations of chrysotile asbestos developed neoplasms believed to be renal cell carcinomas. The results of this work have not been reproduced.

Cook and Olsen (1979) detected asbestos fibers in the urine of Duluth, MN residents drinking unfiltered Lake Superior water that contained low concentrations of amphibole asbestos fibers. The particles in the drinking water and urine were exceedingly short, that is, mean fiber length and breadth were 0.96 and 0.17 μm. Guillemin et al. (1989) evaluated the urine of employees of an asbestos-cement factory. The mean concentration of chrysotile in the urine of the asbestos-exposed workers was twofold greater than in control subjects, but the number of crocidolite particles in the urine of the controls was greater than in those exposed in the cement factory. Again, the fibers were exceedingly short and of no probable pathogenic importance (Mean geometric length/breadth of chrysotile: 0.47/0.068 μm, and crocidolite: 0.68/0.1 μm). Because of the inevitable problems resulting from extraneous contamination in the laboratory, these results must be evaluated with critical skepticism.

In a case-controlled study of 147 cases of renal cell carcinoma, exposure to asbestos was found to be associated with a RR of 1.62 (95% confidence index (CI) = 1.3–16.6) (McCredie and Stewart, 1993). A link with employment in dry cleaning, the iron and steel industry, and possibly petroleum refinery employment was also found in this study. In a similar investigation of more than 700 male cases of renal cell carcinoma in New Zealand stratified by age and smoking background, an association with asbestos exposure was not detected, although painters, glass workers, and firefighters were claimed to be at increased risk (Delahunt et al., 1995). An association with asbestos exposure was not demonstrated in an evaluation of 26 renal cancer deaths occurring in a Texas chemical plant (Bond, 1985). Work by Auperin et al. (1994) yielded a similar conclusion, and a recent comprehensive meta-analysis by Goodman et al. (1999) failed to demonstrate an association of renal cancer with asbestos exposure. It is important to note that in many of the negative studies, there was a paucity of workers whose trades might have been expected to result in heavy exposure to asbestos.

Although a low order of association of asbestos with renal cell carcinoma has been suggested by some investigators, the bulk of the evidence argues against a causative role for asbestos in kidney cancer. It should be recognized, however, that the difficulties one encounters in conducting a definitive study are imposing, considering all the potentially confounding variables. In the writer's view, the finding of minute fibers of asbestos in kidney tissue and urine is of doubtful significance with regard to cancer causation, although it vividly shows that asbestos is distributed widely in the tissues of those who are exposed to industrial aerosols (if not all of us).

Lymphoid Malignancies

Non-Hodgkin's lymphoma, chronic lymphogenous leukemia, and multiple myeloma have as their common denominator an origin in elements of the lymphoid and hematopoietic systems. In general, these are diseases of advancing age. This is a heterogeneous family of sporadically occurring malignancies with a nomenclature that is in a state of flux as the various morphologic types are characterized by molecular approaches and immunocytochemistry (Harris et al., 2000). To a large extent, the etiology is unknown, although experimental and some epidemiological evidence implicate viruses, chemicals, and irradiation (Craighead, 2000; Pearce and Bethwaite, 1992). For reasons that are unclear, the overall incidence of these neoplasms in the general population is increasing (Weisenburger, 1994).

Over the past several decades, case reports and surveys of various occupational groups have documented the occurrence of malignant disease of the lymphoid system in patients with the stigmata of an asbestos-associated disease and among those who claim environmental exposure to asbestos (Table 9.6). Non-Hodgkin's lymphoma of the pleura and lung parenchyma, and immunoblastic lymphadenopathy in the thorax also have been reported in patients with an occupational history of asbestos exposure (Gerber 1970; Maguire et al., 1981; Parisio et al., 1999). And, cases of lymphoblastic leukemia, lymphoma, and

Table 9.6 Literature Review of Malignant Diseases of Lymphoplasmocytic Cells Associated with Asbestos Exposure

Non-Hodgkin's lymphoma

Bengtsson	1982
Dworsky et al.	1982
Elmes and Simpson	1971
Efremidis et al.	1985
Gerber	1970
Kagan and Jacobson	1983
Kang et al.	1997
Lieben	1966
Mancuso and El-Attar	1967
McDonald	1980
Olsson and Brandt	1983
Waxweiler and Robinson	1983

Chronic lymphocytic leukaemia

Bianchi et al.	1979
Epremidis et al.	1985
Kagan and Jacobson	1983
Lieben	1966
Spanedda et al.	1983

Multiple myeloma

DeCarvalho	1973
Gerber	1970
Kagan and Jacobson	1983
Lieben	1966
Linet et al.	1987
Morris et al.	1986
Spanedda et al.	1983
Schwartz et al.	1988

plasmacytoma have been described in a coincidental association with MM presumably caused by asbestos (Efremidis et al., 1985; Perry et al., 1978; Takabe et al., 1997). Many of the reports summarize a cumulated series of cases (Table 9.6; Kagan and Jacobson, 1983; Kagan, 1988). However, in a national survey of more than 1.7×10^4 insulators, Selikoff et al. (1979) found no increase in the incidence of lymphoma or leukemia.

Two case-controlled studies have been carried out. In the report by Schwartz et al. (1988), 4.3×10^2 patients with chronic lymphatic leukemia and almost 7×10^2 with multiple myeloma were studied using controls from the patients' community. Asbestos exposure was assessed on the basis of the job category of the patient, but a critical individual evaluation of exposure was not done. An estimate of the severity of exposure for the patients with lymphoma and leukemia was made, but even when the exposure to asbestos was thought to be heaviest, the RR was only 1.4 with 95% (CI = 0.8–2.3). An association with asbestos exposure was not found for patients with multiple myeloma. A second case-control study was reported by Ross et al. (1982). Patients with large cell lymphomas of the digestive tract were evaluated using a limited number of control subjects and a pair analytical approach. As with the study of Schwartz et al. (1988), the likelihood of asbestos exposure was estimated on the basis of occupation, inasmuch as little objective information was available. In this investigation, the RR proved to be 12, a highly significant result! Unfortunately, additional epidemiological investigations using contemporary approaches and a more critical appraisal of asbestos exposure were not carried out; thus, these intriguing findings have not been confirmed.

A panoply of reports (de Shazo et al., 1983; Dubois et al., 1989; Dworsky et al., 1982; Garcia et al., 1989; Gaurmer et al., 1981; Hartmann et al., 1984; Kagan et al., 1977; Kouzan et al., 1985; Lange et al., 1978; Miller and Kagan, 1981; Rom and Travis, 1992; Warheit et al., 1985; Wilson et al., 1977) argue that chronic stimulation of the immune system by asbestos might result in malignancy. However, concrete support for this thesis, based on experimental or clinical observations, is lacking. And, no compelling mechanistic explanation for malignant transformation of lymphoid elements (that incorporates these diverse experimental observations) has been proposed. Since lymphomas, chronic lymphogenous leukemia, and multiple myeloma occur commonly in the elderly, and overall comprise about 2% of malignancies in this age group, one would anticipate that an inquisitive physician could elicit a history of an actual or alleged asbestos exposure in a sizable proportion of those so affected. Thus, critical skepticism of claims of a disease association is warranted at this time.

References

Acheson ED, Gardner MJ, Winter PD, Bennett C. Cancer in a factory using amosite asbestos. *Int J Epidemiol.* 1984;13:3–10.

Auerbach O, Conston AS, Garfinkel L, Parks VR, Kaslow HD, Hammond EC. Presence of asbestos bodies in organs other than the lung. *Chest.* 1980;77:133–137.

Auperin A, Benhamou S, Ory-Paoletti C, Flamant R. Occupational risk factors for renal cell carcinoma: a case-control study. *Occup Environ Med.* 1994;51:426–428.

Bengtsson NO, Hardell L, Erikson M. Asbestos exposure and malignant lymphoma. *Lancet.* 1982;2:1463.

Berg JW, Howell MA. Occupational and bowel cancer. *J Toxicol Environ Health.* 1975;1:75–89.

Berry G, Newhouse ML. Mortality of workers manufacturing friction materials using asbestos. *Br J Ind Med.* 1983;40:1–7.

Blaser MJ. Hypothesis: the changing relationships of Helicobacter pylori and humans: implications for health and disease. *J Infect Dis.* 1999;179:1523–1530.

Blot WJ. Esophageal cancer trends and risk factors. *Sem Oncol.* 1994;21:403–410.

Blot WJ, Morris LE, Stroube R, Tagnon I, Fraumeni JF Jr. Lung and laryngeal cancers in relation to shipyard employment in coastal Virginia. *JNCI.* 1980;65:571–575.

Blot WJ, Stone BJ, Fraumeni JF Jr, Morris LE. Cancer mortality in US counties with shipyard industries during World War II. *Environ Res.* 1979;18:281–290.

Bolton RE, Davis JMG, Lamb D. The pathological effects of prolonged asbestos ingestion in rats. *Environ Res.* 1982;29:134–150.

Bond GG, Shellenberger RJ, Flores GH, Cook RR, Fishbeck WA. A case-control study of renal cancer mortality at a Texas chemical plant. *Am J Ind Med.* 1985;7:123–139.

Bonelli L, Martines H, Conio M, Bruzzi P, Aste H. Family history of colorectal cancer as a risk factor for benign and malignant tumours of the large bowel. A case control study. *Int J Cancer.* 1988;41:513–517.

Botha JL, Irwig LM, Strebel PM. Excess mortality from stomach cancer, lung cancer and asbestosis and/or mesothelioma in crocidolite mining districts in South Africa. *Am J Epidemiol.* 1986;123:30–40.

Brown DP, Dement JM, Okun A. Mortality patterns among female and male chrysotile asbestos textile workers. *J Occup Med.* 1994;36:882–888.

Brown LM, Mason TJ, Pickle LW, et al. Occupational risk factors for laryngeal cancer on the Texas gulf coast. *Cancer Res.* 1988;48:1960–1964.

Brown LM, Silverman DT, Potern LM, et al. Adenocarcinoma of the esophagus and esophagogastric junction in white men in the United States: alcohol, tobacco and socioeconomic factors. *Cancer Causes Control.* 1994;5:333–340.

Brownson RC. A case-control study of renal cell carcinoma in relation to occupation, smoking, and alcohol consumption. *Arch Environ Health.* 1988;43:238–241.

Brownson RC, Chang JC. Exposure to alcohol and tobacco and the risk of laryngeal cancer. *Arch Environ Health.* 1987;42:192–196.

Burch JD, Howe GR, Miller AB, Semenciw R. Tobacco, alcohol, asbestos, and nickel in the etiology of cancer of the larynx: a case-control study. *JNCI.* 1981;67:1219–1224.

Burt RW, Bishop DT, Cannon LA, Dowdle MA, Lee RG, Skolnick MH. Dominant inheritance of adenomatous colonic polyps and colorectal cancer. *N Engl J Med.* 1985;312:1540–1544.

Cantor KP, Sontag JM, Held MF. Patterns of mortality among plumbers and pipefitters. *Am J Ind Med.* 1986;10:73–89.

Chan CK, Gee BL. Asbestos exposure and laryngeal cancer: an analysis of the epidemiologic evidence. *J Occup Med.* 1988;30:23–27.

Chow W-H, Finkle WD, McLaughlin JK, Frankl H, Ziel HK, Fraumeni JF. The relation of gastroesophageal reflux disease and its treatment to adenocarcinomas of the esophagus and gastric cardia. *JAMA.* 1995;274:474–477.

Clemmesen J, Hjalgrim-Jensen S. Cancer incidence among 5686 asbestos-cement workers followed from 1943 through 1976. *Ecotoxicol Environ Saf.* 1981;5:15–23.

Coggon D, Barker DJ, Cole RB. Stomach cancer and work in dusty industries. *Br J Ind Med.* 1990;47:298–301.

Condie LW. Review of published studies of orally administered asbestos. *Environ Health Perspect.* 1983;53:3–9.

Cook PM, Olson GF. Ingested mineral fibers: elimination in human urine. *Science.* 1979;204:195–198.

Craighead JE, ed. *Pathology of Human Environmental and Occupational Disease.* St. Louis, MO: Mosby Year-Book, Inc.; 1995.

Craighead JE. *Pathology and Pathogenesis of Human Viral Infection.* New York: Academic Press, Inc.; 1999.

Craighead JE. *Pathology and Pathogenesis of Human Viral Disease,* San Diego: Academic Press; 2000.

Cunningham HM, Moodie CA, Lawrence GA, Pontefract RD. Chronic effects of ingested asbestos in rats. *Arch Environ Contam Toxicol.* 1977;6:507–513.

Delahunt B, Bethwaite PB, Nacey JN. Occupational risk for renal cell carcinoma. A case control study based on the New Zealand Cancer Registry. *Br J Urology.* 1995;75:578–582.

de la Provôte S, Desoubeaux N, Paris C, et al. Incidence of digestive cancers and occupational exposure to asbestos. *Eur J Cancer Prev.* 2002;11:523–528.

Dement JM, Brown DP, Okun A. Follow-up study of chrysotile asbestos textile workers: cohort mortality and case-control analyses. *Am J Ind Med.* 1994;26:431–447.

Demers RY, Burns PB, Swanson GM. Construction occupations, asbestos exposure, and cancer of the colon and rectum. *J Occup Med.* 1994;36:1027–1031.

de Shazo RD, Hendrick DJ, Diem JE, et al. Immunologic aberrations in asbestos cement workers: dissociation from asbestosis. *J Allergy Clin Immunol.* 1983;72:454–461.

Dodson RF, O'Sullivan MF, Huang J, Holiday DB, Hammar SP. Asbestos in extrapulmonary sites: omentum and mesentery. *Chest.* 2000;117:486–493.

Doll R, Peto J. Other asbestos-related neoplasms. In: Antman K, Aisner J, eds. *Asbestos-Related Malignancy.* Chap. 4, New York: Grune & Stratton; 1987: 81–96.

Donham KJ, Berg JW, Will LA, Leininger JR. The effects of long-term ingestion of asbestos on the colon of F344 rats. *Cancer.* 1980;45:1073–1084.

Dubois C, Bissonnette E, Rola-Pleszczynski M. Leukotriene B4 and tumor necrosis factor production after in vitro exposure of rat alveoloar macrophages to mineral dust: potential role in fibrogenesis. In: Mossman BT, Begin RO, eds. *Effects of Mineral Dusts on Cells,* New York: Springer-Verlag; 1989: 389.

Dworsky R, Ross R, Nichols P, Paganini-Hill A, Lukes R, Henderson B. *Asbestos exposure associated with large cell lymphomas of the gastrointestinal tract. Proceedings of the 13th International Cancer Congress,* Seattle, WA; September 8–15, 1982: 657.

Edelman DA. Exposure to asbestos and the risk of gastrointestinal cancer: a reassessment. *Br J Ind Med.* 1988;45:75–82.

Edelman DA. Laryngeal cancer and occupational exposure to asbestos. *Int Arch Occup Environ Health.* 1989;61:223–227.

Efremidis AP, Waxman JS, Chahinian AP. Association of lymphocytic neoplasia and mesothelioma. *Cancer.* 1985;55:1056–1059.

Ehrlich A, Gordon RE, Dikman SH. Carcinoma of the colon in asbestos-exposed workers: analysis of asbestos content in colon tissue. *Am J Ind Med.* 1991;19:629–636.

Ehrlich A, Rohl AN, Holstein EC. Asbestos bodies in carcinoma of colon in an insulation worker with asbestosis. *JAMA.* 1985;254:2932–2933.

Elmes C, Simpson MJC. Insulation workers in Belfast. 3. Mortality 1940–1966. *Br J Ind Med.* 1971;28:226–232.

Elwood JM, Pearson JCG, Skippen DH, Jackson SM. Alcohol, smoking, social and occupational factors in the aetiology of cancer of the oral cavity, pharynx and larynx. *Int J Cancer.* 1984;34:603–612.

Englund A. Cancer incidence among painters and some allied trades, In: Vainio H, Sorsa M, Hemminki K, eds. *Occupational Cancer and Carcinogenesis,* New York: Hemisphere Publishing Corp.; 1981: 1267–1273.

Englund A. Cancer incidence among painters and some allied trades. *J Toxicol Environ Health.* 1980;6:1267–1273.

Enterline PE, Hartley J, Henderson V. Asbestos and cancer: a cohort followed up to death. *Br J Ind Med.* 1987;44:396–401.

Enzinger PC, Mayer RJ. Esophageal cancer. *N Engl J Med.* 2003;349:2241–2252.

Flanders WD, Cann CI, Rothman KJ, Fried MP. Work-related risk factors for laryngeal cancer. *Am J Epidemiol.* 1984;119:23–32.

Forastiere A, Koch W, Trotti A, Sidransky D. Head and neck cancer. *N Engl J Med.* 2001;345:1890–1900.

Frumkin H, Berlin J. Asbestos exposure and gastrointestinal malignancy review and meta-analysis. *Am J Ind Med.* 1988;14:79–95.

Fuchs CS, Giovannucci EL, Colditz GA, Hunter DJ, Speizer FE, Willett WC. A prospective study of family history and the risk of colorectal cancer. *N Engl J Med.* 1994;331:1669–1674.

Gammon MD, Schoenberg JB, Ahsan H, et al. Tobacco, alcohol, and socioeconomic status and adenocarcinomas of the esophagus and gastric cardia. *J Natl Cancer Inst.* 1997;89:1277–1284.

Gao Y-T, McLaughlin JK, Blot WJ, et al. Risk factors for esophageal cancer in Shanghai, China. I. Role of cigarette smoking and alcohol drinking. *Int J Cancer.* 1994;58:192–196.

Garabrant DH, Peters RK, Homa DM. Asbestos and colon cancer: lack of association in a large case-control study. *Am J Epidemiol.* 1992;135:843–853.

Garcia JG, Griffith DE, Cohen AB, Callahan KS. Alveolar macrophages from patients with asbestos exposure release increased levels of leukotriene B4. *Am Rev Respir Dis.* 1989;139:1494–1501.

Gardner MJ, Winter PD, Pannett B, Powell CA. Follow-up study of workers manufacturing chrysotile asbestos cement products. *Br J Ind Med.* 1986;43:726–732.

Garewal HS, Sampliner R. Barrett's esophagus: a model premalignant lesion for adenocarcinoma. *Prev Med.* 1989;18:749–756.

Gaumer HR, Doll NJ, Kaimal J, Schuyler M, Salvaggio JE. Diminished suppressor cell function in patients with asbestosis. *Clin Exp Immunol.* 1981;44:108–116.

Gerber MA. Asbestosis and neoplastic disorders of the hematopoietic system. *Am J Clin Pathol.* 1970;53:204–208.

Ghadirian P, Lacroix A, Maisonneuve P, et al. Nutritional factors and colon carcinoma. A case control study involving French Canadians in Montreal, Quebec, Canada. *Cancer.* 1997;80:858–864.

Gibel W, Lohs K, Korn KH, Wildner GP, Hoffmann F. Tierexperimentelle Untersuchungen uber eine kanzerogene Wirkung von Asbestfiltermaterial nach oraler Aufnahme. *Arch Geschwulst.* 1976;46:437–422.

Giovannucci E, Rimm EB, Stampfer MJ, et al. A prospective study of cigarette smoking and risk of colorectal adenoma and colorectal cancer in U.S. men. *J Natl Cancer Inst.* 1994a;86:183–191.

Giovannucci E, Rimm EB, Stampfer MJ, Colditz GA, Ascherio A, Willett WC. Intake of fat, meat, and fiber in relation to risk of colon cancer in men. *Cancer Res.* 1994b:54:2390–2397.

Goodman M, Morgan RW, Ray R, Malloy CD, Zhao K. Cancer in asbestos-exposed occupational cohorts: a meta-analysis. *Cancer Causes Control.* 1999;10:453–465.

Graham S. Future inquiries into the epidemiology of gastric cancer. *Cancer Res.* 1975;35:3464–3468.

Guillemin MP, Litzistorf G, Buffat PA. Urinary fibres in occupational exposure to asbestos. *Ann Occup Hyg.* 1989;33:219–233.

Haenszel W, Correa P. Developments in the epidemiology of stomach cancer over the past decade. *Cancer Res.* 1975;35:3452–3459.

Haggitt RC, Reid BJ. Hereditary gastrointestinal polyposis syndromes. *Am J Surg Pathol.* 1986;10:871–887.

Hartmann DP, Georgian MM, Oghiso Y, Kagan E. Enhanced interleukin activity following asbestos inhalation. *Clin Exp Immunol.* 1984;55:643–650.

Harris NL, Jaffe ES, Diebold J, et al. *The World Health Organization classification of hematological malignancies report of the clinical advisory committee meeting*, Airlie House, Virginia, November 1977. *Mod Pathol.* 2000;13:193–207.

Hartge P, Silverman D, Hoover R, et al. Changing cigarette habits and bladder cancer risk: a case-control study. *JNCI.* 1987;78:1119–1125.

Herity B, Moriarty M, Daly L, Dunn J, Bourke GJ. The role of tobacco and alcohol in the aetiology of lung and larynx cancer. *Br J Cancer.* 1982;46:961–964.

Hill AB. The environment and disease: association or causation? *Proc R Soc Med.* 1965;58:295–300.

Hillerdal G, Lindholm C-E. Laryngeal cancer and asbestos. *ORL.* 1980;42:233–241.

Hilt B, Langard S, Anderson A, Rosenberg J. Asbestos exposure, smoking habits and cancer incidence among production and maintenance workers in an electrochemical plant. *Am J Ind Med.* 1985;8:565–577.

Hinds MW, Thomas DB, O'Reilly HP. Asbestos, dental x-rays, tobacco, and alcohol in the epidemiology of laryngeal cancer. *Cancer.* 1979;44:1114–1120.

Hirsch A, Bignon J, Sebastien P, Gaudichet A. Asbestos fibers in laryngeal tissues. Findings in two patients with asbestosis associated with laryngeal tumors. *Chest.* 1979;76:697–699.

Hodgson JT, Jones RD. Mortality of asbestos workers in England and Wales 1971–81. *Br J Ind Med.* 1986;43:158–164.

Hoey J, Montvernay C, Lambert R. Wine and tobacco: risk factors for gastric cancer in France. *Am J Epidemiol.* 1981;113:668–674.

Homa DM, Garabrant DH, Gillespie BW. A meta-analysis of colorectal cancer and asbestos exposure. *Am J Epidemiol.* 1994;139:1210–1222.

Huang J, Hisanaga N, Sakai K, et al. Asbestos fibers in human pulmonary and extrapulmonary tissues. *Am J Ind Med.* 14:331–339, 1988.

Hughes JM, Weill H, Hammad YY. Mortality of workers employed in two asbestos cement manufacturing plants. *Br J Ind Med.* 1987;44:161–174.

Jakobsson K, Albin M, Hagmar L. Asbestos, cement, and cancer in the right part of the colon. *Occup Environ Med.* 1994;51:95–101.

Jankowski JA, Wright NA, Meltzer SJ, et al. Molecular evolution of the metaplasia-dysplasia-adenocarcinoma sequence in the esophagus. *Am J Pathol.* 1999;154:965–973.

Kagan E. Current issues regarding the pathobiology of asbestosis: a chronologic perspective. *J Thorac Imaging.* 1988;3:109.

Kagan E, Jacobson RJ. Lymphoid and plasma cell malignancies: asbestos-related disorders of long latency. *Am J Clin Pathol.* 1983;80:14–20.

Kagan E, Solomon A, Cochrane JC, et al. Immunological studies of patients with asbestosis. I. Studies of cell-mediated immunity. *Clin Exp Immunol.* 1977;28:261–267.

Kanarek MS, Conforti PM, Jackson LA, Cooper RC, Murchio JC. Asbestos in drinking water and cancer incidence in the San Francisco Bay area. *Am J Epidemiol.* 1980;112:54–72.

Kanazawa K, Birbeck MS, Carter RL, Roe FJC. Migration of asbestos fibers from subcutaneous injection sites in mice. *Br J Cancer.* 1970;24:96–106.

Kang S-K, Burnett CA, Freund E, Walker J, Lalich N, Sestito J. Gastrointestinal cancer mortality of workers in occupations with high asbestos exposures. *Am J Ind Med.* 1997;31:713–718.

Kogan FM, Vanchugova NN, Frasch VN. Possibility of inducing glandular stomach cancer in rats exposed to asbestos. *Br J Ind Med.* 1987;44:682–686.

Kouzan S, Brody AR, Nettesheim P, Eling T. Production of arachidonic acid metabolites by macrophages exposed in vitro to asbestos, carbonyl iron particles, or calcium ionophore. *Am Rev Respir Dis.* 1985;131:624–632.

Lagergren J, Bergstrom R, Lindgren A, Nyrén O. Symptomatic gastroesophageal reflux as a risk factor for esophageal adenocarcinoma. *N Eng J Med.* 1999;340:825–831.

Lange A, Smolik R, Chmielarczyk W, Garncarek D, Gielgier Z. Cellular immunity in asbestosis. *Arch Immunol Ther Exp (Warsz).* 1978;26:899–903.

La Vecchia C, Negri E, Decarli A, et al. A case control study of diet and colo-rectal cancer in northern Italy. *Int J Cancer.* 1988;41:492–498.

La Vecchia C, Negri E, D'Avanzo B, Franceschi S. Smoking and renal cell carcinoma. *Cancer Res.* 1990;50:5231–5233.

Levy BS, Sigurdson E, Mandel, J, Laudon E, Pearson J. Investigating possible effects of asbestos in city water: Surveillance of gastrointestinal cancer incidence in Duluth, Minnesota. *Am J Epidemiol.* 1976;103:362–368.

Liddell FDK. Laryngeal cancer and asbestos. *Br J Ind Med.* 1990;47:289–291.

Lieben J. Malignancies in asbestos workers. *Arch Environ Health.* 1966;13:619–621.

Lieberman DA, Prindiville S, Weiss DG, Willett W, for the VA Cooperative Study Group 380. Risk factors for advanced colonic neoplasia and hyperplastic polyps as asymptomatic individuals. *JAMA.* 2003;290:2959–2967.

Lindor NM, Rabe K, Peterson GM, et al. Lower cancer incidence in Amsterdam. Criteria families without mismatch repair deficiency. *JAMA.* 2005;293:1779–1785.

Linet MS, Harlow SD, McLaughlin JK. A case-control study of multiple myeloma in Whites: chronic antigenic stimulation, occupation, and drug use. *Cancer Res.* 1987;47:2978–2981.

Luce D, Guenel P, Leclerc A, Brugere J, Point D, Rodriguez J. Alcohol and tobacco consumption in cancer of the mouth, pharynx, and larynx: a study of 316 female patients. *Laryngoscope.* 1988;98:313–316.

Maclure M. Asbestos and renal adenocarcinoma. A case-control study. *Environ Res.* 1987;42:353–361.

Maguire FW, Mills RC, Parker FP. Immunoblastic lymphadenopathy and asbestosis. *Cancer.* 1981;47:791–797.

Mancuso T, Coulter E. Methodology in industrial health studies. *Arch Env Health.* 1963;6:36–52.

Mancuso TF, El-Attar AA. Mortality pattern in a cohort of asbestos workers. A study based on employment experience. *J Occup Med.* 1967;9:147–162.

Marsh GM. Critical review of epidemiologic studies related to ingested asbestos. *Environ Health Perspect.* 1983;53:49–56.

McConnell EE, Rutter HA, Urland BM, Moore JA. Chronic effects of dietary exposure to amosite asbestos and tremolite in F344 rats. *Environ Health Perspect.* 1983a;53:27–44.

McConnell EE, Shefner AM, Rust JH, Moore JA. Chronic effects of dietary exposure to amosite and chrysotile asbestos in Syrian golden hamsters. *Environ Health Perspect.* 1983b;53:11–25.

McCredie M, Stewart J. Risk factors for kidney cancer in New South Wales: IV Occupation. *Br J Ind Med.* 1993;50:349–354.

McDonald AD, Fry JS, Woolley AJ, McDonald JC. Dust exposure and mortality in an American chrysotile asbestos friction products plant. *Br J Ind Med.* 1984;41:151–157.

McDonald JC, Liddell FDK, Gibbs GW, Eyssen GE, McDonald AD. Dust exposure and mortality in chrysotile mining, 1910–75. *Br J Ind Med.* 1980;37:11–24.

McDonald JC. Asbestos-related disease: an epidemiological review. In: Wagner JC, ed., *Biological Effects of Mineral Fibres.* Vol. 2. Lyon, France: World Health Organization. International Agency for Research on Cancer; 1980:587–601.

McLaughlin JK, Gridley G, Block G, et al. Dietary factors in oral and pharyngeal cancer. *J Natl Cancer Inst.* 1988;80:1237–1243.

McLaughlin JK, Mandel JS, Blot WJ, Schuman LM, Mehl ES, Fraumeni JF Jr. A population-based case-control study of renal cell carcinoma. *JNCI.* 1984;72:275–284.

Miller K, Kagan E. Manifestations of cellular immunity in the rat after prolonged asbestos inhalation. II. Alveolar macrophage-induced splenic lymphocyte proliferation. *Environ Res.* 1981;26:182–194.

Morgan RW. Meta-analysis of asbestos and gastrointestinal cancer. *Am J Ind Med.* 1991;19:407–411.

Morgan RW, Foliart DE, Wong O. Asbestos and gastrointestinal cancer. A review of the literature. *West J Med.* 1985;143:60–65.

Mork J, Lie AK, Glattre E, et al. Human papillomavirus infection as a risk factor for squamous cell carcinoma of the head and neck. *N Engl J Med.* 2001;344:11125–11131.

Morris PD, Koepsell TD, Daling JR, et al. Toxic substance exposure and multiple myeloma: a case-control study. *JNCI.* 1986;76:987–994.

Muscat JE, Wynder EL. Tobacco, alcohol, asbestos, and occupational risk factors for laryngeal cancer. *Cancer.* 1992;69:2244–2251.

Nam J, McLaughlin JK, Blot JK. Cigarette smoking, alcohol, and nasopharyngeal carcinoma: a case control study among U.S. whites. *J Natl Cancer Inst.* 1992;84:619–622.

Newcomb PA, Storer BE, Marcus PM. Cigarette smoking in relation to risk of large bowel cancer in women. *Cancer Res.* 1995;55:4906–4909.

Newhouse ML, Berry G, Wagner JC. Mortality of factory workers in East London 1933–80. *Br J Ind Med.* 1985;42:4–11.

Newhouse ML, Gregory NM, Shannon H. Aetiology of carcinoma of the larynx. In: Wagner JC, ed. *Biological Effects of Mineral Fibres*. Lyon: International Agency for Research on Cancer, 1980 (Sci Publ No 33).

Nogueira C, Figueiredo C, Carneiro F, et al. Helicobacter pylori genotypes may determine gastric histopathology. *Am J Pathol*. 2001;158:647–654.

Nyrén O, Bergström R, Nystgröm L, et al. Smoking and colorectal cancer: a 20 year follow-up study of Swedish construction workers. *J Natl Cancer Inst*. 1996;88:1302–1307.

Ohlson C-G, Klaesson B, Hogstedt C. Mortality among asbestos-exposed workers in a railroad workshop. *Scand J Work Environ Health*. 1984;10:283–291.

Olsen J, Sabroe S. Occupational causes of laryngeal cancer. *J Epidemiol Comm Health*. 1984;38:117–121.

Olsson H, Brandt L. Asbestos exposure and non-Hodgkin's lymphoma. *Lancet*. 1983;1:588.

Parisio E, Bianchi C, Rovej R, Sparacio F, Ferrari A, Scanni A. Pulmonary asbestosis associated to pleural non-Hodgkin's lymphoma. *Tumori*. 1999;85:75–77.

Parnes SM. Asbestos and cancer of the larynx: is there a relationship? *Laryngoscope*. 1990;100:254–261.

Patel-Mandlik KJ, Millette JR. Chrysotile asbestos in kidney cortex of chronologically gavaged rats. *Arch Environ Contam Toxicol*. 1983;12:247–255.

Pearce N, Bethwaite P. Increasing incidence of non-Hodgkin's lymphoma: occupational and environmental factors. *Cancer Res*. 1992;52(19 Suppl):5496s–5500s.

Perry MC, Solinger A, Farhangi M, Luger A. Plasmacytomas and mesothelioma. *Med Pediatr Oncol*. 1978;5:205–212.

Peto J, Doll R, Hermon C, Binns W, Clayton R, Goffe T. Relationship of mortality to measures of environmental asbestos pollution in an asbestos textile factory. *Ann Occup Hyg*. 1985;29:305–355.

Puntoni R, Vercelli M, Merlo F, Valerio F, Santi L. Mortality among shipyard workers in Genoa, Italy. *Ann NY Acad Sci*. 1979;330:353–377.

Ries LAG, Eisner MP, Kosary C, et al., eds. *SEER Cancer Statistics Review, 1973–1999*. Bethesda, MD: National Cancer Institute; 2002.

Roggli VL, Greenberg D, McLarty JL, Hurst GA, Spivey CG, Heiger LR. Asbestos body content of the larynx in asbestos workers. A study of five cases. *Arch Otolaryngol*. 1980;106:533–535.

Rom WN, Travis WD. Lymphocyte-macrophage alveolitis in nonsmoking individuals occupationally exposed to asbestos. *Chest*. 1992;101:779–786.

Rosen P, Savino A, Melamed M. Ferruginous (asbestos) bodies and primary carcinoma of the colon. *Am J Clin Pathol*. 1974;61:135–138.

Ross R, Nichols P, Wright W, et al. Asbestos exposure and lymphomas of the gastrointestinal tract and oral cavity. *Lancet*. 1982;2:1118–1120.

Rothman KJ, Cann CI, Flanders D, Fried MP. Epidemiology of laryngeal cancer. *Epidemiol Rev*. 1980;2:195–209.

Rubino GF, Piolatto G, Newhouse ML, Scansetti G, Aresini GA, Murray R. Mortality of chrysotile asbestos workers at the Balangero Mine, Northern Italy. *Br J Ind Med*. 1979;36:187–194.

Sanden A, Jarvholm B. Cancer morbidity in Swedish shipyard workers 1978–1983. *Intn Arch Occup Health*. 1987;59:455–462.

Schwartz DA, Vaughan TL, Heyer NJ, et al. B cell neoplasms and occupational asbestos exposure. *Am J Ind Med*. 1988;14:661–671.

Sebastien P, Masse R, Bignon J. Recovery of ingested asbestos fibers from the gastrointestinal lymph in rats. *Environ Res*. 1980;22:201–216.

Seidman H, Selikoff IJ, Gelb SK. Mortality experience of amosite factory workers: dose-response relationships 5 to 40 years after onset of short-term work exposure. *Am J Ind Med*. 1986;10:479–514.

Selikoff IJ, Churg J, Hammond EC. Asbestos exposure and neoplasia. *JAMA*. 1964;188:22–26.

Selikoff IJ, Hammond EC, Churg J. Asbestos exposure, smoking, and neoplasia. *JAMA*. 1968;204:106–112.

Selikoff IJ, Hammond EC, Seidman H. Mortality experience of insulation workers in the United States and Canada, 1943–1976. *Ann NY Acad Sci.* 1979;330:91–116.

Selikoff IJ, Seidman H. Cancer of the pancreas among asbestos insulation workers. *Cancer.* 1981;47(6 Suppl):1469–1473.

Selikoff IJ, Seidman H, Hammond EC. Mortality effects of cigarette smoking among amosite asbestos factory workers. *J Natl Cancer Inst.* 1980;65:507–513.

Shettigara PT, Morgan RW. Asbestos, smoking and laryngeal carcinoma. *Arch Environ Health.* 1975;30:517–519.

Sigurdson EE, Levy BS, Mandel J, et al. Cancer morbidity investigations: lessons from the Duluth study of possible effects of asbestos in drinking water. *Environ Res.* 1981; 25:50–61.

Slattery ML, Sorenson AW, Mahoney AW, French TK, Kritchevsky D, Street JC. Diet and colon cancer: assessment of risk by fiber type and food source. *J Natl Cancer Inst.* 1988;80:1474–1480.

Smith AH, Handley MA, Wood R. Epidemiological evidence indicates asbestos causes laryngeal cancer. *J Occup Med.* 1990;32:499–507.

Søndergaard JO, Bülow S, Lynge E. Cancer incidence among parents of patients with colorectal cancer. *Int J Cancer.* 1991;47:202–206.

Spanedda R, Barbieri D, La Corte R. Response letter to: Waxweiler RJ and Robinson C: asbestos and Non-Hodgkin's lymphoma. *Lancet.* 1983;1:189–190.

Spechler SJ, Goyal RK. Barrett's esophagus. *N Engl J Med.* 1986;315:362–371.

Spiegelman D, Wegman DH. Occupation-related risks for colorectal cancer. *JNCI.* 1985;75:813–821.

Stell PM, McGill T. Asbestos and laryngeal carcinoma. *Lancet.* 1973;2:416–417.

Takabe K, Tsukada Y, Shimizu T, et al. Malignant lymphoma involving the penis following malignant pleural mesothelioma. *Intern Med.* 1997;36:712–715.

Talamini R, La Vecchia C, Levi F, Conti E, Favero A, Franceschi S. Cancer of the oral cavity and pharynx in nonsmokers who drink alcohol and in nondrinkers who smoke tobacco. *J Natl Cancer Inst.* 1998;90:1901–1903.

Thomas HF, Benjamin IT, Elwood PC, Sweetnam PM. Further follow-up study of workers from an asbestos cement factory. *Br J Ind Med.* 1982;39:273–276.

Truhaut R, Chouroulinkov I. Effects of long-term ingestion of asbestos fibers in rats. In: Bignon J, Peto J, Saracci R, eds. IARC Scientific Publication no. 90. Lyon: International Agency for Research on Cancer, 1989;127–133.

Tsai SP, Waddell LC, Gilstrap EL, Ransdell JD, Ross CE. Mortality among maintenance employees potentially exposed to asbestos in a refinery and petrochemical plant. *Am J Ind Med.* 1996;29:89–98.

Tuyns AJ, Esteve J, Raymond L, et al. Cancer of the larynx/hypopharynx, tobacco and alcohol: IARC international case-control study in Turin and Varese (Italy), Zaragoza and Navarra (Spain), Geneva (Switzerland) and Calvados (France). *Int J Cancer.* 1988;41:483–491.

Van Houten VMM, Snuders PJF, van den Brekel MWM, et al. Biological evidence that human papillomaviruses are etiologically involved in a subgroup of head and neck squamous cell carcinomas. *Int J Cancer.* 2001;93:232–235.

Warheit DB, George G, Hill LH, Snyderman R, Brody AR. Inhaled asbestos activates a complement-dependent chemoattractant for macrophages. *Lab Invest.* 1985;52:505–514.

Waxweiler RJ, Robinson C. Asbestos and Non-Hodgkin's lymphoma. *Lancet.* 1983;1:189–190.

Weisburger JH, Raineri R. Dietary factors and the etiology of gastric cancer. *Cancer Res.* 1975;35:3469–3474.

Weisenburger DD. Epidemiology of non-Hodgkin's lymphoma: recent findings regarding an emerging epidemic. *Ann Oncol.* 1994;5(Suppl 1):19–24.

Weiss W. The lack of causality between asbestos and colorectal cancer. *J Environ Med.* 1995;37:1364–1373.

Westlake GE, Spjut HJ, Smith MN. Penetration of colonic mucosa by asbestos particles. An electron microscopic study in rats fed asbestos dust. *Lab Invest.* 1965;14:2029–2033.

Willett WC, Stampfer MJ, Colditz GA, Rosner BA, Speizer FE. Relation of meat, fat, and fiber intake to the risk of colon cancer in a prospective study among women. *N Engl J Med.* 1990;323:1664–1672.

Williams RR, Horm JW. Association of cancer sites with tobacco and alcohol consumption and socioeconomic status of patients: Interview study from the third National Cancer Survey. *J Natl Cancer Inst.* 1977;58:525–547.

Wilson MR, Gaumer HR, Salvaggio JE. Activation of the alternative complement pathway and generation of chemotactic factors by asbestos. *J Allergy Clin Immunol.* 1977;60:218–222.

Wu AH, Henderson BE. Alcohol and tobacco use: risk factors for colorectal adenoma and carcinoma? Alcohol and tobacco use: risk factors for colorectal adenoma and carcinoma? *J Natl Cancer Inst.* 1995;87:239–240.

Wu AH, Wan P, Bernstein L. A multiethnic population-based study of smoking, alcohol and body size and risk of adenocarcinoma of the stomach and esophagus (United States). *Cancer Causes Control.* 2001;12:721–732.

Wu-Williams AH, Tu MC, Mack TM. Life-style, workplace, and stomach cancer by subsite in young men of Los Angeles County. *Cancer Res.* 1990;50:2569–2576.

Young TB, Wolf DA. Case control study of proximal and distal colon cancer and diet in Wisconsin. *Int J Cancer.* 1988;42:167–175.

Yu MC, Garabrant DH, Peters JM, Mack TM. Tobacco, alcohol, diet, occupation, and carcinoma of the esophagus. *Cancer Res.* 1988;48:3843–3848.

Zagraniski RT, Kelsey JL, Walter SD. Occupational risk factors for laryngeal carcinoma: Connecticut, 1975–1980. *Am J Epidemiol.* 1986;124:67–76.

Zhang Z-F, Kurtz RC, Marshall JR. Cigarette smoking and esophageal and gastric cardia adenocarcinoma. *J Natl Cancer Inst.* 1997;89:1247–1249.

Zoloth S, Michaels D. Asbestos disease in sheet metal workers: the results of a proportional mortality analysis. *Am J Ind Med.* 1985;7:315–321.

10

Diagnostic Features and Clinical Evaluation of the Asbestos-Associated Diseases

David Weill

Introduction

Asbestos exposure is associated with a variety of pulmonary manifestations, ranging from mild, asymptomatic changes primarily discovered radiographically, to severe diseases resulting in significant respiratory compromise. Although decreasing in frequency and severity as workplace exposures have been reduced, clinical pulmonologists must be familiar with the many different lung diseases associated with asbestos exposure and understand the diagnostic modalities available today, which differ from those used in the past. In this chapter, the clinical manifestations of asbestos-associated lung problems will be reviewed with particular emphasis on the milder forms of the diseases, which are now more common.

Although Occupational Safety and Health Administration (OSHA) has promulgated regulations since the early 1970s in an effort to reduce asbestos exposure, between 1920 and 1970 the worldwide production of asbestos increased 25-fold. During this period, it was recognized that asbestos exposure could lead to nonmalignant conditions such as the parenchymal fibrotic lung disease known as asbestosis and pleural diseases such as pleural effusion, diffuse pleural fibrosis (DPF), pleural plaques (PP), and rounded atelectasis (RA), but its role in the pathogenesis of malignant conditions, such as lung cancer (LC) and malignant mesothelioma (MM) was uncertain.

Occupational History

As in most aspects of medicine, an appropriate history is necessary to establish a diagnosis. In no area of medicine is this more important than in diagnosing occupation-related disorders. In addition to documenting the chronology of a worker's various jobs, one must accomplish at least a qualitative assessment of workplace exposures. This can, of course, be difficult when a worker has had many occupations spanning a lifetime. Further, recollection can either vary regarding precise duration and types of exposure, or workers may be unaware that asbestos existed in their workplace. Alternatively, because the potential hazard of asbestos exposure has now been brought to the attention of the public through the lay press and as a result of litigation, some workers may be overly concerned about their own asbestos exposure, if only trivial. Therefore, for a variety of reasons, workers may either under- or overestimate their exposure, which can diminish the quality of the occupational history.

In formulating a work history chronology, the physician must determine the type of work performed, the duration of each job, and the type of asbestos-containing products that were used. Because of the inherent latency of the asbestos-related diseases, occupations of more than 15 years' duration in the past should be emphasized. Also, a description of the intensity of each exposure is necessary to, at least qualitatively, estimate exposure. Patients should also be asked about their hobbies, living situation, and other nonoccupational activities that could be associated with exposure to asbestos. Because workers can transport asbestos into the home by means of their work clothes, the physician should ask about relatives who worked in occupations that may have involved exposure to asbestos. Of course, as with any medical history, intensity and duration of tobacco use must be defined, as smoking is associated with lung disease unrelated to pneumoconioses.

Lung Parenchymal Disease

Lung disease related to asbestos exposure is caused by the deposition of asbestos fibers in the alveoli of the lung (Chapters 3 and 6). Although effective defense mechanisms exist to prevent fiber accumulation in the deeper regions of the lung, these defenses can be overwhelmed by heavy exposures. When this happens, there occurs a cascade of events characterized initially by inflammation and, if repair is not successful, later by fibrosis. It is likely that the malignancies associated with asbestos exposure share similar molecular and biochemical pathways with those that lead to fibrosis.

Diagnosis

Asbestosis is a nonmalignant, fibrotic parenchymal lung disease associated with heavy and prolonged asbestos exposure. Clinically, the disease can be static or slowly progressive. When progressive, asbestosis can lead to profound respiratory disability after cessation of exposure. Because histological samples usually are not available for pathological study in suspected cases of asbestosis, the diagnosis customarily is based on clinical parameters alone, such as those established by Committees of the American Thoracic Society in 1986 and 2004. Because of the infrequency with which lung tissue is available for microscopical analysis, clinical parameters were given higher importance in establishing a diagnosis of asbestosis. The findings that were considered helpful in diagnosing asbestosis included:

1. A reliable exposure history
2. An appropriate time interval between exposure and detection of disease (a latency period of a "minimum of 15 years and more often considerably longer"). The Committees also noted several clinical criteria that were thought to be of *recognized value* (emphasis added). Unfortunately, the criteria listed below are often used in the medical-legal setting as being, if present individually, sufficient to establish an asbestosis diagnosis. These criteria include

    a. Chest radiograph evidence of small irregular opacities with a profusion of 1/1 or greater

  b. A restrictive pattern of lung function demonstrated by pulmonary function testing
  c. A diffusion capacity below normal
  d. Bilateral late inspiratory crackles

The consensus view in 1986 was revised by a committee that published a statement in 2004 (ATS Statement; Ohar et al., 2004). Similar diagnostic considerations were included in the updated version, but there was some modification in the manner by which the various clinical parameters were presented. As a result, the more recently described diagnostic criteria are more inclusive and nonspecific and therefore, not especially helpful to the clinician. Of course, as with any set of diagnostic guidelines, the criteria described above should take into account the presence of individual patient variability with the recognition that not all the criteria need be present to establish a diagnosis. The presence of certain combinations of the criteria lends more certainty to a diagnosis of asbestosis.

Physical Signs and Symptoms

A complete physical examination is essential for evaluating patients with suspected pneumoconioses. While the findings are rarely specific for a particular occupationally related lung disease, certain features such as cyanosis in the extremities, finger clubbing, and an abnormal chest examination may at least indicate that lung disease is present. For example, while clubbing can be associated with asbestosis, it is also present in other lung diseases, especially idiopathic pulmonary fibrosis, cystic fibrosis, or LC. Less common causes of finger clubbing include bronchiectasis, cirrhosis, tuberculosis, and lung abscess. Clubbing is rare even in established cases of asbestosis and therefore, relying on its presence or absence is not helpful. However, when present, it is associated with a poor prognosis (Coutts et al., 1987; Ohar et al., 2004).

The symptoms of asbestosis usually have an insidious onset but they initially include dyspnea. Chest pain occurs occasionally in advanced cases when either a significant restrictive defect in function or extensive pleural thickening is present. The presence of persistent chest pain should prompt an investigation designed to detect an asbestos-related pleural effusion, metastatic LC to the chest wall, or a MM. A dry cough is common, particularly as the disease advances, but a productive cough can be present in smokers with chronic bronchitis as well as acute and chronic pulmonary disease. Hemoptysis is not a feature of the disease. If it has occurred, one must exclude concomitant LC or other lung diseases such as tuberculosis, pneumonia, and pulmonary embolization. As with many lung conditions, advanced disease usually results in weight loss, likely due, in part, to the caloric expenditure associated with tachypnea.

The most consistent physical finding in patients with asbestosis is inspiratory crackles. Crackles (or rales) heard on chest auscultation are usually present in asbestosis but can also be found in patients with any one of a variety of interstitial lung diseases, as well as heart failure, bronchiectasis, and pneumonia. Crackles can also be detected in cigarette smokers in the absence of obvious pulmonary disorders. Crackles associated with asbestosis are fine and usually occur with each inspiratory effort, a feature that unfortunately does not distinguish them from crackles due to any diffuse pulmonary fibrotic lung disease. At earlier stages of the disease, crackles are best appreciated in the lower lung zones, but as the disease progresses, they are found throughout the lungs.

Wheezes are not a feature of asbestosis and, if present, lead one to consider airways diseases such as chronic bronchitis in either cigarette smokers or persons with asthma. A pleural rub is occasionally heard in patients with DPF. Cyanosis can be present in any one of a variety of cardiopulmonary disorders that cause hypoxemia; therefore, it is not helpful in distinguishing between asbestosis and several other conditions. In advanced disease, signs of right-sided heart failure (ie, jugular venous distension, ascites, and lower extremity edema) can be found. Perhaps the most important aspect of the examination of exposed workers is the finding of physical signs that suggest another pulmonary disease is present (eg, decreased breath sounds on auscultation and hyperresonance on percussion consistent with emphysema).

Radiological Features

Chest radiographs are essential for the diagnosis of asbestosis. As discussed in Chapter 11, the chest radiograph can determine objectively if there is a lung abnormality and what the finding most likely represents. In this regard, the International Labour Office (ILO) has devised a classification scheme that attempts to semiquantitate the degree and type of radiograph abnormalities using a standardized system. The purpose of the ILO/UICC system is to standardize the interpretation of chest radiographs using descriptions of the size, shape, and degree of involvement (ie, the profusion) of radiographic abnormalities. The schema was developed to systemize the reading of x-rays in the pneumoconiosis, both for epidemiological studies and for the longitudinal monitoring of changes in the lungs in individual patients. It does not serve as a basis for establishing a specific diagnosis such as asbestosis and silicosis. Correlative studies have yet to be conducted comparing the various pathological findings with the indicators of disease in ILO/UICC system, as discussed below. The system organizes the interpretation of the reader into shape (small regular or small irregular) and size assessments (small regular: p, q, r, and small irregular: s, t, u). Further, the extent of radiographic abnormalities (profusion) is numbered from normal to increasingly abnormal. The reader also indicates which of the six lung zones are involved. The presence and type of pleural abnormalities are noted, a consideration that is particularly important in the asbestos-associated disease. The schema is discussed in greater detail in Chapter 11.

With regard to the typical chest radiographic appearance, certain distinct abnormalities exist with asbestosis. Asbestosis is generally characterized by lower lobe involvement with the presence of small irregular opacities. In advanced disease, which rarely occurs now, these parenchymal abnormalities can be found in all lung zones, but the abnormalities seen in lower profusion categories are typically lower zone in distribution. The radiographic changes associated with asbestosis are similar to findings in other diseases in which the radiograph reflects diffuse interstitial reticular infiltrates. There is evidence that cigarette smoking alone can lead to radiographic changes that are similar to those due to asbestosis (ie, the presence of small irregular opacities) (Barnhart et al., 1990; Blanc et al., 1988; Hnizdo et al., 1988). The pulmonary changes attributable to emphysema must also be distinguished from the linear and reticular markings of asbestosis. As the disease progresses, the linear opacities become thicker and may ultimately obliterate the vascular markings and the change known as "honeycombing" can be found, especially in the subpleural areas of the lower lobes. "Large" opacities are not seen in asbestosis, unless heavy silica exposure has also occurred and, if present, should raise for consideration the possibility of a LC.

Commonly, but not universally, pleural abnormalities (DPF or PP) are seen in association with the parenchymal changes. Pleural thickening can either be diffuse or focal (PP). DPF is usually present in the lower and middle third of the chest and is often asymmetric. Pleural thickening often leads to costophrenic angle obliteration, a nonspecific change, and is distinguished from PP by the presence of its costophrenic angle location.

In cases where pleural changes due to asbestos exposure are unable to be differentiated from intercostal adipose deposits in the chest wall, oblique radiographs of the chest can often be helpful.

RA is a radiographic finding unique to asbestos pleural disease (Chapters 6 and 11). It represents a folded area of pleura, which traps the adjacent lung tissue. RA is often mistaken for a lung mass and can lead unnecessarily to further invasive evaluation. Because of its characteristic computed axial tomography (CAT) appearance, RA usually can be confidently diagnosed by experienced radiologists. Serial CAT scanning can help exclude a malignancy.

CAT scanning has dramatically increased diagnostic sensitivity (Lozewicz et al., 1989), particularly when using high-resolution computed tomography (HRCT) is used. CAT can also be helpful in distinguishing *en face* PP seen in a routine chest radiograph from parenchymal lesions and can assist in the identification of parenchymal abnormalities when pleural changes obscure the lung parenchyma on chest radiographs. Unfortunately, CAT rarely assists the physician in distinguishing asbestosis from other types of fibrotic lung diseases such as idiopathic pulmonary fibrosis, collagen-vascular associated interstitial lung disease, and drug-induced lung diseases. Studies that support the higher sensitivity of HRCT in diagnosing asbestosis (Neri et al., 1994, 1996; Staples et al., 1989) are limited by their low specificity. The challenge for the clinician is to determine whether or not to assign clinical significance to marginally abnormal CAT scans, and to distinguish between "true" abnormalities and normal variations.

Pathophysiological Features

The physiologic abnormalities associated with asbestosis are due to the parenchymal fibrosis that characterizes the disease. Classically, when advanced asbestosis is present, reduced lung compliance resulting in a restrictive lung functional defect is the most common pulmonary abnormality. Specifically, a reduction in the residual volume (RV) and the total lung capacity (TLC) is usually seen. However, because many patients with asbestosis have, in addition, emphysema (characterized by an increased RV and TLC), a normal or even increased RV and TLC can be present, depending on the relative contribution of each disease. This situation results in a mixed obstructive-restrictive functional defect. Also, because the gas exchange in the alveoli is altered by the fibrotic process, a reduction of the diffusing capacity (DC) is often seen; some have claimed that a reduction in DC is an early indicator of disease. Further, because of the presence of low lung compliance, increased minute ventilation is observed as the respiratory rate increases and the tidal volume decreases. The ventilation changes are particularly marked at the lung bases, the area of the lung most extensively involved in asbestosis. The abnormalities of respiratory mechanics are exacerbated by exercise. Thus, exercise testing tends to unmask occult disease. The pathophysiologic findings described above for asbestosis are nonspecific and can be found in any of the restrictive lung diseases. Artifactual abnormalities and patient noncompliance are an ever present concern to the pulmonary physiologist.

The role of the small airways in the pathophysiology of asbestosis remains unclear, largely because much of the clinical information is derived from cohorts with a high prevalence of cigarette smoking. While structural abnormalities are demonstrated histologically in the small airways of exposed workers (Churg et al., 1985; Chapter 6), the findings are often confounded by the effects of cigarette smoking. Further, studies which purportedly demonstrated a small-airways effect from asbestos exposure rely on the FEF_{25-75}, which is an effort-dependent test that has large variability. A study by

Begin et al. (1983) analyzed a nonsmoking asbestos-exposed cohort. Airflow resistance predominated in patients who also had restrictive pulmonary function. In the nonsmoking workers who did not have restriction, physiologic abnormalities in the small airways were small. A more detailed discussion of the airway function associated with the asbestos-exposed appears later in this chapter.

Bronchoscopy

Transbronchial lung biopsy (TBB) is generally not required to diagnose asbestosis. Asbestos bodies (AB) can be demonstrated in lung tissue, but the TBB sample is usually small and not sufficiently representative to accomplish pathological diagnosis with confidence. Bronchoalveolar lavage (BAL) performed on patients with asbestosis often demonstrates an alveolar macrophage alveolitis with or without an increase in neutrophils, but these findings are nonspecific (Rebuck and Braude, 1983). It has been suggested that neutrophilia correlates with the severity of disease but the evidence is not compelling (Rom et al., 1991; Xaubet et al., 1986). The number of AB present in a BAL is not a reliable marker of lung fibrosis due to asbestos inhalation (Xaubet et al., 1986). Chapter 6 considers these issues in detail.

Distinguishing among the Diffuse Interstitial Lung Diseases

When confronted with the presence of widespread abnormalities in chest radiographs, pulmonary practitioners attempt to categorize the abnormalities into broad radiographic patterns. As described above, asbestosis presents radiographically with reticular (or linear) abnormalities, but many fibrotic lung conditions have a similar radiographic appearance. In addition to a reticular pattern, many fibrotic lung diseases are characterized radiographically by lower zone predominance, traction bronchiectasis, and honeycombing. Although a thorough discussion of all the causes of diffuse lung disease is beyond the scope of this chapter (there are over 100 causes of diffuse interstitial lung disease), one is able to generate a preliminary differential diagnosis based on the presences of reticular infiltrates on chest radiograph. Although these radiographic patterns hold up fairly well in the early or intermediate stages of diffuse lung disease, they are less reliable as the disease progresses toward end-stage. A partial list of lung diseases that have a reticular radiographic pattern is included as Table 10.1 (Figure 10.1).

Distinguishing among these diseases requires the clinician to consider other nonradiographic factors, most notably a work history and, if available, pathological tissue. Particularly in instances where other causes of diffuse interstitial lung disease need to be excluded, a lung biopsy (preferably by obtaining adequate tissue through a surgical approach) should be considered. Also, the clinical course can give some hint about the etiology of the diffuse lung infiltrates. For instance, one is more confident that the patient does not have asbestosis if there is a rapid clinical progression, which would favor a diagnosis such as idiopathic pulmonary fibrosis. Diagnostic uncertainty can be particularly pronounced when concomitant emphysema or other lung conditions are present, which alter the typical radiographic and pathophysiologic picture. Suffice it to state, the diagnostic possibilities are numerous when confronted with patients who have diffuse lung parenchymal abnormalities. A detailed discussion of the diagnostic approaches to idiopathic diffuse pulmonary disease is provided in recent reviews (Flaherty et al., 2004).

Table 10.1 Diseases Sharing Radiographic Features of Asbestosis

Idiopathic pulmonary fibrosis
Collagen-vascular diseases
Chronic hypersensitivity pneumonitis
Chronic eosinophilic pneumonia
Drug-induced pneumonitis
Radiation pneumonitis

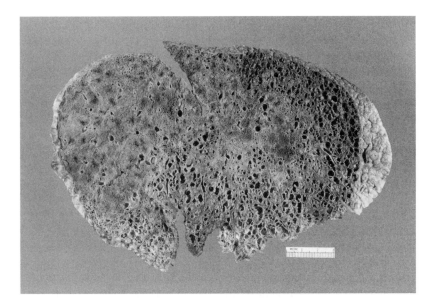

Figure 10.1 Usual interstitial fibrosis of the lungs of a 45-year-old priest. Note the diffuse fibrous obliteration of the lung parenchyma, with extensive "honeycombing." The pleural surface displays a "cobblestone" appearance reflecting the "honeycombing," but it is not thickened and there are no adhesions. These features contrast with asbestosis, a disease characterized grossly by predominantly lower lobe fibrosis and prominent diffuse pleural fibrosis.

Clinical Course (Progression)

Once considered inevitable, progression of asbestosis is no longer certain, particularly when the patient is removed from exposure (Jones et al., 1989; Rubino et al., 1979). The type of exposure is also an important factor in predicting influencing progression. Chrysotile exposure appears to lead to progression in far fewer cases and at a slower rate than when asbestosis is due to amphibole exposure (Churg, 1991; Liddell and McDonald, 1991). Gaensler and his colleagues (1990a,b) also found that progression was more likely to occur when workers smoked cigarettes and when the latency period was short as compared to those who gradually developed fibrosis over a 20-year period after the first exposure. In patients in whom disease stability has been monitored for greater than 10 years, the likelihood of progression is small. There is seldom progression when a patient presents with a low profusion chest radiograph (ILO category 1/0 or 1/1) and further exposure does not occur thereafter. A detailed discussion of progression is found in Chapter 6.

Malignant Mesothelioma

MM should be considered in patients who have an exposure history and latency period and in whom characteristic chest radiographic findings are present (Chapter 11). In patients who present with such findings, the next diagnostic step should be a thoracentesis, which is helpful in excluding other causes of unilateral pleural effusion, but is an infrequent diagnostic basis for MM because definitive cytological assessment is often difficult. High concentrations of hyaluronic acid are found in the pleural fluid in some cases, but its presence is inconsistent and assays are not generally available in clinical laboratories (Chiu et al., 1984). The presence of hyaluronic acid is believed by some to suggest a better prognosis (Frebourg et al., 1987; Thylen et al., 2001). A high serum hyaluronic acid level can help differentiate pleural effusions due to MM from those due to other causes, and may assist the clinician in following an individual patient's clinical course. Other biochemical markers, such as the carcinoembryonic antigen (CEA), have been reported to be helpful, particularly when distinguishing MM from adenocarcinoma, since CEA is only elevated in carcinomas. In a study investigating the role of CEA in assessments of pleural fluid, cytologically confirmed cases of MM were not found when the CEA level was greater than 2.9 ng/mL, while 67% of the adenocarcinoma cases had fluid concentrations above 15 ng/mL (Robinson et al., 1986). More recently, CEA in combination with another tumor marker, CYFRA 21-1, was found to be helpful in distinguishing between MM and metastatic cancers in the pleura. Elevated CYFRA 21-1 in association with a low CEA concentration was found to be highly suggestive of MM, while a high CEA level alone, or a high concentration of both markers, suggested other causes for the malignant effusions (Paganuzzi et al., 2001).

Pleural biopsy, ideally with video-assisted thoracoscopic surgery (VATS), is the diagnostic "gold standard" for the diagnosis of MM. Using VATS, tumor studding of the pleural surface can be appreciated, and the surgeon is able to perform biopsies under direct visualization. Another benefit of this procedure is the ability to mobilize the lung and to perform cytoreductive pleurectomy (Grossebner et al., 1999).

Physical Signs and Symptoms

Patients with MM usually seek medical attention initially because of unilateral chest pain. Commonly, the pain is pleuritic and can be either dull or quite sharp. The chest pain is generally constant and does not change with position. As the disease progresses, the tumor and its associated pleural effusion cause shortness of breath by mechanically limiting lung expansion. Temporary symptomatic relief can be obtained by performing periodic thoracenteses. The reduction in breathlessness provided by multiple drainage procedures, however, has to be weighed against the risk of seeding the needle tract to the pleural space with tumor, a not uncommon complication. When advanced disease is present the utility of repeat pleural space drainage is limited, because the lung essentially becomes encased with fibrous tissue and malignant tumor.

Cough can be a feature of the disease especially when tumor encasement of the lung results in significant atelectasis. Other problems associated with tumor growth include involvement of the pericardium and great vessels of the thorax, both of which may result in cardiac arrhythmias, accompanied by metastasis to the heart and the superior vena cava syndrome.

Peritoneal MM usually presents with ascites and abdominal pain. The cystic variant may cause intermittent bouts of severe abdominal pain but is rarely fatal. Other more aggressive forms of peritoneal MM can spread to the mesenteric lymph nodes and surrounding tissue and through the diaphragm into the chest. On physical examination, an abdominal mass can occasionally be appreciated as it protrudes from the abdominal wall but is more commonly obscured by the large volume of ascitic fluid. If a peritoneal MM is clinically suspected, laparoscopy should be performed and multiple biopsies obtained. Once a diagnosis is confirmed, CAT scans of the chest, abdomen, and pelvis help to rule out systemic disease. If systemic disease is discovered and no intestinal obstruction is present, induction intraperitoneal chemotherapy (CH) is recommended with subsequent restaging and cytoreductive surgery, followed by additional CH. If intestinal obstruction is seen with evidence of only localized disease, cytoreductive surgery should be performed with subsequent CH. If systemic disease is present without evidence of intestinal obstruction, intraperitoneal CH is the preferred treatment.

Radiographic Features

Pleural MM generally present radiographically as a unilateral pleural effusion. In some cases, the pleural effusion is accompanied by the appearance of a pleura-based mass, or masses, which may appear nodular. Mediastinal structures may either be shifted away from the side of the tumor, or toward the tumor side when the predominant tissue reaction to the MM is pleural fibrosis. Pleural MM is usually, but not always, associated with concomitant PP or asbestosis. As the tumor advances, compression of adjacent organs, such as the heart, can distort the central airways and damage adjacent ribs. A detailed, discussion of the radiological features of the disease is found in Chapter 11.

Benign Asbestos-Associated Pleural Diseases

In any individual patient, one or a combination of the pleural findings may be present. While most cases of pleural disease are seen after asbestos exposure in the occupational setting on rare occasions, pleural changes can be found in patients with low levels of exposure, such as changes occurring in environmental or nonoccupational settings. These conditions are discussed in detail in Chapters 6 and 11.

Pleural Plaques

PP are localized, discrete areas of dense fibrosis tissue located on the parietal pleural surface. PP can be either calcified or noncalcified and are generally found on the diaphragmatic pleural surface or along the lateral chest wall. More rarely, fibrous plaques can also be seen on the pericardium. When present along the lateral chest wall, they form a sharp interface with the adjacent lung parenchyma and are termed *in profile* plaques. PP may also exist on the anterior or posterior chest wall and in this position are described as *en face* plaques. PP most closely correlate with the interval of time since first exposure, and are uncommonly seen during the first 20 years of exposure. The pathological and radiological features of PP are described in Chapters 6 and 11.

The effects of asbestos-induced benign pleural conditions on pulmonary function have been controversial since this subject was first studied in the mid-1960s. Firm conclusions have been difficult to reach because of (1) the difficulty of taking into account asbestos exposure, which may have effects on pulmonary function other than those mediated through pleural lesions, (2) the disagreement over the type and extent of radiographic pleural abnormalities, and (3) the many potential confounding factors of reduced pulmonary function, such as cigarette smoking, age, concurrent occupational exposures, and prior chest diseases or trauma.

There is significant disagreement about the functional implications of PP. Although the issue of whether or not PP result in any respiratory disability has been debated for years in the literature, there is little doubt that most individuals with PP are asymptomatic and have no measurable physiologic impairment (Copley et al., 2001; Van Cleemput et al., 2001). Further, in many studies purporting to demonstrate functional impairment due to pleural abnormalities, a distinction was not made between those with localized PP alone and those with concomitant DPF. In the study of Van Cleemput et al. (2001), the authors neither found a relationship between the extent of the PP and lung function, nor was the size of the PP related to either cumulative asbestos exposure, or time since first exposure. In cases where PP are present and where patients are symptomatic and/or have abnormal pulmonary function, one must consider alternative explanations such as either concomitant emphysema or the presence of interstitial lung disease that is either asbestos- or nonasbestos-related. In a study by Schwartz and colleagues (1990), for example, the presence of parietal PP positively correlated with restrictive ventilatory defects, but the authors were unable to exclude the presence of concomitant parenchymal lung disease that was not detected by routine chest radiography. In another study by Sette et al. (2004), the presence of parenchymal lung disease was predictive of gas exchange impairment, but the presence and number of PP failed to provide an additional ability to predict abnormalities of gas exchange above that seen with only parenchymal abnormalities. Reaching a similar conclusion, Gaensler et al. (1990a,b) found no functional impairment in workers with circumscribed PP as compared to those either with no history of exposure or those without PP. Functional abnormalities were observed only in patients with both PP and asbestosis.

Other studies regarding lung function and PP have reached different conclusions. For example, a cohort of almost 400 railroad workers was evaluated for the presence and extent of PP (Oliver et al., 1988). PP were observed in 22.6% of the workers. A decrease in forced vital capacity (FVC) was associated with the presence and the extent of the PP. The DC was similar in the groups with and without PP. The findings supported an association between asbestos-related PP and decremental changes in lung function as measured by FVC. However, the study was limited by the inclusion of more smokers and older workers in the study group. In other investigations (Fridriksson et al., 1981), parenchymal fibrosis in workers with PP was considered to be important in the pathogenesis of restrictive lung changes.

Although many PP slowly progress over time, there is some debate regarding their prognostic implications. While there are no clearly defined mechanisms describing PP as a precursor of MM, some studies have shown a higher risk of MM among those with PP (Hillerdal, 1994; Weiss, 1993). However, it remains unclear whether there is simply an association between PP and MM (because both result from amphibole asbestos exposure). Or, does the presence of PP actually indicate sufficient exposure to increase the risk for MM? Unfortunately, the available data does not answer this question.

The association between PP and LC has also been debated in the medical literature. In the study of Hughes and Weill (1991), the presence of PP was not associated with an increased LC risk. A subsequent meta-analysis performed by Weiss (1993) indicated that, of the 13 studies analyzed, only 3 supported the hypothesis that LC risk is elevated among persons with PP. The positive studies were the most problematic from a methodological standpoint: The Weiss study has been criticized because unrealistically large population studies would be needed to demonstrate a statistical relation between PP and LC. In addition, low-exposure studies were included in the analysis. Nonetheless, the weight of the evidence favors the conclusion that persons with asbestos-related PP do not have an increased risk of LC in the absence of parenchymal asbestosis. A more recent Finnish study evaluated 1.7×10^6 male construction workers for cancer from 1990 to 2000 (Koskinen et al., 2002). Standardized incidence ratios and relative risks (RR) were calculated in a multivariate analysis in comparison to a low-exposure group. Radiographic lung fibrosis indicated a two- to threefold RR for LC, while there was no apparent increase in risk for those with PP.

Although there are some studies that show a positive correlation, very few have controlled for the presence of asbestosis. One such investigation from Sweden evaluated almost 1.6×10^3 men with PP (Hillerdal, 1994). The number of MM and LC were compared with the age- and year-specific expected incidence. The risk of LC for patients with bilateral PP but without asbestosis was increased 1.4 times, which was statistically significant. There were nine MM, while only 0.8 cases were expected. The authors concluded that PP not only implied significant exposure to asbestos but also an increased risk for MM and LC, although the risk for LC was small.

Diffuse Pleural Fibrosis

DPF can be either seen on plain chest radiographs or, more readily by CAT scans (al Jarad et al., 1991). According to the 2000 ILO/UICC radiological classification system, DPF by definition includes involvement of the costophrenic angle. If the costophrenic angle is not involved, pleural fibrosis is classified as localized (ie, PP). Thickening of the visceral pleura can be either unilateral or bilateral. If unilateral, the presence of pleural fibrosis from previous pneumonia with pleural reaction, empyema, or trauma are possible and must be excluded. Of course, the clinician must also consider MM in this circumstance. DPF can be seen in collagen-vascular diseases such as rheumatoid arthritis, scleroderma, or systemic lupus erythematosus. Up to one-third of patients with DPF have experienced a previous benign asbestos-related pleural effusion or pleurisy (Yates et al., 1996; Chapter 6).

Patients with DPF exhibit a restrictive lung defect (Ameille et al., 2004; Kee et al., 1996; Kouris et al., 1991; McGavin and Sheers, 1984). Also, there is considerable evidence that a reduction in the DC is common (Kee et al., 1996). Kilburn and Warshaw (1991) evaluated impairment of lung function associated with different types of asbestos-related disease in almost 1.3×10^3 men. Patients with circumscribed PP, or diffuse pleural thickening but without asbestosis, were compared with men suffering from asbestosis and with men having both pleural abnormalities and asbestosis. Nonsmoking men with pleural disease only exhibited reduced mid expiratory air flow and a reduced FEV_1 (Forced Expiratory Volume in 1 second). These men had normal FVC and TLC. Thus, there was evidence of airways obstruction without restriction. Nonsmoking men with presumptive pulmonary asbestosis (ILO profusion of opacities mostly 1/0 and 1/1) exhibited function similar to men with pleural disease. FEV_1 and FVC and midflow air rates were lower in smokers with asbestosis (after adjustment for duration of smoking) than in nonsmokers with asbestosis. Airflow limitation was worse in the men with both pleural abnormalities and asbestosis among both nonsmokers and current smokers. Men with DPF displayed more airways obstruction and air trapping and lower FVC values than those with circumscribed PP.

Most patients with DPF are asymptomatic. However, there is some evidence that those with DPF have a higher incidence of breathlessness, cough with sputum production, and chest pain (Ameille et al., 2004; Kouris et al., 1991; McGavin and Sheers, 1984) as compared to those without pleural disease or with localized pleural abnormalities. In the relatively few impaired patients, treatment options such as surgical decortication are generally not recommended.

Benign Pleural Effusions

The pathophysiology explaining the effusions is unclear. Inhaled asbestos can also indirectly cause pleural injury by the release of growth factors and inflammatory cytokines from the lung. Whatever the mechanism, most clinical information comes from small series of cases. Some, but not all, effusions are associated with pleuritic chest pain. Regardless of symptomatology, all who present with a pleural effusion should undergo diagnostic thoracentesis with cytological analysis of fluid sediments. If a clear etiology of the effusion is not forthcoming, pleural biopsy should be considered, particularly to exclude the presence of MM.

Robinson and Musk (1981) evaluated 22 patients with benign effusions who had a mean duration of exposure of 5.5 years. The mean interval between exposure and clinical presentation was 16.3 years. Five of the effusions were asymptomatic. The pleural fluid was usually hemorrhagic. The mean duration to clinical resolution of the effusion was 4.3 months. During a follow-up period of 28 years, seven patients had a single recurrence and only one patient had multiple pleural effusions. Three patients experienced persistent pleural pain. It was not possible to predict either the likelihood of recurrence of an effusion, or the persistence of pleural pain from the clinical data. In this series, none of the patients developed MM.

In a report by Epler et al., (1982), 34 patients with benign effusions were recognized clinically among 1.1×10^3 exposed workers. Prevalence was dose related; 7%, 4%, and 0.2% of the patients with effusions, respectively, had what was judged to be either a severe, indirect, or peripheral environmental exposure. The latency period was shorter than for other asbestos-related disorders with effusions being the commonest asbestos-related disease occurring in this worker population during the initial 20 years after exposure. Most effusions were considered to be small; 29% and 66% proved to be asymptomatic. They were detected either by x-ray or physical examination. One of the patients with an apparent benign effusion developed a MM 6 months later, suggesting that the effusion was the first clinical evidence of the malignant disease.

In a study by Hillerdal and Ozesmi (1987), 73 episodes of pleural effusions were discovered in 60 asbestos-exposed patients. The mean latency time from the first exposure to asbestos was 30 years, with a range claimed to be 1–58 years. The effusions lasted from 1 to 10 months, with a median of 3 months. The most common symptoms were pain, fever, cough, and dyspnea. Almost half of the effusions were asymptomatic. Fifty-three percent were hemorrhagic and 26% had an eosinophilic exudate. The authors concluded that a low level of occupational exposure can cause effusions that can occur many years after exposure to asbestos.

In a study of former Wittenoom, Australia crocidolite millers and miners (Cookson et al., 1985), the latency period for benign asbestos pleural effusion was inversely related to total cumulative exposure.

Chronic Airway Obstruction

The role of asbestos exposure to the occurrence of airways disease has been debated for many years. Although asbestos has traditionally been considered to cause a restrictive impairment in the form of asbestosis, some medical literature documents physiological airway obstruction in workers who have normal radiographs and no clinical evidence of asbestosis (Miller et al., 1994; Zejda, 1996). The mechanism by which asbestos may cause airway obstruction is unclear but could be related to the chronic deposition of asbestos in the small airway, leading to an inflammatory response causing airway fibrosis

(Dai et al., 1998; Filipenko et al., 1985; Wright and Churg, 1984; Chapter 6). Whatever the mechanism, the confounding effects of cigarette smoking in blue collar populations limits the values of these studies. Furthermore, the clinical importance of these apparent histologic changes is unknown.

Weill et al. (1975) evaluated radiographic, functional, and dust exposure data on over 800 workers in two asbestos cement plants. Dose-response relationships between increases in the severity of exposure and declining FEF_{25-75} were found. However, the authors failed to show a decrease in the FEV_1/FVC ratio, suggesting that while small-airway physiologic abnormalities may be present, clinically significant obstructive disease (as defined by a reduced FEV_1/FVC ratio) was not.

In a study of over 2.6×10^3 long-term insulators, only 3% of the nonsmokers had obstructive disease, and 6% had a decreased FEV_1/FVC ratio (Miller et al., 1994). Obstruction (judged to be present in 17%) and combined obstructive/restrictive impairment (in 18%) were most common in current smokers. The FEV_1/FVC was decreased in 35% of current smokers and in 18% of exsmokers. As might be expected, normal spirometry findings were most common when the radiograph was normal; almost half the workers with normal radiographs had normal spirometry parameters. Nevertheless, FVC was reduced in 27% of those with normal radiographs and 11% of these workers had restrictive functional parameters. Restrictive and combined restrictive and obstructive impairments of pulmonary function were most frequent when both the parenchyma and pleura were abnormal. A reduced FVC and FEV_1/FVC were both more frequent in insulators who smoked (compared with nonsmoking insulators or smokers in the general population), which suggested an interaction between asbestos exposure and smoking, resulting in these physiologic abnormalities. However, airways obstruction in the absence of radiographic abnormalities and/or cigarette smoking was uncommon.

Other studies examining nonsmoking, asbestos-exposed cohorts have methodological limitations. For instance, when radiographic information is unavailable, the role of asbestos in causing airflow obstruction in workers without radiographic disease cannot be determined. Additionally, it has proven difficult to find differences in the prevalence of obstruction in smokers and nonsmokers (Dossing et al., 1990; Griffith et al., 1993). Studies of nonsmoking asbestos workers for whom radiographs were available found small-airway obstruction as evidenced by a reduction in midflow testing, but decrements in FEV_1 and FVC were not documented. In a study by Kilburn et al. (1985), it was concluded that, in the absence of cigarette smoking and other respiratory diseases, there was a decrease in airflow resulting from asbestos exposure, although the decline was quite small. More recent work by Kilburn and Warshaw (1994) concluded that asbestos exposure alone causes airway obstruction, but there was no difference in lung function between those exposed workers who did and those who did not have asbestosis. Thus, the interpretation of the radiograph was questionable. Furthermore, among the nonsmokers, mean FEF_{25-75} values were higher than 80%, lending doubt to the conclusion that significant airway obstruction resulted from asbestos exposure alone. These and other limitations of this study are discussed by Jones et al. (1995).

In conclusion, studies evaluating the effect of asbestos on airway function are inconclusive. If there is a direct asbestos effect, it likely only involves the small airways and is clinically insignificant, particularly when compared to the effects of cigarette smoke (Wang et al., 1995, 2001). Even though airway scarring associated with asbestos inhalation has been demonstrated in animal models, the clinical impact in humans of these histologic changes, to the extent they occur, remains uncertain. The link between the former and latter appears not to have been established. If asbestos-exposed workers do have significant respiratory disability, the impairment is likely due to a restrictive, rather than an obstructive, process.

Concluding Remarks

For the last several decades, the prevalence of asbestos-related disease has been a matter of considerable debate. A major confounding factor in establishing the true prevalence of these diseases is the proliferation of legal cases based on the presumptive diagnosis of an asbestos-related condition. This has resulted in an unclear picture of true incidence of asbestos-related lung disease, as opposed to individuals who are "diagnosed" without strict adherence to established criteria. Despite polarized viewpoints regarding the true prevalence of these diseases, most would agree that the severity of the diseases, if present, is much less. Further, if one assumes that the severity of disease is less, then clinical presentations of asbestos-related diseases will be different and will likely not follow the classical patterns described in the medical literature. Much of the literature regarding clinical presentations of these diseases was written at a time when exposures were substantially greater and the diseases more prevalent than in recent years.

References

al Jarad N, Poulakis N, Pearson MC, Rubens MB, Rudd RM. Assessment of asbestos-induced pleural disease by computed tomography—correlation with chest radiograph and lung function. *Respir Med*. 1991;85:203–208.

Ameille J, Matrat M, Paris C, et al. Asbestos-related pleural diseases: dimensional criteria are not appropriate to differentiate diffuse pleural thickening from pleural plaques. *Am J Ind Med*. 2004;45:289–296.

American Thoracic Society. Medical Section of the American Lung Association: the diagnosis of nonmalignant diseases related to asbestos. *Am Rev Respir Dis*. 1986;134:363–368.

Barnhart S, Thornquist M, Omenn GS, Goodman G, Feigl P, Rosenstock L. The degree of roentgenographic parenchymal opacities attributable to smoking among asbestos-exposed subjects. *Am Rev Respir Dis*. 1990;141:1102–1109.

Begin R, Cantin A, Berthiaume Y, Boileau R, Peloquin S, Masse S. Airway function in lifetime-nonsmoking older asbestos workers. *Am J Med*. 1983;75:631–638.

Blanc P, Golden J, Garrison G. Asbestos exposure and cigarette smoking. *JAMA*. 1988;259:370–373.

Chiu B, Churg A, Tengblad A, Pearce R, McCaughey WT. Analysis of hyaluronic acid in the diagnosis of malignant mesothelioma. *Cancer*. 1984;54:2195–2199.

Churg A. Analysis of lung asbestos content. *Br J Ind Med*. 1991;48:649–652.

Churg A, Wright JL, Wiggs B, Pare PD, Lazar N. Small airways disease and mineral dust exposure. Prevalence, structure, and function. *Am Rev Respir Dis*. 1985;131:139–143.

Cookson WO, De Klerk NH, Musk AW, Glancy JJ, Armstrong BK, Hobbs MS. Benign and malignant pleural effusions in former Wittenoom crocidolite millers and miners. *Aust N Z J Med*. 1985;15:731–737.

Copley SJ, Wells AU, Rubens MB, et al. Functional consequences of pleural disease evaluated with chest radiography and CT. *Radiology*. 2001;220:237–243.

Coutts, II, Gilson JC, Kerr IH, Parkes WR, Turner-Warwick M. Significance of finger clubbing in asbestosis. *Thorax*. 1987;42:117–119.

Dai J, Gilks B, Price K, Churg A. Mineral dusts directly induce epithelial and interstitial fibrogenic mediators and matrix components in the airway wall. *Am J Respir Crit Care Med*. 1998;158:1907–1913.

Dossing M, Groth S, Vestbo J, Lyngenbo O. Small-airways dysfunction in never smoking asbestos-exposed Danish plumbers. *Int Arch Occup Environ Health*. 1990;62:209–212.

Epler GR, McLoud TC, Gaensler EA. Prevalence and incidence of benign asbestos pleural effusion in a working population. *JAMA*. 1982;247:617–622.

Filipenko D, Wright JL, Churg A. Pathologic changes in the small airways of the guinea pig after amosite asbestos exposure. *Am J Pathol*. 1985;119:273–278.

Flaherty KR, King TE, Raghu G, et al. Idiopathic interstitial pneumonia: What is the effect of a multidisciplinary approach to diagnosis? *Am J Respir Crit Care Med.* 2004;170:904–910.

Frebourg T, Lerebours G, Delpech B, et al. Serum hyaluronate in malignant pleural mesothelioma. *Cancer.* 1987;59:2104–2107.

Fridriksson HV, Hedenstrom H, Hillerdal G, Malmberg P. Increased lung stiffness of persons with pleural plaques. *Eur J Respir Dis.* 1981;62:412–424.

Gaensler E, Jederlinic, PJ, McLoud, TC. *Radiographic Progression of Asbestosis with and without Continued Exposure: Proceedings of the VIIth International Pneumoconiosis Conference,* Part I(Publication 90–108), Pittsburgh, Pennsylvania 1990a:386–392.

Gaensler EA, Jederlinic PJ, McLoud TC. *Lung Function with Asbestos-Related Pleural Plaques: Proceedings of the VIIth International Pneumoconiosis Conference,* Part I(90–108), Pittsburgh, Pennsylvania 1990b:696–702.

Griffith DE, Garcia JG, Dodson RF, Levin JL, Kronenberg RS. Airflow obstruction in non-smoking, asbestos- and mixed dust-exposed workers. *Lung.* 1993;171:213–224.

Grossebner MW, Arifi AA, Goddard M, Ritchie AJ. Mesothelioma—VATS biopsy and lung mobilization improves diagnosis and palliation. *Eur J Cardiothorac Surg.* 1999;16:619–623.

Hillerdal G. Pleural plaques and risk for bronchial carcinoma and mesothelioma. A prospective study. *Chest.* 1994;105:144–150.

Hillerdal G, Ozesmi M. Benign asbestos pleural effusion: 73 exudates in 60 patients. *Eur J Respir Dis.* 1987;71:113–121.

Hnizdo E, Sluis-Cremer GK. Effect of tobacco smoking on the presence of asbestosis at postmortem and on the reading of irregular opacities on roentgenograms in asbestos-exposed workers. *Am Rev Respir Dis.* 1988;138:1207–1212.

Hughes JM, Weill H. Asbestosis as a precursor of asbestos related lung cancer: results of a prospective mortality study. *Br J Ind Med.* 1991;48:229–233.

Jones RN, Diem JE, Hughes JM, Hammad YY, Glindmeyer HW, Weill H. Progression of asbestos effects: a prospective longitudinal study of chest radiographs and lung function. *Br J Ind Med.* 1989;46:97–105.

Jones RN, Glindmeyer HW, 3rd, Weill H. Review of the Kilburn and Warshaw Chest article—airways obstruction from asbestos exposure. *Chest.* 1995;107:1727–1729.

Kee ST, Gamsu G, Blanc P. Causes of pulmonary impairment in asbestos-exposed individuals with diffuse pleural thickening. *Am J Respir Crit Care Med.* 1996;154(3 Pt 1):789–793.

Kilburn KH, Warshaw RH. Abnormal lung function associated with asbestos disease of the pleura, the lung, and both: a comparative analysis. *Thorax.* 1991;46:33–38.

Kilburn KH, Warshaw RH. Airways obstruction from asbestos exposure. Effects of asbestosis and smoking. *Chest.* 1994;106:1061–1070.

Kilburn KH, Warshaw RH, Einstein K, Bernstein J. Airway disease in non-smoking asbestos workers. *Arch Environ Health.* 1985;40:293–295.

Koskinen K, Pukkala E, Martikainen R, Reijula K, Karjalainen A. Different measures of asbestos exposure in estimating risk of lung cancer and mesothelioma among construction workers. *J Occup Environ Med.* 2002;44:1190–1196.

Kouris SP, Parker DL, Bender AP, Williams AN. Effects of asbestos-related pleural disease on pulmonary function. *Scand J Work Environ Health.* 1991;17:179–183.

Liddell FD, McDonald JC. Radiological findings as predictors of mortality in Quebec asbestos workers. *Br J Ind Med.* 1980;37:257–267.

Lozewicz S, Reznek RH, Herdman M, Dacie JE, McLean A, Davies RJ. Role of computed tomography in evaluating asbestos related lung disease. *Br J Ind Med.* 1989;46:777–781.

McGavin CR, Sheers G. Diffuse pleural thickening in asbestos workers: disability and lung function abnormalities. *Thorax.* 1984;39:604–607.

Miller A, Lilis R, Godbold J, Chan E, Wu X, Selikoff IJ. Spirometric impairments in long-term insulators. Relationships to duration of exposure, smoking, and radiographic abnormalities. *Chest.* 1994;105:175–182.

Neri S, Antonelli A, Falaschi F, Boraschi P, Baschieri L. Findings from high resolution computed tomography of the lung and pleura of symptom free workers exposed to amosite who had normal chest radiographs and pulmonary function tests. *Occup Environ Med.* 1994;51:239–243.

Neri S, Boraschi P, Antonelli A, Falaschi F, Baschieri L. Pulmonary function, smoking habits, and high resolution computed tomography (HRCT) early abnormalities of lung and pleural fibrosis in shipyard workers exposed to asbestos. *Am J Ind Med.* 1996;30:588–595.

Ohar J, Sterling DA, Bleecker E, Donohue J. Changing patterns in asbestos-induced lung disease. *Chest.* 2004;125:744–753.

Oliver LC, Eisen EA, Greene R, Sprince NL. Asbestos-related pleural plaques and lung function. *Am J Ind Med.* 1988;14:649–656.

Paganuzzi M, Onetto M, Marroni P, et al. Diagnostic value of CYFRA 21–1 tumor marker and CEA in pleural effusion due to mesothelioma. *Chest.* 2001;119:1138–1142.

Rebuck AS, Braude AC. Bronchoalveolar lavage in asbestosis. *Arch Intern Med.* 1983;143:950–952.

Robinson BW, Musk AW. Benign asbestos pleural effusion: diagnosis and course. *Thorax.* 1981;36:896–900.

Robinson BW, Rose AH, James A, Whitaker D, Musk AW. Alveolitis of pulmonary asbestosis. Bronchoalveolar lavage studies in crocidolite- and chrysotile-exposed individuals. *Chest.* 1986;90:396–402.

Rom WN, Travis WD, Brody AR. Cellular and molecular basis of the asbestos-related diseases. *Am Rev Respir Dis.* 1991;143:408–422.

Rubino GF, Piolatto G, Newhouse ML, Scansetti G, Aresini GA, Murray R. Mortality of chrysotile asbestos workers at the Balangero Mine, Northern Italy. *Br J Ind Med.* 1979;36:187–194.

Schwartz DA, Fuortes LJ, Galvin JR, et al. Asbestos-induced pleural fibrosis and impaired lung function. *Am Rev Respir Dis.* 1990;141:321–326.

Sette A, Neder JA, Nery LE, et al. Thin-section CT abnormalities and pulmonary gas exchange impairment in workers exposed to asbestos. *Radiology.* 2004;232:66–74.

Staples CA, Gamsu G, Ray CS, Webb WR. High resolution computed tomography and lung function in asbestos-exposed workers with normal chest radiographs. *Am Rev Respir Dis.* 1989;139:1502–1508.

Thylen A, Hjerpe A, Martensson G. Hyaluronan content in pleural fluid as a prognostic factor in patients with malignant pleural mesothelioma. *Cancer.* 2001;92:1224–1230.

Van Cleemput J, De Raeve H, Verschakelen JA, Rombouts J, Lacquet LM, Nemery B. Surface of localized pleural plaques quantitated by computed tomography scanning: no relation with cumulative asbestos exposure and no effect on lung function. *Am J Respir Crit Care Med.* 2001;163(3 Pt 1):705–710.

Wang X, Araki S, Yano E, Wang M, Wang Z. Effects of smoking on respiratory function and exercise performance in asbestos workers. *Ind Health.* 1995;33:173–180.

Wang XR, Yano E, Wang M, Wang Z, Christiani DC. Pulmonary function in long-term asbestos workers in China. *J Occup Environ Med.* 2001;43:623–629.

Weill H, Ziskind MM, Waggenspack C, Rossiter CE. Lung function consequences of dust exposure in asbestos cement manufacturing plants. *Arch Environ Health.* 1975;30:88–97.

Weiss W. Asbestos-related pleural plaques and lung cancer. *Chest.* 103:1854–1859, 1993.

Wright JL, Churg A. Morphology of small-airway lesions in patients with asbestos exposure. *Hum Pathol* 1984;15:68–74.

Xaubet A, Rodriguez-Roisin R, Bombi JA, Marin A, Roca J, Agusti-Vidal A. Correlation of bronchoalveolar lavage and clinical and functional findings in asbestosis. *Am Rev Respir Dis.* 1986;133:848–854.

Yates DH, Browne K, Stidolph PN, Neville E. Asbestos-related bilateral diffuse pleural thickening: natural history of radiographic and lung function abnormalities. *Am J Respir Crit Care Med.* 1996;153:301–306.

Zejda JE. Occupational exposure to dusts containing asbestos and chronic airways disease. *Int J Occup Med Environ Health.* 1996;9:117–125.

11

Radiological Features of the Asbestos-Associated Diseases

Haydn Adams and Michael D. Crane

Introduction

In 1897 William Roentgen discovered x-rays, and following this the plain chest radiograph became the main method of radiological assessment of the thorax for the most part of the 20th century. The next major breakthrough in imaging of the chest was the development of body computed tomographin the 1970s. Initially, due to the slow radiological acquisition times of these scanners and the relatively wide collimation used, only relatively crude images of the thorax could be obtained. One of the first reports of the use of CT in the assessment of asbestos related chest disease was by Kreel in 1976 when he described both pleural and parenchymal changes (Kreel, 1976). In the mid-1980s major improvements in scanner technology led to the advent of high-resolution computed tomography (HRCT) of the thorax. Parenchymal images of unprecedented quality were attainable and a large number of scientific papers describing the pleural and pulmonary changes in asbestos-exposed individuals were published. Today HRCT remains the most sensitive tool for radiological assessment of occupational chest diseases. With the introduction of helical or spiral scanning in the 1990s and later development of multidetector scanners, the entire thorax could be imaged with contiguous thin sections during a single breath hold. Such scanners allow reformatting of volumetric data and can provide images in coronal, sagittal, and oblique planes. More recent developments in imaging of the thorax include magnetic resonance imaging (MRI) and positron emission tomography (PET). While these modalities have a useful role in the assessment of selected cases of intrathoracic malignancy, they have virtually no role in the routine assessment of benign asbestos-related chest diseases.

This chapter describes the radiological appearances of benign and malignant asbestos-related chest diseases and the utility of the various imaging modalities for the assessment of each manifestation.

ILO Classification of Radiographs of the Pneumoconioses

The chest radiograph is almost invariably the initial imaging procedure when assessing occupational or environmental respiratory disease due to inhaled dust.

For chest radiography to be useful for epidemiological purposes it is essential that a standard nomenclature be followed to classify the pattern and extent of abnormality. The International Labor Office (ILO) system was initially developed in 1930 for the assessment of silicosis and this has subsequently been modified several times. The 1980 version (ILO, 1980) permits classification of asbestos-associated diseases as well as the other pneumoconioses and includes reference radiographs.

The object of the ILO system is to codify and grade abnormalities objectively in a reproducible manner. It does not define pathological entities, but it allows documentation of the type and extent of disease to allow international comparability. Pulmonary opacities are scored according to their profusion and shape and the presence or absence of pleural thickening can also be recorded.

Several criticisms have been leveled at the ILO system (Rockoff and Schwartz, 1988). It is an arbitrary classification that is based on consensus with no histological correlation. There is intra- and interobserver variation in the assessment of small pulmonary opacities and this is considerable in some series (Impivaara et al., 1998; Welch et al., 1998). The system is imprecise for classification of pleural lesions (Hillerdal, 1991). Radiographic technical factors may also have an influence on the interpretation (Rockoff and Schwartz, 1988). Although it was originally developed for epidemiological purposes, the ILO system is now often applied to individual cases. A recent study has implied that significant bias occurs in interpretation of radiographs in the medicolegal setting by readers retained by attorneys representing plaintiffs alleging respiratory damage from asbestos exposure (Gitlin et al., 2004).

It is well recognized that when studying populations some individuals who do not have occupational dust exposure have a profusion of opacities consistent with the radiographic appearance of pneumoconiosis. The prevalence of such changes varies with gender, age and particularly with differing geographic locations (Meyer et al., 1997). Conversely, it has also been estimated that the ILO reading of a radiograph may be normal in 10%–20% of subjects with asbestosis (Kipen et al., 1987; Rockoff and Schwartz, 1988).

In practice, the vast majority of radiologists do not employ such a semiquantitative classification system when evaluating plain chest radiographs.

Pleural Effusion

Pleural effusion is the earliest manifestation of pleural disease occurring because of asbestos exposure (Peacock et al., 2000) and it was first described by Eisenstadt in 1964 (Eisenstadt, 1964). It usually occurs within 10 years of exposure, but it can also develop later (Peacock et al., 2000). Asbestos related pleural effusion is frequently asymptomatic and the exact prevalence is unknown (Epler et al., 1982; Hillerdal and Ozesmi, 1987; Peacock et al., 2000). Effusions are typically exudates of mixed cellularity and usually do not contain asbestos bodies (Epler et al., 1982). There may be an increased eosinophil cell count (Hillerdal and Ozesmi, 1987). The effusion usually resolves over a few months with a mean duration of 3–4 months, but it can also persist or recur (Epler et al., 1982). Diffuse pleural thickening and in particular blunting of the costophrenic angle is commonly seen after resolution of the effusion (Epler et al., 1982). The development of effusions is thought to be dose related (Epler et al., 1982), but they can occur after even slight exposure (Hillerdal and Ozesmi, 1987). In general medical practice, pleural effusions are a commonly encountered abnormality and the diagnosis of an asbestos related effusion largely relies on exclusion of other explanations in an asbestos exposed patient. The radiological appearances of an isolated asbestos-related benign effusion cannot be differentiated from simple effusions due to other causes (Figure 11.1).

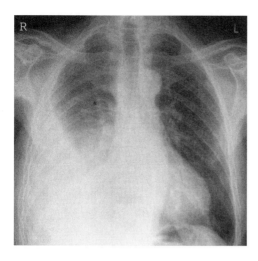

Figure 11.1 PA chest radiograph: large right-sided pleural effusion in an asbestos-exposed individual.

Pleural Plaques

Pleural plaques are well-circumscribed pleural elevations that usually arise from the parietal pleura. They are the commonest radiological finding in asbestos exposed individuals and the presence of multiple discrete calcified plaques during radiological imaging is highly indicative of asbestos exposure (Peacock et al., 2000; Roach et al., 2002; Staples, 1992).

Pleural plaques are usually multiple and bilateral although they can sometimes be unilateral or solitary. Plaques can vary in diameter from just a few millimeters to several centimeters, and in thickness from 1 mm to nodular pleural elevations measuring a centimeter or more in thickness. They may be located on costal, diaphragmatic, or mediastinal pleural surfaces. Costal pleural plaques are classically described as occurring along the postero-lateral chest wall between the seventh and tenth ribs and along the lateral chest wall between the sixth and ninth ribs. However, this may simply reflect the ease with which pleural plaques are seen at these sites on plain radiographs. With the recent widespread use of computed tomography to assess asbestos-related thoracic disease, it has become clear that plaques located anteriorly in the upper thorax and in the paravertebral gutters in the lower thorax are also common (Peacock et al., 2000; Roach et al., 2002). The apical pleura and costophrenic angles are usually free of plaques. Occasionally, plaques may originate from the visceral pleura in which case they can lie in the pulmonary interlobar fissures. They may then be confused with intrapulmonary nodules or masses (Lynch et al., 1988).

Pleural plaques are often partially calcified with frequencies of 10%–15% quoted on plain film studies. Calcification is seen more commonly on computed tomographic studies than on plain films due to the multiplanar capacity and greater contrast resolution of computed tomography (Aberle et al., 1988a).

As they mostly arise from the parietal pleura, simple plaques per se do not usually cause any abnormality of the adjacent lung, unlike diffuse pleural thickening that involves the visceral pleura and may therefore produce changes in the subpleural lung parenchyma (Gevenois et al., 1998).

The radiological manifestations of pleural plaques reflect the characteristics described earlier.

On plain chest radiographs, the appearance of pleural plaques depends on whether they are seen in profile or en face and also on their size and degree of calcification.

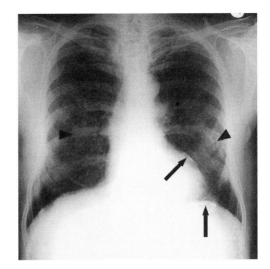

Figure 11.2 PA chest radiograph: calcified pleural plaques. Plaques seen in profile (arrows) appear as dense curvilinear structures. Plaques seen en face (arrowheads) have a typical holly leaf appearance.

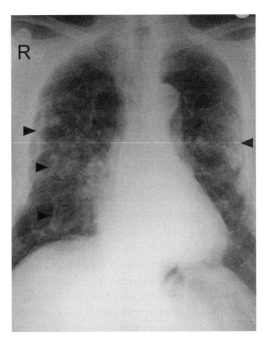

Figure 11.3 PA chest radiograph: calcified pleural plaques seen en face (arrowheads) producing a classic holly leaf appearance.

Small noncalcified plaques or plaques lying in relatively blind positions may produce very subtle appearances or may go totally unrecognized (Cugell, 2004). When seen in profile, plaques appear as localized elevations of the pleura that may indent the underlying lung. If there is extensive calcification the lesions appear as dense curvilinear structures (Figure 11.2) and this is a particularly common manifestation of diaphragmatic plaques that tend to occur on the central tendinous part of the diaphragm. Plaques arising from the costal surfaces of the pleura are often seen to extend along the inner aspects of the underlying ribs.

Pleural plaques seen en face may appear as sharply demarcated lesions with irregular or angular margins and this is best appreciated when the lesions are calcified. Their appearance has been likened to a holly leaf (Figures 11.2 and 11.3; Cugell, 2004).

Plaques may potentially be mistaken for intrapulmonary masses. However, in common with other pleural-based lesions, plaques are generally flat and for their size, they do not have the expected radiographic density of a typically more rounded intrapulmonary mass of similar diameter. Conversely, the presence of multiple pleural plaques may obscure underlying lung detail and focal masses may be missed during plain film interpretation (Lynch et al., 1988).

Several studies have shown that there is a high false positive rate for the detection of asbestos-related pleural disease using plain chest radiography. This occurs due to confusion with normal structures such as subpleural fat or musculature, or other abnormalities such as old rib fractures (Ameille et al., 1993; Friedman et al., 1988; Im et al., 1989). Although the addition of oblique projections to routine postero-anterior views may increase sensitivity for the detection of pleural plaques or thickening, this is at the expense of specificity with one study demonstrating a positive predictive value of only between 13% and 26% (Ameille et al., 1993). On this basis, it has been suggested that the routine use of oblique chest radiographs as a screening test in subjects exposed to low levels of asbestos should be reevaluated. In another study, the use of oblique views increased interobserver variation in the interpretation of plain radiographs for the presence of pleural disease resulting in reduced reliability and validity of the readings (Reger et al., 1982).

Owing to its axial scan plane, computed tomography is well suited for the assessment of the pleura. Plaques appear as localized elevations of the pleura, often separated from rib and extrapleural soft tissue by a layer of fat. The presence of calcification within plaques is easily appreciated (Figures 11.4 and 11.5). Although plaques arising from the costal and mediastinal surfaces are generally easily appreciated on axial images, diaphragmatic plaques may be more difficult to discern unless large or calcified, as they are often orientated in the same axis as the CT scan plane. True pleural diseases including discrete plaques and diffuse thickening can readily be differentiated from subpleural fat that may be a source of confusion during plain film interpretation (Friedman et al., 1988). Whereas pleural plaques and areas of diffuse pleural thickening are of soft tissue density or high CT attenuation when calcification is present, subpleural fat is of low CT attenuation and may only be recognized if appropriate image window settings are used (Figure 11.6).

Computed tomography has a higher sensitivity than plain radiography for the demonstration of pleural plaques, and it also allows differentiation between plaques and diffuse pleural thickening (Aberle et al., 1988a; Al Jarad et al., 1991; Gevenois et al., 1998). It is generally held that HRCT has a higher sensitivity than conventional computed tomography for the detection of plaques due to its greater spatial resolution. HRCT is also more likely than conventional computed tomography to show areas of calcification within plaques (Aberle et al., 1988a,b). However, in one study conventional computed tomography was more sensitive than HRCT for the detection of small plaques, probably because some lesions were missed on HRCT owing to the interspaced sections used (Gevenois et al., 1994). On this basis, it was recommended that where detection of small plaques is medicolegally important, HRCT should be performed initially and if negative for plaques an addition conventional CT study with contiguous slices should also be performed. With the advent of spiral computed tomography, it is now possible to obtain volumetric data of the entire thorax that will ensure that all lesions are included in the radiological acquisition. Narrow collimation axial sections can then be reconstructed at desired intervals from the data to obtain the benefits of higher spatial resolution. In addition, multiplanar reconstruction of images in the sagittal, coronal, or oblique planes will permit easier assessment of problem areas such as the superior sulci or diaphragmatic surfaces.

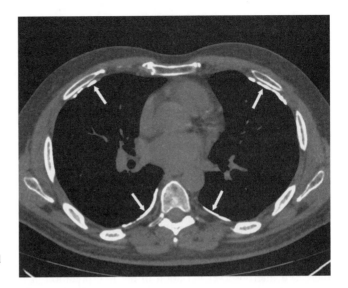

Figure 11.4 CT scan: bilateral densely calcified pleural plaques (arrows).

(A)
(B)

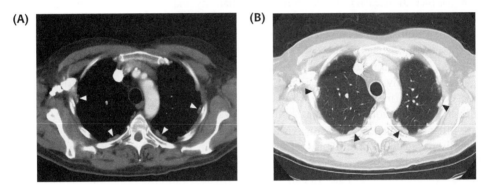

Figure 11.5 CT scan: (A) relatively nodular pleural plaques (arrowheads) viewed on soft tissue settings. There is minimal calcification within some of the plaques (B) on lung settings the plaques are seen to indent the lung surfaces

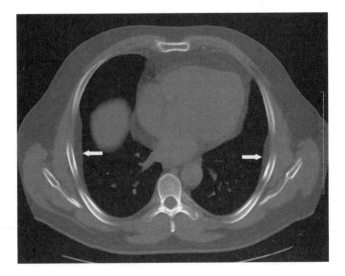

Figure 11.6 CT scan: subpleural fat deposits (arrows). These may be confused for pleural plaques or thickening on plain radiographs.

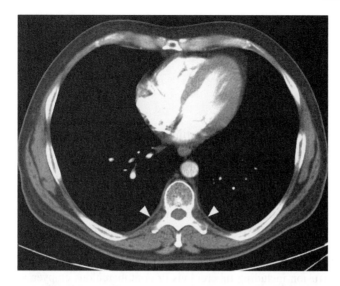

Figure 11.7 CT scan: intercostal veins (arrowheads) may be mistaken for pleural plaques or thickening.

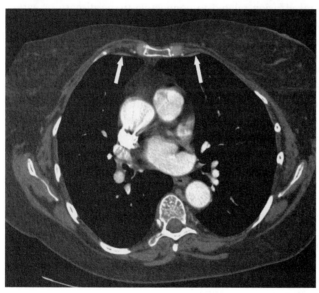

Figure 11.8 CT scan: transverse thoracic muscles (arrows) mimicking pleural plaques.

Despite the sensitivity of computed tomography in the assessment of pleural plaques, considerable interobserver variation may occur in the diagnosis of early lesions (De Raeve et al., 2001). Plaques may be overlooked due to perceptual error. False positive diagnosis of pleural plaques may be made on HRCT, if the appearances of normal structures such as intercostal veins (Figure 11.7) or subcostal muscles posteriorly, or transverse thoracic muscles anteriorly (Figure 11.8) are misinterpreted (Im et al., 1989). Plaques should only be diagnosed in the paravertebral regions if there is continuous thickening of the pleura on several contiguous sections, if the pleural abnormality is separable from underlying intercostal vein by an intervening fat plane, if there is indentation of the adjacent lung by the thickened pleura or if calcification is present. Knowledge of the normal anatomical appearances of the transverse thoracic and subcostal muscles should avoid confusion with plaques in these regions.

Several radiological studies have examined the effect of pleural plaques on lung function and have concluded that simple plaques are functionally insignificant (Copley et al., 2001; Staples et al., 1989).

Diffuse Pleural Thickening

Diffuse pleural thickening is primarily due to thickening and fibrosis of the visceral pleura that is often fused with the parietal pleura. It is seen less frequently than pleural plaques. It may be preceded by a benign pleural effusion (Peacock et al., 2000). In the presence of diffuse pleural thickening due to asbestos exposure, there are often bilateral pleural changes due to either diffuse pleural thickening or contralateral pleural plaques (Aberle et al., 1988; Leung et al., 1990). Calcification can occur within diffuse pleural thickening but it is seldom extensive (Aberle et al., 1988a,b; Friedman et al., 1988).

Diffuse pleural thickening is not specific for asbestos exposure and it may be a sequela of other causes of exudative effusion including tuberculous or nontuberculous empyema, parapneumonic effusion, pleural effusion related to connective tissue disease or earlier haemothorax. Pleural metastases and mesothelioma can occasionally produce a similar appearance. Benign asbestos-related pleural thickening, like other causes of fibrothorax but unlike malignant pleural mesothelioma, seldom involves the mediastinal pleura (Leung et al., 1990; Müller, 1993).

There is no globally accepted definition for the plain film or CT appearances of diffuse pleural thickening. The imaging features are those of a continuous sheet of thickened pleura often involving the costophrenic recesses and apical areas of the affected pleural cavity. Plain film features of diffuse pleural thickening include unilateral or bilateral thickening extending over at least 25% of the chest wall and reaching a thickness of at least 5 mm in at least one site on the radiograph (Figures 11.9 and 11.10; Industrial Injuries Advisory Council, 1996). Others (McLoud et al., 1985; Peacock et al., 2000) have stressed that the radiographic appearance of pleural thickening should be smooth, noninterrupted pleural density extending over at least one quarter of the chest wall internal to the lower ribs. The costophrenic recesses may or may not be obliterated (Figure 11.10). Sargent proposed reserving the term diffuse pleural thickening to those cases where the pleural thickening was associated with ipsilateral costophrenic angle obliteration but this restrictive definition would exclude cases of extensive visceral pleural thickening without costophrenic angle obliteration (Sargent et al., 1978).

Other criteria have been proposed to diagnose diffuse pleural thickening on computed tomography. Lynch (Lynch et al., 1988; Lynch et al., 1989) uses the criteria of a continuous area of pleural thickening more than 5 cm wide, more than 8 cm in craniocaudal extent, and more than 3 mm thick (Figures 11.11 and 11.12). Peacock suggested that diffuse pleural thickening that is less than 3 mm thick or less extensive than that described by Lynch may still be functionally significant and a less rigorous definition may therefore be more appropriate (Peacock et al., 2000).

Purely dimensional criteria do not readily distinguish between extensive confluent parietal plaques and diffuse visceral thickening. Indeed differentiation between diffuse visceral pleural thickening and extensive confluent plaques can be extremely difficult. Extension into the interlobar fissures is indicative of visceral pleural involvement (Fletcher and Edge, 1970; Lynch et al., 1989; McLoud et al., 1985). The major discriminative feature of visceral pleural thickening is that the adjacent lung parenchyma is often affected by the pleural disease. This may be manifested by parenchymal bands or

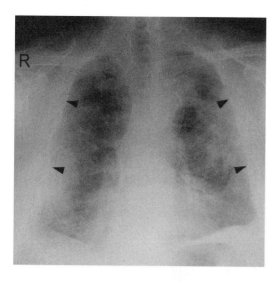

Figure 11.9 PA chest radiograph: bilateral diffuse pleural thickening (arrowheads) with obliteration of the costophrenic angles.

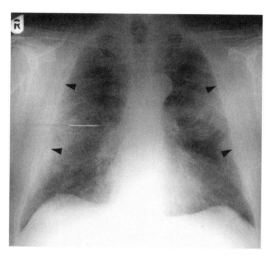

Figure 11.10 PA chest radiograph: bilateral diffuse pleural thickening (arrowheads) with sparing of the costophrenic angles.

rounded atelectasis (Gevenois et al., 1998; Hillerdal et al., 1990). In contrast, with extensive confluent parietal pleural plaques the interface between the pleural thickening and the adjacent lung is usually sharply circumscribed.

Parenchymal bands are linear opacities that are generally 2–5 cm in length and extend from areas of pleural thickening into the adjacent lung (Figures 11.13, 11.14, and 11.15). They tend to be coarse and tapering and they are orientated differently to adjacent vessels. When several parenchymal bands radiate into the underlying lung from an area of pleural thickening they may produce a "crow's foot" appearance (Gevenois et al., 1998; Hillerdal, 1985). These features may be evident on plain chest radiographs or on computed tomography.

The observation of so-called hairy plaques is not unusual and this appearance should be classified among the manifestations of visceral pleural disease. In these cases, numerous short linear interstitial shadows extend into the adjacent pulmonary parenchyma from a focal area of visceral pleural thickening (Figure 11.16). It is important to identify that the localized parenchymal change relates to overlying pleural thickening

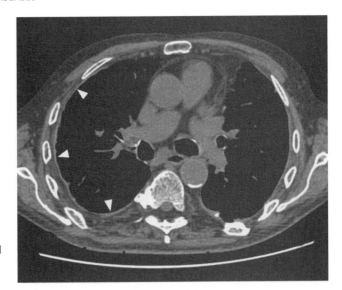

Figure 11.11 CT scan: relatively mild diffuse pleural thickening in the right hemithorax (arrowheads).

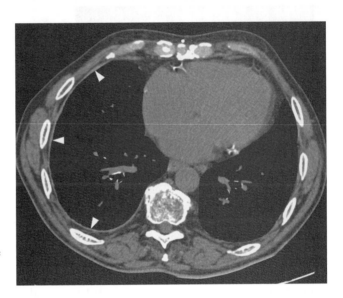

Figure 11.12 CT scan: diffuse pleural thickening of the right hemithorax (arrowheads).

and distinguish it from diffuse interstitial fibrosis seen in areas of lung remote from pleural disease.

Rounded atelectasis, a pulmonary manifestation of diffuse pleural thickening, is discussed later in this chapter.

It is accepted that diffuse pleural thickening can cause significant lung restriction (Al Jarad et al., 1991; Copley et al., 2001; Rosenstock et al., 1988; Yates et al., 1996,). A number of systems for quantification of the extent of pleural thickening have been developed (Al Jarad et al., 1992a; Copley et al., 2001; Hering et al., 2004; Suganuma et al., 2001) but none as yet is in widespread clinical use.

Copley et al. (2001) evaluated several methods for the assessment of pleural thickening on computed tomography and found that there was generally excellent interobserver agreement for both extent of pleural plaques and diffuse pleural thickening. It was

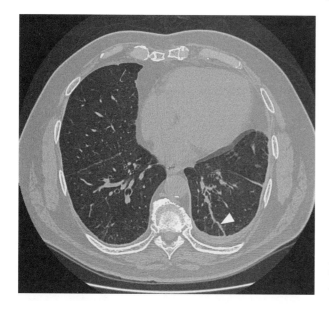

Figure 11.13 CT scan: left sided pleural thickening associated with a parenchymal band (arrowhead) indicating visceral pleural involvement.

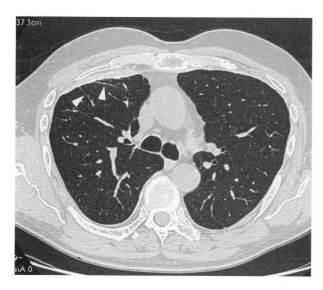

Figure 11.14 CT scan: right sided parenchymal bands (arrowheads) associated with adjacent pleural thickening.

shown that the extent of diffuse pleural thickening strongly correlates with decreasing lung volumes and less strongly with increasing transfer coefficient K(kappa)CO. For a given total extent of diffuse pleural thickening, there was no significant difference between unilateral and bilateral disease. The study confirmed the traditionally held view that pleural plaques are of little consequence regarding impairment of lung function.

Several studies have shown that diffuse pleural thickening may be found in association with asbestosis (Frank and Loddenkemper, 1995; Nishimura and Broaddus, 1998). Fissural visceral pleural thickening may be associated with early pulmonary fibrosis. In one study, this was a strong relationship (Rockoff et al., 1987) but another study failed to confirm this association (McLoud et al., 1985).

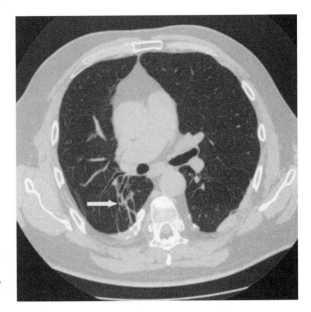

Figure 11.15 CT scan: multiple right-sided parenchymal bands (arrow) associated with partially calcified pleural thickening.

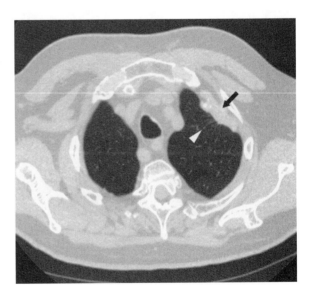

Figure 11.16 CT scan: hairy plaque: fine lines (arrowhead) extend from a left-sided pleural lesion (arrow) indicating visceral pleural involvement.

Rounded Atelectasis

The pathogenesis of rounded atelectasis is not certain (Peacock et al., 2000). It is thought by many to be due to infolding of lung at the thickened visceral pleural surface as described by Blesovsky (1966). Synonyms include Blesovsky's syndrome, folded lung and asbestos pseudotumor. It commonly affects the middle lobe, lingula, and lower lobes (Hillerdal, 1989), but any lobe can be affected and bilateral changes are not uncommon (McHugh and Blaquiere, 1989). It may be associated with the presence of parenchymal bands elsewhere.

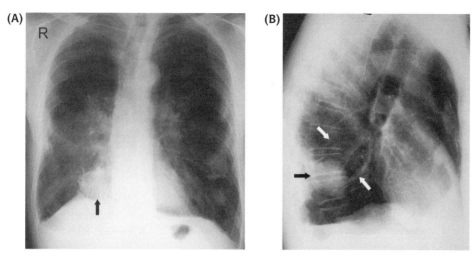

Figure 11.17 Rounded atelectasis, plain radiographic features: (A) a PA chest radiograph demonstrates multiple asbestos-related pleural plaques and a soft tissue mass at the right base (arrow), (B) a lateral chest radiograph shows that the mass lies posteriorly (black arrow). Pulmonary vessels (white arrows) curl into the mass, a characteristic feature of rounded atelectasis.

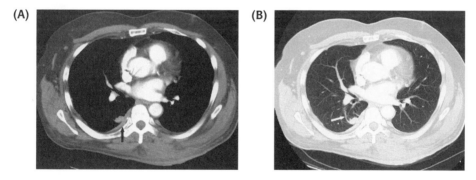

Figure 11.18 Rounded atelectasis, CT features: (A) soft tissue windows show a small ovoid mass lying adjacent to an area of right- sided pleural thickening (arrow), (B) lung windows show bronchovascular structures sweeping into the mass (arrow).

Although there is a strong association with asbestos exposure (Lynch et al., 1988), rounded atelectasis is not specific to asbestos induced pleural thickening and it can follow many causes of an organizing pleural exudate (Peacock et al., 2000).

The chest radiograph typically shows a peripheral round or oval pulmonary opacity that is related to overlying pleural thickening, with or without adjacent lung distortion (Figure 11.17).

The computed tomography features are those of a round or oval opacity abutting thickened pleura. This often has a centrally directed indistinct edge (Peacock et al., 2000). The adjacent bronchovascular structures sweep into the opacity resulting in a "comet-tail" appearance (Figures 11.18 and 11.19; Carvalho and Carr, 1990; McHugh and Blaquiere, 1989). There is often evidence of associated volume loss (Lynch et al., 1988). With the use of intravenous contrast, rounded atelectasis may show some enhancement (Taylor, 1988).

The differential diagnosis of rounded atelectasis includes bronchogenic carcinoma (Figure 11.20). Lack of change in the appearances over the passage of time favors

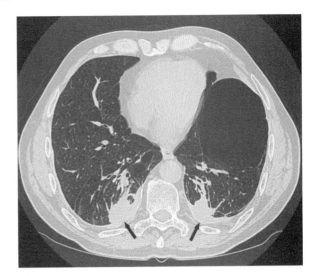

Figure 11.19 CT scan: bilateral rounded atelectasis (arrows). A coincidental emphysematous bulla lies at the left base.

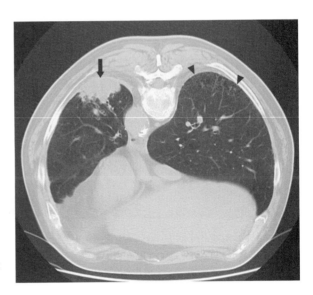

Figure 11.20 Prone CT scan: a peripheral lung cancer at the left base (arrow) in an asbestos exposed individual superficially resembles rounded atelectasis. There is mild subpleural fibrosis at the right base (arrowheads).

a benign aetiology. Careful interpretation of the computed tomographic features combined with surveillance can obviate the need for biopsy in the majority of instances (Lynch et al., 1988). Occasionally, biopsy may be necessary, but percutaneous biopsy may be difficult due to the presence of the thickened, sometimes calcified overlying pleura. Rounded atelectasis is not metabolically active on 2-[^{18}F]fluoro-2-deoxy-D-glucose (FDG) PET. FDG-PET imaging may therefore be useful to differentiate rounded atelectasis from bronchogenic carcinoma (McAdams et al., 1998).

Malignant Mesothelioma

Malignant mesothelioma of the pleura usually, but not invariably, occurs in subjects with a history of asbestos exposure. The disease is often first suspected when a plain chest

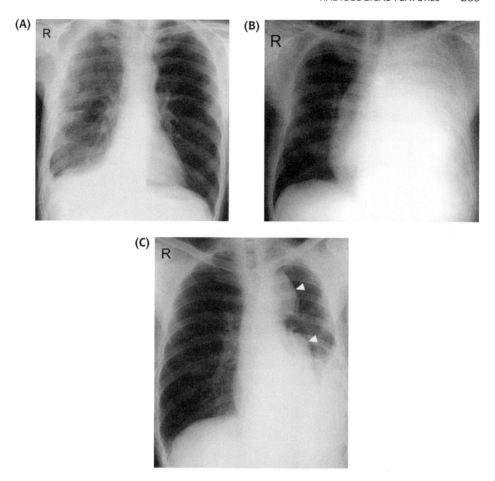

Figure 11.21 Three cases demonstrating the spectrum of plain radiographic appearances in malignant mesothelioma: (A) irregular right-sided pleural thickening (B) massive left-sided pleural effusion due to underlying tumor (C) a combination of left-sided pleural masses (arrowheads) and a basal pleural effusion.

radiograph of an asbestos exposed individual demonstrates evidence of characteristic irregular pleural thickening or a large pleural effusion (Figure 11.21). Once the possibility of malignant mesothelioma is entertained, computed tomography of the thorax and upper abdomen is the mainstay of further investigation.

The characteristic features of malignant mesothelioma can be appreciated on plain chest radiography but computed tomography shows the abnormalities to better effect. The pleural thickening of mesothelioma is typically bulky and irregular, affecting costal, mediastinal, and diaphragmatic pleura and often encasing the entire lung within the affected hemithorax (Figure 11.22). Extension into the interlobar fissures is common. The tumor is often associated with marked contraction of the ipsilateral hemithorax and retraction of the chest wall resulting in rib crowding (Figure 11.23). The mediastinum may be shifted to the involved side but it is often fixed by the tumor, remaining in the midline (Kawashima and Libshitz, 1990; Ng et al., 1999; Sahin et al., 1993).

The characteristic pleural thickening of malignant mesothelioma is often associated with the presence of a pleural effusion of varying size but sometimes pleural effusion

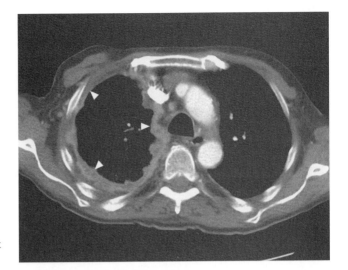

Figure 11.22 CT scan: malignant pleural mesothelioma. Irregular circumferential pleural thickening affects the right hemithorax (arrowheads).

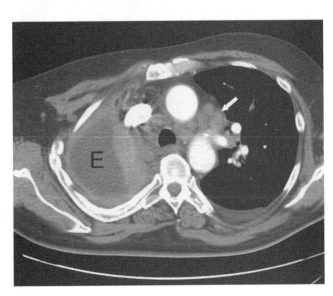

Figure 11.23 Right-sided malignant mesothelioma associated with a pleural effusion (E). CT demonstrates contraction of the affected hemithorax with rib crowding. Contralateral mediastinal lymph nodes are involved (arrow).

is the main radiological manifestation of the disease (Figure 11.21B; Kawashima and Libshitz, 1990; Ng et al., 1999; Sahin et al., 1993). In between 10% and 21% of cases, the effusion may cause enlargement of the affected hemithorax with contralateral mediastinal shift (Kawashima and Libshitz, 1990; Ng et al., 1999; Sahin et al., 1993). The presence of a large effusion may totally obscure underlying pleural thickening on plain chest radiographs (Rusch et al., 1988). In a small number of cases, malignant mesothelioma presents radiologically as a pleural effusion with no radiological evidence of pleural thickening (Figure 11.24; Ng et al., 1999). In such cases, invasive investigation such as thoracoscopy often shows the pleural surfaces to be studded with numerous small tumor deposits (IMIG, 1995; Rusch et al., 1988).

Although malignant mesothelioma usually occurs in asbestos exposed individuals, benign asbestos-related pleural plaques or pleural calcification are usually seen in only about 10%–20% of patients (Figure 11.24; Kawashima and Libshitz, 1990, Ng et al., 1999). However, in one series calcified pleural plaques were evident on computed

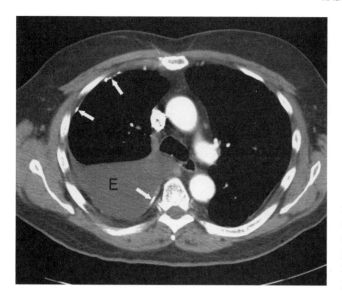

Figure 11.24 Malignant mesothelioma presenting as a large effusion (E). CT shows calcified pleural plaques (arrows) but there is no evidence of malignant pleural thickening.

tomography in 62% of subjects with long-term environmental exposure to asbestos from an early age (Sahin et al., 1993).

A number of clinical staging systems have been applied to malignant mesothelioma but in the past, none has been universally accepted. More recently, an international TNM (Tumor, Node, Metastasis) staging system has been proposed to provide clinical and prognostic information (IMIG, 1995). However, the limitations of cross-sectional imaging in the assessment of malignant mesothelioma mean that accuracies of only around 50%–60% may be achieved for a number of the features of the staging system, particularly local invasion and mediastinal nodal metastases (Heelan et al., 1999).

Involvement of the chest wall may be manifested by invasion of the endothoracic fascia, rib destruction, or an extrapleural soft tissue mass (Heelan, 1999; IMIG, 1995; Kawashima and Libshitz, 1990; Sahin et al., 1993). While advanced chest wall invasion is generally well recognized on computed tomography (Figure 11.25), lesser degrees of invasion may be undetectable and chest wall involvement is often understaged (Heelan, 1999; Rusch et al., 1988; Sahin et al., 1993). The propensity for malignant mesothelioma to spread along needle biopsy or intercostal drain tracks is well recognized and on subsequent cross-sectional imaging differentiation between true tumor infiltration and scarring at these sites may be difficult (Patz et al., 1992). The tumor may breach the diaphragmatic pleura resulting in invasion of diaphragmatic muscle (Figure 11.26), peritoneum, or upper abdominal viscera such as the liver (Kawashima and Libshitz, 1990; Ng et al., 1999). Owing to the orientation of the diaphragmatic disease in the axial scan plane, diaphragmatic involvement is often underestimated (Heelan, 1999; Ng et al., 1999). Assessment may be improved by multiplanar reconstruction of CT data in sagittal or coronal planes or by the use of MRI.

Mediastinal involvement by malignant mesothelioma is common although direct invasion is often difficult to differentiate from overlying malignant pleural thickening (Kawashima and Libshitz, 1990; Sahin et al., 1993). Tumor may extend into the mediastinal fat or invade deeper mediastinal organs including pericardium, the heart, and major vessels, or the oesophagus (Ng et al., 1999). The presence of a soft tissue mass surrounding more than 50% of the circumference of a major mediastinal vessel is highly indicative of direct involvement (Patz et al., 1992). Transmural involvement of the pericardium can be associated with pericardial effusion (Figure 11.27; Kawashima and Libshitz, 1990; Ng et al., 1999).

(A)   **(B)**

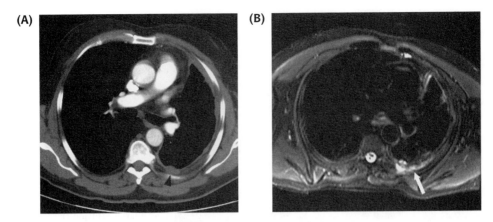

Figure 11.25 Focal invasion of extrapleural fat by malignant mesothelioma. (A) CT demonstrates a small mass extending extrapleurally (arrowhead), (B) MRI STIR sequence confirms extrapleural spread by showing abnormal signal in the chest wall (arrow).

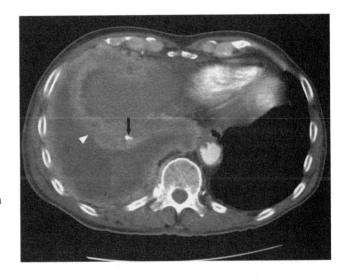

Figure 11.26 CT scan: diaphragmatic involvement by malignant mesothelioma (white arrowhead). A calcified pleural plaque (black arrow) has been engulfed by tumor.

Enlarged intrathoracic lymph nodes are common in malignant mesothelioma, occurring in 34%–58% of unselected patients (Figure 11.23; Kawashima and Libshitz, 1990; Ng et al., 1999; Sahin et al., 1993). The pattern of nodal spread is less predictable than in other thoracic malignancies such as nonsmall cell lung cancer (Heelan, 1999; IMIG, 1995) and ipsilateral and contralateral mediastinal, internal mammary, pericardial and paraoesophageal groups may be affected. Spread to extrathoracic nodal groups including axillary, supraclavicular, scalene, retrocrural, and celiac axis nodes is not uncommon. As malignant mesothelioma often spreads directly along the mediastinal surface in an irregular fashion, separation of the primary tumor from contiguous involved mediastinal lymph nodes may often be difficult (Heelan, 1999; Kawashima and Libshitz, 1990; Patz et al., 1992).

As with many other solid tumors, computed tomography readily demonstrates distant metastases including spread to lung or liver (Wang et al., 2004).

Despite its limitations for evaluation of individual components of the TNM staging system, computed tomography provides a useful overall assessment of the extent of

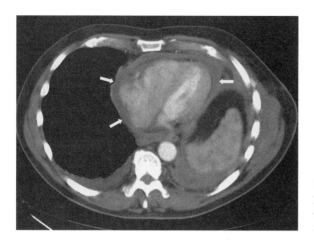

Figure 11.27 CT scan: malignant pericardial effusion (arrows) due to pericardial invasion by malignant mesothelioma.

disease, particularly in the majority of cases who will have clearly advanced tumor at presentation (Patz et al., 1992). In one series, the use of computed tomography upstaged the extent of the mesothelioma in 25% of patients, including a number of those initially considered to have potentially resectable tumor (Sahin et al., 1993).

In a minority of cases with malignant mesothelioma, particularly those being considered for radical surgery, further investigation by MRI (Figure 11.28) or PET (Figure 11.29) may be undertaken (Heelan et al., 1999; Patz et al., 1992; Wang et al., 2004).

Utilizing MRI, images may be obtained using a variety of sequences and contrast enhancement with gadolinium to optimize visualization of the tumor (Heenan, 1999; Patz et al., 1992; Wang et al., 2004). The multiplanar capability of MRI and its high contrast resolution have been shown to allow more accurate assessment of endothoracic fascia involvement, solitary foci of chest wall invasion (Figure 11.25B) and invasion of diaphragmatic muscle (Heelan, 1999). However, for other aspects of the staging of malignant mesothelioma, CT and MRI have been shown to be of equivalent diagnostic accuracy and the addition of MRI to the investigative algorithm often does not affect surgical management. In view of these findings, and for cost reasons, it has been recommended that computed tomography should be considered the standard diagnostic investigation before treatment (Heelan, 1999; Patz et al., 1992).

PET scanning in mesothelioma is based on the principle that malignant tumors often exhibit abnormally high rates of glucose metabolism (Figure 11.29). They will therefore take up radio-labeled analogues of glucose and scanning can provide useful anatomical and functional information. The use of positron emitting FDG for the assessment of malignant mesothelioma has been described (Benard et al., 1998; Benard et al., 1999; Schneider et al., 2000). Uptake of this radionuclide is significantly higher in malignant mesothelioma than in benign pleural thickening (Benard et al., 1998), which may aid differentiation between the two processes in difficult cases. The technique allows whole body imaging and it can be used to identify previously unsuspected nodal and distant metastases, avoiding unnecessary radical surgery in patients with advanced disease (Benard et al., 1998; Schneider et al., 2000). PET imaging has a particular advantage over computed tomography and MRI in that it can demonstrate abnormal uptake in normal sized but metastatic lymph nodes (Benard et al., 1998). The spatial resolution of PET scanning is limited in comparison to computed tomography and anatomical delineation of the tumor is best achieved by fusion of PET and CT images, CT-PET (Clarke, 2004).

(A)   (B)

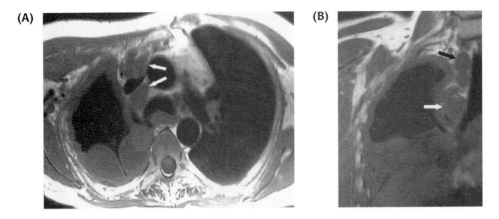

Figure 11.28 MRI scan: (A) axial and (B) coronal T1 weighted images show a bulky right-sided mesothelioma with enlarged mediastinal nodes (arrows).

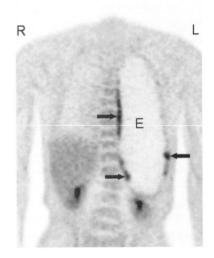

Figure 11.29 PET demonstration of malignant mesothelioma. A massive pleural effusion (E) is causing a large photon deficient area and inversion of the left hemidiaphragm. Metabolically active tumor is represented by foci of increased radionuclide activity (arrows).

Although the radiological appearances are characteristic in many cases, it may be difficult to differentiate malignant mesothelioma from other extensive pleural processes including benign diffuse pleural thickening and in particular metastatic adenocarcinoma (Figure 11.30). Biopsy is often required to establish the correct diagnosis. It is difficult to diagnose malignant mesothelioma from a cytological aspirate and a good sample of material is usually required for histological examination including immunohistochemical techniques. While this can be achieved by more invasive procedures such as thoracoscopy or open surgical biopsy, there is good evidence that radiologically guided biopsy using semiautomated cutting needles is safe and effective with one series reporting sensitivity of 86% and specificity of 100% (Adams et al., 2001)

While malignant mesothelioma usually affects the pleura, it may occasionally arise from the pericardium or peritoneum. Primary pericardial mesothelioma is characterized by pericardial thickening and effusion. The typical features of primary peritoneal mesothelioma include peritoneal infiltration, nodules or masses, and the presence of ascites (Figure 11.31; Guest et al., 1992; Yeh and Chapman, 1980).

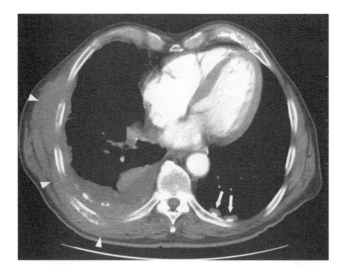

Figure 11.30 CT scan showing extensive chest wall tumor (arrowheads) with coincidental pleural plaques (arrows). Although mimicking malignant mesothelioma, biopsy demonstrated non-Hodgkins lymphoma.

(A)   (B)

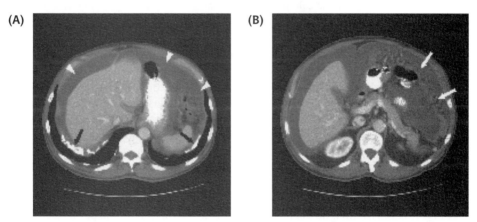

Figure 11.31 Peritoneal mesothelioma. CT scan (A) there are calcified pleural plaques (black arrows) and there is abdominal ascites (white arrowheads), (B) in addition to ascites there is infiltration of the omentum by tumor (white arrows).

Asbestosis

Asbestosis can be defined as diffuse pulmonary parenchymal fibrosis secondary to the inhalation of asbestos fibres (Fraser et al., 1999). It may or may not be associated with pleural fibrosis. There is a dose-response relationship between exposure and the severity of the fibrosis (Dee, 2000). Subjects with asbestosis should give a reliable history of substantial exposure, usually over a long period. The latent interval between exposure and onset of symptoms is usually 20 years or more but can be as little as 3 years with severe heavy exposure (Dee, 2000; Fraser et al., 1999; McLoud et al., 1985). Fibrosis usually begins posteriorly at the lung bases. Peribronchiolar areas adjacent to the visceral pleura are initially affected and the disease then progresses centrally extending to the right middle lobe and lingula (Churg, 1988; Müller et al., 2003). Honeycombing can occur in advanced stages of the disease but is not seen in the majority of patients. Aberle (Aberle et al. 1988a,b) reported honeycombing in 7%–17% of their cases.

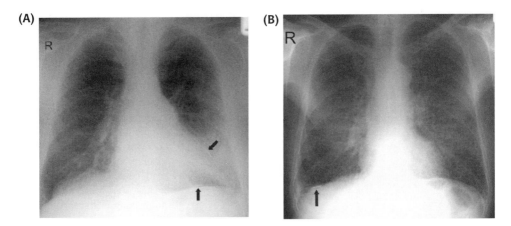

(A)

(B)

Figure 11.32 PA chest radiographs of two cases of asbestosis: (A) ground glass shadowing and fine reticulation is present at both lung bases. Calcified pleural plaques are evident (arrows) (B) bilateral mid and lower zone reticulo-nodular shadowing produces a 'shaggy' cardiac outline. A pleural plaque is again evident (arrow).

Plain chest radiographic features include ground glass opacification, small irregular nodular and reticular opacities, a *shaggy* cardiac silhouette, and ill-defined diaphragmatic outlines. Honeycombing and volume loss are seen in more advanced disease (Figure 11.32; Fraser et al., 1999). Asbestosis can be present but not detectable on plain films. In a study by Gamsu (Gamsu et al., 1995) of histopathologically proven cases of asbestosis, plain chest radiographic findings were suggestive of asbestosis in only 11 of 25 cases. Similarly, asbestosis may be present and may cause physiological impairment when the lung parenchyma appears normal on the chest radiograph (Kipen et al., 1987; Staples et al., 1989). In addition to underdetection of asbestosis, plain chest radiographs may also result in overdiagnosis of asbestosis due to obscuration of the pulmonary parenchyma by overlying pleural plaques, diffuse pleural thickening, or even extrapleural fat deposits. The sensitivity, specificity, and negative predictive value of plain chest radiographs are improved by expert reading (Friedman et al., 1988).

The plain film changes described earlier are not specific for asbestosis, but the diagnosis should be strongly suspected if there are also either pleural plaques or diffuse pleural thickening. Pleural diseases may be evident on plain chest radiographs in around 80% of patients with asbestosis (Figure 11.32; Dee, 2000). The radiological findings should prompt the taking of an in depth occupational history.

Computed tomography, especially high resolution CT, is more sensitive than plain radiography in demonstrating the features of asbestosis (Aberle et al., 1988b; Friedman et al., 1988; Staples et al., 1989). In a study by Aberle (Aberle et al., 1988a), HRCT demonstrated changes of asbestosis in 80% of patients with a clinical diagnosis of asbestosis but no chest radiographic evidence and showed changes of asbestosis in one third of asbestos-exposed individuals with neither clinical nor chest radiographic evidence of asbestosis. Staples (Staples et al., 1989) described similar findings.

The CT criteria for the diagnosis of asbestosis have been described as subpleural curvilinear lines, thickened septal and core lines, subpleural density, parenchymal bands, and honeycombing. These abnormalities are usually seen best in the posterior subpleural area of the lung bases and they persist in the prone position (Aberle et al., 1988a; Staples, 1992). Gamsu subsequently discarded subpleural density as a sign of asbestosis due to its

(A)

(B)

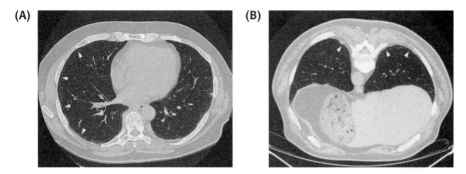

Figure 11.33 Subpleural curvilinear lines: (A) supine CT scan showing right sided subpleural curvilinear line (arrowheads). Less marked changes are present on the left (B) prone CT scan in another individual showing mild bilateral subpleural curvilinear lines (arrowheads).

lack of specificity and substituted subpleural nodules and the useful sign of architectural distortion (Gamsu et al., 1995). Akira et al. have also described ground glass opacities as a feature of asbestosis (Akira et al., 1990, 1991).

Curvilinear subpleural lines consisting of linear opacities of increased density located within 1 cm of the pleura and parallel to the inner chest wall (Figure 11.33; Yoshimura et al., 1986) have been noted in dependent areas of the lungs in not only 30% of patients with asbestosis but also in 9%–35% of the control subjects (Aberle et al., 1988b; Bergin et al., 1991). This radiological sign is nonspecific, may be transient and is only significant when persisting in nondependent areas of lung (Gamsu et al., 1989).

Thickened interstitial septae are represented by linear shadows 1–2 cm in length in the lung periphery and lying perpendicular to the overlying pleura (Figure 11.34; Staples, 1992).

Thickened core structures that comprise of centrilobular bronchovascular bundles are seen as branching linear shadows approximately 1 cm from the pleural surface (Figure 11.34). These opacities are the most frequent finding in patients with asbestosis (Aberle et al., 1988b; Bergin et al., 1991; Gamsu et al., 1989).

Parenchymal bands are linear shadows 2–5 cm long, coursing through the lung and usually contacting the pleura (Figures 11.13, 11.14, and 11.15; Aberle et al., 1988b). They are differentiated from pulmonary vessels by their abnormal orientation within the lung. They occur frequently not only in patients with asbestosis but also in control subjects (Aberle et al., 1988b; Bergin et al., 1991). Parenchymal bands are often closely related to areas of thickening of the visceral pleura. When they occur in the absence of other CT features of asbestosis it is difficult to determine whether they represent foci of atelectasis or fibrosis secondary to the pleural thickening with possible restricted lung movement, or whether they are an early feature of true interstitial fibrosis. (Staples, 1992).

Honeycombing is seen as multiple airspaces less than 15 mm in diameter with discrete thickened walls (Figure 11.35). This change is usually most obvious subpleurally at the lung bases and particularly in the paravertebral gutters.

The subpleural opacities described by Akira et al. (1990) appear as subpleural, isolated, dot-like, and branching opacities related to the most peripheral branches of the pulmonary artery. These opacities may increase in number on sequential scans to produce a reticulonodular interstitial pattern (Akira et al., 1991).

Gamsu et al. (1995) found that interstitial lines due to thickened interlobular septae and centrilobular core structures were the most commonly found abnormality in asbestosis (84% of cases) followed by parenchymal bands (76%), and distortion of secondary pulmonary lobules (56%). Subpleural curvilinear opacities and honeycombing were less frequent.

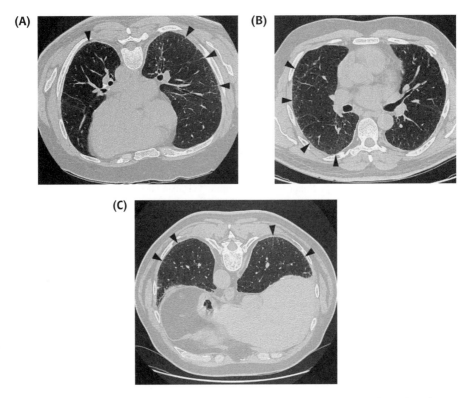

Figure 11.34 (A)–(C) Thickened septae and core structures: three examples of subpleural interstitial shadowing (arrowheads) demonstrated by CT in cases of mild asbestosis.

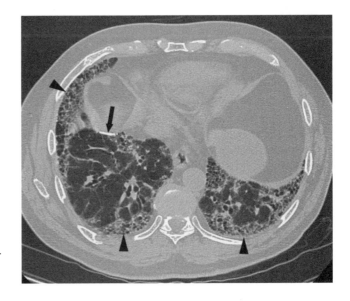

Figure 11.35 CT scan: advanced subpleural honeycomb change (arrowheads). The changes could be due to asbestosis or coincidental usual interstitial pneumonia in an asbestos-exposed individual. A calcified diaphragmatic plaque is present (arrow).

Ground glass opacification has also been described in patients with asbestosis and is the term applied to hazy patches of increased parenchymal attenuation without obscuration of normal lung structures. Subpleural ground glass opacification or reticulation can occur as a gravity dependent effect and on supine scans is seen in the subpleural areas of lung posteriorly.

(A) 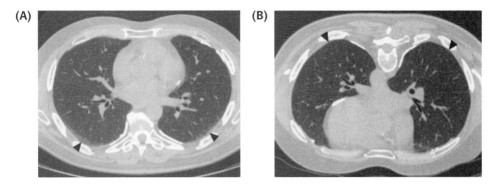 (B)

Figure 11.36 Gravitational effect mimicking early pulmonary fibrosis: (A) on a supine CT scan there are crescents of ground glass opacification in dependent parts of both lungs (arrowheads). (B) these disappear on a prone scan. Note calcified pleural plaques.

(A) 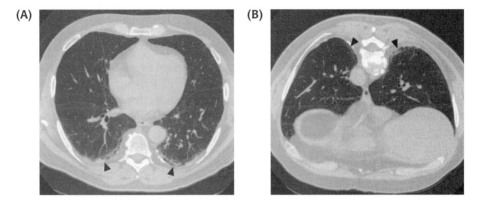 (B)

Figure 11.37 True asbestosis: (A) on a supine CT scan there are areas of increased density posteriorly in both lower lobes (arrowheads) with associated pleural plaques (B) the pulmonary abnormality persists in the prone position indicating true structural disease (arrowheads).

As a true manifestation of asbestosis it is a fixed abnormality and not posture dependent. The use of prone scans allows differentiation between transient gravitational effects (Figure 11.36) and the fixed structural abnormality of asbestosis (Figure 11.37; Aberle et al., 1988b).

There are only very limited studies correlating radiological and histological findings. HRCT-pathological correlation studies have shown that subpleural dots and branching structures correspond to peribronchiolar fibrosis (Akira et al., 1991; Müller et al., 2003). Extension of fibrous tissue into the parenchyma between affected bronchioles results in pleural-based nodular irregularities (Akira et al., 1991). Thickened interlobular septa seen on HRCT correspond either to fibrosis of the septa themselves or to fibrosis in the periphery of the lobule. Ground glass opacities are related to mild alveolar wall fibrosis (Akira et al., 1990, 1991). Parenchymal bands have been shown to correspond to fibrosis along the bronchovascular sheath or interlobular septa with associated distortion of parenchymal architecture (Akira et al., 1990).

HRCT is not infallible (Roach et al., 2002). None of the HRCT signs of asbestosis are diagnostic. Subpleural curvilinear densities, subpleural density in dependent locations, parenchymal bands, and thickened septal lines can all occur as isolated or combined findings in patients with a variety of conditions other than asbestosis. Their occurrence, even in patients with CT evidence of pleural plaques, does not necessarily indicate the presence of asbestosis (Bergin et al., 1994). Gamsu assessed the frequency of five HRCT features of asbestosis in a group of subjects including those with histologically proven asbestosis and a small number of cases without asbestosis. This showed that any one type of abnormality was present in 88% of patients with asbestosis, two types in 78% and three in 56%. To include only cases with proven asbestosis three or more abnormalities had to be present. Abnormalities also needed to be bilateral or multifocal. The HRCT scans were normal or near normal in five cases of histologically proven asbestosis (20%). Gamsu concluded that a combination of the cumulative number of different findings and an assessment of the extent and severity of the various radiographic abnormalities could be complementary (Gamsu et al., 1995).

HRCT is sometimes helpful in distinguishing asbestosis from other causes of lung fibrosis when a history of asbestos exposure is in doubt but differentiation can be difficult as many of the above findings are not specific to asbestosis.

The main differential diagnosis both radiologically and histopathologically is usual interstitial pneumonitis (UIP) or idiopathic pulmonary fibrosis (IPF; Staples, 1992). Studies comparing the HRCT findings in these conditions have found that ground glass opacities are common in IPF and uncommon in asbestosis. The reverse is true for parenchymal bands and subpleural lines. In a study by Al Jarad, parenchymal bands were present in 79% of patients who had asbestosis compared with 11% in patients who had IPF (Al Jarad et al., 1992b). Copley et al. (2003) have shown that patients with asbestosis have coarser fibrosis than those with IPF. However, there was no difference between the radiological appearances of asbestosis and UIP and the difference was largely due to the inclusion of a subset of patients with nonspecific interstitial pneumonitis (NSIP). It was concluded that the HRCT pattern of asbestosis closely resembles that of biopsy proven UIP, but it differs markedly from that of biopsy proven NSIP. A basal and subpleural distribution of disease was usual in all subgroups (asbestosis, UIP, NSIP) but was significantly more prevalent with asbestosis than with UIP or NSIP.

A study by Akira comparing asbestosis and IPF (Akira et al., 2003) has shown that subpleural dot-like or branching opacities, subpleural curvilinear lines, mosaic perfusion, and parenchymal bands were more common in patients with asbestosis than in patients with IPF. Visible intralobular bronchioles, bronchiolectasis within fibrotic consolidations, and honeycombing were more common in patients with IPF. The frequency of interlobular septal thickening, ground glass opacities, fibrotic consolidation, and emphysema were similar in both groups. Parenchymal bands and fibrotic consolidation were more commonly seen in patients with asbestosis associated with pleural disease than in patients with asbestosis without pleural disease.

It is evident that there is considerable overlap in the radiological appearances of asbestosis and IPF.

Lung Cancer

There is increased incidence of bronchogenic carcinoma in subjects with asbestosis (Figure 11.20). There is considerable controversy about whether asbestos exposure without radiological evidence of asbestosis also leads to a higher risk of lung cancer (Figure 11.38; Wilkinson et al., 1995). This is discussed in detail in another section of this book (Chapter 7).

Although there may be radiological features of previous asbestos exposure including pleural plaques, diffuse pleural thickening or pulmonary fibrosis, the radiological manifestations of lung cancer in asbestos-exposed individuals are the same as those seen in nonexposed individuals (Figure 11.20). Radiological diagnostic and staging procedures should therefore be performed according to normal protocols.

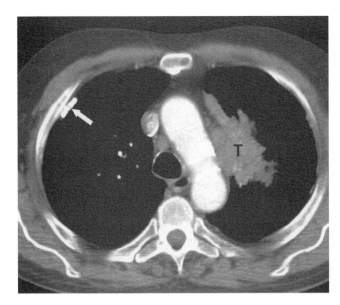

Figure 11.38 CT scan: central left sided bronchogenic carcinoma (T) in an asbestos-exposed subject. A calcified pleural plaque is present on the right (arrow).

Computed tomography has been used to screen for early lung cancer in a high-risk population exposed to asbestos. Although in one series five cancers were detected in 602 workers, there were 111 false positive cases of nonmalignant pulmonary nodules of which 66 required further hospital evaluation. Only one patient with malignancy ultimately underwent surgery (Kivisaari et al., 2002). On the basis of this evidence the value of screening asbestos-exposed individuals for early lung cancer must be doubtful.

References

Aberle DR, Gamsu G, Ray CS. High-resolution CT of benign asbestos-related diseases: clinical and radiological correlation. *Am J Roentgenol.* 1988a;151:883–891.

Aberle DR, Gamsu G, Ray CS, Feuerstein IM. Asbestos-related pleural and parenchymal fibrosis: detection with high-resolution CT. *Radiology.* 1988b;166:729–734.

Adams RF, Gray W, Davies RJ, et al. Percutaneous image-guided cutting needle biopsy of the pleura in the diagnosis of malignant pleural mesothelioma. *Chest.* 2001;120:1798–1802.

Akira M, Yokoyama K, Yamamoto S, et al. Asbestosis: High-Resolution CT-Pathologic correlation. *Radiology.* 1990;176:389–394.

Akira M, Yokoyama K, Yamamoto S, et al. Early asbestosis: evaluation with high-resolution CT. *Radiology.* 1991;178:409–416.

Akira M, Yamamoto S, Inoue Y, Sakatani M. High-resolution CT of asbestosis and idiopathic pulmonary fibrosis. *Am J Roentgenol.* 2003;181:163–169.

Al Jarad N, Poulakis N, Pearson MC, Rubens MB, Rudd RM. Assessment of asbestos-induced pleural disease by computed tomography—correlation with chest radiograph and lung function. *Respir Med.* 1991;85:203–208.

Al Jarad N, Wilkinson P, Pearson M, Rudd RM. A new high resolution computed tomography scoring system for pulmonary fibrosis, pleural disease and emphysema in patients with asbestos related disease. *Br J Ind Med.* 1992a;49:73–84.

Al-Jarad N, Strickland B, Pearson MC, Rubens MB, Rudd RM. High-resolution computed tomographic assessment of asbestosis and cryptogenic fibrosing alveolitis: a comparative study. *Thorax.* 1992b;47:645–650.

Ameille J, Brochard P, Brechot JM, et al. Pleural thickening: a comparison of oblique chest radiographs and high-resolution computed tomography in subjects exposed to low levels of asbestos pollution. *Int Arch Occup Environ Health.* 1993;64:545–548.

Benard F, Sterman D, Smith RJ, Albelda SM, Alavi A. Prognostic value of FDG PET imaging in malignant pleural mesothelioma. *J Nucl Med*. 1999;40:1241–1245.

Benard F, Sterman D, Smith RJ, Albelda SM, Alavi A. Metabolic imaging of malignant pleural mesothelioma with fluorodeoxyglucose positron emission tomography. *Chest*. 1998;114(3):713–722.

Bergin CT, Blank N, Castellino RA. Nonspecificity of high-resolution CT. *Radiology*. 1991;181:117–118.

Bergin CJ, Castellino RA, Blank N, Moses L. Specificity of high-resolution CT findings in pulmonary asbestosis: do patients scanned for other indications have similar findings? *Am J Roentgenol*. 1994;163:551–555.

Blesovsky A. The folded lung. *Br J Dis Chest*. 1966;60:19–22.

Carvalho PM, Carr DH. Computed tomography of folded lung. *Clin Radiol*. 1990;41:86–91.

Churg A. Non-neoplastic diseases caused by asbestos. In: Churg A, Green FHY, eds. *Pathology of Occupational Lung Disease*, New York: Igaku-Shoin Medical Publishers; 1988: 214–217.

Clarke JC. PET/CT 'Cometh the hour, cometh the machine?' *Clini Radiol*. 2004;59:775–776.

Copley SJ, Wells AU, Rubens MB, et al. Functional consequences of pleural disease evaluated with chest radiography and CT. *Radiology*. 2001:220;237–243.

Copley SJ, Wells AV, Sivakumaran P, et al. Asbestosis and idiopathic pulmonary fibrosis: Comparison of thin section CT features. *Radiology*. 2003;229:731–736.

Cugell DW. Asbestos and the pleura. *Chest*. 2004;125:1103–1117.

Dee P. Inhalational lung diseases. In: Armstrong P, Wilson AG, Dee P, Hansell DM, eds. *Imaging of Diseases of the Chest*. 3rd ed. London, UK: Mosby, Harcourt; 2000: 485.

De Raeve H, Verschakelen JA, Gevenois PA Mahieu P, Moens G, Nemery B. Observer variation in computed tomography of pleural lesions in subjects exposed to indoor asbestos. *Eur Respir J*. 2001;17:916–921.

Eisenstadt HB. Asbestos pleurisy. *Dis Chest*. 1964;46:78–81.

Epler GR, McLoud TC, Gaensler EA. Prevalence and incidence of benign asbestos pleural effusion in a working population. *JAMA*. 1982;247:617–622.

Fletcher DE, Edge JR. The early radiological changes in pulmonary and pleural asbestosis. *Clin Radiol*. 1970;21:355–365.

Frank W, Loddenkemper R. Fiber-associated pleural disease. *Semin Respir Crit Care Med*. 1995;16:315–323.

Fraser RS, Müller NL, Colman N, Paré PD. Chapter 60- Inhalation of organic dust (pneumoconiosis). In: *Diagnosis of Diseases of the Chest*, 4th ed. Philadelphia: WB Saunders; 1999: 2386–2484.

Friedman AC, Fiel SB, Fisher MS, Radecki PD Lev-Toaff AS, Caroline DF. Asbestos-Related Pleural Disease and Asbestosis: a comparison of CT and chest radiography. *Am J Roentgenol*. 1988; 50:269–275.

Gamsu G, Aberle DR, Lynch D. Computed tomography in the diagnosis of asbestos-related thoracic disease. *J Thorac Imaging*. 1989;4:61–67.

Gamsu G, Salmon CJ, Warnock ML, Blanc PD. CT quantification of interstitial fibrosis in patients with asbestosis: a comparison of two methods. *Am J Roentgenol*. 1995;164:63–68.

Gevenois PA, de Vuyst P, Dedeire S, Cosaert J, Vande WR, Struyven J. Conventional and high resolution CT in asymptomatic asbestos-exposed workers. *Acta Radiol*. 1994;35:226–229.

Gevenois PA, de Maertelaer V, Madani AC, et al. Asbestosis, pleural plaques and diffuse pleural thickening: three distinct benign responses to asbestos exposure. *Eur Respir J*. 1998;11:1021–1027.

Gitlin JN, Cook LL, Linton OW, Garrett-Mayer E. Comparison of 'B' readers' interpretations of chest radiographs for asbestos related changes. *Acad Radiol*. 2004;11:843–856.

Guest PJ, Reznek RH, Selleslag D, Geraghty R, Slevin M. Peritoneal mesothelioma: the role of computed tomography in diagnosis and follow-up. *Clin Radiol*. 1992;45:79–84.

Heelan RT, Rusch VW, Begg CB, et al. Staging of malignant mesothelioma: comparison of CT and MRI imaging. *Am J Roentgenol*. 1999;172:1039–1047.

Hering KG, Tuengerthal S, Kraus T. Standardisierte CT/HRCT- Klassifikation der Bundersrepublik Deutschland für arbeits—und um- weltbedingte Thoraxerkrankungen. *Radiologe*. 2004;44:500–511.

Hillerdal G. Non-malignant pleural disease related to asbestos exposure. *Clin Chest Med.* 1985;6:141–152.

Hillerdal G, Ozesmi M. Benign asbestos pleural effusion. 73 exudates in 60 patients. *Eur J Respir Dis.* 1987;71:113–121.

Hillerdal G. Rounded atelectasis. Clinical experience with 74 patients. *Chest.* 1989;95:836–841.

Hillerdal G, Malmberg P, Hemmingsson A. Asbestos-related disease of the pleura: Parietal plaques compared to diffuse thickening studied with chest roentgenography, computed tomography, lung function, and gas exchange. *Am J Ind Med.* 1990;18:627–639.

Hillerdal G. Pleural lesions and the ILO classification: the need for a revision. *Am J Ind Med.* 1991;19:125–130.

Im J-G, Webb RW, Rosen A, Gamsu G. Costal Pleura: Appearances at High-Resolution CT. *Radiology.* 1989;171:125–131.

Impivaara O, Zitting AJ, Kuusela T Alanen E, Karjalainen A. Observer variation in classifying chest radiographs for small lung opacities and pleural abnormalities in a population sample. *Am J Ind Med.* 1998;34:261–265

Industrial Injuries Advisory Council in accordance with Section 171 of the Social Security Administration Act 1992: asbestos related diseases. London, UK: Her Majesty's Stationery Office; 1996.

International Labour Office: Guidelines for the use of ILO International Classification of radiographs of pneumoconioses. Geneva: 1980:1–48.

International Mesothelioma Interest Group. A proposed new international TNM staging system for malignant pleural mesothelioma. *Chest.* 1995;108:1122–1128.

Kawashima A, Libshitz HI. Malignant pleural mesothelioma: CT manifestations in 50 cases. *Am J Roentgenol.* 1990;155:965–969.

Kipen HM, Lilis R, Suzuki Y, Valciukas JA, Selikoff IJ. Pulmonary fibrosis in asbestos insulation workers with lung cancer: a radiological and histopathological evaluation. *Br J Ind Med.* 1987;44:96–100.

Kivisaari TM, Huuskonen MS, Mattson K, et al. Computed tomography screening for lung cancer in asbestos-exposed workers. *Lung Cancer.* 2002;35:17–22.

Kreel L. Computer tomography in the evaluation of pulmonary asbestosis. Preliminary experiences with the EMI general purpose scanner. *Acta Radiol Diagn.* 1976;17:405–412.

Leung AN, Müller NL, Miller RR. CT in differential diagnosis of diffuse pleural disease. *Am J Roentgenol.* 1990;154:487–492.

Lynch DA, Gamsu G, Ray CS, Aberle DR. Asbestos-related focal lung masses: manifestations on conventional and high-resolution CT scans. *Radiology.* 1988;169:603–607.

Lynch DA, Gamsu G, Aberle DR. Conventional and high resolution tomography in the diagnosis of asbestos-related diseases. *Radiographics.* 1989;9:S23-S51.

McAdams HP, Erasmus JJ, Patz FF, Goodman PC, Coleman RE. Evaluation of patients with round atelectasis using 2-[18F]fluoro-2-deoxy-D-glucose PET. *J Comput Assist Tomogr.* 1998;22:601–604.

McHugh K, Blaquiere RM. CT features of rounded atelectasis. *Am J Roentgenol.* 1989;153:257–260.

McLoud TC, Woods BO, Carrington CB, Epler JR, Gaensler EA. Diffuse pleural thickening in the asbestos-exposed population. *Am J Roentgenol.* 1985;144:9–18.

Meyer JD, Islam SS, Ducatman AM, McCunney RJ. Prevalance of Small Opacities in Populations unexposed to dusts. A literature analysis. *Chest.* 1997;111:404–410.

Müller NL. Imaging of the pleura. *Radiology.* 1993;186:297–309.

Müller NL, Fraser RS, Lee KS, Johkoh T. Chapter 9, Occupational lung disease. In: *Diseases of the lung. Radiologic and Pathologic Correlations*, Philadelphia, PA: Lippincott Williams and Wilkins; 2003:183–207.

Nishimura SL, Broaddus VC. Asbestos-induced pleural disease. *Clinic Chest Med.* 1998;19:311–329.

Ng CS, Munden RF, Libshitz HI. Malignant pleural mesothelioma: the spectrum of manifestations on CT in 70 cases. *Clinl Radiol.* 1999;54:415–421.

Patz EF, Shaffer K, Piwnica-Worms DR, et al. Malignant pleural mesothelioma: value of CT and MRI in predicting respectability. *Am J Roentgenol.* 1992;159:961–966.

Peacock C, Copley SJ, Hansell DM. Asbestos-related benign pleural disease. *Clin Radiol.* 2000;55:422–432.

Reger RB, Ames RG, Merchant JA, et al. The detection of thoracic abnormalities using posterior-anterior (PA) vs PA and oblique roentenograms. *Chest.* 1982;3:290–295.

Roach HD, Davies GJ, Attanoos R, Crane M, Adams H, Phillips S. Asbestos: when the dust settles- an imaging review of asbestos-related disease. *Radiographics.* 2002;22:S167-S184.

Rockoff SD, Kagan E, Schwartz A, Kriebel D, Hix W, Prashant R. Visceral pleural thickening in asbestos exposure: the occurrence and implications of thickened interlobar fissures. *J Thorac Imaging.* 1987;2:58–66.

Rockoff SD, Schwartz A. Roentgenographic underestimation of early asbestosis by International Labour Organisation classification. *Chest.* 1988;93:1088–1091

Rosenstock L, Barnhart S, Heyer NJ, et al. The relation among pulmonary function, chest roentgenographic abnormalities, and smoking status in an asbestos-exposed cohort. *American Rev Respir Dis.* 1988;138:272–277.

Rusch VW, Godwin JD, Shuman WP. The role of computed tomography scanning in the initial assessment and follow-up of malignant pleural mesothelioma. *J Thorac Cardiovasc Surg.* 1988;96:171–177.

Sahin AA, Coplu L, Selcuk ZT, et al. Malignant pleural mesothelioma caused by environmental exposure to asbestos or erionite in rural Turkey: CT findings in 84 patients. *Am J Roentgenol.* 1993;161:533–537.

Sargent EN, Gordonson J, Jacobson G, Birnbaum W, Shaub M. Bilateral pleural thickening: a manifestation of asbestos dust exposure. *Am J Roentgenol.* 1978;131:579–585.

Schneider DB, Clary-Macy C, Challa S, et al. Positron emission tomography with f18-fluorodeoxyglucose in the staging and pre-operative evaluation of malignant pleural mesothelioma. *Cardiovasc Surg.* 2000;120:128–133.

Staples CA, Gamsu G, Ray CS, Webb RW. High resolution computed tomography and lung function in asbestos-exposed workers with normal chest radiographs. *American Rev Respir Dis.* 1989;139:1502–1508.

Staples CA. Computed Tomography in the evaluation of benign asbestos-related disorders. *Radiol Clin North Am.* 1992;30(6):1191–1207.

Suganuma N, Kusaka Y, Hosoda Y, et al. The Japanese classification of computed tomography for pneumoconiosis with standard films: comparison with the ILO Classification of radiographs for pneumconioses. *J Occup Health.* 2001;43:24–31.

Taylor PM. Dynamic contrast enhancement of asbestos related pulmonary pseudotumors. *Br J Radiol.* 1988;61:1070–1072.

Wang ZJ, Reddy GP, Gotway MB, et al. Malignant pleural mesothelioma: evaluation with CT, MR imaging and PET. *Radiographics.* 2004;24:105–119.

Welch LS, Huntink KL, Balmes J, et al. Variability in the classification of radiographs using the 1980 International Labour Organisation classification for pneumoconiosis. *Chest.* 1998;114:1740–1748.

Wilkinson P, Hansell DM, Janssens J, et al. Is lung cancer associated with asbestos exposure when there are no small opacities on the chest radiograph? *Lancet.* 1995;345:1074–1078.

Yates DH, Browne K, Stidolph PN, Neville E. Asbestos-related bilateral diffuse pleural thickening: natural history of radiographic and lung function abnormalities. *Am J Respir Crit Care Med.* 1996;153:301–306.

Yeh HC, Chapman AP. Ultrasonography and computed tomography of peritoneal mesothelioma. *Radiology.* 1980;135:705–712.

Yoshimura H, Hatakeyama M, Otsuji H, et al. Pulmonary asbestosis: CT study of subpleural curvilinear shadow. *Radiology.* 1986;158:653–658.

12

Mineral Fiber Analysis and Asbestos-Related Diseases

Allen R. Gibbs and Fred Pooley

Introduction

There are several established methods for mineral fiber analysis; they differ in sensitivity, specificity, complexity, and cost. Results of analyses from one laboratory cannot be directly compared with those from a second laboratory since the protocols and equipment are likely to differ. Since a variety of fiber types, including asbestos, are ubiquitous in the air and present in the lungs of nonindustrially exposed populations, results from a specific case(s) should be compared with those for a background population.

Mineral fiber analysis can provide valuable information for both research and the assessment of exposure (Table 12.1; Gibbs and Pooley, 1996). It reflects deposition and biological persistence of fibers. Anecdotal assessments of airborne exposure are beset with difficulties. There are a number of reasons. Airborne fiber measurements using air samplers have been poorly characterized since (1) methods of sampling differ over time; (2) the measurements of fibers 5 μm or greater in length are not broken down into respirable and nonrespirable; and (3) no fiber size distributions are given and generally the published data is based on counts using phase contrast microscopy (PCM). The latter, when compared with transmission electron microscopy (TEM), underestimates the number of fibers by several orders of magnitude. For example, for a given sample, PCM will only detect about 10% of the amosite, and about 1%–2% of crocidolite fibers in lung tissue. Deposition of fibers is critically dependent on fiber size; a small percentage alteration in fiber size distribution, which might follow certain industrial manipulations, can result in a disproportionate effect on deposition in the lung. Information of this type is generally not available when estimating airborne exposures in terms of f/mL-years. This is reflected in a case study of the relation between asbestos fiber lung burdens and estimates of cumulative asbestos exposure in terms of f/mL-years (Fischer et al., 2002).

Mineral fiber analysis of lung samples has clarified the types of fiber exposure in a number of industrial situations. For example, railroad workers in the United States were claimed to have been only exposed to chrysotile, and malignant mesothelioma (MM) occurring in these workers were therefore attributed to this fiber type (Mancuso, 1988). However, many railroad workers were also exposed to lesser quantities of amosite, and on mineral fiber analysis, substantial amounts of amosite were demonstrated in their lungs. And, sometimes crocidolite was found (Churg and Green, 1990; Roggli, 2004). Another example is based on the study of the Rochdale textile plant worker in the United

Table 12.1 Situations where Mineral Fiber Analysis is Useful

1. Correlations between fiber concentrations in tissues and both the patterns and severity of asbestos-related disease in occupational cohorts
2. Clarification of the role of different fiber types in the causation of disease
3. Validation of levels of exposure in different industrial settings and correlation with hygiene assessments such as job exposure matrices
4. Clarification of usage of different materials at a facility
5. Validation of exposure in a given case
6. Attribution of diseases such as MM, diffuse pleural fibrosis (DPF), and lung fibrosis to mineral fiber exposures
7. Assessment of mixed mineral particle exposures

Kingdom. These workers were thought to have been exposed to chrysotile and little or no amphibole. However, lung burden analysis demonstrated considerable quantities of crocidolite in amounts greatly exceeding background population (Wagner et al., 1982).

 Analytical Techniques

Light Microscopy of Tissue Sections

These are technically simple, inexpensive, and widely available but have several limitations.

Routine light microscopy (LM) allows for a basic assessment of fibers retained in the lungs. Ferruginous bodies can be identified in 5 μm thick sections, but detection is improved either by using Perl's iron stain or by the evaluation of thick, unstained (20 μm) thick sections. The pathologist should be able to distinguish ferruginous bodies formed on transparent fibrous cores typical of asbestos bodies (AB) from those formed on nonasbestos minerals such as carbon, iron oxide, rutile, aluminum oxide, chromium oxide, mullite, kaolin, mica, talc, and glass (Crouch and Churg, 1984; Roggli, 2004).

As discussed in Chapter 6 ferruginous body formation is influenced by a number of factors including asbestos fiber type, length, lung fiber burden, and biological factors unique to the host. Therefore, counts of AB do not show a consistent relationship to fibers. For example, the proportion of a given number of amosite fibers forming AB will be higher than that of an equivalent number of crocidolite fibers, while a very small proportion (0.14% on average) of chrysotile fibers form AB (Pooley and Ranson, 1986). Churg and colleagues (1979) have analyzed 600 AB from 82 subjects who were not exposed industrially to asbestos. They found that 98% of the AB had an amphibole core and 2% a chrysotile core. It has therefore been assumed that ferruginous bodies with a thin transparent fibrous core are nearly always amphibole.

Nonfibrous platy silicates such as talc, mica, and kaolin display by LM numerous fine brown particles within macrophages and the interstitium. Numerous strongly birefringent plate-like structures are revealed in polarizing light. Asbestos is not birefringent; it is not seen by light or polarizing microscopy.

Many of the important mineral particles are below the optical resolution of the LM. LM analyses consistently underestimate the retained mineral and their elemental content. As a consequence, there is often a poor correlation with exposure history.

Examination of Lung Tissue Digests

Airborne (environmental) and lung tissue measurements may be undertaken using PCM, scanning electron microscopy (SEM), or TEM. Laboratories performing these examinations should use a well-defined protocol for digestion, and preparation and microscopic examination of the samples because there are numerous steps within the process, which can lead to loss or break up of particles leading to artifactual values (Gibbs and Pooley, 1996; Pooley, 1981).

With respect to analytical techniques, there are a few important general considerations: Laboratories must define control populations and establish reference values for the methods used in order to meaningfully interpret results. Reference values need to be used to define whether the observed particulate concentration indicates abnormal retention of the particle, and to estimate the probability that the disease in question can be attributed to past exposure. A high mineral burden indicates exposure but is not proof of disease. A negative result is not proof of the absence of significant exposure, especially when, for example, chrysotile is a concern. The exposure history should always be correlated carefully with the results obtained by mineral analysis (De Vuyst et al., 1998).

Some investigators only count fibers of certain lengths whereas others count all that are detected. It is our practice to count and type 100–200 fibers of all sizes; although there is compelling evidence to indicate that fibers of >5 μm in length cause asbestos-related diseases.

Intraboratory variations generated by analyses of different tissue samples from the same individual may yield differences of up to threefold using pooled tissue samples, and up to 10-fold if very small tissue samples are used. Consequently, analyses of transbronchial samples of lung should only be undertaken in exceptional circumstances and the results viewed with caution. Ideally, analyses should be carried out on pooled tissue samples from several areas of the lung (De Vuyst et al., 1998).

Phase Contrast Microscopy

PCM analysis is a relatively easy, inexpensive method that allows for basic quantitative assessment of fiber burden. However, the method does not distinguish between fiber types (ie, cannot specifically identify asbestos and nonasbestos particles) and has a resolution limit of approximately 0.2 μm. Thus, a substantial proportion of the fibers in a lung sample will not be detected (Ashcroft and Heppleston, 1973).

Nonasbestiform fibers occasionally represent an important proportion of the total particle burden of the lung. The most common particles are mullite, rutile, silica, aluminum oxide, mica, and kaolin Electron microscopy makes possible discrimination of asbestos fiber types, but light microscopic analytical techniques do not. A comparative study of light to electron microscopic counts has shown a disproportionately high ratio of coated to uncoated fibers when fiber counts are low, so one cannot easily extrapolate from counts of AB to numbers of uncoated fibers (Pooley and Ranson, 1986). Electron microscopic analyses also allow the identification of platy silicates such as talc, mica, kaolin, and other clays (Gibbs et al., 1992; Wagner et al., 1986). Kaolin particles can often be distinguished by their hexagonal shape. Fume particles have a distinctive appearance, being characterized as very small, round particles occurring as aggregates, often with a chain-like appearance.

Scanning Electron Microscopy

SEM is a technical and scientific compromise between LM and TEM. SEM can be used to determine the number and dimension of both fibrous and nonfibrous inorganic particulates as well as to identify qualitatively the types of particles present in the lung and their relative proportions. This method requires minimal tissue preparation and has the advantage of allowing for examination of larger amounts of tissue than is feasible using TEM. Tissue is usually examined at 5×10^3 X magnification and the method has a resolution limit of ~0.05 μm diameter. It does not resolve the finest fibers, in particular, chrysotile fibrils. Energy-dispersive x-ray analyses can be performed, but qualitative information is more limited than for TEM.

Transmission Electron Microscopy

TEM is regarded as the best method available. Tissue counting is usually performed between 1.5×10^4 and 2×10^4 X magnification and therefore, resolution is superior (detecting fibers as small as 1 nm in diameter). Fiber burden counts on the same specimen are usually threefold higher by TEM than by SEM. TEM also allows the study of particle morphology and use of electron diffraction for identification. Diffraction analysis used to determine fiber crystal structure is limited with a SEM and details on internal particle structure are often better appreciated by TEM. Nonfibrous minerals can also be readily identified by this methodology, although reference control ranges are more problematic due to the complexity of the mix of particles inhaled in occupational settings. Therefore, quantification of nonfibrous particles is frequently not carried out.

Control Subjects

All or nearly all individuals from the general population have experienced some background exposure to asbestos. Fiber analysis of lung tissue of nonindustrially asbestos-exposed control subjects regularly reveals chrysotile and amphibole asbestos fibers (Table 12.2; Case and Sebastien, 1987; Churg and Warnock, 1980; Gaudichet et al., 1988; Karjalainen et al., 1994a; Mowe et al., 1985; Roggli et al., 2004; Whitwell et al., 1977). The lung fiber burden tends to be slightly higher in urban than in rural populations (Kohyama, 1989). The general population is also exposed to other types of mineral fiber and generally their lungs contain greater numbers of nonasbestos fibers in a ratio of about 4:1 or 5:1. Therefore, the results of case studies should be evaluated with reference background values determined by the same laboratory using the same protocol. For European laboratories performing counts by TEM, the upper reference values for total

Table 12.2 Asbestos Fiber Concentrations in Control Subjects

Study Reference No.	Number	Location	Method of Analysis	Uncoated f/g dry × 10⁶
Whitwell et al. (1977)	100	UK	PCM	0.007 (ND*-0.521)
Mowe et al. (1985)	28		SEM	0.25 (ND-4.8)
Roggli et al. (2004)	20	USA	SEM	0.031[†]
Gaudichet et al. (1988)	20	France	TEM	11.2
Churg and Warnock (1980)	20	USA	TEM	1.29 (0.26–7.55)
Case and Sebastien (1987)	23	Canada	TEM	0.62

* ND = not detectable.
[†] Only fibers > 5 μm in length counted.

amphibole fibers have been approximately $1\text{--}2 \times 10^6$ f/g dry lung and 1×10^5 f/g for amphibole fibers longer than 5 μm (De Vuyst et al., 1998). Reference values for tremolite have usually been higher in North America than in Europe (Berry et al., 1989; Churg, 1986; Dawson et al., 1993; Dodson et al., 1988; Gibbs et al., 1991; Howel et al., 1999; Karjalainen et al., 1994a; Rodelsperger et al., 1999; Wagner et al., 1988).

As can be seen in Table 12.3, lung burdens of residents of the community of Thetford Mines (a chrysotile mining town located in the Province of Québec, Canada), who had not worked in the asbestos industry showed approximately 10 times the number of chrysotile and tremolite fibers as residents of Vancouver, BC. (Churg, 1986). In addition, there was a higher proportion of long fibers in the Thetford Mines residents than in those from Vancouver. This asbestos fiber burden has not been associated with any pathological effects in the Thetford Mines residents. The ambient chrysotile concentration of lungs of residents in this community are roughly 250–500 times the amount found in the lungs of residents of most North American cities (Siemiatycki, 1983).

Pleural Plaques

Pleural plaques (PP) often develop after relatively brief, low intensity exposures to asbestos. This is reflected in the results of studies of lung mineral fiber content (Table 12.4; Churg and Vedal, 1994; Churg et al., 1993; Churg, 1982; Gylseth et al., 1981; Karjalainen et al. 1994b; Roggli et al., 2004; Roggli, 1990). Gylseth et al. (1981) found an approximately fourfold increase in asbestos fiber concentrations in patients with PP compared to controls (Table 12.4). Churg (1982) studied autopsy subjects of the general public chosen because they had PP and compared them with subjects who had no occupational exposure to asbestos and no PP. The numbers of chrysotile and noncommercial (ie, tremolite and anthophyllite) amphibole fibers were similar in both groups, but the cases with PP showed a marked increase in the number of the commercial amphiboles (amosite and crocidolite). However, half of the PP cases did not appear to be related to amphibole asbestos exposure on the basis of the analysis. It was concluded that in this general autopsy population, two subgroups were present: one subgroup had asbestos-related PP, and in the other subgroup of persons with PP, the etiology was unclear.

Karjalainen et al. (1994b) studied the occurrence of PP in men from autopsies in Finland. PP were seen in 58%, the frequency increased with (1) age, (2) smoking, (3) probability of past exposure to asbestos, and (4) an increase in the lung concentration of asbestos fibers. The median concentrations of asbestos fibers were about threefold greater among cases with widespread PP than among those without PP. More than 80% of cases with lung concentrations greater than 1×10^6 f/g of dry lung had PP. PP were also detected in 43% of persons who had no occupational history of exposure, and in 38% of those with less than 1×10^5 f/g in the dry lungs. In contrast, in a study of 22 cases with PP at postmortem, Gibbs et al. (1994b) found amphibole fiber levels elevated above the reference value in only six patients. There was no correlation between fiber concentrations and the number and size of PP. Orlowski et al. (1994) examined bronchoalveolar lavage fluids for AB and found elevated counts in 40% of subjects with PP, but there was no correlation between the concentration of fibers and the extent of the PP (Chapter 6). Roggli et al. (2004) found an elevated tissue asbestos content in 174 (95%) of 184 subjects with PP.

In summary, the occurrence of PP is associated with increased pulmonary concentrations of commercial amphibole asbestos in the lung but not with increased amounts of chrysotile or noncommercial amphiboles (with the exception of chrysotile miners and millers in Canada where tremolite exposure occurs). The severity and extent of PP

Table 12.3 Asbestos Fiber Concentrations by Mineral in Control Subjects

Study Reference No.	Number	Location	Method of Analysis	Median Uncoated f/g dry × 10⁶
Gibbs et al. (1991)	55	UK	TEM	Chrysotile (1.4* (ND-11.7) Amphibole (0.02 (ND-1.7)
Dawson et al. (1993)	31	UK	TEM	Chrysotile 4.4 (ND-20.1) Amphibole 0.04 (ND-1.0)
Howel et al. (1999)	122	UK	TEM	Chrysotile 0.4 Amphibole < 0.1
Churg (1986)	7	Thetford Canada	TEM	Chrysotile 1.2* (0.3–2.7) Tremolite 1.2b (0.2–20)
Churg (1986)	20	Vancouver Canada		Chrysotile 0.2* (0–1.3) Tremolite 0.2* (0–1.2)
Wagner et al. (1988)	56	UK	TEM	Chrysotile 9.3[†] Amphibole 1.93[†]
Berry et al. (1989)	50	Australia	TEM	Amosite 0.09 (0.04–0.19)[‡] Crocidolite 0.22 (0.11–0.47)[‡]
Berry et al. 1989	56	UK	TEM	Amosite 0.05 (0.01–0.35)[‡] Crocidolite 0.14 (0.02–1.0)[‡]
Berry et al. (1989)	94	UK	TEM	Amosite 0.18 (0.04–0.6)[‡] Crocidolite 0.07 (0.01–0.07)[‡]
Berry et al. (1989)	100	North America	TEM	Amosite 0.03 (0.01–0.2)[‡] Crocidolite 0.01 (0.01–0.07)[‡]
Dodson et al. (1988)	10	USA (East Texas)	SEM	Chrysotile 0.09 (ND-4.2) Amphibole 0.26 (0.05–5.2)
Karjalainen et al. (1994)	120	Finland	SEM	Amphibole 0.16 (ND-2.9)
Rodelsperger et al. (1999)	47M	Germany	STEM	Chrysotile ND[§] Amphibole 0.03[§]
Rodelsperger et al. (1999)	19F			Chrysotile 0.02[§] Amphibole 0.04[§]

ND = Not detectable.
* Geometric mean.
[†] Arithmetic mean.
[‡] Interquartiles.
[§] Only fibers > 5 μm in length counted.
M = Male.
F = Female.

Table 12.4 Asbestos Fiber Concentrations by Type in Subjects with Pleural Plaques

Study Reference No.	Number	Location	Method of Analysis	Uncoated f/g dry $\times$ 10^6 (range)
Gylseth et al. (1981)	14		SEM	2.2 (0.1–13)
Churg (1982)	29	USA	TEM	Chrysotile 5.1*
				Tremolite 1.3*
				Crocidolite 2.4*
				Amosite 2.6*
Churg et al. (1993)	63	Quebec chrysotile miners	TEM	Chrysotile 15† Tremolite 75†
Churg and Vedal (1994)	103	North America	TEM	Chrysotile 0.004† Tremolite 0.049† Amosite 1.4†
Karjalainen et al. (1994)	80 (moderate)	Finland	SEM	0.4‡ (ND-4.7)
Karjalainen et al. (1994)	88 (widespread)			0.57‡ (ND-160)
Roggli et al. (2004)	40	USA	SEM	0.148§ (0.004–1.89)

ND = Not detectable.
* Arithmetic mean.
† Geometric mean.
‡ Apart from one case, only amphibole fibers detected.
§ Only fibers > 5 μm in length counted.

correlate with increasing lung burdens of commercial amphibole fibers. The commercial amphibole asbestos fiber burdens tend to be lower in those with PP compared to subjects with MM (Table 12.5) and, in turn, these values are lower than that in patients with asbestosis. It would appear that PP are not consistently related to asbestos exposure although there might be alternative explanations (De Vuyst et al., 1998). It could be that PP are caused by chrysotile and that fiber burden analyses do not reflect such an exposure (but there is very little epidemiological evidence to support this notion). It is possible that either the amphibole exposure is very low, or the fibers have migrated to the pleura and as a result, elevated lung parenchymal burdens are not found (an improbable explanation; Boutin et al., 1996).

Diffuse Pleural Fibrosis and Rounded Atelectasis

Studies on lung tissue fiber concentrations in cases of diffuse pleural fibrosis (DPF) and rounded atelectasis (RA) are few (Gibbs et al., 1991; Stephens et al., 1987; Voisin et al., 1995). In cases of DPF, commercial amphibole levels in the lung are higher than in control subjects, and generally higher than those seen in patients with PP (Gibbs et al., 1991; Stephens et al., 1987). Voisin et al. (1995) examined the AB content of the lung parenchyma in six cases of RA and found a median AB count of 3 $\times$ 10^3 (CV = 1 $\times$ 10^2–4 $\times$ 10^4) per gram dry lung. Since RA is frequently associated with the presence of PP, it is not surprising that the levels observed in such cases are similar to those seen in association with PP (Roggli, 2004).

Table 12.5 Asbestos Fiber Concentrations by Minerality in Malignant Mesothelioma

Study Reference No.	Number of Subjects	Location	Method of Analysis	Uncoated f/g dry × 10⁶ (range)
Churg et al. (1993)	15	Canada chrysotile miners	TEM	Chrysotile 34* Tremolite 180*
Dawson et al. (1993)	117	UK women	TEM	Chrysotile 7.1* (ND-2506) Crocidolite 5.1* (ND-2888) Amosite 0.09* (ND-2420) Tremolite 0.03* (ND-120)
Churg and Vedal (1994)	15	North America	TEM	Chrysotile 0.004* Tremolite 0.051* Amosite 0.86*
De Klerk et al. (1996)	90	Australia Wittenoom	TEM	Crocidolite 183* (0.8–9.586)
Edwards et al. (1996)	32	UK Acre Mill	TEM	Chrysotile 4.9 (ND-243.0) Crocidolite 144.0 (ND-7195.0) Amosite 14.3 (ND-243.0)†
Dodson et al. (1997)	55	USA	TEM	Chrysotile (ND-0.621) Crocidolite (ND-28.90) Amosite (ND-67.55) Tremolite (ND-0.449)
Howell et al. (1999)	147	UK	TEM	Chrysotile 2.4 Amphibole 5.7
Rodelsperger et al. (1999)	60M 6F	Germany	SEM	Chrysotile 0.02‡ Amphibole 0.33§ Chrysotile ND§ Amphibole 0.31§

ND = not detectable.
* Geometric mean.
† Arithmetic mean.
‡ Apart from one case, only amphibole fibers detected.
§ Only fibers >5 μm in length counted.

Malignant Mesothelioma

Most studies of tissue mineral content have been performed in patients with MM and have provided useful information, often clarifying the nature of the exposure. These studies consistently demonstrate the close correlation between elevated levels of commercial amphibole and risk for MM (apart from a few special exceptions) Wagner et al. (1982b).

Tuomi et al. (1991) evaluated patients with MM using work histories and by determining the fiber burdens of their lung tissue by SEM. Concentrations of amphibole exceeded 1 × 10⁶ f/g dry lung in 65%, whereas 26% showed lesser amounts. They classified occupational exposure into four categories by history: (1) definite; (2) probable; (3) possible; and (4) unlikely or unknown. Patients with a higher probability of exposure tended to have higher lung concentrations of amphibole asbestos. Concentrations of $>1 \times 10^6$ f/g dry lung were found in all group 1 and 2 cases, 50% of group 3, and 38% of group 4.

Churg et al. (1993) found higher concentrations of tremolite than chrysotile in the lungs of chrysotile miners in the Province of Québec, Canada. Risk of MM correlated better with exposure to tremolite than with chrysotile as shown epidemiologically, and by analysis of lung mineral fiber content (McDonald et al., 1997).

Dawson et al. (1993) performed mineral fiber analysis in 117 of 177 women who had died with MM. A higher lung burden of amphibole was found in 98% compared to the mean for control subjects. This striking observation is a reflection of the high proportion of women in their case series with a history of exposure to asbestos relative to other published series. However, 5 of the 14 women with no exposure history had amphibole concentrations in the lungs equal to or lower than the highest counts in the control series. This finding supports the supposition that MM unrelated to asbestos exposure occur.

De Klerk et al. (1996) examined the lungs of 90 former Australian Wittenoom crocidolite miners. The maximum period of exposure was 3 years. Twenty-seven had MM. They found good agreement between the numbers of crocidolite fibers in the lung tissue and the estimated cumulative crocidolite exposure in f/mL-years. The half-life of crocidolite in the lung was estimated to be 92 months.

A total of 73 MM cases occurring in a community in the north of England were studied by Edwards et al. (1996). The majority worked at a factory that manufactured various asbestos products using all commercial types of asbestos. High concentrations of commercial amphiboles were found in the lungs. Interestingly enough, two cases were employed for only 2 months in the textile department. Substantial amounts of crocidolite (3.3×10^7 and 2.56×10^7 f/g dry lung) were found in the tissue.

Dodson et al. (1997) examined the lung tissue of 55 MM cases from the United States Pacific Northwest, the majority of whom were exposed in shipyards. The most common fiber found in the lung was amosite (96.4% of the cases). Tremolite, chrysotile, and crocidolite were demonstrated in 60%, 56%, and 40% of cases, respectively.

Rodelsperger et al. (1999) carried out a case-control study of 66 patients with MM and an equal number of control subjects from 5 towns in Germany. They found a dose-response relationship for concentration of amphibole fibers longer than 5 μm, but not for chrysotile or other mineral fibers.

In a recent case-referent study by McDonald et al. (2001a) of 73 subjects with MM whose age at diagnosis was 50 years or less, it was concluded that 80% of cases could be accounted for by amosite and crocidolite exposures. Tremolite was thought to be responsible for some 7%. The occupations of the members of this cohort comprised mainly carpenters, plumbers, electricians, and insulators in the construction industry (McDonald et al., 2001b). Work in shipbuilding and the manufacture of mineral products was less important than in earlier studies. As much as 90% of cases were in men who had commenced work prior to 1970.

Asbestosis

Asbestosis occurs predominantly in industrial workers with direct, heavy, and prolonged exposures to asbestos (Roggli, 1990). This is corroborated by the finding of high concentrations of amphibole in the lungs of these cases. There have been comparatively

Table 12.6 Mean Amphibole Fiber Concentrations (f × 10⁶ /gm dry weight) According to Grade of Fibrosis

Study	Grade 0	Grade 1	Grade 2	Grade 3	Grade 4
Wagner et al. (1986)	3.9	13.0	30.9	219.6	2167.8*
Wagner et al. (1988)	1.9	34.6	224.0	661.1	1532.5*
Dawson et al. (1993)	3.9	10.4	6.0	25.2	NA[†]

* Arithmetic mean.
† Geometric mean.

few systematic studies of lung fiber burdens in cases of asbestosis, and even fewer in which the fiber concentration was evaluated in relation to grade of fibrosis (Table 12.6). Investigations of this type can only be done reliably in cohorts of workers who have been exposed in the same industrial setting because of the confounding influence of fibrosis unrelated to asbestos exposure. It is remarkable that there is little information concerning the prevalence of various grades of interstitial fibrosis unrelated to asbestos exposure in the general population. A recent study indicates that minor degrees of interstitial fibrosis unrelated to asbestos exposure are not uncommon, being seen in about 40% of patients studied at autopsy. In a study of 254 subjects, the prevalence of diffuse idiopathic fibrosis was: grade 0: 59%; grade 1: 23%; grade 2: 12%; grade 3: 4%; and grade 4: 2%. Therefore, the background prevalence of interstitial lung fibrosis should be taken into account, to a large extent consequent to smoking (Adesina et al., 1991; Hogg et al., 1994).

Churg and Vedal (1994) examined the mineral fiber burden of lung tissue by TEM from 144 shipyard workers and insulators with heavy mixed exposures to both chrysotile and amosite. A high concentration of amosite in the lungs correlated with the presence of airway fibrosis and asbestosis but there was no correlation with the amount of chrysotile and tremolite. In the cases with asbestosis, the geometric mean concentration of amosite was 2.3×10^7 f/g dry lung, whereas in those without disease, the geometric mean concentration was 6.7×10^5 f/g. For the other disease conditions such as MM and PP, the amosite concentrations were lower.

Wagner et al. (1986, 1988) examined the lung mineral fiber concentrations by TEM in two cohorts of workers employed at a naval dockyard and an asbestos products manufacturing facility. Both studies revealed high concentrations of commercial amphibole that increased with the severity of the fibrosis. In addition, the proportions of commercial amphibole retained in the lungs rose with exposure estimated according to the type and duration of work, whereas the amounts of chrysotile decreased. Dawson et al. (1993) performed a similar analysis on the lungs of 116 women with MM. The concentrations of commercial amphibole correlated with increasing grades of fibrosis, but there was no correlation with chrysotile concentrations.

Green et al. (1997) examined, at autopsy, former workers in an asbestos textile plant where chrysotile was the only asbestos processed. However, from the 1950s to 1975, a small amount of crocidolite was woven into a tape or made into a braided packing. Estimates of cumulative exposure and lung fiber burdens strongly correlated with severity of asbestosis. As might be expected, the concentration of tremolite in the lung provided a better estimate of lung fibrosis than did the amount of chrysotile. Interestingly enough, the lungs of both the controls derived from the local population (who had not worked at the plant) and the workers showed concentrations of commercial amphibole fibers in excess of background. The level of commercial amphiboles present would be sufficient to account for the few MM that developed among those working at this plant.

Asbestos Miners

There have been several studies of the lung asbestos content in miners. Consistently, much higher rates of MM occur in workers who have mined or milled commercial amphibole, in contrast to those who mined only chrysotile. Crocidolite miners in Australia and South Africa have higher MM mortality rates than South African amosite and chrysotile miners (de Klerk et al., 1994; Liddell et al., 1997; McDonald et al., 1997; Rees et al., 1999; Sluis-Cremer et al., 1992). TEM fiber examination of lung tissues of the Wittenoom, Australia mine workers showed high levels of crocidolite as might be expected (de Klerk et al., 1996). When the lung tissues of Québec chrysotile miners and millers are examined for fiber content, high concentrations of tremolite are found, which exceed the levels of chrysotile (Liddell et al., 1997; McDonald et al., 1997; Pooley, 1976). This finding has led to a detailed study of workers employed in different mines in Canada. The MM rate differed from one mine to another. It was higher in the mines located around the township of Thetford, PQ than in mines around the town of Asbestos, PQ, which corresponded with a higher level of tremolite contamination of the ore in Thetford (Liddell et al., 1998; Nayebzadeh et al., 2001). The geometric means for tremolite were respectively, 2.9 and 6.4×10^7 million f/g dry lung, and chrysotile concentrations were 0.33 and 3×10^6 million f/g dry lung, for fibers less than 5 μm in length. The mines located around Thetford could be further subdivided; it was found that MM mainly occurred among workers employed in mines that were located near the community of Thetford, not among those who worked in mines near the periphery of the township. Analysis of lung tissue from members of the cohort who worked in and around Thetford showed that workers in the *central* mines had approximately four times as much tremolite as those working in the peripheral mines. Therefore, MM risk was associated with tremolite, rather than chrysotile exposure (McDonald and McDonald, 1997). Asbestosis and lung cancer (LC) cases had a similar distribution (Liddell et al., 1997, 1998; McDonald et al., 1997).

Interestingly enough, among Brazilian and South African chrysotile miners, there is no apparent risk of MM (Case et al., 2002; Rees et al., 1999). And, examination of lung fiber content of those miners reveals low concentrations of tremolite (compared to the Canadian miners; Case et al., 2002; Rees et al., 2001).

Yano et al. (2001), investigators in China, claimed that two MM, one pleural and one peritoneal, occurred in miners of chrysotile which they believed contained negligible amounts of amphibole asbestos. Tossavainen et al. (2001) examined the Chinese ores, and lung tissue burdens of miners. They detected substantial amounts of noncommercial amphibole asbestos fibers, both tremolite and anthophyllite, an indication that the mine was not amphibole free.

An SEM study of the lung mineral content of 24 Russian chrysotile miners, millers, and production workers showed a low mean concentration of tremolite (5.8×10^5 f/g dry) compared to chrysotile (1×10^7 f/g dry lung; Tossavainen et al., 2000). The mean concentration and range for chrysotile were similar to those reported for workers in the Canadian chrysotile mining and milling industry but the mean concentration for tremolite was less by at least an order of magnitude. The mean concentrations were lower (chrysotile—2.6×10^6 f/g and tremolite 0.18×10^6) in the residents of the Russian community lacking occupational exposure to asbestos.

The importance of tremolite as a contaminating fiber in various nonasbestiform ores is exemplified by the results of studies at a Libby, Montana vermiculite mine. This deposit had within it small amounts (4%–6%) of the tremolitic asbestos, lizardite, and antigorite. And, as a consequence, there has been a high rate of respiratory disease, including MM, among the workers (McDonald et al., 1986). In a recent update, a proportionate mortality ratio (PMR) for MM of 4.2% was reported, a risk similar to South African crocidolite miners (McDonald et al., 2002). It is about 10-fold greater than the PMR for MM in the Québec cohort, where the concentrations of the tremolite contamination of the mined ore is about 10-fold greater.

End-Product Users

Studies of the lung mineral content have been performed on workers employed in various industrial settings. On occasion, they have revealed evidence of exposure to asbestos types that were discounted in epidemiological studies. Case series have consistently demonstrated the strong relationship between the risk of MM and the use of commercial amphiboles in a wide diversity of industries (Churg and Vedal, 1994; Dawson et al., 1993; Dodson et al., 1997; Edward et al., 1996; Howel et al., 1999; McDonald et al., 1982; Roggli et al., 2002; Wagner et al., 1982; Chapter 4).

Mineral analysis demonstrated elevated concentrations of crocidolite in the lung tissues of English gas mask workers with MM, many years after cessation of employment. These workers had assembled military gas masks using crocidolite filter pads during World War II (Jones et al., 1996). Amosite was the predominant fiber in the lungs of workers employed at a factory manufacturing asbestos products (Gibbs et al., 1994a). Interestingly enough, workers with MM who had been employed in an asbestos textile plant in the north of England (which predominantly used chrysotile), had substantially elevated levels of crocidolite in their lungs (Wagner et al., 1982a). Similarly, in a study of the lung content of South Carolina textile workers who were thought to have been exposed to chrysotile asbestos, it was found that about a quarter of the work force had elevated levels of commercial amphiboles in their lungs (Green et al., 1997).

Railroad employees who worked on and around steam engines had the potential for exposure to asbestos since locomotives and carriages contained asbestos (Chapter 3). Some developed MM. Mancuso (1988) claimed that these workers were exposed to chrysotile with little or no amphibole exposure, but mineral fiber analyses have disclosed elevated lung concentrations of amosite in the cases from the United States (Roggli, 2004). In contrast, both crocidolite and amosite concentrations were elevated in the lungs of British railroad shop workers.

Friction product workers and garage mechanics, who were potentially exposed to chrysotile, do not have an increased risk of MM, LC, and nonmalignant respiratory disease (Blake et al., 2003; Goodman et al., 2004; McDonald et al., 1984; Newhouse and Sullivan, 1989; Paustenbach et al., 2004, Weir et al., 2001). However, occasional cases of MM have developed in auto mechanics, a not surprising occurrence in view of the very large number of workers involved in these trades (over 2 million in the United States). Obviously, some workers would have been exposed to commercial amphiboles in other jobs. One study of the mineral fiber content of the lungs of 10 brake repair workers with MM showed either an asbestos fiber content within the background range, or elevated levels of commercial amphibole (Butnor et al., 2003).

Paraoccupational Exposures

Paraoccupational (domestic) exposures to asbestos (usually as a consequence of the washing of asbestos-contaminated work clothes) have resulted in PP and MM (Anderson et al., 1979; Newhouse and Thompson, 1965). Occupational groups that have been associated with disease resulting from domestic exposure include insulators and pipe fitters, and workers in power plants, chemical plants, and construction. Lung fiber burden analyses of cases with paraoccupational exposure have been comparatively few but generally, they have shown commercial amphiboles in amounts comparable to workers with light to moderate direct occupational exposure (Dawson et al., 1993; Gibbs et al., 1990; Huncharek et al., 1989; Roggli, 2004; Chapter 4).

Environmental Exposures

In some countries, environmental exposures to naturally occurring deposits of asbestos, particularly tremolite, have occasionally resulted in the development of benign and malignant asbestos-related diseases. Countries where this has occurred are Turkey (Coplu et al., 1996; Zeren et al., 2000), Greece (Constantopoulos et al., 1985), Cyprus (McConnochie et al., 1987), Corsica (Rey et al., 1993), New Caledonia (Luce et al., 2000), and Afghanistan (Voisin et al., 1994). In some, local soils containing tremolite are used to stucco buildings. Accordingly, both outdoor and indoor exposures result. Mineralogical analysis has revealed abundant tremolite in the stucco of houses and in the soil from the roads of villages (Coplu et al., 1996). In Turkey, MM occur in the countryside where there are environmental exposures to tremolite. In a few villages in the Cappadocia region of south central Turkey, the population is exposed to erionite, a nonasbestiform aluminum silicate fibrous mineral that has physical similarities to crocidolite. Residents of this region of Turkey have the highest recorded rates of MM in the world (Baris et al., 1987). Mineral fiber analyses have been conducted on the lungs of a few human cases, and some animals living locally. Erionite was found in the lung tissue of Cappadocian village residents where a high rate of MM has occurred (Baris et al., 1987; Dawson et al., 1993).

In villages in northeast Corsica, a high rate of nonoccupational PP and cases of MM are found. High airborne fiber concentrations were found in indoor and outdoor air samples. In addition, asbestos was found in the pleura of animals. In comparison with a control village the levels of airborne tremolite were increased by an order of magnitude or greater (Rey et al., 1993).

In contrast, although the lung chrysotile and tremolite lung content in residents around Thetford, PQ, was about 10 times that observed in Vancouver residents, epidemiological studies have not shown an increased incidence of respiratory disease (Churg, 1986). However, the concentrations were about 50 times lower than those observed in the mine workers where there is an elevated incidence of asbestos-related disease.

Fiber Dimension

Experimental studies have consistently shown that *short* fibers (ie, less than 5 μm) are cleared more efficiently from the lung than longer fibers. *Short* fibers are unlikely to cause cancer in humans, although they possibly may contribute to the development of pulmonary fibrosis (Agency for Toxic Substances and Diseases, 2003; Berman and Crump, 2004). Studies of lung mineral fiber concentrations have not provided clear-cut evidence on this matter because naturally occurring asbestos has a broad range of fiber dimensions.

A case-referent study by McDonald et al. (2001b) of a series of MM found that a range of fiber lengths (<6, 6–10, and >10 μm) are all associated with MM risk, but those longer than 10 μm manifest the greatest risk followed by those intermediate in length (6–10 μm).

Studies by Churg and Vedal (1994) of Canadian chrysotile miners and millers, as well as Pacific Northwest shipyard workers and insulators, did not disclose a significant relationship of disease with fiber dimension and aspect ratio, although a large number of high aspect ratio amphibole fibers were found in those with PP (Churg et al., 1993; Churg and Vedal, 1994).

References

Adesina AM, Vallyathan V, McQuillen EN, Weaver SO, Craighead JE. Bronchiolar inflammation and fibrosis associated with smoking. *Am Rev Respir Dis.* 1991;143:144–149

Agency for Toxic Substances and Diseases Registry. Report of the expert panel on health effects of asbestos and synthetic vitreous fibers: the influence of fibre length. 2003. US Department of Health and Human Services.

Anderson HA, Lilis R, Daum SM, et al. Asbestosis among household contacts of asbestos factory workers. *Ann NY Acad Sci.* 1979;330:387–399.

Ashcroft T, Heppleston AG. The optical and electron microscopic determination of pulmonary asbestos fibre concentration and its relation to the human pathological reaction. *J Clin Pathol.* 1973;26:224–234.

Baris I, Simonato L, Artvinli M, et al. Epidemiological and environmental evidence of the health effects of exposure to erionite fibers: a four-year study in the Cappadocian region of Turkey. *Int J Cancer.* 1987;39:10–17.

Berman DW, Crump KS. *Final Draft: Technical Support Document for a Protocol to Assess Asbestos-Related Risk.* Washington: EPA; 2004.

Berry G, Rogers AJ, Pooley FD. Mesotheliomas—asbestos exposure and lung burden. *IARC Sci Publ.* 1989;90:486–496.

Blake CL, Van Orden DR, Banasik M, Harbison RD. Airborne asbestos concentration from brake changing does not exceed permissible exposure limit. *Regul Toxicol Pharmacol.* 2003;38:58–70.

Boutin C, Dumortier P, Rey F, Viallat JR, De Vuyst P. Black spots concentrate oncogenic asbestos fibres in the parietal pleura. Thorascoscopic and mineralogic study. *Am J Respir Crit Care Med.* 1996;153:444–449.

Butnor K, Sporn T, Roggli V. Exposure to brake dust and malignant mesothelioma: a study of 10 cases with mineral fiber analyses. *Ann Occup Hyg.* 2003;47:325–330.

Case BW, Dufresne A, Bagatin E, Capelozzi VL. Lung-retained fibre content in Brazilian chrysotile workers. *Ann Occup Hyg.* 2002;46(Suppl 1):144–149.

Case BW, Sebastien P. Environmental and occupational exposures to chrysotile asbestos: a comparative microanalytic study. *Arch Environ Health.* 1987;42:185–191.

Churg A. Asbestos fibres and pleural plaques in a general autopsy population. *Am J Pathol.* 1982;109:88–96.

Churg A. Lung asbestos content in long-term residents of a chrysotile mining town. *Am Rev Respir Dis.* 1986;134:125–127.

Churg A, Green F. Mesothelioma in railroad machinists. *Am J Ind Med.* 1990;17:523–530.

Churg A, Vedal S. Fiber burden and patterns of asbestos-related disease in workers with heavy mixed amosite and chrysotile exposure. *Am J Respir Crit Care Med.* 1994;150:663–669.

Churg A, Warnock ML. Asbestos fibers in the general population. *Am Rev Respir Dis.* 1980;122:669–678.

Churg A, Warnock ML, Green N. Analysis of the cores of ferruginous (asbestos) bodies from the general population. II. True asbestos bodies and pseudoasbestos bodies. *Lab Invest.* 1979;40:31–38.

Churg A, Wright JL, Vedal S. Fiber burden and patterns of asbestos-related disease in chrysotile miners and millers. *Am Rev Respir Dis.* 1993;148:25–31.

Constantopoulos SH, Goudevenos JA, Saratzis N, Langer AM, Selikoff IJ, Moutsopoulos HM. Metsovo lung: pleural calcification and restrictive lung function in northwestern Greece. Environmental exposure to mineral fiber as etiology. *Environ Res.* 1985;38:319–331.

Coplu L, Dumortier P, Demir AU, et al. An epidemiological study in an Anatolian village in Turkey environmentally exposed to tremolite asbestos. *J Environ Pathol, Toxicol Oncol.* 1996;15:177–182.

Crouch E, Churg A. Ferruginous bodies and the histologic evaluation of dust exposure. *Am J Surg Pathol.* 1984;8:109–116.

Dawson A, Gibbs AR, Pooley FD, Griffiths DM, Hoy J. Malignant mesothelioma in women. *Thorax.* 1993;48:269–274.

de Klerk NH, Musk A, Armstrong BK, Hobbs MST. Disease in miners and millers of crocidolite from Wittenoom, Western Australia: a further follow-up to December 1986. *Ann Occup Hyg.* 1994;38(Suppl. 1):647–655.

de Klerk NH, Musk AW, Williams V, Filion PR, Whitaker D, Shilkin KB. Comparison of measures of exposure to asbestos in former crocidolite workers from Wittenoom Gorge, W. Australia. *Am J Ind Med.* 1996;30:579–587.

Dement JM, Brown DP. Lung cancer mortality among asbestos textile workers: a review and update. *Ann Occup Hyg.* 1994;38:525–532.

De Vuyst P, Karjalainen A, Dumortier P, et al. Guidelines for mineral fibre analyses in biological samples: report of the ERS Working Group. European Respiratory Society. *Eur Respir J.* 1998;11:1416–1426.

Dodson RF, O'Sullivan M, Corn CJ, McLarty JW, Hammar SP. Analysis of asbestos fiber burden in lung tissue from mesothelioma patients. *Ultrastruct Pathol.* 1997;21:321–336.

Dodson RF, Williams MG Jr, Corn CJ, Rankin TL. A comparison of asbestos burden in nonurban patients with and without lung cancer. *Cytobios.* 1988;56:7–15.

Edwards AT, Whitaker D, Browne K, Pooley FD, Gibbs AR. Mesothelioma in a community in the north of England. *Occup Environ Med.* 1996;53:547–552.

Fischer M, Gunther S, Muller KM. Fibre-years, pulmonary asbestos burden and asbestosis. *Int J Hyg Environ Health.* 2002;205:245–248.

Gaudichet A, Janson X, Monchaux G, et al. Assessment by analytical microscopy of the total lung fibre burden in mesothelioma patients matched with four other pathological series. *Ann Occup Hyg.* 1988;32(Suppl. 1):213–223.

Gibbs AR, Gardner MJ, Pooley FD, Griffiths DM, Blight B, Wagner JC. Fiber levels and disease in workers from a factory predominantly using amosite. *Environ Health Perspect.* 1994a;102(Suppl 5):261–263.

Gibbs AR, Griffiths DM, Pooley FD, et al. Comparison of fibre types and size distributions in lung tissues of paraoccupational and occupational cases of malignant mesothelioma. *Br J Ind Med.* 1990;47:621–626.

Gibbs AR, Pooley FD. Analysis and interpretation of inorganic mineral particles in "lung" tissues. *Thorax.* 1996;51:327–334.

Gibbs AR, Pooley FD, Griffiths DM. Lung fibrous content of subjects with pleural plaques. *Eur Respir J.* 1994b;7(Suppl. 18):425.

Gibbs AR, Pooley FD, Griffiths DM, et al. Talc pneumoconiosis: a pathologic and mineralogic study. *Hum Pathol.* 1992;23:1344–1354.

Gibbs AR, Stephens M, Griffiths DM, Blight BJ, Pooley FD. Fibre distribution in the lungs and pleura of subjects with asbestos-related diffuse pleural fibrosis. *Br J Ind Med.* 1991;48:762–770.

Goodman M, Teta MJ, Hessel PA, et al. Mesothelioma and lung cancer among motor vehicle mechanics: a meta-analysis. *Ann Occup Hyg.* 2004;48:309–326.

Green FH, Harley R, Vallyathan V, et al. Exposure and mineralogical correlates of pulmonary fibrosis in chrysotile asbestos workers. *Occup Environ Med.* 1997;54:549–559.

Gylseth B, Mowe G, Skaug V, et al. Inorganic fibers in lung tissue from patients with pleural plaques or malignant mesothelioma. *Scand J Work Environ Health.* 1981;7:109–113.

Hogg JC, Wright JL, Wiggs BR, Coxson HO, Opazo Saez A, Pare PD. Lung structure and function in cigarette smokers. *Thorax.* 1994;49:473–478.

Howel D, Gibbs A, Arblaster L, et al. Mineral fibre analysis and routes of exposure to asbestos in the development of mesothelioma in an English region. *Occup Environ Med.* 1999;56:51–58.

Huncharek M, Capotorto JV, Muscat J. Domestic asbestos exposure, lung fibre burden, and pleural mesothelioma in a housewife. *Br J Ind Med.* 1989;46:354–355.

Jones JSP, Gibbs AR, McDonald JC, Pooley FD. Mesothelioma following exposure to crocidolite (blue) asbestos. A fifty year follow-up study. In Antypas G. *Proceedings, 2nd International Congress on Lung Cancer,* Italy: Monzuzzi Editore; 1996: 407–411.

Karjalainen A, Vanhala E, Karhunen PJ, Lalu K, Penttila A, Tossavainen A. Asbestos exposure and pulmonary fiber concentrations of 300 Finnish urban men. *Scand J Work Environ Health.* 1994a;20:34–41.

Karjalainen A, Karhunen PJ, Lalu PK, et al. Pleural plaques and exposure to mineral fibres in a male urban population. *Occup Environ Med.* 1994b;51:456–460.

Kohyama N. Airborne asbestos levels in non-occupational environments in Japan. *IARC Sci Publ.* 1989;90:262–276.

Liddell FD, McDonald AD, McDonald JC. The 1891–1920 birth cohort of Québec chrysotile miners and millers: development from 1904 and mortality to 1992. *Ann Occup Hyg.* 1997;41:13–36.

Liddell FDK, McDonald AD, McDonald JC. Dust exposure and lung cancer in Québec chrysotile miners and millers. *Ann Occup Hyg.* 1998;42:7–20.

Luce D, Bugel I, Goldberg P, et al. Environmental exposure to tremolite and respiratory cancer in New Caledonia. A case-control study. *Am J Epidemiol.* 2000;151:259–265.

Mancuso TF. Relative risk of mesothelioma among railroad machinists exposed to chrysotile. *Am J Ind Med.* 1988;13:639–657.

McConnochie K, Simonato L, Mavrides P, Christofides P, Pooley FD, Wagner JC. Mesothelioma in Cyprus: the role of tremolite. *Thorax.* 1987;42:342–347.

McDonald JC, Armstrong B, Edwards CW, et al. Case-referent survey of young adults with mesothelioma: I. Lung fibre analyses. *Ann Occup Hyg.* 2001b;45:513–518.

McDonald AD, Case BW, Churg A, et al. Mesothelioma in Québec chrysotile miners and millers: epidemiology and aetiology. *Ann Occup Hyg.* 1997;41:707–719.

McDonald JC, Edwards CW, Gibbs AR, et al. Case-referent survey of young adults with mesothelioma. II. Occupational analyses. *Ann Occup Hyg.* 2001a;45:519–523.

McDonald AD, Fry JS, Woolley AJ, McDonald JC. Dust exposure and mortality in an American chrysotile asbestos friction products plant. *Br J Ind Med.* 1984;41:151–157.

McDonald JC, Harris J, Armstrong B. Cohort Mortality study of vermiculite miners exposed to fibrous tremolite. *Ann Occup Hyg.* 2002;46(Suppl. 1):93–94.

McDonald JC, McDonald AD, Armstrong B, Sebastien P. Cohort study of mortality of vermiculite miners exposed to tremolite. *Br J Ind Med.* 1986;43:436–444.

McDonald JC, McDonald AD. Chrysotile, tremolite and carcinogenicity. *Ann Occup Hyg.* 1997;41:699–705.

McDonald AD, McDonald JC, Pooley FD. Mineral fibre content of lung in mesothelial tumours in North America. *Ann Occup Hyg.* 1982;26:417–422.

Mowe G, Gylseth B, Hartveit F, Skaug V. Fiber concentration in lung tissue of patients with malignant mesothelioma. A case-control study. *Cancer.* 1985;56:1089–1093.

Nayebzadeh A, Dufresne A, Case BW, et al. Lung mineral fibers of former miners and millers from Thetford Mines and asbestos regions: a comparative study of fiber concentration and dimension. *Arch Environ Health.* 2001;56:65–76.

Newhouse ML, Sullivan KR. A mortality study of workers manufacturing friction materials: 1941–86. *Br J Ind Med.* 1989;46:176–179.

Newhouse ML, Thompson H. Mesothelioma of pleura and peritoneum following exposure to asbestos in the London area. *Br J Ind Med.* 1965;22:261–269.

Orlowski E, Pairon JC, Ameille J, et al. Pleural plaques, asbestos exposure, and asbestos bodies in bronchoalveolar lavage fluid. *Am J Ind Med.* 1994;26:349–358.

Paustenbach DJ, Finley BL, Lu ET, Brorby GP, Sheehan PJ. Environmental and occupational health hazards associated with the presence of asbestos in brake linings and pads (1900 to present): a "state-of-the-art" review. *J Toxicol Environ Health B Crit Rev.* 2004;7:25–80.

Pooley FD. An examination of the fibrous mineral content of asbestos lung tissue from Canadian chrysotile mining industry. *Environ Res.* 1976;12:281–298.

Pooley FD. Tissue mineral identification. In: Weill H, Turner-Warwick M, eds. *Occupational Lung Diseases: Research Approaches and Methods*, New York: Marcel Decker; 1981: 189–235.

Pooley FD, Ranson DL. Comparison of the results of asbestos fibre dust counts in lung tissue obtained by analytical electron microscopy and light microscopy. *J Clin Pathol.* 1986;39:313–317.

Rees D, Goodman K, Fourie E, et al. Asbestos exposure and mesothelioma in South Africa. *So Afr Med J.* 1999;89:627–634.

Rees D, Phillips JI, Garton E, Pooley FD. Asbestos fibre lung concentration in South African chrysotile mine workers. *Ann Occup Hyg.* 2001;45:473–477

Rey Y, Boutin C, Steinbauer J, et al. Environmental pleural plaques in an asbestos-exposed population of northeast Corsica. *Eur Respir J.* 1993;6:978–982.

Rodelsperger K, Woitowitz HJ, Bruckel B, Arhelger R, Pohlabeln H, Jockel KH. Dose-response relationship between amphibole fiber lung burden and mesothelioma. *Cancer Detect Prev.* 1999;23:183–193.

Roggli V. Asbestos bodies and nonasbestos ferruginous bodies. In: Roggli V, Oury TD, Sporn TA, eds. *Pathology of Asbestos-Associated Diseases.* 2nd ed. New York: Springer; 2004: 34–70.

Roggli VL. Human disease consequences of fiber exposures: a review of human lung pathology and fiber burden data. *Environ Health Perspect.* 1990;88:295–303.

Roggli VL, Sharma A. Analysis of tissue mineral fibre content. In: Roggli VL, Oury TD, Sporn TA, eds. *Pathology of Asbestos-Associated Diseases.* 2nd ed. New York: Springer; 2004: 309–354.

Roggli VL, Sharma A, Butnor KJ, et al. Malignant mesothelioma and occupational exposure to asbestos: a clinicopathologic correlation of 1445 cases. *Ultrastruct Pathol.* 2002;26:55–65.

Siemiatycki J. Health effects on the general population: mortality in the general population in asbestos mining areas. In *Proceedings of the World Symposium on Asbestos, Montreal, 1983.* Montreal, Canada: Asbestos Information Centre; 1983: 337–348.

Sluis-Cremer GK, Liddell FD, Logan WP, Bezuidehout BN. The mortality of amphibole miners in South Africa, 1946–80. *Br J Ind Med.* 1992;49:566–575.

Stephens M, Gibbs AR, Pooley FD, Wagner JC. Asbestos induced diffuse pleural fibrosis: pathology and mineralogy. *Thorax.* 1987;42:583–588.

Tossavainen A, Kotilainen M, Takahashi K, Pan G, Vanhala E. Amphibole fibres in Chinese chrysotile asbestos. *Ann Occup Hyg.* 2001;45:145–152.

Tossavainen A, Kovalevsky E, Vanhala E, Tuomi T. Pulmonary mineral fibers after occupational and environmental exposure to asbestos in the Russian chrysotile industry. *Am J Ind Med.* 2000;37:327–333.

Tuomi T, Huuskonen MS, Tammilehto L, Vanhala E, Virtamo M. Occupational exposure to asbestos as evaluated from work histories and analysis of lung tissues from patients with mesothelioma. *Br J Ind Med.* 1991;48:48–52.

Voisin C, Fisekci F, Voisin-Saltiel S, et al. Asbestos-related rounded atelectasis: radiologic and mineralogic data in 23 cases. *Chest.* 1995;107:477–481.

Voisin C, Marin I, Brochard P, et al. Environmental airborne tremolite asbestos pollution and pleural plaques in Afghanistan. *Chest.* 1994;106:974–976.

Wagner JC, Berry G, Pooley FD. Mesotheliomas and asbestos type in asbestos textile workers: a study of lung content. *Br Med J.* 1982a;285:603–606.

Wagner JC, Moncrieff CB, Coles R, Griffiths DM, Munday DE. Correlation between fibre content of the lungs and disease in naval dockyard workers. *Br J Ind Med.* 1986;43:391–395.

Wagner JC, Newhouse ML, Corrin B, Rossiter CE, Griffiths DM. Correlation between fibre content of the lung and disease in east London asbestos factory workers. *Br J Ind Med.* 1988;45:305–308.

Wagner JC, Pooley FD, Berry G, et al. A pathological and mineralogical study or asbestos-related deaths in the United Kingdom in 1977. *Ann Occup Hyg.* 1982b;26:423–431.

Weir FW, Meraz LB. Morphological characteristics of asbestos fibers released during grinding and drilling of friction products. *Appl Occup Environ Hyg.* 2001;16:1147–1149.

Whitwell F, Scott J, Grimshaw M. Relationship between occupations and asbestos-fibre content of the lungs in patients with pleural mesothelioma, lung cancer and other diseases. *Thorax.* 1977;32:377–386.

Yano E, Wang ZM, Wang XR, Wang MZ. Lan YJ. Cancer mortality among workers exposed to amphibole-free chrysotile asbestos. *Am J Epidemiol.* 2001;154:538–543.

Zeren EH, Gumurdulu D, Roggli VL, Zorludemir S, Erkisi M, Tuncer I. Environmental malignant mesothelioma in southern Anatolia: a study of fifty cases. *Environ Health Perspect.* 2000;108:1047–1050.

13

US Governmental Regulatory Approaches and Actions

John E. Craighead

On April 28, 1971 the Occupational Safety Act of 1970 was implemented by the US Government, establishing the National Institute for Occupational Safety and Health (NIOSH), an agency focused on research, and the Occupational Safety and Health Administration (OSHA), a regulatory body concerned with health in the workplace. Action had been a long time coming!

During the era of the Roman Empire, pulmonary disease consistent with asbestosis developed all too frequently among manual workers, usually slaves exposed to crude asbestos quarried in the foothills of the Alps. Confusion with silicosis, a far more common occupational disease, and a variety of other chronic lung diseases precluded specific clinical diagnoses for centuries thereafter. In 1899, the Annual Report of the Inspector of Factories of the United Kingdom noted "the evil effects of asbestos," first recognized in the form of disabling asbestosis rampant among textile workers.

The report of *Her Majesty's Inspector of Factories* in 1930 (Merewether and Price) recommended dust suppression in asbestos factories as a control measure, although routine governmental monitoring of workplaces was yet to be implemented. Five years later Lanza et al. (1935), a leading American occupational health researcher, recommended the following practices: (1) industries should face the problem of dust control in asbestos plants seriously; (2) industries should sponsor studies of known cases of asbestosis as well as studies on the effects of asbestosis on the heart and circulation; (3) employees be examined physically, preferably every year, but at least every 2 years, this examination to include an x-ray of the chest.

In 1937 simple measures of dust suppression in the granite industry—specifically improved ventilation and wet drilling/cutting—were found to reduce dramatically the occurrence of silicosis among stone polishers working indoors. A similar approach would have been feasible in textile mills even though the aerodynamic properties of silica dust and asbestos differ. In his pathfinding book published in 1942 "*Occupational Tumors and Allied Disease,*" the National Cancer Institute's foremost researcher, W.C. Hueper, again emphasized the importance of dust control in the workplace to protect against the adverse effects of asbestos. Perhaps the most telling impact on environmental and occupational regulation during the 20th century, however, was a provocative series

317

of articles published by Rachael Carlson in the influential *New Yorker* magazine, soon
to be followed by her landmark book *Silent Spring* in 1962. Articles by Paul Brodeur
also published in the *New Yorker* a few years later focused on asbestosis and, to a more—
limited extent, asbestos-related lung cancer (LC), and the newly "discovered cancer"—
malignant mesothelioma (MM). Public outcries followed. President John F. Kennedy
promptly appointed a Scientific Advisory Committee to consider the implications of the
claims of these early environmental activists. Governmental regulations of asbestos and
other environmental air pollutants were soon to follow. Kennedy's initiative was cut short
by his untimely death, but others responded to the national outcry for action. In 1965,
Senator Edward Muskie, the environmentalist candidate for president, initiated legislation
regulating automobile exhaust and in 1969, his actions in the senate served to strengthen
existing air pollution regulations. Public involvement was crystallized by the nationwide
Earth Day demonstrations in the spring of 1970. In July of that year, the Environmental
Protection Agency (EPA) was created by an act of Congress and a year later, the Clean
Air Act (CAA) was implemented. The Toxic Substances Act (TOSCA) followed in 1976.
It provided the EPA with the legal authority to track industrial chemicals produced or
imported into the United States with the authority to ban manufacturing of chemicals
that pose an unreasonable risk for workmen and members of the general population. The
CAA required the EPA to develop and enforce regulations to protect the general public
from exposure to asbestos contaminants known to be hazardous to human health. The
National Emissions Standard for Hazardous Air Pollutions (NESHAP) was designed by
the EPA to protect the public, and asbestos was the first hazardous air pollutant to be
regulated (1971). NESHAP focused on the release of aerosols of asbestos during the
processing, handling, and disposal of asbestos-containing materials. In particular, it dictated work practices during demolition and renovation of buildings, controls that are
now widely implemented and accepted. Later EPA research under the aegis of the Clean
Water Act resulted in the discovery of asbestos in potable water throughout the United
States and the establishment of regulations on water quality. Additional studies by the
State of Minnesota and the EPA demonstrated asbestos in the water of Lake Superior,
the largest of North America's Great Lakes, consequent to the deposition of tailings from
the northern Minnesota iron mines into lake water. Finally, our economically thriving
nation was heeding Albert Schweitzer's prophetically dire warning, "Man has lost the
capacity to foresee and forestall. He will end by destroying the earth."

It would be presumptuous and far beyond the scope of this text to recount the details
of the vast body of regulations and supporting documents promulgated by agencies of the
United States, specifically, the EPA, OSHA, the Consumer's Product Safety Commission
(CPSC), and other US federal agencies (Table 13.1), as well as the World Health Organization (WHO), and individual governmental agencies in countries worldwide. Rather,
in this chapter, the historical evolution of society's efforts to protect workers and the
members of the general public in the United States will be considered in the context of
the existing regulations in major industrial countries of Europe and North America.

Few issues evoke more contentious debate than the establishment of broad-sweeping
environmental regulations that have profound national, economic, and health implications,
often in the context of incomplete and conflicting scientific information. The responsible
governmental agencies and their administrators are confronted with a seemingly impossible task, particularly when few of the countless interested parties will be satisfied with
the outcome. Compromise is inevitable. Industry may be burdened with new, untold and
unproven, costly requirements for environmental controls and incalculable expenses that
threaten their competitive edge, particularly when competing with unregulated industries abroad; workmen are often burdened by cumbersome requirements such as the

Table 13.1 Agencies of the United States Responsible for Monitoring and Controlling Asbestos

Agency	Area of Responsibility
Environmental Protection Agency	Products, emissions, buildings, and water
Occupational Safety and Health Administration	Workplace products
US Department of Transportation	Shipping
Food and Drug Administration	Asbestos in foods, drugs, and cosmetics
Consumer Product Safety Commission	Asbestos in consumer products
Department of Commerce and Customs Service	Import/export of products

compulsory uses of face masks that to them may seem to make little sense; and the general public ponders, wonders, and worries whether in fact their best interests have been served by government, or their health compromised by the avarice of capitalistic industry. Some would claim that the Congress abrogated its responsibility for environmental and occupational regulation, assigning an almost impossible burden of scientific research and control on agencies subject to the influences and criticisms of diverse constituencies. The record shows that the relevant regulatory agencies have found it impossible to "keep up" with evolving science, and the arduous task of establishing and implementing up-to-date realistic and effective regulations. The EPA was born with limited power and an overwhelming burden of responsibilities.

Occupational asbestos regulations were initially implemented as an outgrowth of the comprehensive studies of workers in the textile industry conducted by Dreessen and his associates in 1938 (Chapter 3). They employed a crude but nonetheless quantitative measure of environmental contamination, that is, phase contrast microscopy (PCM). Dust concentrations were calculated in the context of millions of particles per cubic foot of ambient air (mppcf). Few measures could be more imprecise, for it was not an enumeration exclusively of fibrous asbestos particles, 5 μm or longer, but included organic and inorganic dusts of various types and other fibrous materials in the workplace air. Approaches other than PCM for sampling air for dust were largely untested at the time, and quantitative assessments failed to identify the particles assayed, whether they be animal, vegetable, or mineral. It was only some years later that scanning (SEM) and transmission electron microscopy (TEM) supplemented by x-ray spectrometry were introduced as quantitative tools measuring specific types of asbestos in the air.

At the 1964 New York Academy of Sciences conference (Chapter 1), Roach (1965), questioned the suitability of the regulations arising from the Dreessen (1938) study. Similar reservations were voiced by representatives of the textile industry (Lane, 1968) and by a spokesman for the Johns-Manville Corporation, at that time, the major manufacturer and supplier of asbestos products. Clearly, the fine line between "*safe*" and "*hazardous*" had yet to be defined. Nonetheless, the criterion recommended by Dreessen et al. (1938) was adopted as the standard for federal contracts negotiated by the government under the regulatory aegis of the Walsh-Healey Contracts Act that dictated in detail the work practices permitted by contractees of the federal government. Simply stated, the tenets of the Act were designed to protect the health of the workmen, but in retrospect, it is unclear to what extent these requirements were implemented nationwide. It was only years later that the prescient concerns of the scientists and public health officials were justified by research showing that the actual threshold for asbestosis was substantially lower than 5 mppcf.

Enter on the scene the American Conference of Governmental Industrial Hygienists (ACGIH), organized in the 1940s to conduct independent assessments of industrial settings and propose environmental controls for consideration outside of the sphere of the federal regulatory process. This voluntary, nongovernmental organization enjoyed the luxury of a skilled, scientifically trained, and knowledgeable membership of industrial hygienists drawn from academia, the private sector, and industry. They annually consider major health and regulatory issues in open forum. In 1946, the ACGIH initially accepted the 5 mppcf criterion recommended by Dreessen et al. in 1938, only to propose a new guideline of 12 f/mL or 2 mppcf in 1969. This recommendation was interpreted in the construct of an exposure for 8 hours daily, 5 days per week, the so-called Time Weighted Average (TWA). Based on limited science but a concerted attempt to establish regulations on the basis of fibers per unit volume of air, a simplistic multiplication factor of six was proposed to convert mppcf to f/mL, recognizing that a substantial but variable proportion of the dust particles detected by PCM were not asbestos, depending on the industrial and environmental setting.

In 1972, shortly after OSHA was established, the recommendations of ACGIH were adopted as the legal standard with a provision for a 15 minute exposure ceiling of 10 f/mL over a 15 minute period. During the ensuing years, OSHA and the EPA have adopted new and increasingly stringent measures for regulating airborne asbestos, guided in part by the ACGIH (Table 13.2). During this period, parallel regulatory activities have

Table 13.2 Occupational Exposure Standards in the United States

Date	Agency	MAC	TWA	Short-Term Ceiling Concentrations
1938	US Public Health Service	5 mppcf		
1939–1957	States of Texas, Ohio, Oregon, and California			
1946	American Conference of Governmental Industrial Hygienists	5 mppcf		
1951	US Department of Labor	5 mppcf		
1971	Occupational Safety and Health Administration		12 f/mL 2 mppcf	
1972	Occupational Safety and Health Administration		5 f/mL	10 f/mL
1976	Occupational Safety and Health Administration		2 f/mL	10 f/mL
1980	American Conference of Governmental Industrial Hygienists			
	Amosite		0.5 f/mL	1.5 f/mL
	Chrysotile		2 f/mL	4 f/mL
	Crocidolite		0.2 f/mL	0.6 f/mL
	Other Forms		2 f/mL	4 f/mL
1986	Occupational Safety and Health Administration		0.2 f/mL	N/A
1994	Occupational Safety and Health Administration		0.1 f/mL	1 f/mL
1998	American Conference of Governmental Industrial Hygienists		0.1 f/mL	0.5 f/mL

MAC = Maximum Allowable Concentration.
TWA = Time Weighted Average (8 h).
N/A = Not applicable.

been conducted to a variable extent in many developed countries; however, the details defy summarization and will not be considered here.

As noted above, the arduous task of establishing effective regulations to address the stated goal of the enabling legislation, that is, the elimination of occupational and environmental asbestos-related disease, rarely satisfies all interested parties. The outcome proves to be a compromise, in part, dictated by the technical inadequacies of industrial control measures for dust in the work place, and the shortcomings of the available scientific information, particularly data on the long-term outcome of asbestos exposures in humans. Regulations dealing with asbestos are concerned with three distinctively unique disease processes that differ one from another with regard to presumptive thresholds and the potential toxicity of the various mineralogical types of asbestos and the fiber dimensions. The relatively long latency period of these diseases, as well as inadequate exposure data, hampers the use of human epidemiological information to assess risks, both prospectively and retrospectively. Animal and in vitro studies also have consequential limitations, precluding realistic extrapolations to human disease. Thus, regulators are faced with an impossible task juxtaposed between the pleas of industry for economic "sanity" and members of the general population often influenced by inflammatory predictions of the media, worker groups, and environmental activists. The regulatory criteria summarized in Table 13.2 demonstrate that the evolving concerns initially focused on preventing the occurrence of asbestosis, and much later, on MM. Almost all states have regulations addressing asbestos in addition to those promulgated by EPA and OSHA. For example, California has separate air quality control districts; Florida has multiple districts; and the cities of New York and Chicago have their own rules. A complex, ever-changing mirage, however good the intentions.

To address justifiable concerns, regulators have chosen to extrapolate to zero in dose-response analyses, based on the assumption that the diseases under consideration manifest no threshold. Thus, theoretically, a single fiber could induce a MM, although the likelihood of this occurring in a finite population is negligible. Although mathematically suitable, and seemingly rational from a political perspective, the approach is biologically indefensible because it is inconsistent with our understanding of the pathogenesis of the asbestos-associated diseases.

Due to uncertainties regarding the disease-causing potential of so-called short fibers (ie, <5 μm), the issue of fiber dimension has largely been ignored by regulators in rule making. A recent comprehensive evaluation of this question by a committee appointed by the Agency for Toxic Substance and Disease Registration (ATSDR) portends a revised approach to this critical issue based on contemporary scientific information. It would appear that fibers <5 μm are nonpathogenic and the widely circulated 2005 report authored by Berman and Crump under the aegis of EPA, suggests that fibers shorter than 10 μm in length may be nonpathogenic. It should be recalled that an industrial asbestos product is a mixture of countless fibers each differing one from another in length and breadth. Moreover, industrial grades of fiber that are "long" and "short" differ as to the proportion in a product.

Because it is usually impractical to identify the various types of asbestos in environmental sampling exercises (without time-consuming, costly laboratory studies), the commercial asbestos types have not been regulated individually in the United States. In years past, some European countries have done so, recognizing the substantial disease-causing potential of commercial amphiboles in contrast to chrysotile. Alas, the US regulatory agencies have thus far failed to differentiate between the commercial amphiboles and chrysotile, with regard to their capacity to cause disease (even though the amphiboles now have no industrial applications in the United States and other developed countries).

Again, this issue was recently evaluated by an expert committee of scientists at the behest of the EPA and the agency's outdated posture seems likely to be modified at some future date. Finally, the regulatory agencies have understandably chosen to incorporate a significant margin of error in their determinations of permissible levels of exposure, since thresholds are impossible to determine based on epidemiological studies.

As noted elsewhere (Chapter 6), control measures now have largely eliminated the threat of asbestosis from the workplace. It is highly unlikely that asbestos exposure is a contributing factor to the development of LC in most patients at currently permissible levels of exposure (Chapter 7). MM now poses the major hurdle (Chapter 8). Scientific questions abound; the most critical issues relate to a definition of threshold for humans under which disease occurs and the duration of latency period. Today, the disease is developing in septuagenarians and octogenarians whose only recognized consequential documented exposure to amphibole asbestos occurred during or shortly after World War II. Epidemiological evidence suggests that the duration of the latency period is inversely related to the dosage (Chapter 4).

Since abundant epidemiological evidence indicates that chrysotile is either not a cause of MM or is an exceedingly weak carcinogen, should the mineral be regulated differently from amphiboles? The bulk of the scientific information at present supports this contention. It should be emphasized that scientific research has yet to exclude definitively subtle amphibole asbestos exposures as a cause of many of the not uncommon, so-called "idiopathic" MM.

The current OSHA asbestos standard requires products used in the workplace to be labeled if they contain greater than 1% asbestos, assuming they are likely to result in exposures above the permissible limits during their foreseeable use. Material Safety Data Sheets (MSDS) that provide detailed information on a product's composition are now required to be made available to employers and their employees by suppliers of materials containing 0.1% or more of known carcinogens.

The EPA, under the auspices of the CAA, promulgated Asbestos Hazardous Emergency Response Act (AHERA) and NESHAP regulations for asbestos-containing materials according to friability through usage, sanding, grinding, cutting, and abrading. NESHAP is designed to minimize the release of asbestos during the processing, handling, and disposal of asbestos-containing materials such as during demolition and renovation of nonresidential buildings. The November 1990 revised asbestos NESHAP prohibited spray-on application of materials containing more than 1% asbestos to buildings, pipes, and conduits unless the material is encapsulated with a bituminous or resinous binder and the materials are not friable after drying. It allows spray-on application of materials (on equipment and machinery) that contain more than 1% asbestos in sites where the asbestos in the materials is encapsulated.

In 1984 a survey by the EPA indicated that more than 7×10^5 buildings in the United States contained friable asbestos insulation (Chapter 3). It estimated there were 2.7×10^9 sq. ft. of asbestos-containing floor tile in 1.5×10^6 buildings, excluding schools, smaller industrial facilities, and residences. Nonresidential and commercial buildings were subject to the overlapping OSHA asbestos standards, AHERA and NESHAP regulations promulgated by the EPA, as well as regulations based on various individual state and local statutes.

Elementary and secondary schools are covered by the EPA, AHERA, and NESHAP regulations and are obliged to adhere to the OSHA standards with regard to custodians and teachers. Although the AHERA regulations do not apply to commercial, industrial, and other public buildings, owners and consultants often find the AHERA tenets to be a useful guide; thus, they have been widely implemented in industry and commerce.

Table 13.3 The Status of Asbestos Products in the United States (2005)

Prohibited	Authorized
Corrugated paper	Corrugated and flat asbestos cement sheet, pipe and shingles
Commercial paper	
Flooring felt	Vinyl asbestos floor tile
Rollboard	Friction materials such as:
Speciality paper	Brake linings, clutch facings, disc brake pads, and transmission compounds
New uses of asbestos	
	Asbestos clothing and textiles
	Roofing felt and coating
	Gaskets and packing
	Millboard
	Pipeline wrap and sealant tapes
	Acetylene cylinder filler and missile liners
	Asbestos diaphragms
	High-grade electrical paper
	Arc chutes
	Battery separators
	Reinforced plastics

However, facilities such as power plants and oil refineries, no doubt, would find AHERA regulations difficult, if not impossible, to implement.

During the period 1979 through 1990, the EPA published a series of guidance documents for the regulation and remediation of asbestos-containing materials in public buildings. The rules required responsible officials to identify friable asbestos in their buildings and notify employees of its location. Even with the passage of AHERA in 1986 and the subsequent compliance rules, the hazard assessment was still based on visual surveys by an inspector. Assays of fiber type and concentration in the air were not required, although building surveys are now carried out in most jurisdictions using state-of-the-art technical approaches including TEM.

The AHERA goal for satisfactory abatement is an environmental asbestos air concentration of less than 0.005 f/mL as determined by TEM, that is, equivalent to background. This concentration is 20-fold lower than the current permissible occupational (OSHA) level and more than 1×10^5 lower than the occupational concentrations experienced by some asbestos workers in the past.

In the mid-1980s, public panic over asbestos in buildings—which was later discovered to be largely unwarranted—prompted the EPA, in 1989, to issue a final rule banning most, but not all, asbestos-containing products manufactured or imported into the United States (Table 13.3). EPA's proposal resulted in a massive compilation of information on the benefits of asbestos in many products, as well as the potential risk for human exposure in such uses. Upon review of this comprehensive record, the US Court of Appeals for the Fifth District District in 1991 found a ban unwarranted based on the following criteria:

- No significant human exposure to asbestos fibers would occur if the products were produced and used under controlled conditions.
- Substitutes for asbestos-containing products themselves pose potential human health risks that could be more significant than any potential risks from asbestos.
- Asbestos-containing products offered significant benefits not offered by substitute products.

Thus far, federal agencies have not formally addressed and contested the issues raised by the Court, although as noted above, EPA is currently reevaluating its position with regard to chrysotile asbestosis. Nonetheless, use of asbestosis in certain industrial products is prohibited (Table 13.3).

Worldwide, more than 30 countries have banned all forms of asbestos. In 1991, the European Union Commission banned amphibole asbestos and, as of 2003, chrysotile asbestos is to be eliminated from most products (asbestos-cement, friction materials, seals, gaskets, and various specialty uses). The ban does not require in place asbestos-containing products to be removed until the end of their so-called service life. Regardless, on a worldwide basis, chrysotile continues to be used in manufactured products, particularly in developing countries as discussed in detail in Chapter 16.

Approaches to Sampling Air for Asbestos

Methodologies for evaluating airborne asbestos dust in ambient air have evolved over the years. The impinger method for measurement became the standard approach in the 1920s. As noted above, in this assay, airborne particles are collected in a liquid medium, and fibers ≥ 5 μm are counted, and expressed as mppcf. This work was done by optical microscopy.

In the past, the standard method for measuring dust in the United States was the Greenberg-Smith impinger. Later, the midget impinger was employed. This approach was originally designed to assay airborne silica dust but, for practical reasons, it soon became the standard tool for the measurement of asbestos.

The study by Dreessen et al. (1938) used impinger data and rather arbitrary decisions were made concerning the levels of risk that were "acceptable." The standard was applied not only to the textile industry but to other industries. In various countries other assay methods were adopted. In the United Kingdom measurements in the textile industry were made using a thermal precipitator. In South Africa, both konimeters and thermal precipitators were used. Measurements in the former Soviet Union were made gravimetrically. Since the introduction of the membrane filter method in the late 1960s, there have been several changes in the techniques used to render the filters transparent. Methods of counting have also changed. Richards (1994) reported that a concentration of 100 f/mL using the thermal precipitator converted to 400 f/mL with the early membrane filter method. The count changed to 800 f/mL when an eyepiece graticule was the standard approach and 1600 f/mL when triacetin clearing was replaced by acetone clearing of the filter. Obviously, the methodology was less than satisfactory, precluding its use in scientific studies designed to determine risk and threshold levels.

While attempts to correct for these factors in risk estimates have rarely, if ever, been undertaken, the problems should be borne in mind since a risk assessment, based on historical exposure data are overestimates (Borron et al., 1997). Side-by-side assessments using the midget impinger and membrane filter methods in the Québec mines and mills showed that overall there was very poor correlation between these different approaches (Gibbs and LaChance, 1974).

References

Borron SW, Forman SA, Lockey JE, Lemasters GK, Yee LM. An early study of pulmonary asbestosis among manufacturing workers: original data and reconstruction of the 1932 cohort. *Am J Ind Med.* 1997;31:324–334.

Dreessen WC, Dalla Valle JM, Edwards TI, et al. *A Study of Asbestosis in the Asbestos Textile Industry.* Washington: *Publ Hlth Bul*; 1938: No 241.

Gibbs GW, LaChance M. Dust exposure in chrysotile mines and mills of Québec. *Arch Environ Health.* 1974;24:189–197.

Lane RE. Hygiene standards for chrysotile asbestos dust. *Ann Occup Hyg.* 1968;2:47.

Lanza AJ, McConnell WJ, Fehnel JW. Effects of the inhalation of asbestos dust on the lungs of asbestos workers. U.S. Public Health Reports, 1935;50:1.

Merewether ERA, Price CW. Report on Effects of Asbestos Dust on the Lungs and Dust Suppression in the Asbestos Industry. Home Office, HMSO; 1930.

Richards AL. Levels of work of workplace exposure. *Ann Occup Hyg.* 1994;38:469–475.

Roach SA. Measurement of airborne asbestos dust by instruments measuring different parameters. Discussion. Biological Effects of Asbestos; Selikoff IJ and Churg J (eds). *Ann NY Acad Sci.* 1965;132:306–315.

14

Therapeutic Approaches to Malignant Mesothelioma

Harvey I. Pass, Stephen Hahn, and
Nicholas Vogelzang

Natural History

Most patients with pleural malignant mesothelioma (MM) die from complications of
local disease due to (1) increasing tumor bulk causing progressive respiratory compromise, pneumonia or myocardial dysfunction with arrhythmias and/or (2) unrelenting
chest wall pain requiring narcotics leading to pulmonary complications and cachexia,
and (3) dysphagia from tumor compression of the esophagus. Small bowel obstruction from direct extension through the diaphragm develops in approximately one-third,
and 10% die of pericardial or myocardial involvement (Antman et al., 1980). The most
important predictor of survival in nonsurgical studies of MM is performance status (see
Prognostic Indicators below). The median survival of patients treated in 10 clinical trials
was 7 months (Herndon et al., 1998); however, for those with performance status 0, the
median survival was 13–14 months. In various series, the median survival ranges from
4 to 18 months. Extrathoracic metastases occur late in the course of disease and are not
usually the direct cause of death.

Prognostic Indicators

Although the overall prognosis for patients with MM is poor, there are some patients who
do not conform to the norm and live for a considerable period. Retrospective analysis of
prognostic variables to define these outlier cases are usually characterized by differences
in treatment (chemotherapy, surgery, multimodality therapy) and a lack of uniformity in
pathologic staging. Recently, published studies have provided insight into potential prognostic variables. There are, however, no standardized prognostic indices used universally
by all clinicians to guide therapy.

We learned from the European Organization for Research and Treatment of Cancer
(EORTC) experience with over 200 adults that the median survival was 13 months from
diagnosis, and 8 months from trial entry. Poor prognosis was associated with (1) poor
performance status, (2) leukocytosis, (3) male gender, and (4) sarcomatous histologic
subtype (Curran et al., 1998). Among 337 patients in the Cancer and Leukemia Group
B (CALGB) studies, (1) poor performance status, (2) chest pain, (3) dyspnea, (4) platelet

counts greater than 400 000/μL, (5) weight loss, (6) serum lactate dehydrogenase concentrations greater than 500 IU/L, (7) pleural involvement, (8) anemia, (9) leukocytosis, and (10) age over 75 years predict shorter survival (Herndon et al., 1998).

The molecular prognostication of MM has been explored by two groups. Gordon et al. (2003) developed a four-gene expression ratio test that predicted treatment-related patient outcome independent of histologic type of the tumor. Similarly, Pass et al. (2004) reported a 27 gene expression array that was validated using Gordon's data. The gene classifier recapitulated both the actual time to progression, as well as survival with over 95% accuracy. Clinical outcomes were independent of the histological features of the tumor. These data require further validation in larger prospective analyses but imply that gene expression data at the time of initial biopsy may predict clinical outcomes.

Staging

The original staging system relied on pathologic generalizations instead of specific quantitative measures of disease and was designed well before recognition of the different prognostic implications of lymph node involvement (Butchart et al., 1981). The American Joint Commission on Cancer (AJCC) staging system was adopted by the International Mesothelioma Interest Group (IMIG) in 1995, and has been validated in a number of trials (Pass et al., 1997b, 1998; Rusch, 1996; Rusch and Venkatraman, 1999). The proposed Brigham and Women's Hospital Staging System also differs from the AJCC by defining intrapleural adenopathy as Stage II disease, and extrapleural adenopathy as Stage III disease (Sugarbaker et al., 1999; Sugarbaker and Garcia, 1997; Waller, 2004; Zellos and Sugarbaker, 2002). The AJCC system classifies nodal involvement, either intrapleural or extrapleural, as Stage III disease.

Treatment

Overview

No standards exist for the management of resectable pleural MM, and treatment decisions are influenced by the functional evaluation of elderly individuals and the philosophy of the treating physician. In the United Kingdom, only 46% of the physicians surveyed would consider referral of a MM patient to a thoracic surgeon for radical resection (Butchart, personal communication, October 2000). This attitude may have changed recently; however, since a randomized trial of extrapleural pneumonectomy (EPP) compared to nonsurgical treatment is underway in the United Kingdom (Waller, 2004). The French have concentrated on early Stage I disease detection and treatment with intrapleural therapy, including interferon gamma with or without chemotherapy (CH). Surgery is performed after CH only to improve local control either by pleurectomy or EPP. In patients with Stage II or III disease, Boutin et al. (1999) recommends surgery and postoperative radiation.

In the United States a consortium of cancer centers are conducting Phase I/II type trials that involve either novel systemic approaches for the disease or a multimodality approach. The use of surgery in MM with or without intraoperative and/or postoperative innovative adjuvant therapies is being defined.

For unresectable patients who are candidates for CH, Phase III trials have shown a 3–4 months survival advantage for the 2-drug regimen of Pemetrexed and Cisplatin compared to the one drug regimen of Cisplatin (Vogelzang et al., 2003).

Supportive Care

The median survival of patients who select supportive care ranges from 4 (Edwards et al., 2000) to 13 months (Antman et al., 1980), no doubt due to (1) variations in tumor biology, and host responsivity, (2) detection and lead-time bias, and (3) the use of either ad hoc or unreported treatments. There are no published studies that randomize patients to a treatment group.

Control of pleural effusion can be accomplished with (1) repeated thoracenteses, (2) talc pleurodesis, (3) pleuroperitoneal shunting, or (4) placement of a Pleurex catheter. Talc pleurodesis is performed by instilling asbestos-free talc over the lung and the parietal surfaces. Success rates in effusion control approaches 90% (Canto et al., 1997; Viallat et al., 1996). Failure is usually associated with (1) lung entrapment by the tumor, (2) a large solid tumor mass, (3) a long history of effusion with multiple thoracenteses leading to loculations, (4) advanced age, and (5) poor performance status. In such cases, the Pleurex catheter with its one-way valve can be implanted into the fluid collection and the patient encouraged to drain themselves using the available disposable kits (Pien et al., 2001). Alternatively, internal drainage from the pleura to the abdomen can be accomplished using a pleuroperitoneal shunt.

The chest pain of MM frequently requires narcotics and consultation by a dedicated pain management team to assist in the optimization of quality of life. Subcutaneous epidural catheter anesthesia has also been used in selective cases for long-term, out-of-hospital management.

The median survival is 4–5 months (Bissett et al., 1991; de Graaf-Strukowska et al., 1999) when only local palliation has been delivered solely for pain or chest wall tumor nodules.

Surgery

Surgery is only part of the treatment regimen for aggressive therapy of pleural MM. The operations include pleurectomy/decortication or EPP, and the indications for these operations depend on the extent of disease and the performance and functional status of the patient. Operative intervention falls into one of the three categories: (1) primary effusion control as described already for supportive care, (2) cytoreduction before multimodal therapy, and (3) delivery and monitoring of innovative intrapleural therapies.

Preoperative Considerations

The majority of patients are middle to older aged individuals with a long latency period between asbestos exposure and tumor development. A detailed physiological-functional workup to assess the patient's cardiac and pulmonary status must be performed if a surgical intervention is to be considered.

Pulmonary Evaluation

Concomitant smoking history, amount of lung trapped by tumor or fluid, and patient age all influence pulmonary function in these patients. Asbestosis along with a reduced CO_2 diffusion capacity increases dyspnea, and abnormal chest wall motion result in reduced lung volume on the affected side influencing respiratory functional reserve and the extent of surgery. An FEV_1 of less than 1 L/s, a $PO_2 < 55\%$ and hypercapnia are contraindications for EPP (Sugarbaker et al., 1991). An FEV_1 of less than 2 L/s, or a predicted FEV_1 of less than 1.2 L/min mandates quantitative lung perfusion scanning to estimate the pulmonary reserve.

Cardiac Evaluation

Patients with a recent myocardial infarction and/or an ejection fraction of less than 45% are not candidates for EPP. Coronary disease should be considered with angioplasty before operative intervention.

Staging and Operative Therapy

The goal of a surgical resection is a near complete cytoreduction of tumor. Operation can be attempted in all clinically staged individuals with Stages I-III disease, and good performance status, including those with the T3 category of Stage III patients (invasion of the endothoracic fascia or mediastinal fat, a solitary focus of tumor invading soft tissues of the chest wall (eg, at an old thoracoscopy site), or/and nontransmural involvement of the pericardium.

Involvement of lymph nodes by metastatic MM is an ominous prognostic sign. It is unclear whether the prognostic importance of mediastinal nodal involvement is equal to, or greater than, the prognostic importance of those nodes within the visceral envelope of the lung. Positive nodes within the lung may reflect disease at a late time point in its natural history. It is possible that positron emission tomographc PET scanning will help to define patients with node involvement (Schouwink et al., 2003).

Which Operations?

Most MM cannot be surgically removed en bloc with negative histologic margins. Nevertheless, in one of the largest series of EPP, 36% of patients were believed to have negative resection margins. Patients with epithelial MM and no evidence of spread beyond the resection margins, and without nodal involvement, enjoy 2 and 5 year survival rates of 68% and 46%, respectively (Sugarbaker et al., 1999). Since a minority of patients have margin-free resections, and less bulky disease, it may be justifiable to spare functioning lung if the visceral pleura is minimally involved. Such "lung-preserving surgery" can potentially be accomplished by performing a radical parietal pleurectomy instead of EPP. Minimal visceral pleural disease is an undefined clinical entity and there are no criteria to define how many sites should be involved, the size of these involved sites, and to define the importance of involvement of the lung fissures. Some surgeons make the decision regarding the type of operation in an individual patient at the time of the exploration. In general, patients who have pleurectomy decortications have less severe disease, and live longer.

EPP is an extensive dissection and may be more complete than a pleurectomy, chiefly on the diaphragmatic and visceral pleural surfaces. Some surgeons, however, include diaphragmatic resection and pericardial resection with pleurectomy to accomplish removal of "all gross disease." EPP, pericardiotomy, and partial pericardiectomy are performed during the resection since it helps expose vessels and allows intrapericardial control to prevent a surgical catastrophe.

No guidelines exist that assure preoperatively which operation will be necessary. The presence on computer axial tomography (CAT) of irregular, bulky disease that infiltrates into the fissures probably dictates EPP; a large effusion with minimally bulky disease may only call for pleurectomy decortication. Hence, Stage II MM may indeed be an absolute indication for EPP as opposed to pleurectomy.

Some surgeons reserve EPP for patients with bulk disease that prevents simple pleurectomy, while others feel that the greatest chance for complete gross excision will be EPP for the patient with minimal disease. This important factor (preoperative quantitative bulk of disease), not only influences the choice, but may be an important preoperative prognostic factor. Moreover, the selection of the type of resection is influenced by analysis of the regional lung function.

To summarize, the final decision as to whether pleurectomy and decortication or EPP is to be performed, given the above caveats, becomes an intraoperative decision.

Pleurectomy

When performed routinely, pleurectomy has few major complications. The most common complication is prolonged air leaks, and this occurs in 10% of patients. Contemporary mortality is 1.5%–2% with death resulting from either respiratory insufficiency or hemorrhage (Pass et al., 1997a; Rusch, 1997). Pleurectomy and decortication are effective in controlling pleural effusion. In one study, effusions were controlled in 88% of patients by decortication (Law et al., 1984). Ruffie et al. (1989) reported control of effusion in 86%, and Brancatisano et al. (1991) reported 98% control of effusion after pleurectomy.

Many of the published series using pleurectomy for palliative management have added therapies postoperatively (Table 14.1). Mediastinal nodes had not been sampled in the majority and mediastinal dissection was not done. Nevertheless, the overall median

Table 14.1 Survival of Patients with Pleural MM after Pleurectomy

Authors	No. of Patients	Median (Months)	2 Year (%)
Sugarbaker et al. (2003)	44	10–20	—
Aziz et al. (2002)	47	14	—
Lee et al. (2002)	26	18.1	—
Martin-Ucar et al. (2001)	51	7.2	—
Takagi et al. 2001	73		26.1
Pass et al. (1997)*	39	14.5	—
Rusch and Venkatraman (1996)	51	18.3	—
Allen et al. (1994)	56	9	8.9
Brancatisano et al. (1991)	45	16	21
Harvey et al. (1990)	9	11.9	—
Ruffie et al. (1989)	63	9.8	—
Faber (1988)	33	10	12
DaValle et al. (1986)	23	11.2	—
Law et al. (1984)	28	20	32
Brenner et al. (1982)	69	15	—
Chahinian et al. (1982)	30	13	27
Wanebo et al. (1976)	33	16.1	—

Modified from Singhal and Kaiser (2002).

* All patients received intrapleural hyperthermic CH.

(—) Information not available.

survival for patients having solely pleurectomy is approximately 13 months. The patients who receive pleurectomy and decortication alone usually have early effusions with minimal bulk tumor. If these patients have epithelial MM and no lymph node involvement, survival can be significantly longer. A further discussion of multimodality therapy and pleurectomy is found in the *Multimodality* section.

Extrapleural Pneumonectomy

A cohort of patients who are explored with the intent of undergoing an EPP is found to be unresectable at the time of the operation. Out of 46 (63%) patients 29 of them (63%) were eligible for EPP (Butchart et al., 1976), in an operative series at one university hospital, but 33 out of 56 (59%) explored patients over a 27-year period had EPP (Faber, 1986). Sugarbaker et al. (2004) recently reported that 50% of his patients are not eligible for EPP and adjuvant therapy. The Lung Cancer Study Group performed a pilot study of EPP (Rusch et al., 1991b). Eligible patients were required to have disease limited to the hemithorax, a residual FEV_1 after resection of at least 1 L/s, and no significant cardiovascular illness. Only 20 of 83 patients were resected with an EPP. EPP could not be performed due to (1) extent of disease (54%), (2) inadequate respiratory reserve (33%), and (3) concurrent medical illness (10%).

EPP has significantly greater morbidity than pleurectomy, and the major complication was arrhythmia. In a recent report, morbidity occurred in about 60% of patients undergoing EPP (Sugarbaker et al., 2004). The rate for bronchopleural fistula is greater with right-sided EPP with an overall fistula rate of 3%–20%. The bronchopleural fistula can be handled for the most part by establishing open thoracostomy drainage.

Table 14.2 Survival of Patients with Pleural MM after EPP

Author	No. of Patients	Median Survival (Months)	2-Year Survival
Rusch et al. (2001)*	61	17	—
Schouwink et al. (2001)†	28	10	—
Takagi et al. (2001)	116		29.7
Sugarbaker et al. (1999)‡	183	19	38
Pass et al. (1997a)§	39	9.4	—
Rusch and Venkatraman (1996)	50	9.9	—
Allen et al. (1994)	40	13.3	22.5
Harvey et al. (1990)	7	5.4	28.5
Ruffie et al. (1989)	23	9.3	17
Faber (1988)	33	13.5	24
DaValle et al. (1986)		17.8	24
Chahinian et al. (1982)	6	18	33
DeLaria et al. (1978)	11	18	—
Butchart et al. (1976)	29	4.5	10.3

Modified from: Singhal and Kaiser (2002).

* Postoperative hemithorax radiation therapy; all patients; Stages I/II, 33.8; Stages III/IV, 10.

† Intraoperative photodynamic therapy.

‡ Postoperative multimodal therapy.

§ Phase I trials of photodynamic therapy or immunochemotherapy.

(—) information not available.

The mortality rates after EPP were unacceptably high in the 1970s with a 31% (Butchart et al., 1976). Since then, however, there has been a steady decline in the operative mortality to rates less than 10%. Mortality occurs chiefly in older patients from respiratory failure, myocardial infarction, or pulmonary embolus. Rusch et al. (1999, 2001) reported a perioperative mortality of 6%–8% after EPP and Sugarbaker et al. (2004) reports a benchmark perioperative mortality of about 4%.

Although the local control is superior to other modalities, EPP is associated with distant recurrence. Pass et al. (1997a) found that recurrence after EPP was chiefly local. The sites of first recurrence are (1) local (35%), (2) abdominal (26%), (3) contralateral thorax (17%), and (4) distant sites (8%) (Baldini et al., 1997).

Survival after EPP remains disappointing (Table 14.2). Rusch et al. (1991a, 2001) found a median survival of 10 months and Pass et al. (1997a) reported the median survival to be 9.4 months after EPP. All histological types of MM and pathological grades II and III were included in this series. More recently, Sugarbaker et al. (1999) reported a 17 month median survival in a series heavily weighted with Stage I patients with epithelial MM. The 2 and 5 year survivals were 68% and 46%, respectively. In the series published by Rusch and Venkatraman (1999), the 2 and 5 year survivals of Stage I were 65% and 30%, respectively.

Radiotherapy

Curative RT as a Single Modality

It is difficult to administer potentially *curative* RT (Radiotherapy) due to the risks of toxicity in the large volumes of tissue involved. Law et al. (1984) used a rotational technique to deliver 5000–5500 cGy to the pleural space. Survival ranged from 3 to 10 months, with one exceptional long-term survivor. Ball and Cruickshank (1990) treated 12 patients with 5000 cGy to the entire hemithorax resulting in a median survival of 17 months compared to 7 months for those offered palliative treatment only. Selection bias may explain these differences; those fit enough to undergo a full course of RT were likely to have a greater survival regardless of treatment. Moreover, a few patients developed radiation hepatitis and myelopathy that led to death. A larger study of 49 patients resulted in a median survival of 9.8 months for patients treated either with radical RT or palliative RT (Ruffie et al., 1989). Alberts et al. (1988) used a variable schedule, split course of RT with a median duration of response of 133 days. Holsti et al. (1997) reported a 2 year survival rate of 21% and the 5 year survival of 9%.

Combined CH and RT

Poor results with RT alone have led to studies evaluating the combination of CH and RT. Alberts et al. (1988) treated patients with a variety of CH regimens, all concurrent with RT. Although the response rates and durations were increased with the addition of CH compared to radiation alone, the median survival was not significantly increased over those patients who received radiation alone. Ruffie et al. (1989) used doxorubicin-based regimens and other combinations of CH. There was a significant increase in survival (median of 12.3 vs 7.3 months) compared to those who did not receive CH. The CH/RT group had a median survival of 14 months. Linden et al. (1996) treated patients with hemithoracic RT (40 Gy in 20 daily fractions) followed by CH in good performance status patients. The CH consisted of doxorubicin and cyclophosphamide. In this nonrandomized trial, the response rates were no different in patients treated with RT alone, CH alone, or combined treatment. The median survival was highest (13 months) in patients treated with combined modality therapy. The differences in survival among the treatment groups are likely the result of selection bias in favor of combined modality.

Some investigators have evaluated the addition of radiation sensitizers. Herscher et al. (1998) studied the use of a 5 day continuous infusion of paclitaxel with hemithoracic RT delivered initially, followed by RT to the gross tumor volume for a total dose of 5760–6300 cGy. The treatment was well tolerated. Chen et al. (2001) documented a 12% complete response rate and an 88% partial response rate with pulsed paclitaxel delivered during RT in a Phase I trial. It is unlikely that the addition of RT sensitizers to radical RT will be a curative, and as such definitive CH/RT should be considered experimental.

Combined Surgical Resection and *Definitive* RT

Surgical resection, when feasible, is the desired treatment for patients with pleural MM. After an EPP, radical RT can be administered without concern for damage to the underlying ipsilateral lung in the chest since the lung has been removed surgically. However, radical RT after a pleurectomy continues to place the ipsilateral lung at risk for substantial loss of function. Ruffie et al. (1989) and Law et al. (1984) reported no difference in survival when decortication or EPP was followed by RT. Toxicity was minimal.

Some investigators have used brachytherapy or intraoperative external beam RT in combination with surgery. Hilaris et al. (1984) treated patients with pleural MM after a parietal pleurectomy; however, there was residual disease in the majority. Either brachytherapy or radioisotopes were used to eradicate gross residual disease. Permanent ^{125}I brachytherapy implants were used in patients who had measurable gross residual disease. If the residual disease was too diffuse, temporary ^{192}Ir implants were placed 3–5 days after the pleurectomy. If gross disease was noted on the surface of the lung, a solution of ^{32}P was instilled into the pleural cavity 5–7 days after thoracotomy. External beam radiation was delivered to the pleural surface after surgery using a combination of photons and electrons. There was no mortality and minimal toxicity, but 15% of patients developed complications. The median survival was 21 months, with 1 and 2 year survivals of 65% and 40%, respectively. The lungs failed in only 17%, no doubt a reflection of aggressive local therapy. Intraoperative brachytherapy followed by external beam radiation proved to be an effective method for controlling local recurrence, but it is not clear if it translates into improved survival.

Rusch et al. (2001) completed a Phase II trial of surgery followed by postoperative radiation. The most common complications were (1) atrial arrythmia, (2) respiratory failure, (3) pneumonia, and (4) empyema. In general, radiation was well tolerated, with toxicity mainly related to fatigue, nausea, and esophagitis. There were five grade 4 toxicities, the most serious being an esophagopleural fistula. Only the patients who underwent EPP were considered for survival analysis. The median survival was 17 months, with an overall survival of 27% at 3 years. Only 13% had recurrence, with the majority of patients failing with distant metastases. The authors concluded that their approach of aggressive surgery with EPP followed by high-dose radiation to the entire hemithorax provided a favorable outcome for patients who were able to complete the therapy. However, it is difficult to evaluate the relative impact of the treatment regimen because of patient selection factors.

Lee et al. (2002) recently reviewed retrospectively the efficacy and toxicity of surgery with intraoperative RT followed by CH. The median overall survival was 18 months and the median progression-free interval was 12 months. They concluded that this approach was a potential treatment option for adjuvant radiotherapy in patients who were unable to tolerate an EPP.

Intensity Modulated Radiation Therapy offers the potential for administering higher doses of RT to the hemithorax while minimizing normal tissue toxicity. In an MD Anderson Cancer Study, 1-year survival was 65%. These early results were encouraging (Ahamad et al., 2003; Forster et al., 2003).

Prevention of Recurrences of MM in Chest Scars

Malignant seeding along thoracentesis, biopsy and chest tube tracts, and surgical incision sites are common complications of MM observed in approximately 20%–50% of patients (Boutin et al., 1995). Cutaneous recurrences usually present as painful subcutaneous nodules unresponsive to conventional therapies. Boutin et al. (1995) investigated the use of RT to prevent malignant seeding after invasive diagnostic procedures. No patients in a radiation treatment group developed subcutaneous nodules, whereas, 40% of untreated patients developed metastases. This study supports the use of RT to the chest wall after diagnostic procedures to prevent cutaneous tumor recurrences. However, a recent randomized trial failed to confirm a therapeutic advantage to prophylactic RT (Bydder et al., 2004).

Palliation Using RT

RT is commonly used to palliate pain in patients with advanced MM (de Graaf-Strukowska et al., 1999). Unfortunately, pain recurrence within the treated field remains a significant problem. Ball and Cruickshank (1990) reported a 72% rate of symptom improvement using palliative RT. One of the largest studies was reported by Davis et al. (1994). Greater than 60% of patients had some symptomatic benefit from RT, and the authors reported that the palliative response did not vary with dose. Therefore, the standard approach was to offer patients short courses of treatment rather than longer courses of RT.

Adjuvant Therapy for Surgically Cytoreduction

There are no Phase III trials that investigate the impact of adjuvant therapy compared to surgery alone; however, patients treated with surgery and postoperative adjuvant therapy have an apparent improved survival compared to those treated with palliative therapy alone. The importance of the cytoreduction has been quantified by Pass et al. (1998). For patients who have a more complete cytoreduction, the time to progression and survival is longer. For patients who had comparable cytoreduction, the addition of a uniform postoperative adjuvant therapy appears to influence postoperative survival (Pass et al., 1997b).

Multimodality Treatment

Surgery and Standard Agents

The intrapleural route of therapy remains intriguing, but its efficacy is uncertain. Phase II studies with the following design principles continue to be needed: (1) a tolerable regimen without chronic side effects, (2) a standard debulking approach with definition of the extent of residual disease, and (3) careful documentation of recurrence patterns.

Rusch et al. (1991a) used intrapleural CH after surgical debulking followed by systemic CH, and in a subsequent report used an even more aggressive regimen of pleurectomy, immediate intracavitary cisplatin and mitomycin-C with two cycles of these same agents. The most recent trial revealed an overall survival rate of 68% at 1 year and 44% at 2 years, with a median of 17 months (Rusch, 1994). A very similar regimen combining pleurectomy or EPP with cisplatin and mitomycin-C resulted in a disappointing median survival of 13 months. In an Italian study, pleurectomy and diaphragmatic or pericardial resection, combined with intrapleural CH after pleurectomy, followed by systemic CH revealed a median time to disease reappearance of 7.4 months, and median survival of only 11.5 months (Colleoni et al., 1996).

EPP, CH, and RT

A multimodal approach using EPP, postoperative CH and targeted postoperative RT has been ongoing since 1980 (Zellos and Sugarbaker, 2002). Over a 19-year period, 183 patients have been treated with a preoperative mortality of less than 4%. The median survival was approximately 17 months, which is a significant improvement over results from other trials. A large nonrandomized series also demonstrated an apparent increased survival with multimodal treatment compared to best supportive care (Calavrezos et al., 1988). Patients chose either best supportive care or multimodal treatment. Surgery consisted of pleurectomy decortication or EPP followed by systemic CH. Patients in remission at the end of the CH received RT to the hemithorax. Median survival was 13 months compared to 7 months for those receiving best supportive care.

Maggi et al. (2001, 2002, 2003) used the Sugarbaker et al. (2003) protocol of EPP followed by adjuvant CH and concurrent hemithoracic RT up to a total dose of 55 Gy. The results were encouraging with an operative mortality rate of slightly greater than 6%. However, a median survival of only 9.5 months was reported since 50% of the patients were found to be in Stage III after the procedure.

Induction CH followed by Surgery

Induction or neoadjuvant therapy for MM followed by surgery has been patterned after approaches used with nonsmall cell lung cancer. Results have been disappointing due to the inability of the patients to tolerate both the cytotoxic CH and the surgery, as well as increased difficulty in performing the surgical dissection after induction of CH. With the improved efficacy of doublet CH (gemcitabine/cisplatin or pemetrexed/cisplatin), there is renewed interest in investigating a neoadjuvant approach. In a Swiss study, 32% showed a response to therapy and the median survival was 23 months (Weder et al., 2004).

A similar trial was performed by de Perrot et al. (2003). It involved induction CH, surgery, and postoperative hemithorax RT with a 6% operative mortality and 74% 1-year survival.

Novel Intrapleural Approaches: New Techniques with New/Old Agents

Photodynamic Therapy

Photodynamic therapy (PDT) involves the light activated sensitization of malignant cells (Pass et al., 1997b) using a photosensitizer such as Photofrin II that is retained by malignant tissue in vivo. The sensitizer is activated by 630 nm light and interacts with molecular oxygen to produce reactive oxygen species. After a series of Phase I and II trials, a group of 63 patients with localized MM were randomized for surgery in conjunction with or without intraoperative photodynamic therapy. All patients received postoperative CH. There were no differences in median survival (14.4 vs 14.1 months) or median progression-free time (8.5 vs 7.7 months), and sites of first recurrence were similar. Thus, aggressive multimodal therapy incorporating PDT can be delivered to patients with MM, but first-generation PDT does not prolong survival or improve local control for MM. Other Phase II trials of PDT for MM have not demonstrated therapeutic efficacy (Baas et al., 1997; Bonnette et al., 2002; Schouwink et al., 2001). Most recently, preliminary results using intrapleural PDT with Metatetrahydroxy-phenylchlorin after EPP revealed significant toxicity without survival benefit (Friedberg et al., 2003).

Pleural Perfusion

Hyperthermic chemoperfusion of the pleura is based on the hypothesis that the treatment will provide increased local control and avoid systemic CH toxicity. Ratto et al. (1999) delivered cisplatin to the pleural space after pleurectomy or EPP in 10 patients and recorded the pharmacokinetics but did not comment on survival or recurrences. Other small Phase II studies using cisplatin or doxorubicin with cisplatin have documented morbidity rates of 33%–65% using temperatures of 40 °C–42 °C without impacting on survival (van Ruth et al., 2003; Yellin et al., 2001). Sugarbaker et al. (2004) presented a Phase I/II trial using hyperthermic cisplatin (42 °C) to perfuse both the abdomen and the pleura after pleurectomy and decortication. Operative mortality was 11%, and survival of all patients was 10.5 months; however, in the group of patients surviving surgery who received 225 mg/m^2 of cisplatin, the median survival was 22 months and disease free survival was 20 months (Sugarbaker et al., 2003).

Novel Gene and Cytokine-Related Therapies

By transferring the herpes simplex virus thymidine kinase (HSV-tk) gene to a tumor that is then infected with an adenovirus construct containing the TK gene, the investigator attempts to kill the tumor cells by the addition of gancyclovir. A Phase I trial of intrapleural *suicide* gene therapy has been reported (Sterman et al., 1998). More recently, the role of interferon modulation is being explored using adenovirus delivery along with inhibitors of the cycoloxygenase pathway (Cordier et al., 2003; Kruklitis et al., 2004). Immunomodulatory gene therapy is also being investigated by transfecting MM with cytokine genes that activate CD4 T cells or stimulate proliferation of CD8 T cells. The IL-2 gene has been inserted into a replication deficient vaccinia virus and patients have been treated with 1 to 3 weekly injections of vaccinia virus–IL-2 into the tumor (Mukherjee et al., 2000, 2001; Nowak et al., 2002b). Preclinical trials in which interferon β (Odaka et al., 2001, 2002), interleukin 4, and p14 (ARF; Yang et al., 2001, 2003) are transfected into MM are ongoing. An approach that combines *suicide* gene therapy and vaccination strategies uses genetically modified allogeneic irradiated ovarian cancer cells transduced with the HSV-tk gene followed by systemic gancyclovir treatment (Harrison et al., 2000; Schwarzenberger et al., 1998a, 1998b, 1999). Newer trials include the use of adenovirus interferon replacement therapy.

Intrapleural and Systemic Cytokine Therapy

The use of intrapleural cytokine therapy had been documented in early stage MM (Boutin et al., 1994; Driesen et al., 1994). Intrapleural Interleukin-2 (IL-2) based regimens have also been exploited (Astoul et al., 1998).

Chemotherapy and Newer Agents

Early reports in the literature (Antman et al., 1988; Chahinian et al., 1982; Herndon et al., 1998; Samuels et al., 1998; Vogelzang et al., 1984) described the use of a single CH drug based on the hope that a major therapeutic advance would be discovered. The most common single-agent drugs used for MM have been the anthracyclines, platinum agents, and antimetabolites (Janne, 2003). Typically, tumor regression of short duration associated with symptomatic improvement occurred in almost 15% of patients treated with CH but the median survival remained at about 7–9 months. Response rates of 0%–15%, with median survivals of 4.4–9.5 months were found with the anthracyclines, cis-platinum, or carboplatinum have had response rates of 7%–16%, with median survivals of 5–8 months. Antimetabolites as single agents have reported response rates from 0% to 37%, the highest observed in methotrexate (37%) and gemcitabine (31%) (Janne, 2003). Those data lead Ong and Vogelzang (1996) to conclude that there was no CH agent(s) sufficiently active to be called *standard*. Some patients experienced disease stabilization and prolonged survival following CH, but it was unknown whether the improvement or stabilization was due to the therapy or due to indolent tumor behavior.

Combination CH has had higher response rates, and longer median survival times have been documented, than with single-agent regimens. Anthracycline based combinations have response rates from 11% to 32% and median survival times from 5.5 to 13.8 months; platinum-based CH have had response rates of 6%–48% with median survivals of 5.8–16 months (Janne, 2003). A 1998 report from the United Kingdom, however, was encouraging. It suggested that reduction in pain and dyspnea occurred in up to 40%-50% of patients treated with a combination regimen of mitomycin-C, vinblastine, and cis-platin (Middleton et al., 1998). A similar rate of clinical benefit with the single-agent, vinorelbine (Navelbine) has recently been reported (Steele et al., 2000). These findings have resulted in a randomized clinical trial involving treatment of patients with either: (1) a single agent vinorelbine, (2) the mitomycin/vinblastine/cisplatin combination, or (3) active supportive care (Girling et al., 2002).

Byrne et al. (1999) was the first to demonstrate efficacy of the combination of cisplatin combined with gemcitabine. Forty-seven percent of patients had a 30% or greater reduction in the thickness of the pleural rind of tumor and improvement in symptoms. A follow-up multicenter trial, however, demonstrated a 26% rate of activity and a median survival of only 7.5 months (Nowak et al., 2002a). The favorable response rate with gemcitabine and cisplatinum in other multicenter Phase II studies (van Haarst et al., 2002), and in trials including patients earlier treated with other CH (Vogelzang, 1999) and other gemcitabine/carboplatin regimen (Favaretto et al., 2003) has lead to its widespread use. Gemcitabine (Kindler and Van Meerbeeck, 2002; Van Meerbeeck et al., 1999), cisplatin (Mintzer et al., 1985; Planting et al., 1994; Zidar et al., 1988) and carboplatin (Mbidde et al., 1986; Raghavan et al., 1990; Vogelzang et al., 1990) all have independent but modest single-agent activity. Whether the cisplatin/gemcitabine the so-called *doublet* is superior to both single-agent is not known, and no Phase III studies are in progress examining the question.

A role for the antifolates has been suggested since Solheim et al. (1992) reported that methotrexate induced regressions in 37% of MM patients. Other antifolates had consistent but low activity as well (Calvert et al., 1986, 1987; Cantwell et al., 1986; Kindler et al., 1999; Scagliotti and Novello, 2003; Vogelzang et al., 1994). A novel antifolate, pemetrexed, demonstrated broad antitumor activity in Phase I and II trials. When combined with cisplatin, pemetrexed induced regressions in 38% of MM patients in a Phase I trial (Thodtmann et al., 1999). A Phase I study of pemetrexed and carboplatin reported significant radiological improvements in approximately 40% of patients (Hughes et al., 2002). These two trials lead to a Phase II trial of pemetrexed as a single agent in which only 14% of patients responded. While trials were underway, a comprehensive multivariate analysis revealed that folic acid and vitamin B_{12} deficiency states were the major contributors to the toxicity of pemetrexed. Folic acid therapy and B_{12} reduced myelosuppression and gastrointestinal toxicity, while preserving and possibly enhancing efficacy.

Because of the encouraging results in Phase I and II trials, a Phase III trial comparing single-agent cisplatin versus pemetrexed plus the same dose of cisplatin was undertaken. The results showed that the 2-drug regimen was clearly superior to a 1-drug regimen as assessed by median survival time (12.1 vs 9.3 months, respectively). Response rates as measured by an average 30% reduction in the thickness of the pleural rind were 41.3% versus 16.7% in the Cisplatin alone arm. Quality of life also improved in a significant manner in the pemetrexed/cisplatin-treated patients. Treatment with pemetrexed and cisplatin, supplemented with folic acid and vitamin B_{12}, appears to provide an improved risk-benefit ratio in treatment. However, other 2-drug regimens have been studied in Phase II trials (gemcitabine/cisplatin, etc.) and appear to be associated with response rates and median survivals comparable to findings with pemetrexed/cisplatin.

Another antimetabolite, raltitrexed, when combined with oxaliplatin, also has activity (Fizazi et al., 2003) and a Phase III trial recently compared cisplatin to raltitrexed plus cisplatin. A trend toward improved survival of patients treated with the combination of drugs was found (Van Meerbeeck et al., 2004).

Ranpirnase was reported in 2000. On the basis of an encouraging Phase II experience (Mikulski et al., 2002), a Phase III trial compared the median survival after treatment with either a single-agent doxorubicin or ranpirnase, a ribonuclease. No difference in the median survivals (seven to 8 months in each group) was found. But, the randomization failed to equally distribute poor risk patients. When those patients were omitted from the analysis, the median survival favored rapirnase. The trial has now been extended to compare doxorubicin to doxorubicin plus ranpirnase. Ranpirnase has recently been granted *orphan* drug status for the treatment of MM by the European Union.

In spite of these modestly heartening results, effective agents with unique mechanisms of action against MM are still desperately needed. Vascular endothelial growth factor signal transduction inhibitors are being tested and have clinical activity.

CH agents have historically had little effectiveness against MM. Newer agents seem to be somewhat more effective and the pemetrexed and cisplatin combination alters the natural history of the disease. Second-line CH may also alter the biology of these neoplasms.

Peritoneal (Abdominal) MM

Virtually all MM of the abdominal cavity initially present with local symptoms. Thus, the presenting complaints are commonly pain, abdominal distention, due to local ascites and invasive disease in the peritoneal cavity and omentum. Although a tumor *rind* several centimeters thick is not an uncommon finding on CT scan, frequently there is no easily measurable disease. Owing to the early dissemination of the neoplasm throughout the abdomen, loops of bowel seen on CT scan are often thickened and *tented* around the root of the mesentery. With advancing disease, the ascites becomes loculated and difficult to drain, eventually leading to massive intraabdominal carcinomatosis. In the absence of effective therapy, death occurs within a median time of 6–15 months as a result of some combination of intestinal obstruction, cachexia, and perforation. Overt metastatic disease is rarely the cause of death, although at autopsy, 50% of patients have microscopically demonstrable lymphatic and hematogenous metastases.

The treatment of peritoneal MM was recently reviewed at several conferences in the United States. In centers that treat more than 20–30 cases per year, a sequence of maximal surgical debulking followed immediately by intraperitoneal CH is the general approach. This is a technically demanding complex of procedures. Systemic CH given before or after surgery is less common. For patients who are not surgical candidates or for whom previous surgical approaches were unsuccessful, systemic CH with a combination of cisplatin and pemetrexed is a clearly effective regimen (Janne et al., 2005).

Conclusions

MM remains an orphan disease which, when detected early, can be treated with a multidisciplinary approach leading to prolonged survival. Unfortunately, the majority of patients are detected in a late stage. Future directions must concentrate on the development of biomarkers for the potential screening of high risk, asbestos exposed individuals, and a greater understanding of the pathways involved in mesothelial carcinogenesis. By detecting the disease earlier and leading to greater local control with better, therapeutic options, investigators may be able to offer less invasive therapies with greater chances for long-term survival.

References

Ahamad A, Stevens CW, Smythe WR, et al. Intensity-modulated radiation therapy: a novel approach to the management of malignant pleural mesothelioma. *Int J Radiat Oncol Biol Phys.* 2003;55:768–775.

Alberts AS, Falkson G, Goedhals L, Vorobiof DA, Van der Merwe CA. Malignant pleural mesothelioma: a disease unaffected by current therapeutic maneuvers. *J Clin Oncol.* 1988;6:527–535.

Allen KB, Faber LP, Warren WH. Malignant pleural mesothelioma. Extrapleural pneumonectomy and pleurectomy. *Chest Surg Clin NAM.* 1994;4:113–126.

Antman K, Shemin R, Ryan L, et al. Malignant mesothelioma: prognostic variables in a registry of 180 patients, the Dana-Farber Cancer Institute and Brigham and Women's Hospital experience over two decades, 1965–1985. *J Clin Oncol.* 1988;6:147–153.

Antman KH, Blum RH, Greenberger JS, Flowerdew G, Skarin AT, Canellos GP. Multimodality therapy for malignant mesothelioma based on a study of natural history. *Am J Med.* 1980;68:356–362.

Astoul P, Picat-Joossen D, Viallat JR, Boutin C. Intrapleural administration of interleukin-2 for the treatment of patients with malignant pleural mesothelioma: a Phase II study. *Cancer.* 1998;83:2099–2104.

Aziz T, Jilaihawi A, Prakash D. The management of malignant pleural mesothelioma; single centre experience in 10 years. *Eur J Cardiothorac Surg.* 2002;22:298–305.

Baas P, Murrer L, Zoetmulder FA, et al. Photodynamic therapy as adjuvant therapy in surgically treated pleural malignancies. *Br J Cancer.* 1997;76:819–826.

Baldini EH, Recht A, Strauss GM, et al. Patterns of failure after trimodality therapy for malignant pleural mesothelioma. *Ann Thorac Surg.* 1997;63:334–338.

Ball DL, Cruickshank DG. The treatment of malignant mesothelioma of the pleura: review of a 5-year experience, with special reference to radiotherapy. *Am J Clin Oncol.* 1990;13:4–9.

Bissett D, Macbeth FR, Cram I. The role of palliative radiotherapy in malignant mesothelioma. *Clin Oncol.* 1991;3:315–317.

Bonnette P, Heckly GB, Villette S, Fragola A. Intraoperative photodynamic therapy after pleuropneumonectomy for malignant pleural mesothelioma. *Chest.* 2002;122:1866–1867.

Boutin C, Monnet I, Ruffie P, Astoul P. Malignant mesothelioma: clinical and therapeutic study. *Rev Mal Respir.* 1999;16(6 Pt 2):1317–1326.

Boutin C, Nussbaum E, Monnet I, et al. Intrapleural treatment with recombinant gamma-interferon in early stage malignant pleural mesothelioma. *Cancer.* 1994;74:2460–2467.

Boutin C, Rey F, Viallat JR. Prevention of malignant seeding after invasive diagnostic procedures in patients with pleural mesothelioma. A randomized trial of local radiotherapy. *Chest.* 1995;108:754–758.

Brancatisano RP, Joseph MG, McCaughan BC. Pleurectomy for mesothelioma. *Med J Aust.* 1991;154:455–457, 460.

Brenner J, Sordillo PP, Magill GB, Golbey RB. Malignant mesothelioma of the pleura: review of 123 patients. *Cancer.* 1982;49:2431–2435.

Butchart EG, Ashcroft T, Barnsley WC, Holden MP. Pleuropneumonectomy in the management of diffuse malignant mesothelioma of the pleura. Experience with 29 patients. *Thorax.* 1976;31:15–24.

Butchart EG, Ashcroft T, Barnsley WC, Hoden MP. The role of surgery in diffuse malignant mesothelioma of the pleura. *Semin Oncol.* 1981;8:321–328.

Bydder S, Phillips M, Joseph DJ, et al. A randomised trial of single-dose radiotherapy to prevent procedure tract metastasis by malignant mesothelioma. *Br J Cancer.* 2004;91:9–10.

Byrne MJ, Davidson JA, Musk AW, et al. Cisplatin and gemcitabine treatment for malignant mesothelioma: a phase II study. *J Clin Oncol.* 1999;17:25–30.

Calavrezos A, Koschel G, Husselmann H, et al. Malignant mesothelioma of the pleura. A prospective therapeutic study of 132 patients from 1981–1985. *Klin Wochenschr.* 1988;66:607–613.

Calvert AH, Alison DL, Harland SJ, et al. A phase I evaluation of the quinazoline antifolate thymidylate synthase inhibitor, N10-propargyl-5,8-dideazafolic acid, CB3717. *J Clin Oncol.* 1986;4:1245–1252.

Calvert AH, Newell DR, Jackman AL, et al. Recent preclinical and clinical studies with the thymidylate synthase inhibitor N10-propargyl-5,8-dideazafolic acid (CB 3717). *NCI Monogr.* 1987;213–218.

Canto A, Guijarro R, Arnau A, Galbis J, Martorell M, Garcia AR. Videothoracoscopy in the diagnosis and treatment of malignant pleural mesothelioma with associated pleural effusions. *Thorac Cardiovasc Surg.* 1997;45:16–19.

Cantwell BM, Earnshaw M, Harris AL. Phase II study of a novel antifolate, N10-propargyl-5,8 dideazafolic acid (CB3717), in malignant mesothelioma. *Cancer Treat Rep.* 1986;70:1335–1336.

Chahinian AP, Pajak TF, Holland JF, Norton L, Ambinder RM, Mandel EM. Diffuse malignant mesothelioma. Prospective evaluation of 69 patients. *Ann Intern Med.* 1982;96:746–755.

Chen Y, Pandya K, Keng PP, et al. Schedule-dependent pulsed paclitaxel radiosensitization for thoracic malignancy. *Am J Clin Oncol.* 2001;24:432–437.

Colleoni M, Sartori F, Calabro F, et al. Surgery followed by intracavitary plus systemic chemotherapy in malignant pleural mesothelioma. *Tumori.* 1996;82:53–56.

Cordier KL, Valeyrie L, Fernandez N, et al. Regression of AK7 malignant mesothelioma established in immunocompetent mice following intratumoral gene transfer of interferon gamma. *Cancer Gene Ther.* 2003;10:481–490.

Curran D, Sahmoud T, Therasse P, van Meerbeeck J, Postmus PE, Giaccone G. Prognostic factors in patients with pleural mesothelioma: the European Organization for Research and Treatment of Cancer experience. *J Clin Oncol.* 1998;16:145–152.

DaValle MJ, Faber LP, Kittle CF, Jensik RJ. Extrapleural pneumonectomy for diffuse, malignant mesothelioma. *Ann Thorac Surg.* 1986;42:612–618.

Davis SR, Tan L, Ball DL. Radiotherapy in the treatment of malignant mesothelioma of the pleura, with special reference to its use in palliation. *Australas Radiol.* 1994;38:212–214.

de Graaf-Strukowska L, van der ZJ, van Putten W, Senan S. Factors influencing the outcome of radiotherapy in malignant mesothelioma of the pleura—a single-institution experience with 189 patients. *Int J Radiat Oncol Biol Phys.* 1999;43:511–516:.

de Perrot M, Ginsberg R, Payne D. A phase II trail of induction chemotherapy followed by extrapleural pneumonectomy and high dose hemithoracic radiation for malignant pleural mesothelioma. *Lung Cancer.* 2003;41(Suppl. 2): S59.

DeLaria GA, Jensik R, Faber LP, Kittle CF. Surgical management of malignant mesothelioma. *Ann Thorac Surg.* 1978;26:375–382.

Driesen P, Boutin C, Viallat JR, Astoul PH, Vialette JP, Pasquier J. Implantable access system for prolonged intrapleural immunotherapy. *Eur Respir J.* 1994;7:1889–1892.

Edwards JG, Abrams KR, Leverment JN, Spyt TJ, Waller DA, O'Byrne KJ. Prognostic factors for malignant mesothelioma in 142 patients: validation of CALGB and EORTC prognostic scoring systems. *Thorax.* 2000;55:731–735.

Faber LP. Surgical treatment of asbestos-related disease of the chest. *Surg Clin North Am.* 1988;68:525–543.

Faber LP. Extrapleural pneumonectomy for diffuse, malignant mesothelioma. Updated in 1994. *Ann Thorac Surg.* 1986;58:1782–1783.

Favaretto AG, Aversa SM, Paccagnella A, et al. Gemcitabine combined with carboplatin in patients with malignant pleural mesothelioma: a multicentric phase II study. *Cancer.* 2003;97:2791–2797.

Fizazi K, Doubre H, Le CT, et al. Combination of raltitrexed and oxaliplatin is an active regimen in malignant mesothelioma: results of a phase II study. *J Clin Oncol.* 2003;21:349–354.

Forster KM, Smythe WR, Starkschall G, et al. Intensity-modulated radiotherapy following extrapleural pneumonectomy for the treatment of malignant mesothelioma: clinical implementation. *Int J Radiat Oncol Biol Phys.* 2003;55:606–616.

Friedberg JS, Mick R, Stevenson J, et al. A phase I study of Foscan-mediated photodynamic therapy and surgery in patients with mesothelioma. *Ann Thorac Surg.* 2003;75:952–959.

Girling DJ, Muers MF, Qian W, Lobban D. Multicenter randomized controlled trial of the management of unresectable malignant mesothelioma proposed by the British Thoracic Society and the British Medical Research Council. *Semin Oncol.* 2002;29:97–101.

Gordon GJ, Jensen RV, Hsiao LL, et al. Using gene expression ratios to predict outcome among patients with mesothelioma. *J Natl Cancer Inst.* 2003;95:598–605.

Harrison LH Jr, Schwarzenberger PO, Byrne PS, Marrogi AJ, Kolls JK, McCarthy KE. Gene-modified PA1-STK cells home to tumor sites in patients with malignant pleural mesothelioma. *Ann Thorac Surg.* 2000;70:407–411.

Harvey JC, Fleischman EH, Kagan AR, Streeter OE. Malignant pleural mesothelioma: a survival study. *J Surg Oncol.* 1990;45:40–42.

Herndon JE, Green MR, Chahinian AP, Corson JM, Suzuki Y, Vogelzang NJ. Factors predictive of survival among 337 patients with mesothelioma treated between 1984 and 1994 by the Cancer and Leukemia Group B. *Chest.* 1998;113:723–731.

Herscher LL, Hahn SM, Kroog G, et al. Phase I study of paclitaxel as a radiation sensitizer in the treatment of mesothelioma and non-small-cell lung cancer. *J Clin Oncol.* 1998;16:635–641.

Hilaris BS, Nori D, Kwong E, Kutcher GJ, Martini N. Pleurectomy and intraoperative brachytherapy and postoperative radiation in the treatment of malignant pleural mesothelioma. *Int J Radiol Oncol Biol Phys.* 1984;10:325–331.

Holsti LR, Pyrhonen S, Kajanti M, et al. Altered fractionation of hemithorax irradiation for pleural mesothelioma and failure patterns after treatment. *Acta Oncol.* 1997;36:397–405.

Hughes A, Calvert P, Azzabi A, et al. Phase I clinical and pharmacokinetic study of pemetrexed and carboplatin in patients with malignant pleural mesothelioma. *J Clin Oncol.* 2002;20:3533–3544.

Janne PA. Chemotherapy for malignant pleural mesothelioma. *Clin Lung Cancer.* 2003;5:98–106.

Janne PA, Wozniak AJ, Belani CP, et al. Open-label study of pemetrexed alone or in combination with Cisplatin for the treatment of patients with peritoneal mesothelioma: outcomes of an expanded access program. *Clin Lung Cancer.* 2005;7:40.

Kindler HL, Belani CP, Herndon JE, Vogelzang NJ, Suzuki Y, Green MR. Edatrexate (10-ethyl-deaza-aminopterin) (NSC #626715) with or without leucovorin rescue for malignant mesothelioma. Sequential phase II trials by the cancer and leukemia group B. *Cancer.* 1999;86:1985–1991.

Kindler HL, Van Meerbeeck JP. The role of gemcitabine in the treatment of malignant mesothelioma. *Semin Oncol.* 2002;29:70–76.

Kruklitis RJ, Singhal S, Delong P, et al. Immuno-gene therapy with interferon-beta before surgical debulking delays recurrence and improves survival in a murine model of malignant mesothelioma. *J Thorac Cardiovasc Surg.* 2004;127:123–130.

Law MR, Gregor A, Hodson ME, Bloom HJ, Turner-Warwick M. Malignant mesothelioma of the pleura: a study of 52 treated and 64 untreated patients. *Thorax.* 1984;39:255–259.

Lee TT, Everett DL, Shu HK, et al. Radical pleurectomy/decortication and intraoperative radiotherapy followed by conformal radiation with or without chemotherapy for malignant pleural mesothelioma. *J Thorac Cardiovasc Surg.* 2002;124:1183–1189.

Linden CJ, Mercke C, Albrechtsson U, Johansson L, Ewers SB. Effect of hemithorax irradiation alone or combined with doxorubicin and cyclophosphamide in 47 pleural mesotheliomas: a nonrandomized phase II study. *Eur Respir J.* 1996;9:2565–2572.

Maggi G, Casadio C, Cianci R, Rena O, Ruffini E. Trimodality management of malignant pleural mesothelioma. *Eur J Cardiothorac Surg.* 2001;19:346–350.

Maggi G, Casadio C, Giobbe R, Ruffini E. The management of malignant pleural mesothelioma. *Eur J Cardiothorac Surg.* 2003;23:255–256.

Maggi G, Giobbe R, Casadio C, Rena O. Palliative surgery for malignant pleural mesothelioma. *Eur J Cardiothorac Surg.* 2002;21:1128–1129.

Martin-Ucar AE, Edwards JG, Rengajaran A, Muller S, Waller DA. Palliative surgical debulking in malignant mesothelioma. Predictors of survival and symptom control. *Eur J Cardiothorac Surg.* 2001;20:1117–1121.

Mbidde EK, Harland SJ, Calvert AH, Smith IE. Phase II trial of carboplatin (JM8) in treatment of patients with malignant mesothelioma. *Cancer Chemother Pharmacol.* 1986;18:284–285.

Middleton GW, Smith IE, O'Brien ME, et al. Good symptom relief with palliative MVP (mitomycin-C, vinblastine and cisplatin) chemotherapy in malignant mesothelioma. *Ann Oncol.* 1998;9:269–273.

Mikulski SM, Costanzi JJ, Vogelzang NJ, et al. Phase II trial of a single weekly intravenous dose of ranpirnase in patients with unresectable malignant mesothelioma. *J Clin Oncol.* 2002;20:274–281.

Mintzer DM, Kelsen D, Frimmer D, Heelan R, Gralla R. Phase II trial of high-dose cisplatin in patients with malignant mesothelioma. *Cancer Treat Rep.* 1985;69:711–712.

Mukherjee S, Haenel T, Himbeck R, et al. Replication-restricted vaccinia as a cytokine gene therapy vector in cancer: persistent transgene expression despite antibody generation. *Cancer Gene Ther.* 2000;7:663–670.

Mukherjee S, Nelson D, Loh S, et al. The immune anti-tumor effects of GM-CSF and B7–1 gene transfection are enhanced by surgical debulking of tumor. *Cancer Gene Ther.* 2001;8:580–588.

Nowak AK, Byrne MJ, Williamson R, et al. A multicentre phase II study of cisplatin and gemcitabine for malignant mesothelioma. *Br J Cancer.* 2002a;87:491–496.

Nowak AK, Lake RA, Kindler HL, Robinson BW. New approaches for mesothelioma: biologics, vaccines, gene therapy, and other novel agents. *Semin Oncol.* 2002b;29:82–96.

Odaka M, Sterman DH, Wiewrodt R, et al. Eradication of intraperitoneal and distant tumor by adenovirus-mediated interferon-beta gene therapy is attributable to induction of systemic immunity. *Cancer Res.* 2001;61:6201–6212.

Odaka M, Wiewrodt R, Delong P, et al. Analysis of the immunologic response generated by Ad.IFN-beta during successful intraperitoneal tumor gene therapy. *Mol Ther.* 2002;6:210–218.

Ong ST, Vogelzang NJ. Chemotherapy in malignant pleural mesothelioma. A review. *J Clin Oncol.* 1996;14:1007–1017.

Pass HI, Kranda K, Temeck BK, Feuerstein I, Steinberg SM. Surgically debulked malignant pleural mesothelioma: results and prognostic factors. *Ann Surg Oncol.* 1997a;4:215–222.

Pass HI, Liu Z, Wali A, et al. Gene expression profiles predict survival and progression of pleural mesothelioma. *Clin Cancer Res.* 2004;10:849–859.

Pass HI, Temeck BK, Kranda K, Steinberg SM, Feuerstein IR. Preoperative tumor volume is associated with outcome in malignant pleural mesothelioma. *J Thorac Cardiovasc Surg.* 1998;115:310–317.

Pass HI, Temeck BK, Kranda K, et al. Phase III randomized trial of surgery with or without intraoperative photodynamic therapy and postoperative immunochemotherapy for malignant pleural mesothelioma. *Ann Surg Oncol.* 1997b;4:628–633.

Pien GW, Gant MJ, Washam CL, Sterman DH. Use of an implantable pleural catheter for trapped lung syndrome in patients with malignant pleural effusion. *Chest.* 2001;119:1641–1646.

Planting AS, Schellens JH, Goey SH, et al. Weekly high-dose cisplatin in malignant pleural mesothelioma. *Ann Oncol.* 1994;5:373–374.

Raghavan D, Gianoutsos P, Bishop J, et al. Phase II trial of carboplatin in the management of malignant mesothelioma. *J Clin Oncol.* 1990;8:151–154.

Ratto GB, Civalleri D, Esposito M, et al. Pleural space perfusion with cisplatin in the multimodality treatment of malignant mesothelioma: a feasibility and pharmacokinetic study. *J Thorac Cardiovasc Surg.* 1999;117:759–765.

Ruffie P, Feld R, Minkin S, et al. Diffuse malignant mesothelioma of the pleura in Ontario and Quebec: a retrospective study of 332 patients. *J Clin Oncol.* 1989;7:1157–1168.

Rusch VW. Trials in malignant mesothelioma. LCSG 851 and 882. *Chest.* 1994;106:359S–362S.

Rusch VW. A proposed new international TNM staging system for malignant pleural mesothelioma from the International Mesothelioma Interest Group. *Lung Cancer.* 1996;14:1–12.

Rusch VW. Indications for pneumonectomy. Extrapleural pneumonectomy. *Chest Surg Clin N Am.* 1999;9:327–38.

Rusch VW. Pleurectomy/decortication in the setting of multimodality treatment for diffuse malignant pleural mesothelioma. *Semin Thorac Cardiovasc Surg.* 1997;9:367–372.

Rusch VW, Figlin R, Godwin D, Piantadosi S. Intrapleural cisplatin and cytarabine in the management of malignant pleural effusions: a Lung Cancer Study Group trial. *J Clin Oncol.* 1991a;9:313–319.

Rusch VW, Piantadosi S, Holmes EC. The role of extrapleural pneumonectomy in malignant pleural mesothelioma. A Lung Cancer Study Group trial. *J Thorac Cardiovasc Surg.* 1991b;102:1–9.

Rusch VW, Rosenzweig K, Venkatraman E, et al. A phase II trial of surgical resection and adjuvant high-dose hemithoracic radiation for malignant pleural mesothelioma. *J Thorac Cardiovasc Surg.* 2001;122:788–795.

Rusch VW, Venkatraman E. The importance of surgical staging in the treatment of malignant pleural mesothelioma. *J Thorac Cardiovasc Surg.* 1996;111:815–825.

Rusch VW, Venkatraman ES. Important prognostic factors in patients with malignant pleural mesothelioma, managed surgically. *Ann Thorac Surg.* 1999;68:1799–1804.

Samuels BL, Herndon JE, Harmon DC, et al. Dihydro-5-azacytidine and cisplatin in the treatment of malignant mesothelioma: a phase II study by the Cancer and Leukemia Group B. *Cancer.* 1998;82:1578–1584.

Scagliotti GV, Novello S. Pemetrexed and its emerging role in the treatment of thoracic malignancies. *Expert Opin Investig Drugs.* 2003;12:853–863.

Schouwink H, Rutgers ET, van der Sijp J, et al. Intraoperative photodynamic therapy after pleuropneumonectomy in patients with malignant pleural mesothelioma: dose finding and toxicity results. *Chest.* 2001;120:1167–1174.

Schouwink JH, Kool LS, Rutgers EJ, et al. The value of chest computer tomography and cervical mediastinoscopy in the preoperative assessment of patients with malignant pleural mesothelioma. *Ann Thorac Surg.* 2003;75:1715–1718.

Schwarzenberger P, Byrne P, Kolls JK. Immunotherapy-based treatment strategies for malignant mesothelioma. *Curr Opin Mol Ther.* 1999;1:104–111.

Schwarzenberger P, Harrison L, Weinacker A, et al. The treatment of malignant mesothelioma with a gene modified cancer cell line: a phase I study. *Hum Gene Ther.* 1998a;9:2641–2649.

Schwarzenberger P, Lei D, Freeman SM, et al. Antitumor activity with the HSV-tk-gene-modified cell line PA-1-STK in malignant mesothelioma. *Am J Respir Cell Mol Biol.* 1998b;19:333–337.

Singhal S, Kaiser LR. Malignant mesothelioma: options for management. *Surg Clin North Am.* 2002;82:797–831.

Solheim OP, Saeter G, Finnanger AM, Stenwig AE. High-dose methotrexate in the treatment of malignant mesothelioma of the pleura. A phase II study. *Br J Cancer.* 1992;65:956–960.

Steele JP, Shamash J, Evans MT, Gower NH, Tischkowitz MD, Rudd RM. Phase II study of vinorelbine in patients with malignant pleural mesothelioma. *J Clin Oncol.* 2000;18:3912–3917.

Sterman DH, Treat J, Litzky LA, et al. Adenovirus-mediated herpes simplex virus thymidine kinase/ganciclovir gene therapy in patients with localized malignancy: results of a phase I clinical trial in malignant mesothelioma. *Hum Gene Ther.* 1998;9:1083–1092.

Sugarbaker D, Richards W, Zellos LS. Feasibility of pleurectomy and intraoperative bicavitary hyperthermic cisplatin lavage for mesothelioma: a phase I-II study. *Proc Am Soc Clin Oncol.* 2003;22.

Sugarbaker DJ, Flores RM, Jaklitsch MT, et al. Resection margins, extrapleural nodal status, and cell type determine postoperative long-term survival in trimodality therapy of malignant pleural mesothelioma: results in 183 patients. *J Thorac Cardiovasc Surg.* 1999;117:54–63.

Sugarbaker DJ, Garcia JP. Multimodality therapy for malignant pleural mesothelioma. *Chest.* 1997;112:272S-275S.

Sugarbaker DJ, Heher EC, Lee TH, et al. Extrapleural pneumonectomy, chemotherapy, and radiotherapy in the treatment of diffuse malignant pleural mesothelioma. *J Thorac Cardiovasc Surg.* 1991;102:10–14.

Sugarbaker DJ, Jaklitsch MT, Bueno R, et al. Prevention, early detection, and management of complications after 328 consecutive extrapleural pneumonectomies. *J Thorac Cardiovasc Surg.* 2004;128:138–146.

Takagi K, Tsuchiya R, Watanabe Y. Surgical approach to pleural diffuse mesothelioma in Japan. *Lung Cancer.* 2001;31:57–65.

Thodtmann R, Depenbrock H, Blatter J, Johnson RD, van Oosterom A, Hanauske AR. Preliminary results of a phase I study with MTA (LY231514) in combination with cisplatin in patients with solid tumors. *Semin Oncol.* 1999;26:89–93.

van Haarst JM, Baas P, Manegold C, et al. Multicentre phase II study of gemcitabine and cisplatin in malignant pleural mesothelioma. *Br J Cancer.* 2002;86:342–345.

Van Meerbeeck JP, Baas P, Debruyne C, et al. A Phase II study of gemcitabine in patients with malignant pleural mesothelioma. European Organization for Research and Treatment of Cancer Lung Cancer Cooperative Group. *Cancer.* 1999;85:2577–2582.

Van Meerbeeck JP, Manegold C, Gaafar R, et al. A randomized phase III study of cisplatin with or without raltitrexed in patients (pts) with malignant pleural mesothelioma (MPM): An intergroup study of the EORTC Lung Cancer Group and NCIC. *Proc Am Soc Clin Oncol.* 2004;22:14S.

van Ruth S, Baas P, Haas RL, Rutgers EJ, Verwaal VJ, Zoetmulder FA. Cytoreductive surgery combined with intraoperative hyperthermic intrathoracic chemotherapy for stage I malignant pleural mesothelioma. *Ann Surg Oncol.* 2003;10:176–182.

Viallat JR, Rey R, Astoul P, Boutin C. Thoracoscopic talc poudrage pleurodesis for malignant effusions. A review of 360 cases. *Chest.* 1996;110:1387–1393.

Vogelzang NJ. Gemcitabine and cisplatin: second-line chemotherapy for malignant mesothelioma? *J Clin Oncol.* 1999;17:2626–2627.

Vogelzang NJ, Goutsou M, Corson JM, et al. Carboplatin in malignant mesothelioma: a phase II study of the Cancer and Leukemia Group B. *Cancer Chemother Pharmacol.* 1990;27:239–242.

Vogelzang NJ, Rusthoven JJ, Symanowski J, et al. Phase III study of pemetrexed in combination with cisplatin versus cisplatin alone in patients with malignant pleural mesothelioma. *J Clin Oncol.* 2003;21:2636–2644.

Vogelzang NJ, Schultz SM, Iannucci AM, Kennedy BJ. Malignant mesothelioma. The University of Minnesota experience. *Cancer.* 1984;53:377–383.

Vogelzang NJ, Weissman LB, Herndon JE, et al. Trimetrexate in malignant mesothelioma: a cancer and leukemia group B phase II study. *J Clin Oncol.* 1994;12:1436–1442.

Waller DA. Malignant mesothelioma—British surgical strategies. *Lung Cancer.* 2004;45(Suppl 1):S81-S84.

Wanebo HJ, Martini N, Melamed MR, Hilaris B, Beattie EJ Jr. Pleural mesothelioma. *Cancer.* 38:2481–2488, 1976.

Weder W, Kestenholz P, Taverna C, et al. Neoadjuvant chemotherapy followed by extrapleural pneumonectomy in malignant pleural mesothelioma. *J Clin Oncol.* 2004;22:3451–3457.

Yang CT, You L, Lin YC, Lin CL, McCormick F, Jablons DM. A comparison analysis of anti-tumor efficacy of adenoviral gene replacement therapy (p14ARF and p16INK4A) in human mesothelioma cells. *Anticancer Res.* 2003;23:33–38.

Yang CT, You L, Uematsu K, Yeh CC, McCormick F, Jablons DM. p14(ARF) modulates the cytolytic effect of ONYX-015 in mesothelioma cells with wild-type p53. *Cancer Res.* 2001;61:5959–5963.

Yellin A, Simansky DA, Paley M, Refaely Y. Hyperthermic pleural perfusion with cisplatin: early clinical experience. *Cancer.* 2001;92:2197–2203.

Zellos LS, Sugarbaker DJ. Diffuse malignant mesothelioma of the pleural space and its management. *Oncology.* 2002;16:907–913.

Zidar BL, Green S, Pierce HI, Roach RW, Balcerzak SP, Militello L. A phase II evaluation of cisplatin in unresectable diffuse malignant mesothelioma: a Southwest Oncology Group Study. *Invest New Drugs.* 1988;6:223–226.

15

Asbestos Exposure and the Law in the United States

Kevin Leahy

Historical Overview

The modern asbestos industry originated in the late 19th century. At that time, asbestosis was an unnamed disease, and malignant mesothelioma (MM) was a rare tumor with no known cause. When the asbestos product industry began in the 1860s and 1870s, lawsuits had not yet been filed claiming asbestos-related injury. One hundred years later, a series of cases (filed against asbestos mining and manufacturing companies in the United States) claimed asbestos-related injury. They coincided with an era of growing environmental awareness and heightened scrutiny of workplace safety. However, due to both an incomplete knowledge of the health effects of asbestos dust during the first half of the previous century, and the latent nature of asbestos-related illness, improvements in environmental controls came too late to stop illness from occurring in some individuals who had been exposed to respirable fibers. Likewise, the early lawsuits that started in the 1930s and resurfaced in the 1960s did not prevent others from being filed; instead, they laid the ground work for an avalanche of asbestos-related filings that continue unabated to this day.

What transpired after the first successful claims against companies in the late 1960s and early 1970s was unprecedented in the history of common law—a massive influx of claims overwhelmed court dockets from New York to Hawaii. Commentators have invoked the term *mass tort* to identify the asbestos-related litigation because of the sheer number of cases claiming asbestos exposure. In the 1999 *Report on Mass Tort Litigation*, prepared at the request of US Supreme Court Chief Justice William Rehnquist, the authors provide the following working definition of a mass tort: "Mass tort litigation emerges when an event or series of related events allegedly injure a large number of people or damage their property, giving rise to a large number of cases" (Report on Mass Tort Litigation, 1999). In the words of Justice Helen Friedman, who has presided over thousands of asbestos-related actions filed in New York City: "When a summary judgment motion in a tort action brings hundreds of lawyers into the courtroom, a judge should suspect that a mass tort has arrived" (Freedman, 1999). Aside from its *mass tort* status, asbestos litigation has also been called an *elephantine mess* by jurists and *out-of-control* by legislators. The number of lawsuits filed in state and federal courts has eclipsed every prediction made to date.

This chapter discusses the historical development of asbestos litigation and the current state of relevant legal affairs in the United States. Depending on one's vantage point, the history of asbestos-related lawsuits reveals either a series of unwitting failures to understand the gravity of the problem, or a knowing disregard and avoidance of the health concerns faced by workers and their families. Whether it is lack of knowledge or reckless disregard, responsibility for fault has become the paramount issue for assigning blame during American trials involving asbestos exposure and disease. However, jurors and jurists have simply been unable to identify any one entity or organization that is fully responsible for asbestos disease. The result over time has shifted blame for asbestos-induced injury that has fueled four decades of active lawsuits with an ever widening scope of defendant participation.

Blame is the fundamental theme of many texts describing the asbestos litigation. Perhaps the most notable book outlining blameworthy corporate conduct is *Outrageous Misconduct: The Asbestos Industry on Trial* by Paul Brodeur (Brodeur, 1985a). In that text, Brodeur explores the groundbreaking lawsuit filed by Clarence Borel in the late 1960s that was tried to jury verdict by Ward Stephenson in the Federal District Court in Beaumont, Texas. In summarizing that book, one commentator offered:

> Brodeur's narrative establishes successfully, if incidentally, that the tort system emerged as *the* uniquely effective and indispensable means of exposing and defeating the asbestos conspiracy, providing compensation to victims, and deterring future malfeasance. The book vividly describes the failure of every other institutional safeguard: the asbestos companies, of course, but also the medical and legal professions, the unions, the insurance carriers, and all manners of regulatory and legislative bodies.

> *Rosenberg, 1986*

Ronald Motley, a well-known plaintiffs' lawyer who was successful at discovering critical historical documents early in the litigation, along with his then-associate Susan Nial, offered insight in whom not to blame: "The government is not to blame. The labor unions are not to blame" (Motley and Nial, 1992). Whom to blame and whom not to blame has continued to shift over time as trends fell in and out of favor, with government and military branches at times defending their interests in court along side mining companies, associations, product manufacturers, distributors, and premise owners. The effort to sort out the truly blameworthy is complex. In many states, common law does not permit responsibility to be placed on bankrupt or otherwise unavailable parties. As a result, the deflection of blame from more responsible parties, such as Johns Manville Corporation, to less responsible parties, such as the local hardware store that sold a Johns Manville product, is now commonplace as plaintiffs seek untapped resources to recover for alleged asbestos-related injury.

The litigation that so successfully punished the prime manufacturers with corporate bankruptcy and encouraged appropriate regulatory reform has continued and now progresses with an insatiable appetite for new sources of cash. In the absence of the early and obvious targets, the links between injury, disease, causation, and responsibility have become increasingly tenuous over time. Yet the litigation marches on into this new century and continues to shroud the landscape of American jurisprudence with massive jury verdicts, unmanageable court dockets, and no single solution that will satisfy all parties.

Notwithstanding a 70-year legacy, therefore, the course of asbestos litigation remains in uncharted territory. Blame, economics, and uncertainty have all played significant roles in the history of this litigation. The story that unfolds is a complicated one, and one that continues to develop and reinvent itself, year after year. This chapter details some of the highlights of how lawsuits alleging asbestos injury arose, and how the litigation has progressed into the current century.

The Early Years: Tort versus Workers' Compensation Laws

Black's Law Dictionary (1999) defines *personal tort* as "[a] tort involving or consisting in an injury to one's person, reputation, or feelings, as distinguished from an injury or damage to real or personal property." The origin of tort law is based on an observable injury due to a direct action or cause. The notion of an unseen latent effect acting in concert with other similar effects over several years to inflict injury was completely foreign to the common law.

Not surprisingly, the legal system was ill prepared to adequately address the occurrence of latent diseases as they began to appear with the increased production of the industrial revolution. This was particularly true with asbestos disease because the medical and scientific fields were still attempting to understand the causal mechanisms and diagnostic indicators even as the number of potentially related injuries and lawsuits continued to increase. The uncertainties of diagnosis and an inability to identify the exact cause of injury prevented the timely adjudication of asbestos-related injuries and stalled the appropriate redress to prevent future injury.

The early history of asbestos-related lawsuits is not well documented; scant records remain. Undoubtedly, early cases alleging asbestos injury involved employees who sought relief from their employers due to direct exposure on the job—either in connection with the mining or milling of raw asbestos or, in some instances, manufacturing asbestos-containing products. However, legal theories for addressing workplace injury due to asbestos were novel or nonexistent in the first part of the previous century. The term *legal theories* used here refers to one of several approaches a plaintiff's counsel can rely upon to recover damages from a defendant due to a claimed harm. For example, the legal theory of negligence provides that the defendant had a duty to act reasonably under the circumstances to avoid causing an asbestos-related injury, which it knew or should have known would occur with an excessive exposure to asbestos fibers from the defendant's product. As more injuries occurred over the years, lawyers developed several additional legal theories to bring defendants to court including strict liability, nuisance, and breach of implied warranty.[1]

The earliest references to asbestos-related claims alleging negligence coincided with the development of the workers' compensation system, which was backed by industry to alleviate the pressure placed on it by the growing body of personal injury tort law. Although well-intentioned, workers' compensation laws resulted in a missed opportunity early on to address and possibly avoid some of the later problems that would lead to the demise of asbestos use and the asbestos product industry.

Workers' compensation laws developed as a response to job-related injury generally and eventually encompassed workplace disease, as well. However, these laws were slow to identify and permit recovery for dose-response diseases such as asbestosis because the most obvious priority was compensation for traumatic injury. The first compensation law for occupational diseases in this country was passed in 1908 by congress for US civil service employees. But even laws permitting compensation for traumatic accidents took a long time to develop and only began gaining prominence in the early 1900s (Brown, 1940). From 1910 through 1913, New York, Minnesota, and Wisconsin were the first states to enact workers' compensation laws (Goldberg, 1939).

---

1 The concept of legal theories are discussed further in the Appendix to this chapter. Unlike scientific theories, which are tested in the laboratory, legal theories are tested in the court room and on appeal.

As conceived, workers' compensation laws dealt almost exclusively with accidental injuries that occurred at a definite time and place and due to a sudden and unexpected event. Occupational diseases were not initially compensable (Lanza, 1938). For example, in *Adams v Acme White Lead and Color Works*, 182 Mich. 157 (Mich. 1914), decedent Augustus Adams was employed at the Acme White Lead and Color Works and was exposed on the job to extreme levels of lead. He eventually died of lead poisoning; however, compensation was not awarded because the court held poisoning was an *occupational disease* and not an *accident*.

By 1919, six states had enacted workers' compensation laws that covered asbestosis. At the start of the Great Depression, 10 States and 3 Territories had enacted laws making occupational disease compensable and by the end of the 1930s, 11 more states offered some form of occupational disease compensation, and a total of 16 states included silicosis and other dust diseases as compensable.

However, it was not until 1927 that exposed workers made their first claims for compensation in the United States because of asbestos-related illness (Corn and Starr, 1987). During that time period, claimants began filing asbestos-related lawsuits alleging negligence and tort on the part of some asbestos product manufacturers. Anthony Lanza (1938), a prominent researcher of dust diseases in America from the 1930s through the 1950s, reported on the early occurrence of asbestos-related lawsuits: "Asbestosis was first described in the United States by Pancoast, Miller, Smyth and Landis in 1918, but its importance was not realized until it was introduced into the damage suit situation which led to the first comprehensive study of this disease in the United States."

The appearance of lawsuits alleging dust disease tracked improvements in the diagnosis of those diseases and research linking a particular disease to a specific cause. It was not asbestos-related illness, however, that initially drew serious attention to the concerns faced by workers who performed tasks in dusty conditions. Instead, by the 1930s silica exposure was the predominant concern among the dusty trades. Confirmed cases of silicosis in significant numbers of miners and millers throughout America induced an onslaught of lawsuits during the Great Depression.

During the same time period—although in significantly fewer numbers—workers began pursuing damages associated with asbestos exposure. For example, in 1932 and 1933, American asbestos manufacturers including Johns Manville Company and the Raybestos-Manhattan Corporation settled their first lawsuits brought by individuals claiming asbestos-related illness. Little remains of the history of those earliest lawsuits alleging asbestos injury. It is also unclear if other asbestos industry employers experienced similar filings and actively played down the asbestos-related injuries occurring in their worker populations.

The early lawsuits did draw the attention of medical researchers. In a 1938 book entitled *Silicosis and Asbestosis*, Lanza wrote:

> Silicosis and asbestosis burst upon the amazed consciousness of American industry during the period 1929–1930. Previously, the terms "silicosis," "asbestosis," "pneumoconiosis," were practically unknown to industrialists except that in the hard rock mining industry, silicosis, under its various colloquial designations, was well recognized. Knowledge of these conditions was limited to the small number of those whose investigations of pulmonary dust diseases had made them conversant with the subject.
>
> Arising out of the period of economic depression, the situation with respect to silicosis and asbestosis became manifest as a medico-legal phenomenon of a scope and intensity that was at once preposterous and almost unbelievable. Damage suits, under the common law, were instituted against employers by employees, alleging pulmonary dust disease, in industrial centers all over the United States, to an amount in excess of 1×10^8 dollars.

In his book, Lanza offers concrete evidence for when asbestosis claims arose on the national scene. He also acknowledges that by the 1930s, legal action presented itself as an obvious recourse for asbestos-related injury. Lanza's publication suggests that fibrosis in American workers brought about by chrysotile fibers was less severe than similar cases of asbestos-related fibrosis occurring in England and France, where crocidolite and then amosite had been imported decades before those fibers were shipped in significant quantities to America.

The dust-related litigation of the 1930s referenced by Lanza resulted in part from the failure of the federal and state governments to include dust diseases as compensable injuries under the various workers' compensation statutes. As workers' compensation coverage expanded to include dust diseases such as asbestosis, fewer lawsuits alleging asbestos illness were filed. Those laws successfully stopped lawyers and their potential clients from seeking recourse under the torts system for asbestos-related injury. The laws did not, however, prevent injury. Instead, the compensation system reduced the likelihood that companies and researchers would address the root cause of the increase of asbestos illness during the 20th century, that is, the unchecked use of asbestos-containing products in the workplace.

The workers' compensation system was an imperfect solution to the problem of dust disease. Goldberg (1939) identified one primary concern that foreshadowed an increasing dissatisfaction with workers' compensation that would fuel a search for alternative compensation in the courts 25 years later:

> Even under the new system, workmen are called upon to bear a considerable portion of the entire damage, as compensation is only provided to the extent of from one-half to two-thirds of the wage loss. Victims of industrial accidents, even under the present system, go without full compensation, though undoubtedly in the aggregate much greater benefits are now realized for them.

And the reduced compensation recoveries were not matched by a corresponding ease of proof. Instead, even in a system where compensation resulted without an award for pain and suffering, insurance carriers and their insured challenged claims based on diagnosis and uncertainties regarding causation, and often, claim processing required legal aid (Adam, 1979). The diagnosis of nonmalignant asbestos illness is shifting even today—especially in the context of litigation—and was even more so 50 years ago when diagnostic tools and areas of specialization were not as advanced as they are today. The workers' compensation system itself was simply incapable of properly addressing occupational disease:

> Workers' compensation in most cases is a totally inadequate remedy. In the vast majority of cases, the benefits are far too meager. Successful workers' compensation claims for occupational disease are practically nonexistent. And perhaps most significant, the workers' compensation system seldom provides a sufficient incentive for an employer to attempt seriously to rid the workplace of hazards, particularly long-term toxic substance hazards.
>
> *Provost, 1982*

The legacy of workers' compensation as the exclusive recourse for workers against the dust-related problems brought about by their employer's lack of knowledge and failure to address excessive dust levels in the workplace is now evident. The workers' compensation system funded by the asbestos industry effectively reduced the incentive to remove known hazards from the workplace (eg, high levels of asbestos dust) and unwittingly set the stage for the increase in malignant diseases beginning in the 1960s.

1940s and 1950s: Reasons for the Delay in Court Filings

In hindsight, the workers' compensation system played a significant role in halting court filings that otherwise might have drawn more attention to asbestos exposure and disease.

An indicator of that fact is that although lawsuits involving asbestos-exposure claims arose in the late 1920s and early 1930s, record of continued filings disappeared by the mid-1930s. Indeed, there is virtually no record of lawsuits alleging asbestos exposure from the 1940s through the early 1960s. This is a gap in the asbestos litigation history that is partially explained by World War II and increased use of asbestos. The acceptance of asbestos disease, and compensation for it, delayed more careful monitoring of end-product use and the identification of acceptable dust levels.

The compensation laws mandate that workers' compensation serve as the exclusive remedy for dust injury. As a consequence, workers' compensation laws drew attention away from the continued presence of asbestos illness in worker populations. As with traumatic injury, asbestosis became a known and accepted hazard in primary asbestos industries, such as mining and manufacturing. Therefore, the workers' compensation system masked the impact of harm resulting from less intense asbestos exposure experienced over longer periods of time by individuals not traditionally identified as persons at risk of asbestos-related disease.

The acceptance of occupational diseases as compensable under workers' compensation statutes explains in part why legal claims for asbestos injury did not reoccur in earnest until the 1960s. And, while the impact of asbestos exposure may have been inadvertently obscured by the structure of the workers' compensation system, a second reason asbestos-related lawsuits did not resurface until the 1960s was the result of a more deliberate tactic. As the litigation matured, it became evident that the direct actions of a few companies kept information relating to asbestos illness claims out of the public eye. For example, evidence suggests that Johns Manville entered into a sizable settlement agreement with several attorneys who brought workers' compensation claims alleging asbestos-induced injury in the 1930s on the condition that those lawyers never bring similar actions in the future (Brodeur, 1985a).

That conscious effort to stifle legal recourse for asbestos injury and similar conduct on behalf of the major industry participants eventually would give rise to massive punitive damage awards. Evidence of that type of conduct also served to outrage the jurors and permitted the plaintiffs' lawyers to implicate all defendants in the misdeeds of a select few companies. The trial tactics focused on identified disease concerns from the 1920s forward and emphasized the lack of action on the part of significant players in the asbestos industry. In each case, therefore, the plaintiffs' lawyers were able to put the entire industry on trial. In doing so, they drew attention away from the actual state of knowledge of the particular defendants involved in favor of a general sense of what the industry knew or was capable of knowing and failed to do.

An alternative explanation for a lack of filing during the 1940s and 1950s is the reduction of disease due to a better understanding of the dose-response nature of asbestosis. The dust lawsuits of the 1930s and a better awareness of occupational disease and its causes gave rise to industrial hygiene recommendations and practices designed to reduce asbestos exposure in the workplace. The literature of the time supports the conclusion that the introduction of threshold limit values and rudimentary industrial hygiene procedures had solved the asbestos problem beyond the mines and asbestos textile mills (Chapters 3 and 13).

Early conclusions by researchers about acceptable asbestos-exposure levels and the reduction of any associated harm below a certain level of exposure undoubtedly contributed to the reduction of lawsuits through mid-century. For example, a lawyer who considered filing suit alleging asbestos injury would run counter to the findings of Dreessen and his colleagues (1938) with regard to asbestos exposure and disease.

Dreessen and his coauthors reached the conclusion that disease would not occur if levels of dust were kept below a certain level by studying an American textile facility in the Carolinas that relied almost exclusively on chrysotile asbestos.[2] Since chrysotile is much less carcinogenic than amphibole, their conclusion surely provided undue comfort when applied to general asbestos exposures. At the end of World War II, Fleischer and colleagues reached a similar conclusion about disease that occurred in the pipe-covering trade based on research conducted on workers in US Navy shipyards (Fleischer et al., 1946).

The results of these studies and their miscalculation of disease rates demonstrate the confounding effects of the long latency period of asbestos-related disease. (Fleischer et al. 1946) presented their results as the importation of asbestos began to skyrocket in the United States, but they could not predict the impact of heavy naval exposures experienced during World War II because they were studying many workers who were not far enough away from their first exposure to have developed the disease. The predominant exposure was to chrysotile among those men who had significant lifetime exposure to asbestos insulation products prior to the war. The tragedy is that these workers were the first to encounter large-scale amphibole exposures in America; appropriately designed studies of this very cohort would have revealed the "modern" asbestos problem much sooner than when it actually occurred. As matters transpired, the design of the so-called Fleischer-Drinker study and the lack of appreciable amphibole exposure in the United States prior to the 1940s led to a false sense of security when compared with the European asbestos experience.[3]

The difference in disease prevalence attributable to different fiber types is borne out by researchers as well as court filings. MM cases were not identified in the US literature until the mid-1960s—approximately 20–30 years after government specifications resulted in significantly more imports into America of amphibole asbestos, predominately amosite. By contrast, researchers in Germany and England began identifying MM cases in the 1930s, approximately 20–30 years after the increased importation of South African fiber to Europe. Both time spans satisfy the latency requirements for MM due to asbestos. Accounts of a rise in nonmalignant health concerns by the American asbestos insulators' union did not appear until the 1950s, again consistent with expected latency periods from the time of earliest large-scale importation of amphiboles.[4]

Lanza (1938) noted the disparity between disease occurrence in the United States in contrast to Europe, surmising, "Asbestosis has not appeared to be as serious a disease in the United States as it has in England, judging from the various reports from the latter

2 Some US manufacturing plants relied on amphibole fibers as early as the 1920s. One of them is the Manheim, Pennsylvania plant of Raybestos-Manhattan, which made specialized products for the US Navy, among other customers. The disease occurrence at that facility is startlingly different from that experienced by other facilities, including the occurrence of MM cases prior to other American facilities.

3 The British experience with amphibole fibers and their deleterious health effects is well documented. From the earliest reports, amphibole fibers were more capable of causing asbestosis in a shorter period of time. The European research also presented the hypothesis earlier in time than in the United States that LC and MM were associated with heavy asbestos exposure. As an example of different disease rates and their impact, the British government mandated visible inspection of asbestos exposure in 1931. Britain has always maintained a different exposure level as between the different fibers.

4 In 1956, the Asbestos Worker, a magazine published by the Heat and Frost Worker's Union, identified a rise in pulmonary complaints from its members. The same union magazine had first identified a concern for asbestos exposure and disease in 1930, but at that time relied on British reports instead of their own American experience. Although the union had been organized since the late 1800s and its members had been exposed to chrysotile fibers from thermal insulation installation since that time, no appreciable disease occurrence resulted until approximately 15–20 years after the US Government's mandated use of amphibole asbestos.

country." Lost to history is this observation that the fibrosis resulting from exposure to chrysotile in America into the 1940s resulted in a less severe disease process with fewer cases being reported than case reports from Britain and other European countries due to mixed exposures to amphiboles as well as chrysotile. The assessment reached by Fleischer-Drinker contributed to a perception—certainly made false by the importation of amphibole in the second half of the 20th century and the massive increase in asbestos importation in general—that in "relation to public health, asbestosis is not nearly as serious a problem as silicosis."

According to Lanza (1938) "'Eating dust' was looked upon by the hard rock miner as a natural danger of his trade." Hoffman (1918), writing on behalf of the US Department of Labor, discussed the casual, matter-of-fact manner with which worker health and the occurrence of diseases such as tuberculosis were being dealt with by insurance companies: "It may be said, in conclusion, that in the practice of American and Canadian life insurance companies asbestos workers are generally declined on account of the assumed health-injurious conditions of the industry." Just as traumatic injury was an unavoidable risk of the workplace, dust diseases were also considered a known hazard of the mine and mill workers. The lack of significant asbestos-induced fatalities in the American asbestos products industry linked clearly with the delayed attention asbestos exposure would receive in the 1960s and 1970s.

As a consequence, the asbestos industry experienced a false sense of security with respect to nonmalignant and often nonfatal disease claims by maintaining workers' compensation insurance. The asbestos mining and manufacturing companies did not, however, provide similar premium payments to insure laborers beyond their own work force, such as end-product users like insulators or boilermakers. It was those workers who would eventually take direct legal action to recover for the harms brought about by the companies supplying the asbestos. Legal approaches to these issues would take time to develop and were initially not well suited for the scenario presented by asbestos injury.

Underdeveloped legal theories of monetary recovery for asbestos-induced personal injury may also explain the small number of court filings. Although negligence law had ancient underpinnings, it did not receive wide application as a recovery theory against asbestos product manufacturers during the early part of the previous century. Product liability, including strict liability for defective products, developed decades after asbestos illness first appeared and did not offer tangible returns for claimants as a distinct basis for recovery until the 1960s. On the other hand, expanded theories of recovery followed quickly upon the heels of the *rediscovery* of asbestos health issues at the New York Academy of Sciences 1964 symposium "Biological Effects of Asbestos"; they may well have arisen earlier if the science and medicine had also done so (Selikoff and Gilson, 1965; Chapter 1).

Claims directed against nonemployer parties were virtually unknown until the latter part of the 20th century. This is in part due to the almost-exclusive recourse for dust disease in the workplace through the compensation systems. Nonemployer suits were also reduced due to select industry leaders' determination to keep claims from the public. An additional factor influencing the lack of claims against nonemployer parties was the flawed research results regarding asbestos exposure and disease, and the prevalent legal climate. The 1940s and 1950s saw few, if any, references to lawsuits based on asbestos exposure aside from workers' compensation claims.[5] This is attributable in part to the

---

5 Discovery from a lawsuit involving 30 workers from a Johns Manville plant in Pittsburg, California revealed in the 1970s that Johns Manville had settled two lawsuits in 1957 and 1961 for negligence and breach of warranty against Johns Manville by insulators.

legacy in America of almost-exclusive use of chrysotile fibers until World War II. In addition, average life spans long enough to satisfy disease latency requirements and improvements in medical diagnostic techniques likely contributed to the eventual increase in asbestos-related health claims in the latter years of the previous century. As the occurrence of asbestos-related illness increased into the 1960s, it is no surprise that workers and their lawyers looked to sources other than their own employers for compensation from debilitating asbestos-related disease (Provost, 1982).[6] The link between MM and asbestos, established in 1960 by Wagner and his colleagues from review of data from the crocidolite-mining region of South Africa, was far more ominous for asbestos producers, and eventually asbestos consumers, than they could ever have foretold.

1960s: Emerging Tort Theories and the *Borel* Case

Although case reports of lung cancer (LC) and MM in asbestos exposed populations appeared sporadically from the 1930s through the 1950s, the causal association between asbestos exposure and cancer remained unclear through the 1960s. As evidence mounted that asbestos could cause MM and contribute to the development of LC, legal developments brought about improvements in a claimant's ability to survive legal challenges involving duty and responsibility and encouraged workers and their lawyers to bring suit.

The 1960s ushered in a court-driven movement to expand tort theories. Some of the earliest efforts to establish liability absent fault occurred in California, where the State's Supreme Court championed the theory of strict liability for product defects. Justice Traynor set forth the formative elements in *Escola v Coca Cola Bottling Co. of Fresno*, 24 Cal. 2d 453, 150 P.2d 436 (1944), and *Greenman v Yuba Power Products Inc.*, 377 P.2d 897 (Cal. 1962) (Tuytel, web document). In *Escola*, Justice Traynor set forth the underpinnings of strict liability in his concurring opinion:

> Manufacturing processes, frequently valuable secrets, are ordinarily either inaccessible to or beyond the ken of the general public. The consumer no longer has means or skill enough to investigate for himself the soundness of a product, even when it not contained in a sealed package, and his erstwhile vigilance has been lulled by the steady efforts of manufacturers to build up confidence by advertising and marketing devices such as trade-marks.

Thus, the courts were seeking to shift responsibility for the reasonable use and enjoyment of products to the manufacturer, rather than the end user. In *Greenman* (1962), Justice Traynor affirmatively identified strict liability for a manufacturer's placement of a product on the market.

These early efforts formed the underlying premise of strict liability law. The court-driven initiative was a response to the increasing production of materials in American society, many of which were prone to design, marketing, or warning defects.

With the codification of the Restatement of Torts (2nd) in 1965, the theory of strict liability for product manufacture proposed by the California Supreme Court of the 1940s and 1950s became a national standard. Section 402A of the Restatement placed strict liability upon sellers of defective or unreasonably dangerous products.

---

6 "To more adequately compensate workers, especially those with permanent work disabilities, workers and their lawyers often look to someone other than the employer and the employer's compensation carrier for relief. The result is referred to in legal circles as third-party litigation, and potential third-party defendants are numerous."

Although the California courts were the first to actively apply the new product liability theories to real-world situations, the federal courts in Texas were the site of the first monumental shift in the courtroom approach to asbestos lawsuits. The seminal case upon which all asbestos-related lawsuits have been patterned involved an asbestos worker from East Texas named Clarence Borel.[7]

Borel worked as an asbestos insulation worker from 1936 through the 1960s along the gulf coast of Texas. He was diagnosed with asbestosis, and eventually died of LC. Prior to his death, Borel sought the assistance of Ward Stephenson, a lawyer with a small legal practice in Beaumont, Texas, to file suit on his behalf against the manufacturers of pipe insulation products with which he worked during his career (Brodeur, 1985b). At the time, no law firms specialized in asbestos litigation on either side of the *bar*. Stephenson took on the Herculean task of developing an understanding of the scientific and medical aspects of the case, specifically, the association of asbestos exposure with disease. In doing so, he established himself as an innovator whose style and tenacity set a high standard for his successors.[8]

Against impressive odds, Stephenson pursued Borel's lawsuit to jury verdict, a decision that was affirmed for the plaintiffs on appeal. Success was based on a matrix of legal assertions, some of which incorporated advances in product liability law. In his initial pleading, Borel alleged claims of strict liability, negligence, and breach of warranty. The new theory of *strict liability* for product defects was ultimately the deciding factor in the *Borel* suit. During trial, Stephenson presented evidence that the manufacturers of asbestos-containing thermal insulation failed to warn of the dangers of asbestos dust—dangers they had been aware of since the 1930s and earlier. Further, the products were not tested to determine if the dust release was within prescribed levels. The evidence satisfied the prima facie elements of a strict liability claim against the manufacturers of asbestos-containing thermal insulation products.

The defendants countered with defenses of contributory negligence, sophisticated user, state-of-the-art, assumption of risk, and product misuse. Some of these defenses were novel and arose in direct response to the changes in the law. They have since served as standard approaches taken by the defense bar over the course of the litigation to the present day. Notwithstanding the carefully crafted defenses, the federal court applied *strict liability* during trial and identified a standard that would reverberate throughout the country's courtrooms—the defendant manufacturers were held to the standard of an expert with knowledge of asbestos-fiber health risk. Moreover, the court determined that the defendants had an independent duty to warn of the dangers associated with the use of asbestos-containing products and imposed joint and several liability[9] on all unsettled defendants. These findings were also upheld on appeal.

---

7 Prior to Mr Borel's case, Claude Tomplait filed a similar action in the same court at the end of 1966. That case also served as a template for cases that followed, but to a much lesser degree than the Borel case, in part due to its conclusion in favor of the defendants remaining at trial. P. Brodeur, The Asbestos Industry on Trial, 50–57, *The New Yorker* (June 10, 1985b).

8 Stephenson was a 40-year-old general practitioner with a regional firm out of Beaumont, Texas when he first agreed to represent Tomplait in a federal action against the manufacturers of thermal insulation products. Later, he agreed to take other asbestos-related matters, including the case filed by Borel. Stephenson successfully tried to jury verdict the first major lawsuit alleged by an end user of a product against the product manufacturers. He aggressively pursued the case and obtained critical deposition testimony and discovery responses that formed the basic template of most asbestos litigation that followed. See, P. Brodeur, The Asbestos Industry on Trial, 79, *The New Yorker*, June 10, 1985b, generally.

9 Joint and several liability is a legal concept that places the burden of proving separate liability upon the defendants in a suit rather than the plaintiff. The concept arose due to the courts' belief that defendants

The impact of the *Borel* decision was immediate. For example, John Karjala filed a lawsuit in a Minnesota federal court shortly after his attorney talked to Ward Stephenson about Borel's case. The *Karjala* case (*Karjala v Johns-Manville Products Corp.*, 523 F. 2d 155 (8th Cir. 1975) resulted in a jury verdict that was also upheld on appeal. The case demonstrated that the ability to successfully bring an asbestos-exposure claim to court was not restricted to one particular venue. Soon, additional attorneys began cases in other forums. Predominantly, cases arose in states where industry brought about the massive increase of asbestos product use and where asbestos-manufacturing facilities and shipyards were located.

Notwithstanding Stephenson's early success and the favorable case law he obtained for future claimants, the number of cases filed was manageable even into the late 1970s. The leading industry players continued to assert that they had engaged in no wrongdoing and believed that the number of suits would decrease over time. The 1978 annual report of the Johns Manville Corporation is instructive because it addressed the litigation facing the company in bold language filled with assertions that would eventually prove false and become very costly in the courtroom.[10]

1970s: Trade, Shipyard, and Factory Lawsuits

Armed with the knowledge that they could prevail at trial, plaintiff lawyers in the post-*Borel* environment were willing to litigate cases that previously had been disregarded as too risky (Rosenberg, 1986). Indeed, the realization that asbestos-related trials could be won fundamentally changed the landscape of occupation-related claims in general. It also gave rise to a generation of plaintiff lawyers whose personal wealth places them on lists identifying the wealthiest citizens in the country.[11]

The passage of the Occupational Health and Safety Act (OSHA) in the early 1970s was a pivotal event (Chapter 13). OSHA was enacted "to assure so far as possible every working man and woman in the Nation safe and healthful working conditions and to preserve our human resources" (Kirkland, 1989). OSHA required businesses to place warnings on products to ensure that exposures were below the reduced and now federally mandated threshold exposure levels, and to provide proper work conditions in

were in a better position to sort out who or what caused the harm rather than the plaintiff. In jurisdictions that apply the concept, the plaintiff need only prove one defendant's liability to recover from that defendant 100% of the damages. It is up to the defendants to produce evidence that decreases their liability when compared to other responsible parties.

10 1978 Annual Report, Johns Manville Corporation ("What is inexcusable is the manner in which many lawyers, the media, and even some in the 'public interest' arena have sought to exploit the tragedy of asbestos-related disease through the repetition of inaccuracies, half-truths and exaggerations.") The discovery of several thousand pages of correspondence, memos, and other documentary evidence in a locked safe maintained by the Raybestos-Manhattan Corporation would eventually crack the assertions made by Manville that it had limited knowledge of disease and had acted appropriately under the circumstances. This points to a little noted but critical aspect of the litigation; the people actually accused of wrongdoing are usually not around to defend themselves or the organizations for which they acted, or even to pass their knowledge on to their successors and their lawyers. Thus, some defendants have unwittingly defended cases with incomplete information. Since every misstep in an individual case can be replayed by plaintiffs in every subsequent case involving that defendant, the result can be disastrous.

11 By 2003, one commentator noted that more than "half the total amount spent on litigation by insurers and defendants goes to lawyers and expert witnesses." P. Hanlon, Asbestos Legislation: Federal and State, SJ031 ALI-ABA 549, 554 (2003).

keeping with sound industrial hygiene principles. The act was intended to—and did—reduce disease in the workplace.

The act also increased the awareness of the individual workers. Provost, writing in 1982 and reflecting on the passage of the act, commented:

> [D]uring this period workers learned a great deal. They learned about acknowledged workplace hazards, and they learned how to look for hazards. They also learned what they could expect from OSHA and NIOSH and what not to expect from their employers.

At the same time, plaintiffs' lawyers were beginning to comprehend the impact that OSHA could have on their ability to represent their clients' interests. OSHA promulgations would be referenced frequently in courtrooms as the essential standard by which the conduct and actions of defendants were judged, whether or not that conduct occurred before or after OSHA standards were adopted. Plaintiffs could now rely on the OSHA standards as a measure of reasonable conduct; if the product manufacturer did not test its products to keep the dust release below the prescribed levels, or if the employer never tried to keep exposures below the prescribed levels, then liability (if not causation) was all but established.

Lawsuits in the 1970s were predominantly filed by asbestos insulators, asbestos factory workers, and shipyard laborers. These suits were based on direct exposure to asbestos. In almost all instances, the claims involved massive exposure histories and often, indisputable disease. The suits tended to involve workers who experienced similar exposures, for similar lengths of time, at similar locations. Often, one set of workers would join together and file a consolidated case that might eventually incorporate well over 100 individual claims.

For example, in 1974 Fred Baron, a well-known plaintiffs' lawyer based in Dallas, filed one of the high-profile cases involving asbestos product factory workers.[12] The case involved workers at a Pittsburgh Corning thermal insulation facility located in Tyler, Texas and sought $100 million in damages—an astronomical figure for the time.

The lead plaintiff was Herman Yandle who, together with several others, retained Mr Baron to represent claims arising out of work at the Pittsburgh Corning plant. Eventually, Fred Baron filed a class action on behalf of nearly 570 plaintiffs, although class status was eventually denied (*Yandle v PPG*, 65 F.R.D. 566 (E.D. Tex. 1974). At its conclusion, the case involved several plaintiffs' firms who jointly represented the factory workers' interests and achieved a settlement of $20 million, including contribution from the plaintiffs' union and the US government, as well as foreign mining companies (Provost, 1982).[13]

Still, the number of suits brought during the 1970s seemed manageable to the asbestos industry, which thought the cases were defensible based on several factors—including latency of disease, limited knowledge of corporate conduct, inexperience with trying lawsuits, and a limited awareness of the availability of a legal remedy. Victory for the

---

12 Fred Baron has had a reputation for tenacious lawyering since he first appeared in the asbestos lawsuit arena by filing a claim against entities responsible for asbestos-related disease at a Pittsburgh Corning Unibestos facility located in Tyler, Texas. Provost (1982), paraphrased Mr Baron's approach: "If you want to keep me and other lawyers like me out of your plants, away from your records, and out of your pockets, you are going to have to make an honest effort to clean up the workplace, to tell workers what they are being exposed to, to tell workers where you see spots on their lungs or abnormalities in their blood." Whether such behavior would actually have made much difference for the asbestos industry at that point is doubtful, given that most of the asbestos exposures were significantly curtailed or over by then.

13 The North American Asbestos Corporation (NAAC), a distributor of raw amosite and crocidolite since 1953, dissolved itself soon after the Yandle decision and thereby avoided further liability.

plaintiff was never assured because of uncertainty as to what products injured the plaintiff, questionable exposure histories, and potential errors in diagnosis. At the time, industry observers attempted to quantify how many claims would arise out of past asbestos exposure, but those early predictions woefully underestimated the volumes of claims to follow (Macchiarola, 1996).

The task of marshalling the evidence involved in understanding the scientific and medical history of asbestos exposure and disease and the corporate knowledge of asbestos-related health hazards was daunting. To better prepare themselves for courtroom battles during the early years, plaintiffs' lawyers formed a loose coalition to obtain and share discovery materials (McGovern, 2002). An organization of plaintiff lawyers known as the Asbestos Litigation Group developed out of a 1978 meeting of various plaintiffs' counsel. This group began to share information on product identification, fabrication, use, and exposure.

The plaintiffs' lawyers' collective efforts succeeded. By the end of the 1970s, enough evidence had surfaced to demonstrate that certain industry participants—such as Johns Manville and Raybestos-Manhattan—knew substantially more about the potential for disease among workers than they had publicly acknowledged. A collection of previously undisclosed corporate documents was unearthed in the late 1970s from the personal documents of Sumner Simpson, the one time president of Raybestos-Manhattan from the 1920s through the 1950s. It revealed much about the conduct of some industry participants. During that time, Simpson participated in numerous industry meetings and was actively involved in industrial organizations. In 1979, the Raybestos-Manhattan Corporation produced more than 5000 documents relating to conversations and interactions Simpson had with officials of Johns Manville and other companies and organizations, including Johns Manville's general counsel, Vandiver Brown.

These documents highly incriminated Simpson and his company, as well as Johns Manville, because they detailed extensive knowledge of asbestos disease from the 1930s onward and indicate an intent to keep that information away from public scrutiny. Those documents are generally referred to in the asbestos litigation as the "Sumner Simpson documents." The plaintiffs' bar relied on that information to question the veracity of other companies, under the theory that what was available to one company was available to the others.[14] The notion of industry participants working together in collusion to prevent a full realization of the known and knowable hazards of asbestos, as exemplified by Simpson and his colleagues, became standard fare in all jury trials. Plaintiffs' lawyers shared these and other discovered documents with one another to further present this story of conscious disregard for employee and worker safety.

For their part, defendants and their lawyers also attempted to form defense groups to handle various issues. For example, defendants from time to time entered into agreements to share information and protect that shared information from disclosure by way of a "joint defense agreement." Such agreements have been short-lived, and coordinated efforts by the defense bar to align in a fashion similar to the plaintiffs' bar have failed more often than not. McGovern, commenting on the problems arising from a lack of a coordinated effort on the part of the defense bar, asserted: "Their lack of strategic cooperation has been a major factor in the success of the asbestos plaintiffs" (McGovern, 2002).

Coordination and cooperation required money, time, and a willingness to work through ethical and business conflicts. Although the defense bar did not invest in something as

14 A series of cases published in the 1980s address the ability for plaintiffs to rely on the internal documents of Johns Manville to incriminate the behavior of other members of the industry. In many instances the plaintiffs prevailed, with devastating impact on the remaining defendants.

specific as the plaintiffs' bar's Asbestos Litigation Group, the lawyers for the defense have been active for many years in collecting common thoughts and assisting one another where possible. In addition, the defense bar has been able to rely on one organization, the Defense Research Institute, to assist in collecting thoughts on the trends in the litigation and issues that have arisen through the years.

From the 1960s forward, plaintiffs and defendants identified and engaged experts to set forth the various aspects of asbestos lawsuits. Courts define expert witnesses as individuals who have special knowledge or skill in an area that is relevant to the case being litigated and is beyond the scope of the average juror.[15] Plaintiffs' lawyers focused primarily on diagnostic experts and favored pathologists to confirm diagnosis and cause. Plaintiffs' lawyers also cultivated experts to speak about corporate knowledge.[16] Defense lawyers responded by identifying experts to provide alternative assessments of the diagnostic and causal claims. The defense bar also retained experts to expound on industrial hygiene, exposure levels, and risk assessment.[17] Interestingly enough, with notable exceptions, experts in this litigation are customarily sought by one side of the bar but not the other. This phenomenon has created a distinctly "black and white" view of the underlying substance of the claims.

Many corporations were unprepared to deal with the amount of historical information that was available. Due in large part to the perceived lack of knowledge and impugned failure to act, these companies were portrayed as reckless and wanton in their disregard of the available information on asbestos health risks. Ultimately, the failure to adequately address what was known about asbestos exposure and disease would propel the asbestos litigation to a level of jury outrage rarely seen in other contexts.

The plaintiffs' bar, through discussions with jury panels following successful verdicts, learned that many jurors did not accept the industry's antiquated approach to asbestos use. The lack of an adequate warning on asbestos-containing products became a cornerstone of plaintiff victories over the next several decades. Juries also paid close attention to the lack of industry-wide product testing. Further, juries were inclined to find that information available to one sector of the industry should have been reviewed and understood by another sector. The rule of law that developed from the *Borel* case—that the manufacturer is held to the standard of an expert—was consistent with the commonsense logic of the jury and was a difficult burden for the defense bar to overcome.

To correct the perception of disinterest with respect to asbestos illness, corporations developed an approach known as the "state-of-the-art" defense. The "state-of-the-art"

---

15 Over the years, both sides of the bar have tested the qualifications, relevance, and reliability of experts offering opinions relating to asbestos disease and exposure. Whereas initially the standard by which a court would review the propriety of expert opinion was based on reliability and general acceptance in the field, modern courts have considered additional factors including rates of error, peer-review evaluation, and repeatability.

16 Early in the litigation the plaintiffs were able to rely on Dr Barry Castleman, a researcher from Baltimore. Dr Castleman reviewed documents obtained from his own research and that of Ron Motley and other plaintiffs' lawyers to piece together the complex story of the asbestos industry and its knowledge of hazards due to asbestos exposure. He published the first edition of his book, *Asbestos: A Legal and Medical Analysis*, in 1986. The book has since generated five editions, and Dr Castleman has addressed literally hundreds of juries on the subject of the asbestos industry and its conduct.

17 Many of the defense experts had lived through the history of asbestos exposure and the increasing knowledge of the severity of the problem. For example, Dr Clark Cooper spoke at the Borel trial about the lack of appreciation of the lower levels of asbestos exposure that could bring about cancer during his trial testimony. Transcript of Court Proceedings, *Borel v. Fibreboard Paper Products, Inc. et al.*, US Dist. Ct. Eastern Dist. TX, Civ. Action No. 6449.

defense is not unique to cases alleging asbestos illness but it is well suited because knowledge of asbestos exposure and illness increased over time, and during that same time, the disease did not manifest itself immediately, that is, latency. Therefore, defendants argued that it was reasonable for industry to take actions only when they became knowable of adverse health effects. Since the severity of asbestos exposure and disease could not have been known when the highest levels of industrial exposures were occurring, there is no fault on the part of the defendants.

This defense involved the review of scientific and medical knowledge available at the time a product was marketed and relies on expert witnesses to discuss the manner in which medical and scientific knowledge accumulated. The defense also demonstrates through expert testimony and a review of appropriate documents that the defendant company could not have known about the dangers associated with asbestos at the time it manufactured and distributed its products. The defense further asserted that when the defendant sold the products, knowledge of asbestos and health was such that it was *reasonable* for them to believe that the products were safe.

For example, at trial certain experts—either industrial hygienists or individuals trained in occupational disease and safety—spoke to the jury about specific asbestos exposure levels that were thought to be acceptable over time. They also discussed work practices and industry standards that governed workplace safety during the years at issue. Other experts, often possessing medical degrees, discussed when medical knowledge about particular diseases became available and what impact that knowledge had on work practices. Standard sets of documents and published literature were relied upon by both sides of the bar to reach conclusions about what was known about asbestos exposure and hazards, at the time the subject of the litigation was exposed.

By the end of the 1970s, the litigation was branching out beyond personal injury suits and actions regarding insurance coverage began. Lawsuits between insured industrial concerns and their insurance carriers continued for decades, and the recurring issues of exclusion language and available coverage would often impact on the ability of defendants to present their side adequately in personal injury cases. Rumblings of property damage suits also appeared at this time and would eventually result in additional strain on the financial wherewithal of the industry to pay to those individuals injured as a result of past events.

The late 1970s saw renewed efforts to resolve repetitive issues by filing class actions. These attempts invariably met with failure because the courts were reticent to grant class status for such a diverse groups of claimants, although a variety of efforts at asserting class status would continue well into the latter part of the 20th century. Suits against the US government—based on its involvement with asbestos use and exposure—also began to surface at the end of the 1970s. Most of those cases ended favorably for the government, often based on an underlying understanding of government immunity from tort claims (*Johns Manville v U.S.*, 1988).

1980s: Johns Manville's Bankruptcy, Defense Coordination, and Law Firm Dominance

By early 1980, the caseload of asbestos-related lawsuits was growing and straining the resources of the defendants. The business magazine *Forbes* reported that as of 1980, 1.5×10^4 claims against 300 companies were pending in the federal and state courts (Gibson, 1981). About half of the cases pending in the early 1980s involved shipyard workers (*Johns Manville Corp. v U.S.*, 13 Cl. Ct. at 78). Court dockets bulged with new filings, the insurance industry gasped at liability projections, and the asbestos-industry reeled in disbelief at their shattered corporate footing. The startling rise in lawsuits within less than 5 years brought about the first sincere efforts to solve the growing *asbestos crisis* through national legislation.

Congresswoman Millicent Fenwick began the first major effort to remove asbestos-related claims from the tort system in 1979; thereafter, nine separate bills were introduced through 1985 (Amundson, 2003). However, efforts to solve the growing drain on resources resulting from the mass filing of asbestos lawsuits by politicians such as Fenwick of New Jersey and Senator Hart of Colorado did not succeed. A true national solution appeared untenable because congress, commentators, and claimants alike had conflicting beliefs as to how to address each individual's right to his or her day in court.

Not surprisingly, with mounting caseloads and an ever-growing accumulation of documents damning industry from a select few corporate repositories, asbestos industrialists began turning toward bankruptcy court for economic relief. In 1976, 159 lawsuits were filed against Johns Manville; by 1982, approximately 6000 cases were being filed per year (Macchiarola, 1996). From 1981 through 1982, Johns Manville went to trial approximately 65 times, and in 10 of those cases, punitive damages were awarded.[18] Juror outrage regarding Johns Manville's knowledge and failure to act was on the rise as plaintiffs' experts became increasingly aware of internal documents, such as the Sumner Simpson documents, now in the possession of plaintiffs' lawyers.

With no end in sight to case filings and punitive damages looming large on the horizon, Johns Manville filed for bankruptcy protection by the end of 1982 (White, 2002). The bankruptcy shocked the asbestos-manufacturing industry, which had always looked to Johns Manville for industry leadership and guidance (Macchiarola, 1996).[19] At the time of the bankruptcy filing, the company had settled more than 3000 claims but had over 16 000 unresolved claims on file. It had assets of $2.25 billion, a net worth of $830 million, and commanded a 40% market share of all asbestos-containing materials produced and used in the United States. When Johns Manville sought bankruptcy protection, the burden of defending cases shifted to the remaining defendants.

The Johns Manville bankruptcy reorganization plan called for the establishment of the Manville Personal Injury Settlement Trust, later known as the Manville Trust (White, 2002). The Trust has since identified its purpose and mission:

> The Trust was created as an independent organization to distribute funds as equitably as possible while balancing the rights of current claimants against those of future, unknown claimants. The Trust's mission is to "enhance and preserve the Trust estate" in order to "deliver fair, adequate and equitable compensation to (claimants), whether known or unknown." The Trust was established as a negotiation based settlement organization pursuant to Plan provisions which made it clear that claimants did not need to litigate or threaten to litigate in order to negotiate a fair settlement.

Johns Manville Trust Web, www.mantrust.org

18 Punitive damages are damages that arise separately from those damages that compensate the injured party for medical expenses or pain and suffering. Punitive damages penalize the defendant for reckless or wanton conduct and are designed to inflict enough financial impact to send a message and prevent the behavior moving forward.

19 Johns Manville was proud of its heritage as the largest producer of asbestos-containing products in America, with involvement in every sector of the industry, from mining and manufacturing, to distributing and selling. *Asbestos*, issue from September, 1970 (containing the following advertisement: "Johns Manville participates in almost every facet of the Asbestos Industry and is the largest producer of asbestos-based products in the United States.")

As a result of the formation of the Trust, all tort claims against the Manville Corporation were discharged, and personal injury claims were channeled to the Trust. The Trust's assets were valued at $3 billion.

The Trust was supposed to satisfy the claims for liability asserted by those injured due to Manville's conduct and products; however, the Trust's funds were depleted within 2 years of operation (In re Joint Eastern & Southern Dist. Asbestos Litigation, 129 B.R. 710, 1991). The Trust's creators had grossly underestimated the number of claims. A second reorganization was imposed and resulted in a further reduction of available funds to claimants, from 10% of the original liquidated value set up at the Trust's inception based on disease claimed to 5% of that value in 2004 payouts (White, 2002).

Litigation did not end with Manville bankruptcy, as might have been thought given the dominant position Johns Manville played in the market. Instead, asbestos litigation witnessed the first great shift of focus—from the liability of Johns Manville to those companies that also maintained significant asbestos product market shares, including successors to the Philip Carey Corporation, the Owens Corning Fiberglas Corporation, and the Pittsburgh Corning Corporation, among others. The shift was driven by economics because other companies were held liable in court for the shares of bankrupt companies such as Johns Manville. Therefore, with Manville out of the picture, it became much easier to focus the attention on the remaining defendants.

However, due to the gaps in proofs left in the wake of the Manville bankruptcy, trial victory during this period was not assured. Of the asbestos trials that had gone to verdict by early 1983, 90 resulted in plaintiffs' favor, 51 in defendants' favor, 38 settled during trial, and 3 resulted in mistrials; the remaining verdicts resulted in resolutions that were not easily categorized (Mark, 1983). It did not take long for the plaintiffs bar to realign their offense toward the remaining defendants. In many ongoing claims, Manville became an afterthought in the eyes of plaintiffs who gained with pinpoint precision the ability to identify the remaining solvent defendants by name and trade brand.

All of the early asbestos trials that reached a jury verdict alleged personal injury claims, but the 1980s also brought about an expansion of asbestos-related lawsuits to property damage litigation. A series of cases were brought seeking abatement of property containing asbestos, and in various forms they have continued to the present day. These suits were generally orchestrated by lawyers specializing in personal injury cases who had existing knowledge about the asbestos-manufacturing companies based on prior litigation. The cases, filed on behalf of landowners and organizations with large real estate and physical plant holdings, demanded the removal of asbestos products in place to prevent future asbestos-related personal injuries to the occupants.[20]

By the 1980s, several different strategies arose for those companies that remained as defendants (McGovern, 2002). A small number of defendants pursued a strategy of no settlements because their products were generally considered to release little, if any, asbestos dust. That said, the majority of litigation approaches involved resolving the cases out of court. Some companies chose a hybrid approach; most cases were settled, but certain suits were presented to the jury.

20 For example, in 1984 the US Gypsum Co. paid almost 7.5×10^5 to settle a case involving the removal of asbestos from schools in Lexington County, South Carolina. The first jury verdict was returned in a school property damage case in favor of the defendants. *Anderson County Board of Education v. National Gypsum Co.*, 821 F.2d. 1230 (6th Cir. 1987) (discussing jury verdict below). However, in *Spartanburg County School District No. 7 v. National Gypsum Co.*, 805 F.2d 1148 (4th Cir. 1986), the jury's defense verdict was overturned on appeal. Jury cases since then have resulted in significant recoveries for governmental agencies, school systems, and owners of large, multiuse buildings.

The economics of a massive docket of claims presented very few alternatives for those companies embroiled in them. As a result, settlement strategies have played a significant role since the inception of asbestos lawsuits and rose in prominence as the numbers of claims skyrocketed. For example, certain defendants have been able to retain a *low profile* and are noticeably absent from the courtroom through careful consideration of the cost of settlement in comparison with the corporation's potential liability in a jury trial. Such companies rely on longstanding relationships with plaintiff firms and reach understandings based on prior and future commitments. Defendants, such as boiler manufacturers and gasket materials makers, were able to maintain a *low profile* in the litigation despite the presence of asbestos in their products, in large part because of national efforts to coordinate settlement and arrive at a standard settlement. Those settlement positions have consistently been put to the test over the years as more and more companies seek bankruptcy protection and leave the remaining defendants as the dwindling source to fund the accustomed large revenue stream of asbestos filings.

In their article, Schwartz and Lorber (2000) discuss how Owens Corning Fiberglas Co. sought to address the issue of the national resolution of a massive amount of lawsuits:

> Owens-Corning Fiberglas sought to manage its asbestos claims in several ways: first, through individual, our-of-court settlements; second, by seeking judicial and legislative relief; and finally, through an innovative program called the National Settlement Program (NSP).

Owens Corning Fiberglas ultimately failed, and it declared bankruptcy in 2000. Owens Corning Fiberglas was not alone in seeking *creative solutions*; many defendants attempted similar steps in an effort to avoid bankruptcy. Too often *innovative* solutions have proven inadequate to stave off bankruptcy (Schwartz and Lorber, 2000).

Notwithstanding the early trial successes of some defendants, increasingly during the 1980s, the defendant tended to fare poorly (McGovern, 2002). The plaintiffs' bar became increasingly skilled at honing the case against the various defendants. They had plenty of practice since they brought the same defendants to trial on a repeated basis. The repetitive trials resulted in lawyers and experts alike honing their skills and excelling at their ability to speak clearly to the juries about the issues involved. For instance, state-of-the-art experts such as Barry Castleman and David Ozonoff prepared detailed reports on the major events in the acquisition of knowledge by some industry participants over time, and became adept at telling the asbestos story. Their courtroom commentary focused on the misdeeds of a few no longer viable entities or no longer living individuals. As a consequence of these repeat trials, the plaintiffs' bar began collecting a standard arsenal of approaches to be used against a given company, including specific corporate documents and the cross examination of its corporate representatives.

Individuals representing the knowledge of the corporation, known as corporate representatives, were particularly susceptible to the repetitive nature of the litigation because what they said in any one deposition, or at trial, would remain with them (particularly if it was unfavorable to the defendant) for the balance of their time as the company representative. The pressure was enormous on these individuals to maintain their presence and consistency in discussing the actions of companies that took place in prior decades. Furthermore, as time moved on, fewer and fewer representatives actually had personal knowledge of the events leading up to asbestos use and product distribution. Companies were placed in the unenviable position of defending actions without access, either through death or unavailability, to the individuals involved in the decisions so many decades earlier.

By the mid- to late 1980s, expert witnesses became very effective at discussing the industry and corporate conduct in a manner that resoundingly turned the tide against the nonsettling defendants. In many instances, the expert witness served as a surrogate fact witness who offered testimony about what a company knew or did not know, and what it did or did not do, in response to that knowledge. By the late 1980s it became increasingly more difficult for the defense bar to obtain defense verdicts.

The threat of bad results in the courtroom further emphasized the need for resolution before trial. Generally speaking, resolution of claims out of court was beneficial, particularly in the short term, for defendant companies and their insurance carriers. In 1985, several insurers and asbestos producers entered into an "Agreement Concerning Asbestos Related Claims," or the "Wellington Agreement," named after the mediator responsible for its crafting, Harry Wellington, Dean of the Yale Law School (*North River Ins. Co. v Cigna Re*, 52 F.3d 1194 [3rd Cir. 1995]; Jones, 2001). As a result of the agreement, the Asbestos Claims Facility (ACF) was created and served as a nonprofit claims-handling center that coordinated claim payments on behalf of the asbestos producers. It was formed to combine information regarding claims and resolution schedules and thereby reduce transaction costs. The agreement encouraged settlements in place of costly litigation and established arbitration procedures to adjudicate claims that producers and their insurers could not settle.

Reception to the ACF was mixed. While it offered some beneficial results, it incurred significant costs. By establishing a known income stream, select plaintiff lawyers were afforded a sound economic footing from which to recruit more claims and take advantage of a rolling accounts receivable system to bankroll the research and costs required to bring new defendants to the litigation (McGovern, 2002). The economies of scale of so many repetitive claims reduced transaction costs so that plaintiffs could bring cases that might otherwise not be filed (Report on Mass Tort Litigation, 1999).

In any case, the group's existence was short-lived because Owens Corning, Inc. dropped out of the ACF by the close of 1988, followed closely by Eagle-Picher Industries. The ACF officially dissolved shortly thereafter, leaving some of the original members to re-form into the Center for Claims Resolution (CCR; Jones, 2001). The CCR continued to exist well into the 1990s, at which time membership became strained and the group disbanded.

Such defense-oriented groups were a direct response to the bargaining power of a few very highly organized plaintiff law firms that took on massive numbers of cases because of their special knowledge of the asbestos industry and litigation.[21] In hindsight, what appeared to be an appropriate and economical solution to the ever-growing number of claims likely fueled the fire of increasingly "out-of-control" litigation. Had defendants focused on *product identification* and appropriate medical proof and dissociated themselves from the industry leaders whose incriminating documents were relied on to condemn the entire group, the outcome of 30 years of asbestos lawsuits might have been startlingly different. The most powerful plaintiffs' lawyers in the country eventually *steamrolled* all defendants involved, including those who, for a short time, were able to maintain a *safe harbor* from the courtroom.

The lawyers' power directly correlated with their success in the courtroom and their relationships with trade unions. The misdeeds of some industry leaders made for compelling stories that successful plaintiffs' lawyers learned to tell well. By the 1980s, the plaintiffs' bar squarely placed the asbestos industry on trial. As long as they *peaked*

---

21 M. White, Fifteenth Annual Corporate Law Symposium: Corporate Bankruptcy in the New Millennium—Why the Asbestos Genie Won't Stay in the Bankruptcy Bottle, 70 *U. Cin. L. Rev.* 1319, 1330 (2002) (noting that more than half the claims with the Manville Trust are filed by 10 law firms).

the jury's outrage with general corporate misconduct and industry-wide disregard, the plaintiffs' success was secured. Across the country, lawyers for plaintiffs and union representatives formed alliances to bring lawsuits against an ever-expanding pool of defendants. Pioneer lawyers all seized the opportunity to maximize recoveries for their clients by aggressively influencing the system of trial and resolution over the years through case management orders, strategic preparation of cases, and targeting particular defendants as needed.[22] On the *flip side*, the defense bar also began to witness some *standout* performances by excellent trial lawyers. More senior lawyers lead the charge at the national level and in *hot spots* of litigation around the country. Younger lawyers capable of employing advances in science and medicine to defend these complex cases began to increase their role in the defense.

1990s: Mass Torts and the Explosion of the Plaintiff Pool

By the early 1990s, there were nearly 1×10^5 cases pending in federal and state courts that alleged asbestos-related injury (Zimand, 1991). In 1991, the federal courts established a court to hear all asbestos-related matters, which has been presided over since that time by Judge Charles Weiner. One outcome of that court was a decrease in federal court filings, thereby increasing the burden of asbestos filings in the state courts. Since that time, some states have taken the lead of the federal system and established their own *consolidated* dockets.

The early 1990s observed a brief calm of litigation efforts by the plaintiffs bar. A notable exception was an effort to develop a "fear of cancer" claim in order to increase recovery potential in cases claiming only nonmalignant illness. In some instances, for example, the claimants conceded no impairment, but sought relief in the form of required periodic medical monitoring. These cases were generally denied by the courts as resulting in high costs for uncertain gains.

The advent of settlement groups by the 1990s and the consolidation of power into a few plaintiff firms brought about an unusual détente among the parties to the litigation and encouraged unions, screening companies, and certain law firms to conduct extensive searches for more claimants (Hensler, 2002).[23] Administrative agreements and rules of conduct reduced the notion of an individual plaintiff controlling the course of his or her lawsuit to an archaic feature of previous decades (Hensler, 2002).

One of the most significant developments in the 1990s was the increase in screenings of chest x-rays to identify potential claimants for suspected asbestos-related disease,

22 One of the more influential personalities in the plaintiffs' bar is Ronald Motley, named partner of the now-disbanded Ness Motley law firm based out of Charleston, South Carolina. Mr Motley became involved in the asbestos litigation in 1976 when he served as local counsel in a series of personal injury lawsuits brought on behalf of insulation workers. Motley was instrumental in relying on documents in the possession of Sumner Simpson, the former president of Raybestos-Manhattan, in order to demonstrate corporate wrongdoing. He was a leader in organizing the documentary evidence that would propel the litigation into the next several decades and result in the bankruptcies of several of the largest corporations in America.
23 Professor Hensler eloquently identifies one of the phenomena of the litigation: "One of the anomalies of asbestos litigation has long been its concentration among a small number of law firms. As the litigation became less risky and evidence of product distribution and defendant practices was more widely disseminated, one might have expected more competition among plaintiffs' firms for cases. But, although some new firms entered the litigation in the early 1990s, the leading firms remained those who had shaped its course in the preceding decades."

primarily asbestosis. As a result, the number of nonmalignant claims rose at an *astronomical* rate. Often times, the screenings were supported by lawyers who merely referred positive claims to others rather than trying those cases themselves. An entire subindustry arose employing marketers, laboratory technicians, radiologists and pulmonologists, paralegals and lawyers to help assist these potential claimants in finding their way to the courthouse.

The efforts of plaintiffs' law firms to consolidate and stream line their operations, which the plaintiffs' law firms had converted from trial teams to settlement staffs, were astonishingly successful, and the numbers of filed claims increased many times over the predictions of a few years earlier. By the end of the 1990s, screening for claims was commonplace. This decade also saw the aggressive pursuit of another asbestos litigation trend—venue-shopping (see Appendix). The search for jury pools favorably inclined towards plaintiffs and sympathetic jurists drove most new filings to a few select states, including Mississippi, Illinois, Louisiana, and Texas (Brickman, 2002). The massive influx of claims introduced new pressures on the fragile system of case resolution.

From 1982 through 1999, 48 companies filed for bankruptcy as a result of asbestos claims (White, 2002). In 1994, congress adopted a special set of provisions designed to encourage companies with asbestos liabilities to seek reorganization. Those changes were looked upon favorably by companies that became weary of the ever-present trial threat. In a real sense, bankruptcy court offered a welcome respite for companies tired of staving off uncertain claims. Once a company declares bankruptcy, provisions of the US federal bankruptcy rules permit an automatic freeze on further litigation pending either resolution of the bankruptcy status of the company or permission to lift the stay.

Without question, bankruptcies were the direct result of corporate America's inability to predict claim-filing rates. That unpredictability came about because of the increasing reliance on screenings to identify potential claimants—many of whom demonstrated minimal or no impairment on examination. The shift in the plaintiff population from the seriously ill claimants of the 1970s to a majority of unimpaired claimants by the year 2000 has resulted in some plaintiffs' lawyers denouncing their fellow bar members for unwarranted abuses to the system:

> [T]here are gross abuses to our system. We have lawyers who have absolutely no ethical concerns for their own clients that they represent—we have untrammeled screenings of marginally exposed people and the dumping of tens of thousands of cases in our court system, which is wrong and should be stopped.
>
> *Brickman, 1992*

The 1990s gave rise to interesting developments in both the plaintiffs' bar and the defense bar. On the plaintiffs' side, law firms began to balkanize, with many lawyers splitting off to form their own firms. On the defense side, bankruptcy caused some law firms to consolidate, while others removed themselves from the litigation altogether. Ultimately, these conditions led to an increase in the number of active plaintiff firms filing asbestos-based lawsuits and a decrease in the number of defense firms that had experience in trying asbestos lawsuits.

One method that both plaintiffs and defendants explored to deal with the extent of potential filings was mass filings. Relying on class action law, a series of cases were filed in the 1990s to establish some certainty and payment schemes. This is not the first time class actions had been attempted in asbestos lawsuits; however, given the mature state of the litigation, class actions were once again brought to alleviate some of the pressure arising from the proliferation of mass claims. For example, the collection of defendants known as the CCR participated in an involuntary *class action* that would take their claims out of the court system and force plaintiffs to settle for varying amounts under a preapproved schedule of payments. The defense group's efforts, known as the *Georgine* class action, were favored by some plaintiffs' attorneys but experienced staunch opposition from many others of those representing plaintiffs due to the perceived unequal treatment of some claims. Ultimately, the US Supreme Court rejected the class action, a decision discussed further below. Although well-intentioned, efforts at massive court-sanctioned resolution of large numbers of cases were perceived by the appellate courts as overreaching.

In general, the 1990s witnessed a far more vocal bench than was present in previous decades. The courts throughout the 1990s identified the need for legislative intervention. As early as September 1990, Chief Justice Rehnquist appointed an ad hoc committee to address the strain of asbestos lawsuits on the federal bench. By 1991, that group concluded that "the situation has reached critical dimensions and is getting worse" (Report of the US Judicial Conference Ad Hoc Committee on Asbestos Litigation, 1991). Further, the committee "recognize[d] that virtually all of the issues relating to a so-called 'national solution' are primarily matters of policy for the Congress" and stated that it "firmly believes that the ultimate solution should be legislation recognizing the national proportions of the problem. " The report (1991) also stated:

> The committee firmly believes that the ultimate solution should be legislation recognizing the national proportions of the problem both in federal and state courts and creating a national asbestos dispute resolution scheme that permits consolidation of all asbestos claims in a single forum—whether judicial or administrative—with jurisdiction over all defendants and appropriate assets.

Congress did not act, and the courts continued to vocalize their concerns. In 1993, the Third Circuit commented that "both state and federal courts have recognized that no single court can fashion an effective response to the national problem flowing from mass exposure to asbestos products." (*Dunn v HOVIC*, 1 F.3d 1371, 1386 [3d Cir. 1993]). In 1996, the Third Circuit repeated its message in the *Georgine* class action lawsuit: "But reform must come from the policy-makers, not the courts.... The most direct and encompassing solution would be legislative action." (*Georgine v Amchem Prods., Inc.,* 83 F.3d 610, 633 [3d Cir. 1996]).

In *Georgine,* the Third Circuit overturned the trial court's certification of a proposed nationwide settlement class involving hundreds of thousands of class members and manufacturer defendants who formed the CCR. The Third Circuit struck the class because it failed to meet the commonality and predominance requirements of Federal Rule 23(a) and 23(b)(3)—it was simply too massive a group to fall within the structure set out by the federal rules.

In June 1997, the Supreme Court affirmed the Third Circuit's decision. Writing for the Court, Justice Ruth Bader Ginsburg suggested that congress might be the most appropriate body to resolve the asbestos litigation crisis:

> The argument is sensibly made that a nationwide administrative claims processing regime would provide the most secure, fair and efficient means of compensating victims of asbestos exposure. Congress, however, has not adopted such a solution.

Amchem Prods., Inc. v Windsor, 117 S. Ct. 2231, 2253, 1997

The courts were not through with their message. In 1998, while striking down efforts by the federal trial court to establish mass consolidation of asbestos lawsuits, the Fifth Circuit noted:

> [T]here is no doubt that a desperate need exists for Federal legislation in the field of asbestos litigation. Congress' silence on the matter however, hardly authorizes the federal judiciary to assume for itself the responsibility for formulating what essentially are legislative solutions.

Cinuno v Raymark Industries, Inc., 151 F.3d 297, 313, 5th Cir, 1998

The message was repeated in 1999, when the Supreme Court published a similar opinion rejecting an asbestos class action in its *Ortiz* decision (*Ortiz v Fibreboard Corp.,* 527 U.S. 815, 827, 1999). Both *Amchem* and *Ortiz* made clear that the Supreme Court would not permit Federal Rules of Civil Procedure 23 to generate mass settlements in asbestos-related cases. The *Ortiz* case brought about the now-famous legal reference:

> [T]his case is a class action prompted by the elephantine mass of asbestos cases, ... this litigation defies customary judicial administration and calls for national legislation.

Ortiz v Fibreboard Corp., 119 S. Ct. 2295, 2302, 1999

Chief Justice Rehnquist also adopted the visual cue of a massive laboring beast unable to cope with its own girth, stating:

> Under the present regime, transactional costs will surely consume more and more of a relatively static amount of money to pay these claims...the "elephantine mass of asbestos cases," cries out for a legislative solution.

Ortiz v Fibreboard Corp., 119 S. Ct. 2295, 2324, 1999

These sentiments underline the frustration felt by both bar and bench with the system and its inability to adequately serve the needs of all interested parties. They foreshadowed yet another foray into a legislative solution to the continuing problems with asbestos-related filings.

The end of the decade saw the creation of another review and report requested by Chief Justice Rehnquist (Report on Mass Tort Litigation, 1999). Again, the all too familiar problems were considered and concerns with the size and scope of the asbestos litigation were emphasized. Simultaneously, trials increased and another rash of bankruptcies resulted.

2000 and Beyond: Uncharted Territory and Legislative Aid

In the 21st century, filings have continued to increase, proving incorrect yet again the actuarial data on disease rates and potential claims. Trials began again in earnest at the turn of this century, and the CCR disbanded under the pressure (Hensler, 2002). Heightened efforts to try cases to verdict resulted in an additional series of bankruptcies, which have continued at an alarming rate in the first several years after 2000 (White, 2002). At least 5×10^5 suits have been filed by workers and their family members claiming asbestos exposure (Hensler, 2002). Diligent efforts to find new sources of compensation have brought first-time defendants to the courthouse in droves (Schwartz and Lorber, 2000). In turn, the new millennium is marked by one of the highest rates of bankruptcy filings the litigation has seen (Hanlon, 2003).[24]

---

24 "Since 1982, [asbestos litigation] has forced almost 70 companies into bankruptcy. Over 60% of all asbestos bankrupticies have occurred in the past 5 years."

Schwartz and Lorber (2000) summarized the sentiment fermenting from the latter part of the previous century, stating:

> Most people, including us, thought the asbestos liability cases were a relic of the 1980s, along with the Rubik's Cube. The truth is that the asbestos lawsuits are booming. The number of pending cases doubled in the six years from 1993 to 1999, from 100,000 cases to more than 200,000 cases throughout the country.

As of late 2003, an estimated 3×10^5 claims were pending in federal and state court (Hanlon, 2003).

The massive nature of the problem, described as *elephantine mass* by Justice Ginsberg again caught the attention of the federal government. Previous efforts to resolve concerns at the federal level in the early 1980s had fallen apart. Another round of congressional activity began in earnest in 1998 and 1999 during the collapse of the parties' efforts to resolve the disputes through class action (Amundson, 2003). Although not the first time, current efforts to solve the asbestos litigation crisis through legislative intervention have many hoping that the end to the litigation may be at hand.

The new millennium has also brought about an increase in inactive dockets for unimpaired claimants throughout the country. State courts have abided by new legislation or forged their own creative solutions to deal with the bulk of the cases now clogging their dockets. Although it is too early to determine the ultimate impact of these *deep freeze* dockets, it is likely these dockets will reduce the overall court burdens associated with asbestos claims and focus attention on those claimants who present with life-threatening illness.

Conclusion

The history of asbestos-related litigation tracks approximately 75 years of developing science, medicine, and law. Considered *mature*, the litigation has resulted in such astronomical costs that its entire structure is yet again being heavily scrutinized by congress. Perhaps with legislative intervention this chapter in mass tort litigation will come to a close. In its passing, the litigation will have left an extensive legacy of case law and fundamental shifts in the manner in which parties, jurists, and legislatures look at issues of mass disease and personal injury claims.

Appendix: Anatomy of an Asbestos Lawsuit

An asbestos lawsuit begins when a plaintiff asserts causes of action against a defendant or defendants in a pleading (termed the petition or complaint) filed with the court. The plaintiff pleads the theoretical basis for recovery and alleges that some action or inaction on the part of the defendant or defendants caused the damages alleged. The defendant, in turn, answers the plaintiff's petition or complaint and asserts various defenses. The parties proceed with discovery, which is an organized investigation into the facts of the case that may involve interrogatories, depositions, and other legal investigatory devices to determine the exact facts supporting the claims. At the close of discovery, the parties marshal their evidence, prepare various motions and other procedural maneuvers, and, eventually, arrive at trial to try the case. A jury verdict will result at the conclusion of the plaintiff's case and the defendant's or defendants' affirmative case and presentation of defense arguments.

Recovery Theories

The primary recovery theories available to claimants alleging asbestos injury are negligence and strict liability.[25] To prove negligence, the plaintiff must present evidence that a duty was owed by the defendant to the plaintiff, that the defendant breached the duty, and that the breach caused damage.[26] For example, a premise owner could be liable to a claimant visiting the site if the claimant presents evidence that the premise owner owed a duty to keep the premises safe from a known or obvious asbestos exposure hazard, breached that duty by permitting exposure to occur, and proximately caused or contributed to an asbestos illness.

By contrast, a claim based on strict liability relieves the plaintiff of proving duty and breach. The plaintiff must prove that a defect in the product caused damage. While states may have slightly different versions of strict liability actions, most base their strict liability statutes on Restatement (2d) of Torts Sec. 402a, which indicates that if you sell a product in a "defective" condition and it injures someone, then you are liable for the injuries. There are generally three ways that a product can be defective: due to either a manufacturing flaw, a product design flaw, or a marketing flaw. When asserting a strict liability theory, asbestos claimants invariably prove a marketing defect existed due to an ineffective or nonexistent warning label. In many jurisdictions, the plaintiff relies on the consumer expectations test to qualify the claim.[27] In some states, a failure-to-warn defect case can rely on a "state-of-the-art" defense to demonstrate that the defendant did not and could not have known of the danger requiring a warning. Design and manufacturing defects are much less commonly asserted in asbestos lawsuits.

Causation

Regardless of the theory of recovery asserted, a claim will not succeed without proof of medical causation. There are two distinct approaches adopted by US courts to prove medical causation: substantial contributing factor and producing cause. Substantial contributing factor generally requires proof of a sufficient intensity, proximity, and duration of exposure to contribute to disease. Producing cause also requires identification of an exposure that contributed to the disease.

Defenses

Defendant companies rely on several distinct defenses, including challenges to diagnosis, a failure to prove medical causation, an inability to identify the product, an

25 Other theories of recovery include breach of warranty, nuisance, misrepresentation, conspiracy, fraud, and battery. There are also specialized recourses available for railroad and maritime workers that rely on special federal statutes.

26 Specific negligence theories against manufacturers include: negligence in the design of defendant's asbestos-containing products; negligence in the testing and marketing of defendant's asbestos-containing products; and negligent failure to warn or to warn adequately of the hazards of defendant's asbestos-containing products. Negligence action against property owners and general contractors is that the controlling entity negligently failed to supervise the work done by subcontractors or the environment in which subcontractors worked. The claim against subcontractors is a simple negligence claim. The plaintiff alleges that the subcontractor failed to act in a reasonable manner, violating a standard of due care to others, and thereby caused the plaintiff to be exposed to asbestos.

27 Under the consumer expectation test, the plaintiff alleges that the defendant's product failed to perform as safely as a reasonable consumer would expect when it was used in a foreseeable manner. The "consumer expectation defect" depends on the expectation of the ordinary consumer at the time of alleged exposure.

insufficient exposure to cause disease, lack of any wrongdoing based on the state-of-the-art knowledge available at the time of exposure, the government contractor defense,[28] and lack of control over the workplace. More recently, tort reform in many states has permitted defendants to identify other sources of potential exposure and thereby allocate any jury verdict among multiple sources.

Damages

Damages are determined by the jury. There are two primary components, economic and noneconomic damages. Jurisdictions also vary in their rules for apportioning damages. Damages in some jurisdictions are governed by several liability, meaning each defendant pays only the damages associated with its share of liability. However, over the four decades of active asbestos litigation, the vast majority of jurisdictions have assessed damages under joint and several liability principles, meaning that each defendant is potentially responsible for the entire damages award if certain requirements are met, regardless of assessed liability.

Although tort reform is altering joint and several liability, its preservation in many jurisdictions and dominance during the tenure of the litigation has resulted in clear inequities in many instances. The inequity of apportioned liability is exacerbated by the inability of experts and jurors alike to agree on the appropriate method for apportioning liability among diverse asbestos exposures. In those jurisdictions that apply joint and several liability, bankruptcy filings by asbestos defendants almost always have a negative effect on the remaining defendants because the nonbankrupt defendants are required to assume the potential liability of the bankrupt companies (White, 2002).

Jury verdicts in asbestos lawsuits have historically been inflated, likely due to the perception of conscious fault attributable to the defendants. In the 1980s, evidence uncovered during prior cases of the defendants' knowledge of the dangers of asbestos and concealment of this information from plaintiffs resulted in substantial rewards of punitive damages against the manufacturers. This evidence included information (which later became known as the "Sumner Simpson Papers") from the 1930s compiled by Sumner Simpson, former head of the Raybestos-Manhattan company. Other inflammatory documents were produced from an organization known as the Asbestos Textile Institute. Also, corporate documents, such as those from Johns Manville, added to the cumulative outrage occurring in courtrooms across the country. This knowledge formed the basis of large recoveries in the form of punitive damages for past corporate conduct.

Trial Management Techniques

To deal with the sheer volume of cases, several courts have significantly altered the procedural approach to the litigation. Some of the methods include bifurcation of the trial into discrete issues. Other methods involve consolidating similarly situated claimants for one combined trial (Zimand, 1991). Class actions have also been forwarded as a method to deal with the asbestos litigation crisis, but, as discussed above, they have been rejected by the appellate courts. Other trial management techniques include assigning one judge to all asbestos cases in a particular jurisdiction, putting forward test

---

28 The government contractor defense is an assertion by a defendant that its actions were directly attributable to work it performed for the US government at the government's request and according to the government's strict requirements.

cases, and issuing general or master pretrial orders. In some instances, both federal and state courts have cooperated to achieve judicial economy and simultaneously resolve similar disputes, primarily during the discovery phase (Macchiarola, 1996). As a general rule, as the number of asbestos mass tort cases have increased, mechanisms for processing those claims have been more vigorously pursued. For example, courts have required master complaints and answers, instituted standard sets of interrogatories, permitted the use of depositions from other cases, and, in several instances, mandated document depositories."[29]

Several members of the bench have taken significant steps to organize their asbestos dockets into a manageable and workable form.[30] Special masters are given wide-ranging responsibility and authority to help cases move more efficiently through the system.

Another method for dealing with mass filings of asbestos exposure claims is the transfer of all such cases to one central court for processing. The Judicial Panel on Multidistrict Litigation consists of several circuit and district court judges appointed by the Chief of the Supreme Court (Dutcher, 1993). The panel conducts hearings, considers motions, and decides whether to consolidate cases for pretrial proceedings. Commonly referred to as the multidistrict litigation court, or MDL court, this vehicle for dispute resolution was available for many years prior to its application to asbestos suits in 1991. At that time, all federal court cases involving asbestos exposure claims were transferred to one court for handling. More than 3.5×10^4 cases are currently on file in this court.

Recently, several states have formed their own versions of the federal MDL. For example, in New York City Justice Helen Freedman presides over thousands of asbestos cases consolidated for adjudication (Freedman, 1999). In Texas, legislation enacted in 2003 gave rise to a Judicial Panel on Multidistrict Litigation, which recently appointed Judge Mark Davidson to preside over Texas' version of an MDL court for asbestos litigation. These courts are attempting to deal with the mass filings head-on to reach solutions that are acceptable to members of both sides of the bar and their clients.

"Venue Shopping"

Asbestos litigation has given rise to an unprecedented effort to preselect the particular court where the dispute will be heard to secure favorable rulings (Report on Mass Tort Litigation, 1999). Particularly suitable jurisdictions (or venues) to sue asbestos defendants

---

29 Judge Jack Weinstein, sitting on the federal bench in the Eastern District of New York, earned a reputation for employing creative management of mass torts. He has presided over asbestos lawsuits, Agent Orange claims, and other "mass tort" filings. Judge Weinstein identified several factors that have forced the bench to rely on creative solutions to manage the mass filings: (1) the lack of an effective national administrative regulatory scheme capable of controlling the undesirable conduct of manufacturers; (2) the absence of a comprehensive social welfare-medical scheme; and (3) the lack of adequate state or federal legislation controlling these cases. V. Dutcher, "The Asbestos Dragon: The Ramifications of Creative Judicial Management of Asbestos Cases," 10 Pace Envtl. L. Rev. 955, 959 (1993).

30 One early innovator was Judge Robert Parker, out of the East District of Texas. Other innovators include Jack Weinstein from the New York Federal Court; Helen Freedman from the New York City Supreme Court (the state's trial-level court); Judge Ken Kawaichi from Alameda County, California; Judge John Nagle of the Eastern District of Missouri; Judge Marshall Levin of the Maryland Circuit Court, Baltimore; Judge Lambros of the Ohio Federal District Court; Judge James MeHaffy of Orange County, Texas; and Judge Charles Weiner from the Federal MDL Court in Philadelphia. These judges, in turn, engaged certain special masters that contributed in large measure to the handling of these cases, such as Kenneth Fineberg in New York City.

have arisen since the inception of the litigation. As a result, it is now common to see out-of-state plaintiffs presenting their cases in such familiar asbestos venues as Madison County, Illinois; Pascagoula, Mississippi; Brazoria County or Orange County, Texas; and West Virginia (White, 2002).[31] Some courts have attempted to clear their dockets by requiring mass consolidation and enforcing similar creative judicial management solutions. This has resulted in unintended consequences and a further segmentation of favored venues: "Judges who move large numbers through the litigation process at low transaction costs create the opportunity for new filings. They increase the demand for new cases by their high resolution rates and low transaction costs" (McGovern, 1997). The bench is aware of the unintended consequence of their management skills: "Increased efficiency may encourage additional filings and provide an overly hospitable environment for weak cases" (Freedman, 1999).

References

Adam JA. Proper compensation for the damaged worker. *Ann NY Acad Sci.* 1979;330:597–600.

Amundson J. How a Congressional answer to asbestos litigation would help litigants, courts, and the American economy. *44 S Tex L Rev.* 2003;925:935–936.

Brickman L. On the theory class's theories of asbestos litigation: the disconnect between scholarship and reality. *Pepperdine Law Rev.* 2002;31:33, 62–102.

Brickman L. The asbestos litigation crisis: Is there a need for an administrative alternative? *13 Cardozo L. Rev.* 1992;58:1819, 1889. (quoting Ronald Motley).

Brodeur P. *Outrageous Misconduct: The Asbestos Industry on Trial.* New York: Pantheon Books; 1985a.

Brodeur P. The Asbestos Industry on Trial, *79. The New Yorker*; 1985b.

Brown EW. "Industrial Hygiene and the Navy in National Defense," War Medicine, p. 4. Paper presented at: 5th Annual Meeting of the Air Hygiene Foundation of America, November 13, 1940.

Corn J. Starr J. Historical perspective on asbestos: policies and protective measures in World War II shipbuilding. *Am J Ind Med.* 1987;11:359–373.

Dreessen W, Dallavalle J, Edwards T, Miller J, Sayers R. A study of asbestosis in the asbestos textile industry, Public Health Bulletin 241, United States Government Printing Office, August, 1938; 117.

Dutcher VS. The asbestos dragon: the ramifications of creative judicial management of asbestos cases, *10 Pace Envtl. L. Rev.* 1993;955, 972.

Fleischer W, Viles J Jr., Gade R, Drinker P. A health survey of pipe covering operations in constructing Naval vessels. *28 J Ind Hygiene Tox.* 1946;28.

Freedman H. Product liability issues in Mass Torts: a view from the bench. *15 Touro L. Rev.* 1999;685.

Garner B, Black H, eds. *Black's Law Dictionary*, 7th ed. West Group; 1497, 1999.

Gibson P. When lawyers prosper. *Forbes.* March 30, 1981;43–44.

Goldberg J. *Problems in Workmen's Compensation.* Lanza AJ, Goldberg J, eds. Oxford University Press; 1939;632.

Hanlon P. *Asbestos Legislation: Federal and State.* SJ031 ALI-ABA 549, 552, 2003.

Hensler D. As time goes by: asbestos litigation after *Amchem* and *Ortiz. 80 Tex. L. Rev.* 2002;1899, 1920–1921.

Hoffman FL. Mortality from respiratory diseases in dusty trades (inorganic dusts), U.S. Dept. of Labor, Bureau of Labor Statistics, Bulletin No. 231, Industrial Accidents and Hygiene Series, No. 17, June 1918.

---

31 "Asbestos lawsuits, in addition to being very numerous, are concentrated in a few jurisdictions. Pennsylvania has 26% of asbestos trials and New York and Texas each have 14%."

Jones R. Searching for solutions to the problems caused by the "elephantine mass" of asbestos litigation. *14 Tul. Envtl. L. J.* 2001;549, 551–552.

Kirkland J. What's current in asbestos regulations, *23 U. Rich. L. Rev.* 1989;375, 392, quoting 29 U.S.C. § 651(b).

Lanza AJ, ed. *Silicosis and Asbestosis 408.* New York: Oxford University Press; 1938.

Macchiarola F. The Manville personal injury settlement trust: lessons for the future. *17 Cardozo L. Rev.* 1996;583, 595, 598.

Mark G. Issues in asbestos litigation. *34 Hastings L.J.* 1983;871, 901.

McGovern F. The tragedy of the asbestos commons. *88 Va. L. Rev.* 2002;1721, 1747.

McGovern FE. The defensive use of Federal class actions in mass torts. *39 Ariz. L. Rev.* 1997;595, 606.

Motley R, Nial S. A critical analysis of the Brickman Administrative Proposal: Who declared war on asbestos victims' rights? *13 Cardozo L. Rev.* 1992;1919, 1921.

Provost G. Legal trends in occupational health. *J Occup Med.* 1982;24:2, 116.

Report on Mass Tort Litigation. Joint report prepared by the Advisory Committee on Civil Rules and the Working Group on Mass Torts to the Chief Justice of the United States and to the Judicial Conference of the United States; February 15, 1999; 10.

Report of the US Judicial Conference Ad Hoc Committee on Asbestos Litigation. (March 1991).

Rosenberg D. The Dusting of America: A Story of Asbestos—Carnage, Cover Up, and Litigation (Book review). *99 Harv. L. Rev.* 1986;1693, 1695 (emphasis in original).

Schwartz V, Lorber L. A letter to the nation's trial judges: how the focus on efficiency is hurting you and innocent victims in asbestos liability cases. *24 Am. J. Trial Advoc.* 2000;247, 261.

Selikoff I, Gilson J, eds. Asbestos and disease. *Ann NY Acad Sci.* 1965;132:1–766.

Tuytel N. Asbestos litigation in British Columbia. (web-based version) *Can Insur Law Rev.* 2(2);125–266; *Can Insur Law Rev.* 8(1–3):1–48.

White M. Fifteenth Annual Corporate Law Symposium: Corporate Bankruptcy in the New Millennium—Why the Asbestos Genie Won't Stay in the Bankruptcy Bottle. *70 U. Cin. L. Rev.* 2002;1319, 1322–1323.

Zimand P. Note, national asbestos litigation: Procedural problems must be solved. *69 Wash. U. L. Q.* 1991;899, 902.

16

Asbestos Exposure and Disease Trends in the 20th and 21st Centuries

Bertram Price and Adam Ware

Introduction

This chapter discusses the population characteristics of asbestos-associated diseases in the 20th century and presents a view of these characteristics for the 21st century. We consider the three principal asbestos-associated diseases: malignant mesothelioma (MM), lung cancer (LC), and asbestosis. Other malignant diseases that have been associated with asbestos are cancers of the gastrointestinal tract and larynx. These cancers have not been addressed because studies over the past 10 years indicate that asbestos is an unlikely cause (Chapter 9).[1] In addition to asbestosis, other nonmalignant respiratory conditions are associated with asbestos exposure (Chapter 6). These conditions principally are indicators of asbestos exposure. As such, they may be predictors of future asbestos-associated cancer, but have limited clinical consequences.

We focus on trends in MM incidence and broadly defined asbestos exposure sources to chart the pattern of asbestos-associated disease. MM is a rare disease and, although not all MM are caused by asbestos, a significant population time-trend in MM incidence is associated with a time-trend in population exposure to asbestos. Neither LC nor asbestosis would be effective as a basis for describing asbestos-associated disease patterns. LC has been identified with exposure to a variety of workplace agents and has a strong causal relationship with smoking. Attempting to differentiate asbestos-associated LC from LC due to smoking or other causes involves significant uncertainty (Chase, 1985; Guidotti, 2002).

---

1 Other malignant diseases initially associated with exposure to asbestos have since been shown to be unlikely consequences of asbestos exposure. Selikoff's report noted the first cases of asbestos-related gastrointestinal cancer (Selikoff, in a 1964 study of 1.78×10^4 insulation workers who were members of the Heat and Frost Workers Union, found unexpected numbers of men who die of cancer of the stomach, colon, or rectum). However, later studies (Gamble, 1994) found no evidence of a causal link between asbestos exposure and gastrointestinal cancers. In particular, a review of the scientific and medical literature indicated no scientifically reliable relationship between gastrointestinal cancer and asbestos exposure. Among various studies, the consensus is that the most significant asbestos-associated diseases are asbestosis, lung cancer, and mesothelioma of the pleura and peritoneum (Castleman, 1996; Roggli et al., 2004). (Refer to Chapters 6–9 of this book for a complete discussion of asbestos-related disease.)

Asbestosis incidence trends are not well developed and asbestosis death rates can be misleading because it often is not the principal cause of death in many patients.

Dividing exposure sources into two broad categories, occupational exposure and nonoccupational exposure, provides a useful framework for analyzing and projecting asbestos-associated diseases. Before the 1970s, when industrialized countries first established formal occupational asbestos exposure limits or tightened existing limits, workplace exposures could be extremely high. For example, insulators and shipyard workers experienced exposure intensities sometimes exceeding 50 f/mL and cumulative lifetime exposures of 500 f/mL-yrs or more (EPA, 1986).[2] It is undisputed that heavy occupational exposures have been the basis of a worldwide MM epidemic. However, these exposures have all but been eliminated in most countries of the industrialized world. The resulting trend from this lack of exposure has been one that declines over the next 20–30 years. The extent to which heavy occupational exposures persist in developing countries will be a major factor determining the incidence of asbestos-associated diseases in the second half of the 21st century.

Nonoccupational exposures, aside from a few notable exceptions, continue to be much lower than historical occupational exposures. Low-level nonoccupational exposures currently are widespread and will continue for the foreseeable future, but are unlikely to be responsible for an upward trend in MM or other asbestos-associated diseases. This assessment follows in part from the historic MM incidence trend for women in North America, Western Europe, and the United Kingdom (Greenberg et al., 2002; Hodgson et al., 2005; Price and Ware, 2004). The substantial increases in asbestos consumption that began in the 1930s were responsible not only for heavy occupational exposure, but also increased nonoccupational exposure albeit at much lower levels.[3] Nonoccupational exposures—environmental and domestic exposures[4]—were the only exposures for most women. MM "incidence among women in North America and Western Europe has shown little or no increase during the last 20–30 years, despite the contribution of occupational and household exposure, and the greater diagnostic awareness of physicians and pathologists in the same period" (Greenberg et al., 2002). It follows that low-level nonoccupational exposure is not a significant contributor to MM incidence.

However, some nonoccupational sources that can produce relatively high exposures are linked to diseases in the 20th century, and may have a bearing in the 21st century. These sources are heavy environmental exposures in communities located adjacent to asbestos mines and mills, manufacturing facilities, or waste dumps, where pollution controls were not employed. Examples are asbestos mining in South Africa and Australia, cement manufacturing in Italy, and the manufacturing plant at Manville, New Jersey in the United States.

We discuss the characteristics of diseases separately for industrialized countries and for developing countries. For industrialized countries, asbestos exposure increased substantially during the first three quarters of the 20th century and then decreased rapidly. The increase

2 In the regulatory and scientific literature, airborne concentrations of asbestos are reported both as fibers per cubic centimeter of air (f/mL) and fibers per milliliter of air (f/mL). These are identical units. We use "f/mL" throughout this report.

3 For example, in the United States, the increase in asbestos exposure is a consequence of the increased use of asbestos from 100 000 metric tons in 1930 to a peak of approximately 800 000 in the late 1970s (Virta USGS, 2003a,b).

4 Take-home exposure is defined as the exposure of household members to asbestos brought home on workers' clothes. Environmental exposure consists of outdoor ambient asbestos exposure from nearby factories, shipyards, mines, and other similar outdoor and indoor sources.

in exposure was a consequence of the growth in the use of asbestos in products. The buildup began in the 1930s, and continued at high levels through the 1970s. In some countries consumption doubled every decade until the peak worldwide in 1980 (Virta USGS, 2003a,b). Increasing awareness of the disease consequences of occupational exposure to asbestos in the 1960s and 1970s led to interventions such as mandated exposure limits and voluntary reductions in the use of asbestos in manufacturing. However, since asbestos-associated diseases have long latencies, reductions in disease incidence resulting from exposure reductions in the 20th century will not be fully realized until the middle of the 21st century. The pattern of disease in the second half of the 21st century will depend on whether, how soon, and how well asbestos control regulations are implemented in developing countries.

Background—Review by Country

We describe here trends in the asbestos-associated diseases in various countries, including both industrialized and developing countries. This discussion is not a complete accounting, but a sufficient sampling to develop a view of the types of exposures that have resulted in diseases, the extent of diseases in the population, and the time-pattern of diseases. The results for industrialized countries combined with information about asbestos use in developing countries provide an outlook for asbestos-associated disease in the 21st century.

Developed (Industrialized) Countries

United States

We base our discussion on disease incidence and exposure sources from government data, and from epidemiology and industrial hygiene studies of occupational cohorts and their workplaces. The National Cancer Institute compiles national statistics on cancer incidence, including MM through its Surveillance, Epidemiology, and End Results (SEER) system. SEER data, first reported for year 1973, currently includes data from 11 cancer registries covering approximately 14% of the US population. The registry populations are considered to be approximately representative of the US population (SEER Registries, 2004).

   We use analyses of the SEER data to describe the historical time-pattern and projections of MM in the United States. The age-adjusted time-pattern of MM for males and females in the United States for the years 1973 through 2001 is seen in Figure 16.1, The figure also displays consumption of asbestos in the United States from 1930 through 2001. Figure 16.2 projects the number of cases for males and females through 2050 against the backdrop of asbestos consumption.

   A substantial increase and then a leveling of male MM incidence tracks asbestos use with a shift of 30–40 years. Male exposures generally were very high during the 1930s through the 1960s; for example, cumulative exposures were as great as 500 f/mL-yrs, sometimes higher (EPA, 1986; HEI-AR, 1991).[5] The MM trend reflects these heavy occupational exposures after accounting for latency. The female MM rate remained constant, unaffected by the growth and subsequent decline in asbestos use. From the 1930s to the 1970s, except for the World War II years 1940–1945, few women worked in the industries where high-level exposure to asbestos was likely. As a group, women's

5 These reports are reviews of the epidemiological studies of occupational cohorts in the United States and elsewhere.

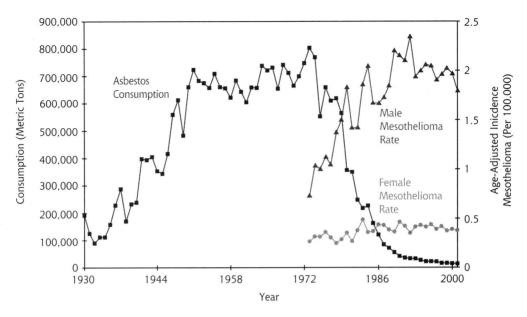

Figure 16.1 Asbestos use in the United States and the 2001 age-adjusted mesothelioma rates for males and females.

principal asbestos exposures were domestic and environmental. As such, the trend data for women indicate that the increase in exposure between 1930 and 1970 did not trigger a corresponding increase in MM incidence. Therefore, it is reasonable to conclude that typical domestic and environmental exposures alone were insufficient to cause MM.

If women's principal sources of asbestos exposure were not the cause of their MM, then their incidence rate would approximate the spontaneous background rate of MM. This rate in the year 2000 was judged to be four per million (Price and Ware, 2004; NCI—Ries et al., 2004; http://seer.cancer.gov/csr/1975_2001/results_single/sect_01_table.07.pdf). The spontaneous background rate for women may not apply directly to men. The ratio of pleural to peritoneal MM in women in this country is approximately 3.4 to 1; the ratio of pleural MM to peritoneal MM for men is about 11.7 to 1 (SEER, 2003). Further, women with peritoneal MM survive longer than men with peritoneal MM. Weill et al. (2004) suggest that peritoneal MM in women have unique features. Therefore, if the female spontaneous background MM rate were to be applied to males, it would need to be adjusted to account for the discrepancy between the sexes. For example, the male spontaneous background MM rate could be estimated by excluding all female peritoneal MM.

Figure 16.2 displays the projected number of MM cases through 2050–2054 for the United States. In 2004, the annual number of male cases was estimated to be approximately 2000; the annual number of female cases is approximately 550.[6] Female cases increase slightly corresponding to population growth and a shifting age-distribution toward older ages. As with most cancers, MM risk increases with age; therefore the aging population of women will show a slight increase in MM over time until either population growth stabilizes or the currently unknown causes of MM are discovered and eliminated. The peak for male cases is indicated in the 2000–2004 time-period and the decline to the spontaneous background level is projected to occur over the next

6 Predictions are from Price and Ware (2004).

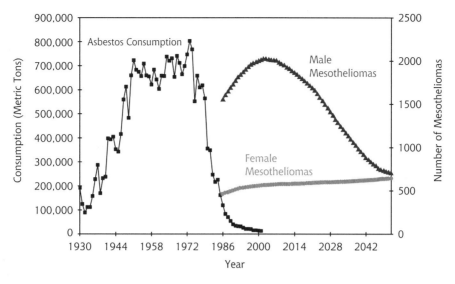

Figure 16.2 Asbestos use in the United States by year and mesotheliomas projected for males and females to the year 2050.

50 years. The decline is a consequence of the reduction in asbestos use in manufacturing and tightening of workplace exposure limits initially imposed in 1971 by OSHA. Weill et al. (2004) argue that the increase in male MM in the United States was influenced by exposure to amphibole asbestos (amosite and crocidolite) in manufacturing. Amphibole use in US industry was introduced in the early 1930s for shipbuilding among other heat insulation applications and peaked around 1960.

In the United States, the MM epidemic principally reflects disease in males who were exposed to high levels of airborne amphibole asbestos in their jobs. Female trends in the United States suggest that sources such as domestic and environmental exposure, with few notable exceptions are, on average, too low to be major concerns. Therefore, the outlook for MM in the United States during the 21st century should follow the pattern described in Figure 16.2.

The future pattern for asbestos-associated LC and asbestosis should follow the MM trend, but should decrease at a faster rate. In the United States, there is no historical trend data for asbestos-associated LC because, as discussed earlier, asbestos-associated LC cannot be separately identified. Nevertheless, two facts support a rapid decline for asbestos-associated LC. First, the rate of asbestos-associated LC is assessed as an increment to background LC, which is dominated by smokers. In this country, male smoking and the male LC rate are declining. The reduction in the background LC rate for men implies a reduction in the asbestos-associated LC rate for men. Second, it is believed to require higher cumulative asbestos exposures than MM (Chapter 7). The reduction in occupational exposure to asbestos starting in the early 1970s makes it much less likely that many surviving men would have had sufficient cumulative exposure to induce LC. For women, the smoking rate and background LC rate are not declining as rapidly as for men. However, women generally did not experience the types of occupational exposures that would be sufficient to increase the risk of LC.

Asbestosis data collected in the United States by the National Center for Health Statistics (NCHS) addresses asbestosis mortality. The data indicate approximately 1.5×10^3 deaths due to asbestosis in 2002, slightly over the 2001 total (CDC-HUS, 2004).

Although there may be many more cases of asbestosis, mortality data will not reveal the number because asbestosis may not be the cause of death for many cases.[7] Asbestosis requires a high cumulative exposure, at least 25–100 f/mL-yrs. Few, if any, of the surviving male former asbestos industry workers and no females would have experienced this level of exposure. Therefore, the number of asbestosis cases in the United States should decline much faster than the number of asbestos-associated LC (Chapter 7).

In summary, asbestos-associated disease in the United States is declining. The slowest decline will be MM which should reach its background rate around the year 2050. The current regulatory structure in the United States and voluntary reductions in asbestos use have been effective over the past 30 years in reducing asbestos-associated diseases, and will continue to be effective in the future.

Canada

The population characteristics of asbestos-associated disease in Canada are best described by considering the Provinces Quebec and Ontario, separately from the remainder of the country. Quebec is unique because it is the home of the Canadian mining industry, one of the principal producers of chrysotile. In the 1970s, the mines shipped approximately 1×10^6 tons of chrysotile asbestos. In the year 2000, shipments totaled 3.5×10^5 tons, which was exceeded only by Russia and China.

McDonald and McDonald (1980) estimated MM incidence separately for men and women for each of the three areas based on data for 1966–1975. The MM incidence rates per million males in the Province of Quebec, Ontario, and the rest of Canada were 4.9, 2.6, and 2.2 respectively; for women the rates were 2.2, 1.1, and 0.7. The annual number of male cases increased during the 9-year period; the annual number of female cases remained "fairly steady at a much lower level." Forty-four percent of the male cases and 50% of female cases occurred in the Province of Quebec.

In July 2004, the Ministry of Health and Human Services and the National Institute of Public Health of Quebec published its review of epidemiological data on MM, LC, and asbestosis in Quebec. It found the average annual incidence rate for male MM in Quebec for the period 1982–1996 to be 14.9 per million population; the rate for females was 3.2 per million. This male rate is three times the average rate for 1966–1975. The Committee reported an average annual growth rate for men of 5% for the years 1982–1996. The female rate for 1982–1996 was 1.5 times the rate for 1966–1975. The average annual growth rate for women for the years 1982–1996 did not achieve a statistically significant trend.

The cohort of males born between 1930 and 1939 had higher cancer rates than other cohorts of Quebec men. It also estimated a reduced risk among cohorts born after 1940 and suggested a peak in MM cases in the year 2010. Because the men in these groups are still young, the projection has a high degree of uncertainty. Quebec men and women have a significantly higher rate of MM than residents in the rest of Canada. As considered in Chapters 1 and 8, asbestiform tremolite in the Quebec ore bodies accounts for the disease which occurs almost exclusively in miners and, to a lesser extent, millers in the Province of Quebec.

---

7 Stallard et al. tabulated the number of asbestosis claims filed by former employees of the Johns-Manville Corporation to be approximately 43 000 for 1995 through 1999 (Stallard et al., 2004). But these are claims, not confirmed asbestosis cases. Moreover, 50% of asbestosis claims against Johns-Manville could not be confirmed as actual asbestosis cases (Carroll et al., 2002).

United Kingdom

In the United Kingdom, the Health and Safety Executive has maintained a register since 1968 of MM deaths mentioned on death certificates. Peto et al. (1995) used these data for the years 1968 through 1991 to analyze trends in MM incidence for males aged 20–89. The historical data indicated 154 MM deaths in 1968, increasing to 1000 in 1991. The projections showed a continuing increase to a peak in 2020 at between 2700 and 3300 deaths. The authors discussed a possible diagnostic trend that would have inflated the annual rate of increase. Adjusting for one proposed characterization of the diagnostic trend, the peak year was reestimated to be 2010 and the peak number of MM projected at 1300. In an update of the 1995 study, Hodgson et al. (2005) projected the peak of MM deaths 10 years earlier than suggested in the previous study. Between 1950 and 2450 MM deaths per year are projected to occur between 2011 and 2015, (at least 10 years later than the peak in the United States). A rapid decline will follow. This result is unexpected because heavy occupational exposure occurred in both countries in ship-yards, especially during World War II, from 1940 to 1945. Peto et al. (1995) analyzed job categories in the United Kingdom and concluded that the highest exposures were in the construction trades (eg, plumbers, gas fitters, carpenters, and electricians) during the 1970s. In the United States, the highest exposures occurred between the 1930s and the 1960s. Weill and Hughes (1995) offer an explanation for the different patterns by considering the use of amphibole versus chrysotile asbestos in the two countries. They show that the amount of amphibole asbestos used in the United States through 1969 exceeds the amount used in the United Kingdom for the same time-period, but after 1969 the trend reversed. These authors note the following: the total amount of amphibole asbestos used in the United Kingdom exceeded the amount used in the United States; the population of the United Kingdom was about 25% of the US population; and amphibole asbestos is significantly more potent as a cause of MM than chrysotile (if chrysotile is a cause at all), the asbestos fiber-type most widely used in commercial applications. On the basis of these considerations, Weill and Hughes (1995) propose the amphibole-to-chrysotile exposure difference between the United Kingdom and the United States as the explanation for the different disease trends. The Health and Safety Executive (2004) projects total male MM in the United Kingdom for the period 2002 through 2050 to be 5.5×10^4. For the United States, Price and Ware project approximately 7.1×10^4 male MM for roughly the same period.

Concerning women, Peto et al. (1995) did not attempt projections because there were too few deaths at younger ages to make stable predictions. The MM death rates in British women for 1968–1971 were similar to the incidence rates in Los Angeles in the 1970s for both men and women with no suspected asbestos exposure (which suggest a spontaneous background risk unrelated to asbestos). Peto and coauthors (1999) allow, however, that some cases in both sexes may be due to environmental exposure unrelated to occupation.

Regulations in the United Kingdom banning products containing asbestos became effective in 2005, ensuring a continuing downward trend in diseases beyond the 2011–2015 peak.

Western Europe

For most countries in western Europe, the only data that reflect MM are death rates for cancer of the pleura. The historical ratio of mesothelioma cases from mesothelioma registers and mortality from pleural cancer often varies from the ideal value of 1:1.

In the United States based on ICD-10 coding the ratio was 1.2:1 (Pinheiro et al., 2004); in the United Kingdom, the ratio was 1.6:1; in France the ratio was at least 1:1, which also would be expected for other European countries (Peto et al., 1999). Peto et al. (1995) and La Vecchia et al. (2000) used male pleural cancer mortality data from the World Health Organization database for 1970 through 1994 to analyze trends in MM for the United Kingdom and six other European countries—France, Germany, Italy, the Netherlands, Switzerland, and Hungary.

The analysis indicated the trends for the six countries were similar to the trend in the United Kingdom. Specifically, age-standardized mortality rates for pleural cancer were increasing from 1970 through 1994. Males born between 1940 and 1950 had the highest risk of pleural cancer, and mortality was projected to peak around the year 2020. The total number of male pleural cancer deaths for Western Europe between 1995 and 2020 would be approximately 250 000.

The projections based on WHO data through 1994 have now been shown to overstate the number of cancers. Analyses of WHO data through 1999 for France, Germany, and Italy indicate that the age-standardized rates have stabilized and the number of pleural cancers projected for 1995–1999, although higher than the number of cancers in the 1990–1994 time frame, were too high by percentages ranging from 2% to 11% (Pelucchi et al., 2004). These findings support the hypothesis that the rising trend in male deaths from MM should level off in the near future. They suggest as one reason for the overestimation an assumption in their original work that the mortality rate for the 1950 birth cohort was the same as the rate for the 1945 cohort, which had the highest historical rate. It now appears that the 1945 cohort was a turning point toward lower rates. The pattern of birth cohort rates is not sufficient to explain the projection errors, but factors such as fiber-type, duration of exposure, and time since exposure occurred, which vary across individuals and may vary on average across countries, also affect the future number of MM. It appears that the number of asbestos-related deaths for Western Europe will fall short of the previously projected 250 000 based on data through 1994 (Pelucchi et al., 2004).

Australia

Whereas the characteristics of asbestos exposure and MM incidence in the United States and United Kingdom indicate that the majority of asbestos-associated disease was from occupational exposures, in Australia, the risk reflects both occupational and environmental exposure (Leigh and Driscoll, 2003). The high rate of MM in Australia is a consequence of an active asbestos mining industry for 100 years and a high level of per capita consumption of asbestos. Chrysotile and amphibole asbestos were mined in Australia. Starting in 1937, crocidolite mining at Wittenoom, Western Australia dominated production until the mine was closed in 1966. On the basis of the Australian Mesothelioma Surveillance Program, which began compiling data in 1980, 6349 cases have been identified through the end of 2001. An analysis of 530 of these cases indicates that the most common exposures were repair and maintenance of asbestos materials (18%), shipbuilding (11%), asbestos-cement production (7%), asbestos-cement use (7%), railways (6%), Wittenoom crocidolite mining/milling (6%), insulation manufacture/installation (4%), wharf laboring (3%), power station work (3%), boiler making (2%), paraoccupational, hobby, and environmental (15%).

During the final 20 years of the 20th century, Australia had the world's highest reported incidence of MM. In 1999, the male rate for ages 20 or older was 53.3 per million; the female rate was 10.2 per million. For comparison, the corresponding US rates in 2001 were approximately 14 and 4 per million. The trend in total cases has been increasing for men over the full period of data collection from 1980 to 2001 and also for women but at a lower rate. Among men, 94% of the MM cases were pleural; 5% were peritoneal. Among women, the percentages were 86% and 14%, respectively. In 2001, the annual number of male cases was approximately 555 and the number of female cases 123. Age-specific incidence patterns for males are similar to the patterns in the United States. In recent years, the "Age 80+" category has been increasing whereas all other age categories have been flat or decreasing. This pattern is a likely reflection of exposure controls introduced in the 1970s. An analysis of a subset of 530 cases indicated that 55% had mixed amphibole-chrysotile exposures, 13% amphibole only, 7% amphibole plus possible chrysotile, 6% chrysotile with possible amphibole, 4% chrysotile only, and 15% unknown.

Overall, the Australian historical high rates of MM are not unexpected due to widespread environmental exposures to high levels of amphibole asbestos including crocidolite. Leigh and Driscoll (2003) projected a peak in MM cases in 2010. Approximately 1.1×10^4 more cases are expected by 2020 in addition to the 700 cases reported through 2001.

Leigh's analysis is based on an extrapolation of MM cases projected by Berry (1991) for workers formerly employed in Wittenoom. Leigh assumed that Wittenoom, which is located in Western Australia, has produced 5% of all Australian cases. Berry provided a range for the number of Wittenoom cases for the years 1987–2020: 250, 500, and 680. Leigh's projection for all of Australia employed a projection of approximately 600 for the Wittenoom workers. On the basis of more recent data through 2000, Berry (1991) revised his Wittenoom projection for 2001 through 2020 to 110 new MM cases. Also, the data for the year 2000 indicate that MM cases among former mine employees account for 3.95% of Australian MM cases, not 5%, a figure that was previously used by Leigh. Employing Leigh's projection approach, the expected number of MM in Australia for the period 2001–2020 would be 2785 (=110/0.0395), not 1.1×10^4.[8]

Hansen et al. (1998) studied former residents of Wittenoom who lived there between 1943 and 1993 for at least 1 month, the years of crocidolite mining, but were not employed in the industry. This cohort of former residents of Wittenoom was used to analyze the relationship between nonoccupational exposure to asbestos and MM. On the basis of MM cases, the age-standardized incidence of MM was approximately equal for males and females at 260 per million. This rate is remarkably high for an environmentally exposed cohort even when compared to rates for all of Australia of 53.3 per million for males and 10.2 per million for females.[9] But this Wittenoom cohort experienced remarkable exposures. The fiber-type was crocidolite, the most potent for MM among the three commercial fiber-types of asbestos, and the environmental exposure levels were much higher than typically expected for environmental exposures. According to Hansen et al. (1998), the majority of cases had cumulative exposures greater than 7 f/mL-yrs and a third had cumulative exposures greater than 20 f/mL-yrs.

Hansen's analysis investigated risk factors for this environmentally exposed cohort. The variables "length of stay in Wittenoom" and "cumulative asbestos exposure" were

8 Berry's results indicate that earlier projections of mesothelioma for Australia were overstated. Therefore, Australia is similar to the United Kingdom and Western Europe in this respect. Berry identified one qualification for the updated projection for Wittenoom, specifically that some portion of the reduction for former ABA workers may have been due to an intervention, a beta carotene and retinol trial, intended to reduce the incidence of mesothelioma and other cancers. However, Berry states that the effect of the trial was minimal, possibly 10 cases between 1990 and 2000. Accounting for the 10 cases, the projected number of mesotheliomas for Australia between 2001 and 2020 would be 3038.

9 The latter rates are annual rates for 1999.

significant considerations. The environmental exposure at Wittenoom was unique and the observations should not be used to extrapolate the consequences of environmental exposures in other circumstances or countries.

South Africa

Crocidolite asbestos deposits were discovered in South Africa in the early 1800s and mining began in 1893. The demand for crocidolite from South Africa increased enormously during World War II. It is reasonable to conclude that both mining and environmental exposures were substantial prior to, and including, this time-period. In 1998, the government of South Africa convened a summit to identify areas of concern and to explore strategies for solving problems related to asbestos and its effects on health. A report by the Deputy Minister of Environmental Affairs in South Africa stated that asbestos would no longer be mined in South Africa as of February 2001 and rehabilitation of the mines...was in progress. On the basis of the available information, it is impossible to project a trend, peak, or total numbers of cases of MM or other asbestos-related diseases that have occurred. It appears, however, that environmental exposure still occurs and current concerns about the number of asbestosis cases suggest that environmental exposures were, at least in the past, heavy. The pattern of asbestos-associated diseases in South Africa during the 21st century will depend on how quickly the problems are resolved and solutions implemented.[10]

Russia

Russia[11] today is a major producer of chrysotile asbestos—currently three operating mills have a capacity of 9×10^5 tons per year. In 2001, its chrysotile mining and milling operations produced 7.5×10^5 tons (approximately 50% of worldwide production). Chrysotile was discovered near Asbest City in the Sverdlovsk region in the late 1800s and by 1889, twenty-four thousand tons of chrysotile asbestos had been produced. Analyses of the chrysotile ore indicate that there are few fibrous impurities. Although no asbestiform tremolite has been identified in the raw chrysotile, traces of tremolite have been found in environmental air samples.

Health monitoring of workers in the largest chrysotile mining and milling complex in the world, was initiated in 1946. Uncontrolled exposures appear to have been associated with high incidences of asbestosis and LC, but MM was rare among these workers. Shcherbakov et al. (2001) show a declining trend in asbestosis associated with a decreasing trend in dust levels due to modernization and industrial hygiene practices. The percentage of new asbestosis cases in the late 1940s approached 30%, but has dipped to approximately 0.5% based on data for 1994. For LC, the relative risk (RR) for males was reported as 4.1 for the period 1948–1967; the RR decreased to 1.5 for the period 1987–1991. For females, the RR decreased from 3.4 to 1.2.

Shcherbakov et al. (2001) estimated MM rates for the Sverdlosk region and its localities. For 10 years during the 1970s, they reported an average annual MM rate of 2.4 per million. For Asbest City, the center of the asbestos mining industry, seven cases occurred during

10 The description of early mining operations in South Africa is based on Wagner et al. (1960) and http://www.asosh.org/TopicSpecific/asbestos.htm and http://www.pmg.org.za/viewminute.php?id=2370
11 This section relies on *The Health Effects of Mining and Milling Chrysotile: The Russian Experience*, Shcherbakov et al., Canadian Mineralogist, Special Publication 5 (2001).

the 5 years from 1978 to 1982, which, based on a population of 1.14×10^5, is an average annual MM rate of 12.3 per million. Moving forward in time, the authors present results for 41 cases diagnosed over the 16 years from 1981 to 1996. The average annual MM rate based on these data is 0.5 cases per million. Five cases were miners and millers, one was from commerce, 11 from occupations with no recognized asbestos exposure, 10 were from other occupations where the workers may have been exposed to asbestos, and 14 could not be classified. Thus, mining and milling is not the only occupation associated with a rise in MM rates in Sverdlosk. However, in the absence of information about numbers of workers in these various occupations the relative importance of occupation cannot be evaluated.

The MM data described above suggest a downward trend over time both for the Sverdlosk region and for Asbest City. Also, data indicate a reduction in asbestosis and LC for the region.

Sweden

Using data from the Swedish Cancer Registry covering years 1961–2000, Hemminki and Li (2003a,b) analyzed the age-adjusted pattern of MM in Sweden. The pattern shows an increase for males beginning in the early 1970s and a leveling-off in the early 1990s (Hemminki and Li, 2003a,b; Hillerdal, 2004). The total number of MM cases was 2×10^3 up to the year 2000 and is continuing at about 20 per year. The pattern for females appears to have increased slightly starting around 1976 and has remained relatively constant since that time.

Asbestos importation and use began to increase in Sweden following World War II and peaked in the 1970–1974 time-period. Most of the asbestos used in Sweden was chrysotile from Canada, although crocidolite from South Africa and anthophyllite from Finland also were used. Sweden banned asbestos in 1976. The principal occupationally exposed groups were construction workers, asbestos-cement plant workers, and shipyard workers. MM incidence became level or slightly reduced in Sweden only 17 years after asbestos use in industry was banned (Hemminki and Li, 2003a). This may be an indication that the incidence of MM cases in Europe may begin to decline sooner than the 2020–2030 time frame typically projected as the peak (which in turn suggests the possibility that the projection of 2.5×10^5 cases in Western Europe is much too high).

Hemminki and Li (2003b) addressed MM risk associated with environmental exposure in Sweden. They found the MM standard incidence rate (SIR) for males in urban areas who were thought to have had no occupational exposure to asbestos to be 2.6 times the SIR for rural farmers. (Men with asbestos-related jobs had a SIR that was six times the rate for farmers). On the basis of these results, it can be concluded that typical urban environmental exposure to asbestos is a significant risk factor for MM in Sweden. However, urban women with the same environmental exposure have an SIR that is less than the urban male SIR by a factor of five. This difference between urban male and female environmental exposures is puzzling and has not been satisfactorily explained. However, urban men are likely to have worked in other jobs that had a higher level of asbestos exposure than the job they were in at the time the survey was taken (Jockel, 2003). Therefore, the discrepancy between MM risks for urban men relative to rural farmers could be explained by their respective levels of occupational exposure.

Norway

Norway began importing asbestos in 1920. Imports increased after World War II and peaked at an average of 600 tons per year in the 1970s. The asbestos was used in the manufacture of cement products beginning in 1942 and thermal insulation for ships and industry. Ulvestad et al. (2003) analyzed data collected in the Cancer Registry of Norway to determine MM incidence for males and females by 5-year intervals from 1965 through 1999. Age-adjusted incidence rates increased during this time interval; in males, the rate increased from 4.3 to 26.1 per million; the female rate increased from 1.4 to 4.3 per million with most of the increase coming after 1990. Looking to the future, Ulvestad et al. (2003) point out *cohort-specific risks* showing that exposed populations born up to 1935 had an increased risk, which *stabilized* thereafter. The latency period for the onset of MM for these birth cohorts, coupled with declining occupational use of asbestos, will have their "greatest effects on the MM rates" around 2010 and the following two decades.

Denmark

Kjaergaard and Andersson (2000) used data for the 1.9×10^3 cases of MM reported during 1943–1993 to the Danish Cancer Registry to describe current MM incidence rates for males and project future rates. From 1973 forward, the age-adjusted MM incidence rates increased to a peak of approximately 14 per million in the late 1980s and then began to decline; in contrast, the female rates were constant during this time-period at an average of 3 per million. The authors project a peak in male MM cases in or around year 2015 at 93 cases among men born before 1955.[12]

Italy

Between 1969 and 1994, mortality due to pleural malignant tumors increased by 15% every 5 years with 500–900 deaths occurring each year (Degiovanni et al., 2004; Gorini et al., 2002).[13] The principal sources of exposure were the shipbuilding, cement, and textile industries. (eg, industries in Casale Monferrato) A mixture of chrysotile and crocidolite asbestos apparently was used. Pelucchi et al. (2004) analyzed the change in the age-standardized pleural cancer rate in three Western European countries including Italy for 1990–1994 versus 1995–1999. Previous projections prepared by Peto et al. (1999; based on a statistical model derived from historical data) were believed to be too high; and the pleural cancer mortality rate had stabilized.

Environmental and domestic exposures as a cause of MM were investigated by Magnani et al. (2001) in Casale Monferrato, which is the former location of Italy's largest asbestos-cement factory. It produced cement pipe and other asbestos-cement products from a mixture of chrysotile and crocidolite asbestos, operating from 1907 to 1985. In a population-based case-control study, Magnani et al. (2001) identified residents with MM over the period 1987–1993. Environmental air samples were collected shortly before the factory shut down in 1985, but no environmental measurements were available from the approximately 70 years of maximum production. The measurements for the mid-1980s generally indicated a range of airborne asbestos levels from 0.001 to 0.011 f/mL.

---

12 The authors state that the model used for the projections was not a good fit to the data, but the peak at 10–15 years nevertheless is reasonable.

13 The number of deaths due to pleural malignant tumors may differ from the number of deaths due to mesothelioma. Gorini et al. (2002) calculated the ratio of male pleural malignant mesothelioma mortality to pleural cancer deaths in Tuscany for the years 1994–1999 equal to 0.73:1. An national mesothelioma registry that will lead to more reliable projections of mesothelioma in the future was initiated in Italy in 1997 (Nesti et al., 2004).

Odds ratios calculated to assess sources of exposure were adjusted for occupational exposure, which not surprisingly was the strongest risk factor. The odds ratios for residential exposure decreased with distance from the cement plant, but remained high indicating other sources of airborne asbestos. The analysis confirmed the association between MM and environmental asbestos exposure, with a greater risk factor than domestic exposure. Given that the pleural cancer rate in Italy has stabilized (Pelucchi et al., 2004) and the cement plant has not operated for more than 15 years, it is unlikely that environmental exposure will contribute to asbestos-associated diseases in the future.

Japan

Japan began importing asbestos in the 1880s, and during World War II developed asbestos mines domestically as well as in Korea and China (Furuya et al., 2003). Thus, Japan is similar to other industrialized countries where asbestos use began early in the 20th century, peaked in the 1970s, and continued until the beginning of the 21st century. Chrysotile is the only type of asbestos that is still imported; crocidolite asbestos imports halted in 1987 and amosite in 1992. Japan banned crocidolite and amosite in 1995. Imports of chrysotile in 2003 represented less than one quarter of the total in the 1970s.

Most asbestos in Japan was used in construction products; about 3% was used in friction materials. Since the 1950s Japan relied on *controlled use* policies enforced under Labor Standards and Industrial Health Laws. In 1988 specific levels were defined—0.2 f/mL for crocidolite, and 2 f/mL for other asbestos types. Japan also has an air pollution control law, revised in 1989 to classify asbestos as a *specified dust* and established 10 f/mL for environmental air concentrations around asbestos manufacturing facilities. After an earthquake in 1996, the law was clarified to regulate the removal of sprayed asbestos (which had been banned for installation since 1995).

Morinaga et al. (2001) conducted a review of asbestos-related LC and MM cases in Japan. They note that due to high smoking rates in Japan (over 50%), "lung cancer deaths caused by the interaction between smoking and asbestos exposure will be continuing." Although pleural mesothelioma in Japan is increasing, Morinaga notes that less asbestos exposure in the future due to regulations will help limit deaths. Japanese Ministry of Health, Labor and Welfare monitoring of diseases, as outlined by Furuya et al. 2003, should help to assess how regulations affect asbestos-associated diseases.

Korea

Korea represents a bridge between industrialized and developing countries. Asbestos use started in the 1920s, later than in most industrialized countries. By the end of World War II, mining had all but stopped until the 1960s when the asbestos-cement industry was established. Mining continued until the mid-1980s. The asbestos textile and friction products industries started in the 1970s fueling asbestos imports that peaked at over 9×10^4 tons in 1992. Korea banned the use of crocidolite and amosite in 1997, and limited occupational chrysotile exposure to 0.1 f/mL in 2003.

Data on asbestos-related diseases in Korea is limited; a surveillance system was not in place until the 1980s, with a more systematic approach initiated 10 years later (Paek, 2003). MM incidence in Korea has increased steadily over the past 20 years. LC cases have tripled since the 1980s, but only a few cases were considered to be occupational in origin. Paek (2003) estimated that Korea had at least 7000 asbestos workers, with about

8% exposed for more than 20 years. These workers are employed in subway renovations (Yu et al., 2004), as well as the manufacturing of friction products and textiles for the shipbuilding and the automobile industry. Given current trends and the time-pattern of increased consumption, Paek (2003) predicts that asbestos disease will dramatically increase in Korea in the near future. This forecast is similar to projections for other developing nations.

Developing Countries

At the beginning of the 21st century, the vast majority of asbestos production and consumption has shifted from industrialized countries to those classified as *developing*. Table 16.1 displays asbestos production and consumption data for the year 2000. With

Table 16.1 Worldwide Raw Asbestos Production, Imports, Exports, and Consumption for Major Production and Consumption Countries—2000

Country	Production	Imports	Exports	Consumption
Argentina	254	2079	—	2333
Australia	—	1246	—	1246
Azerbaijan	—	8252	—	8252
Belarus	—	25301	65	25236
Brazil	209332	35491	63134	181689
Canada	320000	125	315326	4799
Chile	—	1460	—	1460
China	350000	72004	11814	410190
Colombia	—	12189	—	12189
Ecuador	—	4393	—	4393
ElSalvador	—	1678	—	1678
France	—	16	46	–30
Germany	—	189	—	189
Greece	—	501	8946	–8445
Hungary	—	3558	—	3558
India	14516	110000	—	124516
Indonesia	—	54891	—	54891
Iran	2000	—	—	2000
Ireland	—	1007	—	1007
Italy	—	87	—	87
Japan	—	98595	—	98595
Kazakhstan	178400	—	174000	4400
Korea (South)	—	28972	—	28972
Kyrgyzstan	—	17307	—	17307
Latvia	—	857	—	857
Lithuania	—	1356	643	713
Mexico	—	26880	—	26880
Oman	—	2347	—	2347
Pakistan	—	4160	—	4160
Panama	—	1280	—	1280

continued

Table 16.1 Continued

Country	Production	Imports	Exports	Consumption
Poland	—	19	14	5
Portugal	—	4710	—	4710
Romania	—	10244	—	10244
Russia	752000	27259	332417	446842
S. Africa	18910	10217	16627	12500
Saudi Arabia	—	—	9733	−9733
Senegal	—	1784	—	1784
Spain	—	15568	126	15442
Swaziland	12690	—	10000	2690
Taiwan	—	5421	—	5421
Thailand	—	120563	—	120563
Turkey	—	19455	—	19455
United States	5260	14637	18765	1132
United Kingdom	—	246	2	244
Uruguay	—	809	—	809
Venezuela	—	2727	—	2727
Yugoslavia	563	607	—	1170
Zimbabwe	151954	—	140000	11954

Data table adapted from British Geological Survey, World Mineral Statistics 1996–2000. Her Majesty's Stationery Office, 2002, London, pp. 25–28. published in Virta, USGS "Worldwide Asbestos Supply and Consumption Trends from 1900–2000" Confirmed with British Geological Survey, European Mineral Statistics 1998–2002: Her Majesty's Stationery Office, 2003, London.

the exception of Canada, a major producer of chrysotile, and Japan, a consumer of large amounts of asbestos, all other large producers and consumers are developing countries. While industrialized countries in Western Europe currently are approaching peak incidence rates of MM, most developing countries in Africa, Central and South America, and Asia, where asbestos is used, still have low rates (Ulvestad et al., 2003). Ladou (2004) refers to a *shift* in asbestos production and use from industrialized countries to developing countries, a trend likely to translate into increasing asbestos-associated disease rates in developing countries during the 21st century.

However, the pattern may be somewhat muted relative to the historic patterns in industrialized countries for two reasons. First, at the beginning of the 21st century, the difference in disease potential between chrysotile and amphibole asbestos was recognized, and the production or use of amphiboles in many countries is limited or banned. Second, developing countries have access to information about industrial hygiene practices for asbestos. Either they are implementing regulations or are influenced by regulations from developed nations that limit asbestos imports, exports, and consumption (WTO, 2000). Regulations are being established in developing countries at a more rapid pace than in industrialized countries during the 20th century. Thus, the peak and decline in asbestos-associated diseases in developing countries should be abbreviated relative to the pattern in the industrialized countries.

India

India has become one of the major countries using asbestos today (Joshi and Gupta, 2004). Native Indian asbestos primarily is of three mineral types—amosite and two varieties of anthophyllite. As of 2003, India's annual consumption of asbestos was approximately 1×10^5 metric tons, although only a fifth of that is produced in India. The remainder is met through imports, mainly chrysotile from Canada. Over the last 10 years, Indian imports of asbestos have risen in response to consumption demands and declining domestic production.

In developing countries including India, data for asbestos-associated diseases is sketchy due to poor occupational health and safety systems and difficulties of disease detection (Joshi and Gupta, 2004). Aside from finances and knowledgeable health and safety experts being in short supply, development and progress take priority often over worker safety. Experts that are investigating India's asbestos health issues have tried to implement stricter regulations or even a ban, but viewed as a potential hindrance to progress, neither has occurred. Epidemiological studies conducted by the Indian National Institute of Occupational Health found "lung impairment and radiological abnormalities in asbestos milling workers (55%) and miners (20%)." Given latency times and India's still developing asbestos industry and regulatory framework, the time-pattern for disease rates is uncertain. However, Joshi and Gupta indicate that disease rates in India will continue to increase through 2010 and 2020.

China

China (where chrysotile asbestos has been used and mined for over 60 years) was second in worldwide production in 2000 (Shiqu et al., 1990; Table 16.1). Amphibole asbestos, including tremolite, is also mined in China. A small amount of crocidolite reportedly was used in a Shanghai asbestos factory in the 1960s.

Over 4×10^3 cases of asbestosis were reported between 1949 and 1986 (Cai et al., 2001). The prevalence of asbestosis is believed to have decreased after 1980 due to improved working conditions. Currently, there is no organization in China that summarizes incidence data for purposes of projecting disease trends (Cai et al., 2001; Shiqu et al., 1990).

In the 1980s, working conditions improved in asbestos processing industries. New machinery and improved dust control in mines and factories since the 1980s may lead to better air quality and decreased asbestos exposure. The prevalence of asbestosis decreased in the 1980s to less than 10% of the previously higher levels. Very little data has been gathered that might indicate trends in MM, but disease incidence in China apparently has not peaked.

Thailand

As asbestos use in industrialized nations continues to decline, developing countries such as Thailand have become major importers of asbestos for over 30 years (Joshi and Gupta, 2003). There is no domestic production in Thailand. Current levels of use in Asia range from 0 in Singapore to 1.9 kg/capita/yr in Thailand, which has followed an increasing trend over the past few years (Siriruttanapruk, 2003; Takahashi and Karjalainen, 2003). Thailand has banned crocidolite and amosite asbestos, but not chrysotile. Current occupational exposure limits are 5 f/mL, but a reduction to 0.5 f/mL has been proposed (Takahashi and Karjalainen, 2003).

In 2001, 17 asbestos factories employ over 1700 workers. Asbestosis is among eight occupational diseases "under an active health surveillance scheme" run by the government for the past 10 years, but little data are available. Thailand's government expects the use of asbestos to increase and predicts disease incidence to be high in the near future (Takahashi and Karjalainen, 2003).

Brazil

Brazil is one of the five largest producers of asbestos worldwide and is a major consumer and exporter as well. In 2000, Brazil mined approximately 2.1×10^5 tons and exported 6.3×10^4 tons (Table 16.1). Consumption and manufacture of asbestos-containing products were ongoing in Brazil until the 1980s without any regulation or control of occupational and environmental exposures. During the 1990s Brazil signed a voluntary agreement with the Canadian Asbestos Industry stipulating that companies that fail to use asbestos *safely* will have their supplies terminated (Cauchon, 1999). In 1991, the workplace limit in Brazil was 4 f/mL, and the current workplace limit is 0.4 f/mL.

Brazil has no national system for recording disease or occupational deaths. In 1996, an epidemiological study was conducted in a 3500-worker cement plant. The study found a high rate of asbestos-associated health complications, including asbestosis (Giannasi, 2003). More comprehensive studies (Pinheiro et al., 2003) covered MM mortality from 1979 to 2000 but health records were not found to be an accurate accounting of the cause of death (34% were misclassified). Algranti et al. (2001a,b) studied LC among asbestos workers and found the trends for male mortality to be similar to United States. The author could not adequately separate the effect of asbestos exposure from smoking. Given Brazil's historical asbestos production pattern, it appears to be one of the developing countries where asbestos-associated disease rates have not yet peaked.

Other Developing Countries

A number of other developing countries are notable producers or consumers of asbestos, but maintain little information about diseases among their workers or members of the general populations. Kazakhstan and Zimbabwe are major producers of asbestos. In the year 2000, Kazakhstan mined approximately 1.8×10^5 tons and Zimbabwe produced approximately 1.5×10^5 tons (Table 16.1). These countries export almost all of the asbestos they produce. Kazakhstan and three other developing nations, China, Brazil, and Zimbabwe, combined with Canada, export roughly 74% of the world's chrysotile.

Mexico's asbestos workforce numbered approximately 1.2×10^4 in the year 2000 (Aguilar-Madrid et al., 2003). From 1979 through 2000, there were almost 800 deaths attributable to MM. No trends have been developed from these data, but Mexico's experience with asbestos-associated diseases is only now beginning. Apparently, some of the MM cases may have been a result of environmental exposure because many of Mexico's asbestos manufacturing facilities are located in metropolitan areas. Data on rates of asbestos-associated diseases in Kazakhstan, Zimbabwe, Indonesia, and Argentina are not sufficiently developed for analyzing trends.

Indonesia is a major importer of asbestos (Table 16.1) and its current consumption is increasing (Takahashi and Karjalainen, 2003). Information on occupational exposure limits in Indonesia is not available. However, even with exposure limits, the health consequences would be uncertain because Indonesia, "in contrast to other [Asian] countries, does not have specific schemes of medical follow-up" and does not have asbestos-related disease compensation information (Takahashi and Karjalainen, 2003). Given Indonesia's pattern of asbestos importation and use, and the lack of regulations and health measurement, it appears to be still another developing country where asbestos-associated disease rates have not yet peaked.

In Zimbabwe, asbestos is among a group of natural resources considered vital to economic recovery. However, over the past year, Zimbabwe has "seriously considered" banning the mineral (Financial Gazette-Zimbabwe, 2004; PMG, 2003). The asbestos industry booms in Zimbabwe, producing around 1.3×10^5 tons of asbestos for foreign exchange per year (Virta USGS, 2003a,b). Zimbabwe mines chrysotile, 93% of which is exported to over 50 countries worldwide (*Herald*-Harare, 2003). Domestically, a large part of the Zimbabwean population uses asbestos in roofing materials, cement, and other construction products. The local production industry employees 7×10^3 direct workers and 1.2×10^5 workers who indirectly deal with asbestos products (*Herald*-Harare, 2003).

Although the data are limited, the few health studies of Zimbabwe's asbestos industry have found MM and asbestos-associated diseases among miners and workers (Cullen and Baloyi, 1991). Given Zimbabwe's pattern of asbestos mining, it appears to be among the developing countries where asbestos-associated disease rates have not yet peaked.

Asbestos of several types was mined and used in Argentina from the 1960s until it was banned in 2002. The asbestos produced at mines included anthophyllite and chrysotile. No data on exposure or disease have been reported. Limits on asbestos exposure were not established until the early 1990s (Rodriguez, 2004).

Lung Cancer and Asbestosis

We have not attempted to quantify the population patterns of asbestos-associated LC or asbestosis historically or during the 21st century because population data for these diseases either are nonexistent or of highly uncertain accuracy. LC cases attributable to asbestos exposure are difficult to project because the principal cause of LC is smoking and many workers who were exposed to occupational levels of asbestos were smokers. Separating asbestos-associated LC cases from the smoking-dominated background LC cases has proved to be difficult. Although we cannot enumerate the number of asbestos-associated LC, we can project that the incidence in industrialized countries will decline rapidly for the following reasons. First, the number of survivors from the birth cohorts that would have experienced the high-level occupational exposures that occurred before the 1970s is small and declining. Second, workplace exposures for individuals who began work after the 1970s are relatively low and are going downward. Third, the background LC rate is falling. Taken together, these factors suggest that asbestos-associated LC will not be a health issue in the 21st century, although disease related to smoking will not abate.

Asbestosis mortality, but not incidence, is more readily counted than asbestos-associated LC. The incidence of asbestosis may be greater than the number of deaths, but there are no national surveillance systems for asbestosis and many asbestotics have a cause of death other than asbestosis. Cases in industrialized countries will drop off quickly principally because asbestosis requires heavy cumulative exposures (Churg and Green, 1998). Given the current worldwide regulatory environment, it is almost certain that future cumulative exposures in industrialized countries will not approach these levels. Therefore, the incidence of asbestosis should not increase except when exposures in developing countries have recently been high, or may continue to be high into the early part of the 21st century.

Summary

Increases in the incidence of asbestos-associated diseases in the industrialized world during the 20th century were a consequence of heavy occupational exposure mostly occurring before the early 1970s. Industrialized countries established asbestos exposure limits or tightened existing limits during the 1970s. However, due to their long latency periods, disease incidence trends in these countries will not reach their peaks until early in the 21st century.

At the beginning of the 21st century, asbestos production and consumption has shifted from industrialized countries to developing countries. This is likely to translate into increasing disease rates in developing countries during the 21st century.

However, the pattern of asbestos-associated diseases in developing countries may be somewhat muted relative to the historic patterns in industrialized countries because: (1) the difference in disease potential between chrysotile and amphibole asbestos has been fully recognized and production and use of amphiboles is limited or its use has been banned; and (2) developing countries have access to information about modern industrial hygiene practices. Therefore, the peak and period of decline in diseases in developing countries may be moderate relative to the peak and period of decline for industrialized countries. But the asbestos industries and regulatory programs in developing countries have yet to fully mature making the magnitude and time-pattern of asbestos diseases in the 21st century uncertain.

References

Aguilar-Madrid G, Juarez-Perez CA, Markowitz S, Hernandez-Avila M, Sanchez Roman FR, Vazquez Grameix JH. Globalization and the transfer of hazardous industry: asbestos in Mexico, 1979–2000. *Int J Occup Environ Health*. 2003;9:272–279.

Algranti E, Mendonca EM, DeCapitani EM, et al. Non-malignant asbestos-related diseases in Brazilian asbestos-cement workers. *Am J Ind Med*. 2001a;40:240–254

Algranti E, Menezes AM, Achutti AC. Lung cancer in Brazil. *Semin Oncol*. 2001b;28:143–152.

Berry G. Prediction of mesothelioma, lung cancer, and asbestosis in former Wittenoom asbestos workers. *Br J Ind Med*. 1991;48:793–802.

Cai SX, Zhang CH, Zhang X, Morinaga K. Epidemiology of occupational asbestos-related diseases in China. *Ind Health*. 2001;39:75–83.

Carroll SJ, Henslef DR, Abrahamse A, et al. *Asbestos Litigation Costs and Compensation: An Interim Report*. Santa Monica, CA: RAND Institute for Civil Justice; 2002.

Castleman, BI. *Asbestos: Medical and Legal Aspects*. 4th ed. Englewood Cliffs, NJ: Aspen Law and Business; 1996.

Cauchon D. The asbestos epidemic—a global crisis. *U.S.A Today*, August, 1999.

CDC/National Center for Health Statistics. Health, United States, 2004 Report. Available at: http://www.cdc.gov/nchs/hus.htm. Accessed March 25, 2005.

Churg, A, Green, FH. *Pathology of Occupational Disease*. 2nd ed. Williams & Wilkins: Baltimore, MD; 1998.

Cullen MR, Baloyi RS. Chrysotile asbestos and health in Zimbabwe: I. Analysis of miners and millers compensated for asbestos-related diseases since independence (1980). *Am J Ind Med*. 1991;19:161–169.

Degiovanni D, Pesce B, Pondrano N. Asbestos in Italy. *Int J Occup Environ Health*. 2004;10:193–197.

EPA (United States Environmental Protection Agency), 1986, Airborne Asbestos Health Assessment Update, EPA/600/8-84-003F.

Financial Gazette-Zimbabwe. National Report: Shabanie & Mashaba Mines gets $20 billion lifeline from Reserve Bank of Zimbabwe. June, 2004.

Furuya S, Natori Y, Ikeda R. Asbestos in Japan. *Int J Occup Environ Health*. 2003;9:260–265.

Gamble JF. Asbestos and colon cancer: a weight-of-the-evidence review. *Environ Health Perspect*. 1994;102:1038–1050.

Giannasi P. Ministry of labour and employment, Brazil. Asbestos in Brazil. European Conference "Asbestos," 2003.

Greenberg AK, Lee TC, Rom WN. The North American experience with malignant mesothelioma. In: Robinson BWS, Chahinian AP, eds, *Mesothelioma*. London: Martin Dunitz Ltd; 2002.

Gorini G, Merler E, Chellini E, Crocetti E, Costantini AS. Is the ratio of pleural mesothelioma mortality to pleural cancer mortality approximately unity for Italy? Considerations from the oldest regional mesothelioma register in Italy. *Br J Cancer*. 2002;86:1970–1971.

Hansen J, de Klerk NH, Musk AW, Hobbs MS. Environmental exposure to crocidolite and mesothelioma: exposure-response relationships. *Am J Respir Crit Care Med*. 1998;157:69–75.

HEI-AR (Health Effects Institute—Asbestos Research). Asbestos in Public and Commercial Buildings: A Literature Review and Synthesis of Current Knowledge, 1991.

Health and Safety Executive Discussion of Asbestos-Related Disease. Available at: http://www.hse.gov.uk/statistics/causdis/asbestos.htm. Accesed November 17, 2004.

Hemminki K, Li X. Mesothelioma incidence seems to have leveled off in Sweden. *Int J Cancer*. 2003a;103:145–146.

Hemminki K, Li X. Mesothelioma is a killer of urban men in Sweden. *Int J Cancer*. 2003b;105:144–146.

Herald, The (Harare). Asbestos production critical to the economy. October, 2003.

Hillerdal G. The Swedish experience with asbestos: history of use, diseases, legislation, and compensation. *Int J Occup Environ Health*. 2004;10:154–158.

Hodgson JT, McElvenny DM, Darnton AJ, Price MJ, Peto J. The expected burden of mesothelioma mortality in Great Britain from 2002 to 2050. *Br J Cancer*. 2005;92:587–593.

Jockel KH. Re: Mesothelioma is a killer of urban men in Sweden by Kari Hemminki and Xinjun Li. *Int J Cancer*. 2003;107:685.

Joshi TK, Gupta RK. Asbestos-related morbidity in India. *Int J Occup Environ Health*. 2003;9:249–253.

Joshi TK, Gupta RK. Asbestos in developing countries: magnitude of risk and its practical implications. *Int J Occup Med Environ Health*. 2004;17:179–185.

Kjaergaard J, Andersson M. Incidence rates of malignant mesothelioma in Denmark and predicted future number of cases among men. *Scand J Work Environ Health*. 2000;26:112–117.

Ladou J. The asbestos cancer epidemic. *Environ Health Perspect*. 2004;112:285–290.

La Vecchia C, Decarli A, Peto J, et al. An age, period and cohort analysis of pleural cancer mortality in Europe. *Eur J Cancer Prev*. 2000;9:179–184.

Leigh J, Driscoll T. Malignant mesothelioma in Australia, 1945–2002. *Int J Occup Environ Health*. 2003;9:206–217.

Magnani C. Pleural malignant mesothelioma and environmental exposure to asbestos associated with asbestos cement production: The case of Casale, Monferrato, Italy. *Can Mineral*. 2001;Special Publ. #5, p. 29.

McDonald AD, McDonald JC. Malignant mesothelioma in North America. *Cancer*. 1980;46:1650–1656.

Morinaga K, Kishimoto T, Sakatani M, Akira M, Yokoyama K, Sera Y. Asbestos-related lung cancer and mesothelioma in Japan. *Ind Health*. 2001;39:65–74.

National Center for Health Statistics (NCHS). Death rates for selected causes by 10-year age groups, race, and sex: death registration states, 1900–32, and United States, 1933–98. Available at: http://www.cdc.gov/nchs/datawh/statab/unpubd/mortabs/hist290.htm. Page last Reviewed by NCHS/CDC May 7, 2004.

National Cancer Institute (NCI) 2002. Cancer Facts—How is mesothelioma diagnosed? Available at: http://cis.nci.nih.gov/fact/6_36.htm. Accessed March 25, 2005.

Nesti M, Marinaccio A, Chellini E. Malignant mesothelioma in Italy (1997). *Am J Med.* 2004;45(1):55–62.

Paek D. Asbestos problems yet to explode in Korea. *Int J Occup Environ Health.* 2003;9:266–271.

Pelucchi C, Malvezzi M, La Vecchia C, Levi F, Decarli A, Negri E. The Mesothelioma epidemic in Western Europe: an update. *Br J Cancer.* 2004;90:1022–1024.

Peto J, Hodgson JT, Matthews FE, Jones JR. Continuing increase in mesothelioma mortality in Britain. *Lancet.* 1995;345:535–539.

Peto J, Decarli A, La Vecchia C, Levi F, Negri E. The European mesothelioma epidemic. *Br J Cancer.* 1999;79:666–672.

Pinheiro GA, Antao VC, Bang KM, Attfield MD. Malignant mesothelioma surveillance: a comparison of ICD-10 mortality data with SEER incidence data in nine areas of the United States. *Int J Occup Environ Health.* 2004;10:251–255.

Pinheiro GA, Antao VC, Capelozzi VL, Terra-Filho M. Mortality from pleural mesothelioma in Rio de Janeiro, Brazil, 1979–2000: estimation from death certificates, hospital records, and histopathologic assessments. *Int J Occup Environ Health.* 2003;9:147–152.

PMG (Parliamentary Monitoring Group), Environmental Affairs Committee, Parliamentary Asbestos Summit: South Africa and Zimbabwe. Transcript of Minutes, 2003.

Price B, Ware A. Mesothelioma trends in the United States: an update based on surveillance, epidemiology, and end results program data for 1973 through 2003. *Am J Epidemiol.* 2004;159:107–112.

Rodriguez EJ. Asbestos banned in Argentina. *Int J Occup Environ Health.* 2004;10:202–208.

SEER Registries, 2004; Described, Mapped, and Comparable to the general United States Population. Available at: http://seer.cancer.gov/registries/http://seer.cancer.gov/registries/characteristics.html. Accessed March 25, 2005.

Roggli VL, Oury TD, Sporn TA. *Pathology of Asbestos-Associated Diseases.* 2nd ed. New York: Springer-Verlag; 2004.

SEER—Surveillance, Epidemiology, and End Results Program (www.seer.cancer.gov) SEER*Stat Database: Incidence—SEER 9 Regs Public-Use, November 2003 Sub (1973–2001), National Cancer Institute, DCCPS, Surveillance Research Program, Cancer Statistics Branch, released April 2004, based on the November 2003 submission.

Shcherbakov SV, Kashansky S, Domnin SG, et al. The health effects of mining and milling chrysotile: the Russian experience. *Can Mineral.* 2001; Special Publ. #5

Shiqu Z, Yongxian W, Fusheng M, Hongshuen M, Wenzhi, S, Zhenhuan, J. Retrospective Mortality Study of Asbestos Workers in Laiyuan, Dept of Occup Health, Beijing Medical University, China 1990.

Siriruttanapruk T. Asbestos in Thailand. European Conference: Asbestos, 2003.

Stallard E, Manton KG, Cohen JE. *Forecasting Product Liability Claims: Epidemiology and Modeling in the Manville Asbestos Case (Statistics for Biology and Health).* Springer Publ. November, 2004.

Takahashi K, Karjalainen A. A cross-country comparative overview of the asbestos situation in ten Asian countries. *Int J Occup Environ Health.* 2003;9:244–248.

Ulvestad B, Kjaerheim K, Moller B, et al. Incidence trends of mesothelioma in Norway, 1965–1999. *Int J Cancer.* 2003;107:94–98.

Virta RL. USGS. US Dept of the Interior. Worldwide Asbestos Supply and Consumption Trends from 1900 to 2000. 2003 USGS Open Report 03-83, 2003a.

Virta RL. USGS. "Asbestos 2003" from the US Geological Survey Minerals Yearbook, 2003b.

Wagner JC, Sleggs CA, Marchand P. Diffuse pleural mesothelioma and asbestos exposure in the north western cape province. *Br J Ind Med.* 1960:17;260–271.

Weill H, Hughes JM. Mesothelioma. *Lancet.* 1995;345:1234.

Weill H, Hughes JM, Churg AM. Changing trends in U.S. mesothelioma incidence. *Occup Environ Med.* 2004;61:438–441.

WTO-World Trade Organization. European Communities—measures affecting asbestos and asbestos-containing products. 2000 September 18; WT/DS135/R.

Yu IJ, Yoo CY, Chung YH, et al. Asbestos exposure among Seoul metropolitan subway workers during renovation of subway air-conditioning systems. *Environ Int.* 2004;29:931–934.

Index

Note: Page numbers in *italics* refer to figures and tables

Abrasive grinding wheel workers, effects of
    asbestos on, 79
Actinolite asbestos, 37
Adenomatoid tumors, 214
Air pollution, major sources of urban and
    industrial, 26
Airborne asbestos concentration, 62
Alveolar epithelium, 128, 130
Alveolitis, 150
American Conference of Governmental
    Industrial Hygienists (ACGIH),
    96, 319–320
American Society for Testing Materials, 24
Amosite asbestos, 4, 102, 128, 132, 139
Amphibole contamination, 100
Amphibole minerals, 5, 24, 102, 132, 139
  crystalline structures of, 34
  occurrence and physical-chemical
    properties of, 34–38
  rock-forming minerals, 34
  scanning electron micrograph of, *35*
Anthophyllite, 34, 37, 98
Anthophyllite mine, 80, 87
Anti-oxidant defenses, 122
Antigorite, 29
AP-1 and cell cycle progression, 124–126
Apoptosis-inducing factor (AIF), 126
Asbestiform tremolite, 100
Asbestos:
  aerodynamic properties of, 27
  air concentrations in textile factories, *42*
  asbestosis, 8–10
  associated diseases, and trends in 20th and
    21st centuries:
    in Australia, 382–384
    in Brazil, 391
    in Canada, 380
    in China, 390
    in Denmark, 386
    in developed (industrialized)
      countries, 377–388
    in developing countries, 388–392
    in India, 390
    in Italy, 386–387
    in Japan, 387
    in Korea, 387–388
    in Norway, 385–386
    in Russia, 384–385
    in South Africa, 384
    in Sweden, 385
    in Thailand, 390–391
    in United Kingdom, 381
    in United States, 377, *378*, *379*, 380
    in Western Europe, 381–382
    worldwide asbestos production, imports,
      exports and consumption, *388–389*
  associated lesions, in industrial workers, *162*
  bioactivity of, 122
  cell autonomous effects of, 130
  cement pipe, 58
  containing construction material, 58
  containing felts, 74
  deposits, 24
  discovery and beginning, 6–8
  exposure:
    and bronchiolar wall fibrosis, 148
    and malignancy, 10–11
    and respiratory diseases, 139–140
  exposure effects:
    on abrasive grinding wheel workers, 79
    on automotive mechanics, 63–68
    on building interior workmen, 53–54
    on cement manufacturers and end-product
      users, 55–58
    on chemical, petrochemical, and refinery
      workers, 71–72
    on construction workers, 51–53
    on electricians, 62–63

Asbestos (*contd.*)

on floor tile and linoleum installers and removers, 55

on household and community residents, 79–82

on insulators, 47–51

on iron, steel and foundry workers, 76–78

on jewelry and dental laboratory technicians, 78–79

on occupants of public and commercial buildings, 58–60

on paper and pulp mill workers, 74–76

on plumbers and pipe fitters, 51

on railroad workers, 68–70

on sheet metal workers, 70–71

on shipbuilders and navy/merchant marine personnel, 43–47

on textile mill workers, 40–43

on thermoelectric power and chemical plant workers, 72–74

on workmen using gaskets and packing, 60–62

fiber dry lung content, of amosite factory workers, *145*

and generation of Reactive Oxygen Species (ROS), 127–128

health effects of, 3

hypothetic interaction, with airways mucosa, *152*

incombustible properties of, 23

induced cancers, 120

insulation, 49

law in US:

defense coordination, 360–365

emerging Tort Theories and Borel Case, 354–356

historical overview of, 346–347

Johns Manville's bankruptcy, 360–365

law firm dominance, 360–365

lawsuit, 369–373

mass Torts and explosion of plaintiff pool, 365–368

in 1940s and 1950s, 350–354

in 1980s, 360–365

in 1990s, 365–368

in 1970s, 356–360

in 1960s, 354–356

Tort *versus* Workers' Compensation Laws, 348–350

trade, shipyard and factory lawsuits, 356–360

trial management techniques, 371–372

in 2000 and beyond, 368–369

venue shopping, 372–373

markers, 45

mineralogical and geological features of, 23–26

mines and miners, 5, 23, 309–310

naturally occurring fibrous silicates, 4

occupational risk, 9

ROS-dependent effects of, 128–129

surface activity of, 128

Asbestos bodies, 139–143, 258

"bare" asbestos fibers, 143

biologically inert, 143

developing on chrysotile core, *142*

developing on amphibole cores, 140, *141*

and interstitial fibrosis, *146*, 148

in lung samples, *147*

morphologic hallmark of asbestos exposure, 140

and nonspecific pulmonary fibrosis, 148

and phagocytic macrophages, 143

Asbestos control and US governmental regulatory actions, 321, 324

Clean Air Act (CAA), 318

dust suppression measures, 317

National Emissions Standard for Hazardous Air Pollutions (NESHAP), goals of, 318, 322

occupational asbestos regulations, 319, 320

Occupational Safety Act of 1970, 317

Occupational Safety and Health Administration (OSHA), 317, 320

sampling air for asbestos, 324

Toxic Substances Act (TOSCA), 318

Asbestos etiology, and malignant mesothelioma, 191–193

Asbestos Hazardous Emergency Response Act (AHERA):

and asbestos control, 322

goals of, 323

Asbestosis, 266, 289

advanced subpleural honeycomb change, *292*

and asbestos exposure, 139–140

benign pleural disease, 156–157, 261–265

benign pleural effusion, 158

and bronchogenic carcinoma, 295

clinical diagnosis, 10, 140, 251–264

clinical latency of, 143

diffuse fibrotic pulmonary disease, 143, 154, 254–259

diffuse pleural fibrosis, *144*

and fiber burden analysis, 147

grading schema, 164, *165*

gravitational effect mimicking early pulmonary fibrosis, *293*

and Helsinki criteria, 147

and "honeycombing", 143, *144*

latency period for, 8

and lung cancer, 172–186

in nonsmokers, 149

occupational history of, 253–254

pathogenesis of:

benign pleural effusion, 158

host factors in lungs, 150–151

hypothetical cumulative series of injuries, *153*

mesomorphic body configuration, 150

in respiratory bronchiole, 150

pathologic grading of, 163–165

pneumoconiosis assessment, 163

progression, 154–155

in respiratory bronchioles, 147, *148*

risk evaluation, 94–97

in smokers, 149

sputum and bronchoalveolar lavage (BAL) fluid, cytology of, 155–156

subpleural curvilinear lines, *291*
in textile industry, 140–146
Asbestosis and mineral fiber analysis, 299–312
Asbestosis and radiologic features of:
    diffuse pleural thickening (DPT), 276, *277–280*
    diffuse pulmonary parenchymal fibrosis, 289,
        290–292, 293–294
    ILO classification of pneumoconioses, 269–270
    lung cancer, 294–295
    malignant mesothelioma, 282, *283–289*
    pleural effusion, 270, *271*
    pleural plaques (PP), 271, *272*, 273, *274–275*, 276
    rounded atelectasis, 280, *281–282*
Atypical mesothelial cell, *208*
Automotive mechanics, effects of asbestos on, 63

"Bare" asbestos fibers, 143
Basic fibroblast growth factor (bFGF), 123
Benign asbestos-associated pleural diseases:
    chronic airway obstruction, 264–265
Benign pleural disease, 156–157, 261–264
Benign pleural effusions, 158, 264
Biphasic malignant mesothelioma, 201, *203*
Blesovsky's Syndrome, 159–160
Bronchoalveolar lavage (BAL), 258
Bronchiolar-alveolar junctions, 129
Bronchoalveolar carcinoma, 11

Calcifying fibrous pseudotumor of pleura, 216
Carcinoembryonic antigen (CEA), 260
Carcinogenesis, multistage nature of, *131*
Cell cycle kinetics, 131
Cell proliferation, 123–124
Cell signaling, 122–123
Cell-signaling pathways, 121–122
Cellular metabolism, 120
Chronic airway obstruction and
        asbestosis, 264–265
Chronic bronchial irritation, 11, 133
Chronic diseases, 52, 122, 193
Chrysotile, 4, 7, 139
    in brake shoe dust, *66*
    and crocidolite with hamster tracheal mucosa,
        interaction, *185*
    dehydroxylation of, 64
    occurrence and physical-chemical properties
        of, 29–34
    types of, 29
Chrysotile asbestos, 109, 127
Clinical asbestosis, development of, 44
Colinga asbestos, 30
Colorectal carcinoma:
    and asbestos exposure, 239–240
Construction workers, effects of asbestos on, 51–53
Crocidolite, 4, 102, 132, 139
    and chrysotile with hamster tracheal mucosa,
        interaction, *185*
    health effects due to inhalation of, 76
    with hamster trachea epithelium, interaction, *149*
    in lymphatics of parietal pleura of rat, *157*

squamous metaplasia in, *185*
"Crow's foot" lesion, 160
Cummingtomite-grunerite, 35
Curious bodies, 139
Cyclin-dependent kinases (CDK), 123
Cytoskeleton, organization of, 121
Cytosolic enzymes, 122

Desmoplastic malignant mesothelioma:
    extensive infiltration of adipose, *203*
    nodularity at low magnification, *202*
Desmoplastic round cell tumor, 210
Diffuse pleural fibrosis (DPF), 305
Diffuse pleural thickening (DPT) and
        asbestosis, 158–159, 276, *277–280*
DNA:
    fragmentation, 126
    tumor virus, 132
Doll and Peto formula, 57
Dolomites, thermal metamorphism of, 37

Ebstein-Barr virus, 14
Elastosis bodies, 141
Endothelioma, 15
Environmental exposures and asbestosis, 311
Environmental Protection Agency (EPA), 49, *51*, 55,
        60, 61, 100, 111, 150, 192–193, 240,
        318, 323–324
Epidermal growth factor (EGF), 123
Epidermal growth factor receptor (EGFR), 128
Epithelial lining cells, 31
Epithelioid malignant mesothelioma, 198, 201
    adenomatoid differentiation, *199*
    cell pattern, *200*
    cytoplasmic immunopositivity for mesothelin
        antibody, *205*
    decidua in pregnant uterus, *200*
    and differential diagnosis, 209
    immunohistochemical panel, *205*
    pleomorphism with tumor giant cells, *199*
    reactive *versus* malignant lesions, 208–209
    trabecular arrangement simulating
        hepatoma, *200*
    tubulopapillary differentiation, *199*
Erionite etiology, and malignant mesothelioma, 193
Esophageal cancer:
    and asbestos exposure, 235–236
Extracellular signal-regulated kinases
        (ERK), 124–130
Extrapleural pneumonectomy (EPP), 331–332

Fenton-type reactions, 127
Ferruginous bodies, 140–141
    with carbon-black fibrous core, *142*
Fiber burden analyses, 66
Fiber burden hypothesis, 179–180
Fibrosis/cancer hypothesis, studies
        supporting, 177–179
Fibrous cummingtonite granite, 36
Fibrous dust particles, carcinogenic potential of, 26

Fibrous fluoredenite amphibole, 100
Fibrous glass, 47
Fire resistant fabric, 40
Fluoredenite, 38
Foundry workers, effects of asbestos on, 76–78

Gastric cancer:
    and asbestos exposure, 237–238
    etiology, 236
    and *Helicobacter pylori*, 237
    risk in cross-sectional cohorts of asbestos
        workers, *238*
    risk in inception cohorts of asbestos workers, *237*

Gastroesophageal Reflux Disorder (GERD), 235
Gene and cytokine-related therapies, 336
Gene expression profiling, 120–122
Genetic factors etiology, and malignant
    mesothelioma, 195–196
Glutamate cysteine ligase, 131

Hamster tracheal epithelial (HTE) cells, 129
Heating system insulation, 52
High-Resolution Computed Tomography (HRCT), 269
Honeycombing, and asbestosis, 143, *144*
Household and community residents, asbestos
    exposures of, 79–82
Hyalinosis complicata, 158
Hyalinosis simplex, 158
Hydroxyl radicals (OH) production, 127

Idiopathic etiology, and malignant
    mesothelioma, 196
Idiopathic Pulmonary Fibrosis (IPF), 294
International Agency for Research on Cancer
    (IARC), 4, 130
Intracellular metabolism, 122
Intrapleural and systemic cytokine therapy, 337
Iron, effects of asbestos on, 76–78
Iron-rich fibrous silicates, 4
Iron stone formations, 36

Jewelry and dental laboratory technicians, effects of
    asbestos on, 78–79
c-Jun N-terminal kinase (JNK), 124

Laryngeal carcinoma, 232
    with asbestos exposure, association, 233–234
    tobacco smoking, 235
Lipid hydroperoxides, 127
Lipid phosphatase, 121
Lipopolysaccharide, 124
Lizardite, 29
Long running thermal precipitator, 95
Lung cancer (LC), 6, 41
    clinical observation, 185–186
    dose-response analysis, 105
    fiber burden hypothesis, 179–180
    fibrosis/cancer hypothesis, 177–179
    among foundry workers, 78

in friction product workers, 67
Helsinki criteria, 174, 181–183
historical perspective, 172–173
induction of, 131
mechanistic consideration, 173–176, 183–184
mortality from, *47*
risk for development of, 94
risk of, 101–105
standard mortality rate for, 49
synergistic interaction between tobacco
    smoking, *176*, 177–180
Lung parenchymal disease and asbestosis:
    bronchoscopy, 258
    clinical course (progression), 259
    diagnosis of, 254–255
    diffuse interstitial, 258
    interstitial fibrosis, *259*
    pathophysiological features of, 257–258
    physical signs and symptoms of, 255–256
    pneumoconioses, 255–256
    radiological features of, 256–257, *259*
Lymphohistiocytoid malignant mesothelioma, *203*
Lymphoid malignancies:
    asbestos exposure, *243*, 244
    etiology of, 242–243
Lytic cell death, 122

Magnesio-riebeckite, 36
Magnetic resonance imaging, 269
Malignant mesothelioma (MM):
    and asbestosis, 282, *283–289*
        biphasic, 201, *203*
        chronic inflammation etiology, 195
        differential diagnosis of, 208–211
        epithelioid, 198, *199*, *200*, 201
        erionite etiology, 193
        etiology, 191–193
        genetic factors etiology, 195–196
        idiopathic etiology, 196
        man-made mineral fibers etiology, 193–194
        organic fiber etiology, 193
        pathogenesis of, 216–219
        pathologic features, 196–208
        physical signs and symptoms, 260–261
        prognosis and treatment, 191
        radiographic features of, 261
        sarcomatoid, 201, *202*
        therapeutic irradiation etiology, 194
        viral etiology, 194
    biomarkers, 207–208
    cytopathology, 206–207
    and epithelioid malignant mesothelioma, 209
    lesions:
        adenomatoid tumors, 214
        calcifying fibrous pseudotumor of pleura, 216
        multicystic mesothelioma, 213, *214*
        solitary fibrous tumor, 214, 216
        well-differentiated papillary
            mesothelioma, 212, *213*
    mineral fiber analysis and asbestosis, *306*, 307

multimodality treatment:
    induction chemotherapy followed
        by surgery, 335
    surgery and standard agents, 334–335
occurrence in selected study populations, *98*
operations, 329
    extrapleural pneumonectomy, 331–332
    pleurectomy, 330–331
    cytopathology and, 206–207
    electron microscopy, 206
    gross features of, 196–198
    histo- and immunohistochemistry, 204, 206
    light microscopy and, 198, 201, 204
prevalence of, 58
radiotherapy:
    combined chemotherapy and radiation
        therapy, 332–333
    combined surgical resection and radio
        therapy, 333–334
    curative radio therapy, 332
reactive *versus* malignant lesions, 208–209
risk for development of, 94
risk of, 97
and sarcomatoid, 209–210
and serosal sites:
    gonads, 212
    hernial sacs, 212
    pericardial, 212
    peritoneal, 211–212
surgery:
    cardiac evaluation, 329
    operations to be performed, 329–332
    preoperative considerations, 328
    pulmonary evaluation, 328–329
    staging and operative therapy, 329
therapeutic approaches:
    adjuvant therapy for surgically
        cytoreduction, 334
    chemotherapy and newer agents, 337–338
    intrapleural and systemic cytokine therapy, 337
    multimodality treatment, 334–335
    natural history, 326
    novel gene and cytokine-related therapies, 336
    peritoneal (abdominal), 338–339
    pleural perfusion, 336
    prevention of malignant mesothelioma
        recurrences in chest scars, 334
    prognostic indicators, 326–327
    radiotherapy, 332–334
    staging system, 327
    surgery, 328–332
    treatment, 327–328
treatment:
    overview of, 327
    supportive care, 327
Malignant solitary fibrous tumors, 210
Mammalian cells, 121
Man-made mineral fibers etiology, and malignant
        mesothelioma, 193–194
Material Safety Data Sheets, 322

Membrane filter method, 96, 106
Membrane filter phase contrast microscopy
        equivalents, 94
Metamorphic geologic activity, 37
Mineral fiber analysis and asbestosis, 299–300,
        307–308
    asbestos miners, 309–310
    control subjects, 302–303, *302, 304*
    diffuse pulmonary fibrosis (DPF), 305
    end-product users, 310
    environmental exposures, 311
    fiber dimension, 311–312
    malignant mesothelioma, *306*, 307
    paraoccupational (domestic) exposures, 310–311
    pleural plaque, 303, *305*
    rounded atelectasis, 305
Mitochondrial dysfunction, 130
Mitochondrial outer membrane permeabilization
        (MOMP), 126, 130
Mitogen-activated protein kinases (MAPKs), 125,
        128, 129
Multicystic mesothelioma:
    cystic, 213
    from peritoneal cavity, *214*
    peritoneal inclusion cysts, 213

NADPH oxidases, 123
National Emissions Standard for Hazardous Air
        Pollutions (NESHAP), 49, 318, 322
National Institute for Occupational Safety and Health
        (NIOSH), 147, 317
Natural mineral deposits, 4, 26
Neoplastic transformation, 129, 133
New York Conference of 1964, 16–19
Nonasbestiform fibers, 78
Nonmalignant chest disease, 73
Nonspecific Interstitial Pneumonitis (NSIP), 294
Nonthoracic cancers, from asbestos:
    Bradford Hill's criteria, 230–231
    colorectal carcinoma, 238–240
    esophageal cancer, 235–236
    gastric cancer, 236–238
    laryngeal carcinoma, 232–235
    lymphoid mlignancies, 242–244
    oral and nasopharyngeal carcinoma, 231–232
    pancreatic carcinoma, 241
    renal cell carcinoma, 241–242

Occupational cancer, study of, 13
Occupational exposure standards, in US, *320*
Occupational Safety Act of 1970, 317
Occupational Safety and Health Administration
        (OSHA), 4, 23, 41
Oral and nasopharyngeal carcinoma, 231–232
Organic fiber etiology, and malignant
        mesothelioma, 193

Pancreatic carcinoma:
    epidemiological studies showing asbestos
        exposure with, *241*

Pancreatic carcinoma (*contd.*)
    etiology, 241
Paper and pulp mill workers, effects of
    asbestos on, 74–76
Papillary mesothelioma, 212, *213*
Paraoccupational (domestic) exposures, 310–311
Pericardial malignant mesothelioma, 212
Peritoneal (abdominal) malignant
    mesothelioma, 338–339
Peritoneal cancers, 13
Peritoneal mesotheliomas, *50*
Peritoneal malignant mesothelioma, 211–212
Permissible exposure level (PEL), 62
Positron emission tomography (PET), 269, 287
Phagocytosis, 128
Phase contrast membrane filter method, 95
Phase contrast microscopy (PCM), 23, 61, 299,
    301, 319
    mineral fiber analysis and asbestosis, 301
Photodynamic therapy (PDT), 335–336
Phythis, 139
Platelet-derived growth factor (PDGF), 123, 154
Pleural and lung parenchymal disease, 45
Pleural asbestosis, 10, 156–157
Pleural cancer, 11
Pleural effusions, 158
    and asbestosis, 270, *271*
Pleural mesotheliomas, 15, *50*, 129
Pleural plaques (PP), 10, 45
    and asbestosis, 143, *160*, 160–163, 261–263, 271,
        272, 273, *274–275*, 276
    formation in parietal pleura, *162*
    mineral fiber analysis and asbestosis, 303, *305*
    pleural surface of diaphragm, *160*
Pleural tumors, 10, 79
Pleurectomy, 330–331
Plumbers and pipe fitters, effects of asbestos on, 51
Pneumoconiosis, 13, 15, 52, 78
Polycyclic aromatic hydrocarbons, airborne
    concentrations of, 78
Portland-Pozzolan cement, 55
Posttranslational protein, 120
Primitive Neuroectodermal Tumors (PNET), 210
Programmed cell death, 126
Proportional mortality ratio (PMR), 52, 100, 239,
    309–310
    for lung cancer, *175*
    for pleural and peritoneal cancers in men
        in UK, *211*
Protein kinase C (PKC), 128
Protein tyrosine phosphatase 1B (PTP1B), 123
Pseudomesotheliomatous tumor, 198
Pulmonary asbestosis, 9
Pulmonary epithelial cell death, 129
Pulmonary functional abnormalities, 69
Pulmonary interstitial fibrosis, 10

Railroad workers:
    effects of asbestos, 68–70
    radiological abnormalities among, *69*

Reactive nitrogen species (RNS), 120
Reactive oxygen species (ROS), 120, 121, 124
Redox-responsive transcription factor, 125
Redox-sensitive signaling proteins, 130
Relative risk (RR) for lung cancer, *174*
Renal cell carcinoma:
    asbestos exposure, 242
    etiology and pathogenesis, 241
Residential radon exposure, 105
Respiratory diseases:
    and asbestos exposure, 139–140
    occurrence of, 27
Respiratory symptomatology, 57
Respiratory tract, defense mechanisms of, 27
Richerite, 38
RNA synthesis, 121
Rounded atelectasis, 159–160, 305
    and asbestosis, 280, *281–282*

Sarcomatoid malignant mesothelioma, 201
    atypical spindle cells, *202*
    desmoplastic round cell tumor, 209, 210
    immunohistochemical panel, *206*
    malignant solitary fibrous tumors, 210
    malignant spindle cells stroma, *202*
Scanning electron microscopy (SEM),
    mineral fiber analysis and
    asbestosis, 301–302
Serpentine minerals, 24, 29, 30, 31
Sheet metal workers, effects of asbestos on, 70–71
Silicosis, 8, 13
Sodic-calcific amphibole. *See* Richerite
Solitary fibrous tumor, 214, 216
    bland spindle cells displaying "patternless"
        features, *215*
    hypercellular areas of spindle cells with
        mitoses, *215*
    in visceral pleura of lung, *215*
Spray-on asbestos, *51*
Standard membrane filter method, 96
Standard Mortality Rate (SMR), 49, 62
    for friction product worker, *67*
Standardized Mortality Ratio (SMR), 232
    for lung and colorectal cancer, *239*
Steel workers, effects on, 76–78
Sumner Simpson documents, 358
Superoxide dismutases (SOD), 123
SV40 T-antigen, 132
Synovial sarcoma, 209
    dense "blue" staining spindle cells, 210

Therapeutic irradiation, 194
Thermal insulation products, mineral
    composition of, *59*
Thermoelectric power and chemical plant
    workers, effects of asbestos, 72–74
Threshold limit values (TLV), 96
Time weighted average (TWA), 64
TNF-α (tumor growth factor alpha), 154
TNF-β (tumor growth factor beta), 154

Tort theories, and asbestos exposure in US:
    Borel Case, 354–356
    explosion of plaintiff pool, 365–368
    versus Workers' Compensation Laws,
        348–350
Toxic byproducts, 120
Toxic minerals, 5
Toxic Substances Act (TOSCA), 318
Transbronchial lung biopsy (TBB), 258
Transcription factor complexes, 124–125
Transmission electron microscopy (TEM), 299
    mineral fiber analysis and asbestosis, 302
Tumor antigens, 132

Tumor development, 15
Tumor necrosis, 130
TUNEL staining, 129

Ultramafic rock. *See* Anthophyllite
Upper respiratory and digestive tract associated
        cancers, *232*
US Public Health Services (USPHS), 95
Usual interstitial pneumonitis (UIP), 294

Viral etiology, and malignant mesothelioma, 194

Zenker, 139